Chapter 3

Basic physics

Physics is the fundamental science that deals with matter in general and energy in particular. For convenience it is subdivided into several branches, the traditional subdivisions including mechanics, heat, sound, magnetism, electricity, and light, and to these we must now add atomic and nuclear physics ("atomics" and "nucleonics"). We must not forget, however, that these subdivisions are closely related to one another; that is, the principles and laws developed in one area cut across other areas. Moreover, there is one principle that connects all subdivisions of physics—the *law of conservation of energy* (Chapter 4).

MOLECULE

Classic physics is predicated upon the molecule as the "ultimate" particle of matter. Although we know today that the molecule is composed of atoms and that the atom is composed of subatomic particles (a subject that will be explored in the next chapter), the general physical behavior of matter is usually best understood if we go along with the classic view. This is more than just convenience, however, for the basic physical characteristics of molecules have been shown to be unrelated to their *kind*. For instance, oxygen and nitrogen, two entirely different substances, respond in exactly the same way to changes in pressure and temperature.

Size and number. To say that molecules are "small" is a cosmic understatement. In 1 c.c. of air there are roughly 30 billion billion molecules!! Need more be said other than that scientists are convinced that molecules exist because they provide the only plausible explanation for observed natural phenomena.

Avogadro's law. In 1811 the Italian physicist Amedeo Avogadro made the startling announcement that *equal volumes of all gases at the same temperature and pressure contain the same number of molecules.* The idea was so "fantastic" and so far ahead of its time that it took almost 100 years for other scientists to pass judgment, but when that judgment came, it proved that Avogadro was indeed right. What intelligent guesswork!

But modern science has gone beyond the confines of the gaseous state, for we now know that the *gram-molecular weight* (Chapter 4) *of any compound always contains the same number of molecules* (6.02

$\times 10^{23}$). This figure, appropriately called *Avogadro's number,* is one of the basic fibers of our physical and chemical knowledge.

Molecular motion. Aside from their fantastic number and size, all available experimental data tell us that molecules are always in constant motion, a revolutionary statement known formally as the *kinetic theory of matter.* We do not even have to enter the laboratory for evidence; it surrounds us. For instance, perfume from a freshly opened bottle soon reaches the nostrils of all in the room for the simple reason that the energetic molecules "jump out" and diffuse through the air. And what about the dancing dust particles caught in a sunbeam streaming through a hole in a drawn shade? Here, however, we must be careful, for the dust particle is *not* moving under its own power, but is simply being pushed around by the molecules in the air. This phenomenon, which the Scottish botanist Robert Brown first observed while looking through his microscope at dancing pollen grains suspended in water, is aptly referred to as *brownian movement* (Fig. 3-1). Diffusion and brownian movement, then, almost in themselves, offer sufficient proof of molecular motion.

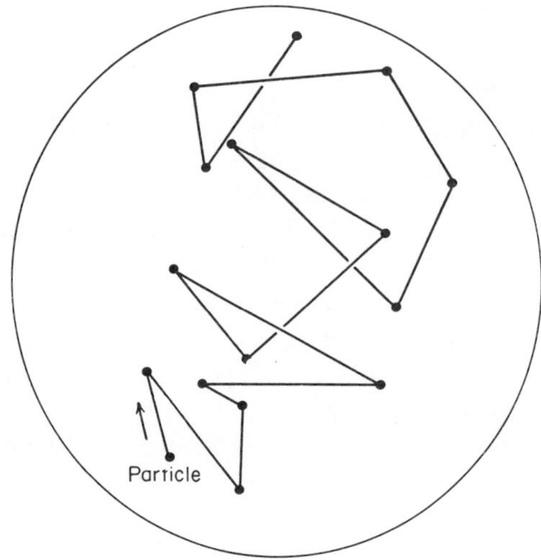

Fig. 3-1. Brownian movement.

Now, since molecules have both mass and motion, they must have *kinetic* energy. Although the energy possessed by a single molecule is beyond our comprehension, the energy that molecules possess *en masse* is considerable, *particularly* in the gaseous state. We can prove this quite simply by heating a little water in a stoppered flask. The formula for kinetic energy (KE) of a single molecule of a gas is

$$KE = \frac{1}{2} mv^2$$

where m is equal to mass and v the velocity. Total kinetic energy of a given mass, therefore, would essentially be this amount multiplied by the number of molecules (an astronomical figure).

Adhesion and cohesion. Another cardinal feature of molecules is their ability to "stick together." As a matter of fact, without this property a piece of matter could conceivably "just fly away." Apparently, then, between the molecules there must exist an attractive force somewhat analogous to the force of gravity between large bodies. We call this attraction between like molecules *cohesion* and the attraction between unlike molecules *adhesion.* For example, a piece of chalk is held together by cohesion, whereas the writing on a blackboard is held there by adhesion.

MECHANICS

Mechanics deals with the behavior of various types of bodies (for example, particles, rigid bodies, liquids, and gases) when subjected to the action of external forces. Some of the more commonly encountered topics under this heading are discussed herewith.

Vectors. In physics a vector is a line, drawn to some convenient scale, that denotes magnitude and direction. In contrast to scalar quantities (for example, temperature, energy, and volume), vector quantities (for example, forces, velocities, and

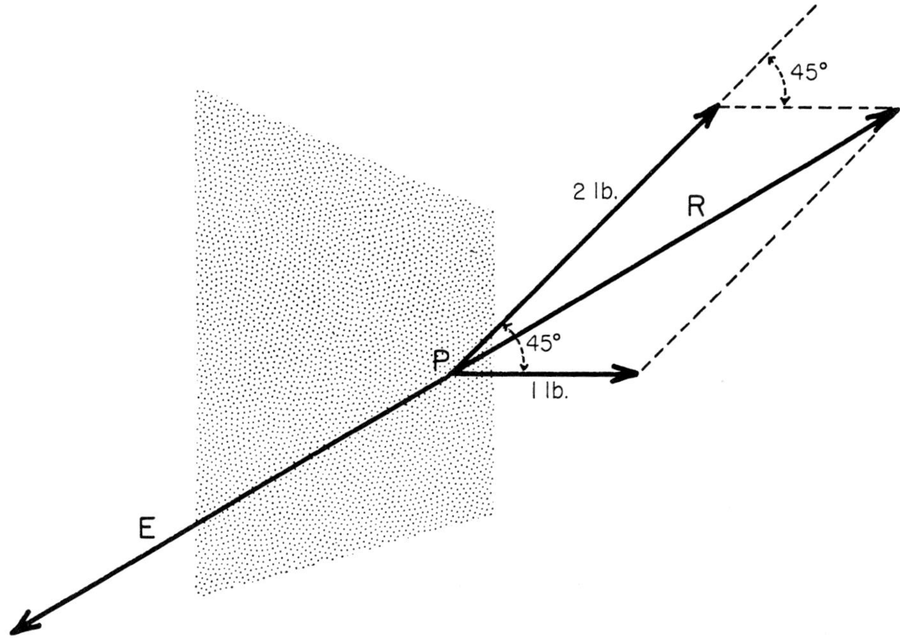

Fig. 3-2. Parallelogram of forces. (See text.)

magnetic and electrical fields) can be expressed and dealt with via the use of vectors.

Let us illustrate the use of vectors by a simple but practical example. If a force of 1 pound and a force of 2 pounds were acting on a point at an angle of 45 degrees, in what direction would the point be pulled? And with what force? In short, what is the resultant vector? One method of solution, and a highly dramatic one, is the parallelogram of forces. In this instance, if we adopt a scale of 1 pound per inch, a 1-inch line and a 2-inch line are drawn at an angle of 45 degrees (Fig. 3-2). Now, with a compass used in the manner shown, a parallelogram is constructed and a diagonal line drawn between its two acute angles. This diagonal line is the *resultant;* its arrowhead shows the direction in which the point will travel, and its length (2¾ inches) shows the amount of pull (2¾ pounds).

Equilibrant. The so-called equilibrant is a vector quantity that is equal in magnitude but opposite in direction to the resultant. It is easily constructed by extending the resultant line through the point acted upon for a distance exactly equal to the length of the resultant. Now, by attaching an arrowhead to the end of this line, we have an equilibrant vector. In the situation illustrated in Fig. 3-2, if an equilibrant force (E) were brought to bear upon the point P, the latter would not move because it would be in equilibrium.

Motion. The subject of motion is a keystone of classic physics, dealing with situations ranging from "a fast ball to first base" to the movement of celestial bodies. We owe what we know of this physical way of life to Newton, perhaps the greatest scientist who ever lived.

Newton's first law. Newton's first law of motion, sometimes referred to as the *law of inertia,* is the epitome of physical common sense. It states that a body *tends to remain at rest or in uniform motion in a straight line unless acted upon by an external force.* An ashtray resting on a table, for example, will not move unless somebody or something moves it. Or a ball rolling along a "frictionless surface" (in the absence of air) will continue to go on and on in a straight line.

Newton's second law. Newton's second law states that when an *unbalanced force acts on a body the change in motion (acceleration) is directly proportional to the magnitude of the force and in the same direction.* On the other hand, acceleration varies inversely to the mass. If we measure the accelerations produced by different forces on the same mass, doubling the force will double the acceleration. The elegance of Newton's second law resides mainly in the fact that the vague and intuitive feeling about the effects of force gives way to a definite quantitative statement; that is, *force* (F) *equals mass* (m) *times acceleration* (a), or $F = ma$.

Speed, velocity, and acceleration. For the beginner, speed, velocity, and acceleration are perhaps best discussed together. Speed, or velocity (s), equals the distance (d) that a moving object travels divided by the time interval (t), or

$$s = \frac{d}{t}$$

For example, if a car travels 120 miles in 3 hours, its speed is 40 miles per hour (40 mph). However, it is important to remember that this is the *average* speed, because in all probability there will be times when the car goes faster or slower than 40 mph. If the direction of this particular car is not stated, we are correct in referring to the 40 mph as *speed.* If, on the other hand, the direction is stated, for example, 40 mph due east, we employ the term *velocity.* Thus, speed is a *scalar* quantity and velocity a *vector* quantity.

In addition to dealing with acceleration in terms of force and mass, we can also describe it in terms of speed or velocity. In this respect we define acceleration as the rate at which speed changes, or

$$\text{Acceleration} = \frac{\text{Change in speed}}{\text{Time to change speed}}$$

or

$$a = \frac{\triangle s}{t}$$

For example, suppose a motorist steps on the gas and jumps his speed from 30 to 45 mph in 10 seconds. His *average* acceleration is

$$a = \frac{\triangle s}{t}$$

$$a = \frac{45\text{-}30}{10 \text{ sec.}}$$

$$a = 1.5 \text{ mph/sec.}$$

Of course, there is also *deceleration,* or negative acceleration. In the instance just cited, for example, if the motorist let up on the gas and dropped his speed from 45 to 30 mph, the car would be slowing down 1.5 mph per second.

Momentum. Momentum (M) is another important feature relating to motion. Defined as the "quantity of motion," it is equal to the product of the mass of a body (m) multiplied by its velocity (v), or $M = mv$.

For example, a 100-pound boy running down the street at a speed of 5 mph has a momentum of 500 pounds mph (that is, pounds miles per hour).

It is interesting to note that Newton's second law can also be stated in terms of momentum; that is, when an unbalanced force acts on a body, the rate of change of momentum is in the direction of the force and proportional to the force.

Newton's third law. The third great law of motion states that *forces always come in pairs, and that for every force there is an equal and opposite force.* When we step on the scales to weigh ourselves, for instance, the reading on the dial means not only that the body is bearing down with a force, say, of 150 pounds, but also that

INTEGRATED BASIC SCIENCE

STEWART M. BROOKS

An introductory science textbook for nursing and allied health programs

THIRD EDITION

INTEGRATED BASIC SCIENCE

STEWART M. BROOKS, M.S.

Visiting Lecturer in Basic Science, Newton Wellesley Hospital, Newton Lower Falls, Massachusetts; formerly, Instructor in Science and Pharmacology, Lasell Junior College, Auburndale, Massachusetts, and Boston City Hospital School of Nursing, Boston, Massachusetts

With 316 illustrations

Saint Louis

The C. V. Mosby Company

1970

Third edition

Printed in the United States of America

Standard Book Number 8016-0804-X

Library of Congress Catalog Card Number 78-99560

Distributed in Great Britain by Henry Kimpton, London

VH/VH/VH 9 8 7 6 5 4

In Memory of

Harold G. Paynton

Columnist
Industrialist
Inventor
Public servant
and
Sportsman

Preface

The purpose of *Integrated Basic Science* is to put the essence of physics, chemistry, microbiology, anatomy, and physiology under "one roof" in an integrated way; that is, the *applications* of physics, chemistry, and microbiology to the human body—the book's central concern—are presented under the appropriate body system. For example, the chemistry of digestion and infections involving the digestive tract are brought together in the chapter on the digestive system. Some, I hasten to state, do not look upon this approach as true integration, apparently because *basic* physics, *basic* chemistry, and *basic* microbiology are presented in *separate* chapters. That is to say, these people would have me "mix it all up"; for instance, intermingle the electron theory with the muscles of the big toe. To some, perhaps, this sounds good on paper, but I know that the student questions the sanity of such a course. Interestingly, but not surprisingly, of all the many outlines and manuscripts of this character floating about, not one has ever found a publisher.

Integrated Basic Science has been addressed primarily to the nursing curriculum, but the response to the first and second editions clearly indicates that it suits the needs of a wide variety of allied medical and basic biologic science programs. In the present edition every effort has been made to perfect the contents of the second, and in this connection I wish to thank a great many instructors across the land for their thoughtful comments and suggestions. Also, I wish to thank Arthur C. Guyton, M.D., Barry G. King, Ph.D., Mary Jane Showers, Ph.D., Carl C Francis, M.D., Catherine P. Anthony, M.S., and the W. B. Saunders Company and The C. V. Mosby Company for their permission to reproduce and modify a great many illustrations.

Stewart M. Brooks

Contents

Chapter 5

Basic organic chemistry, 92

Chapter 6

Basic medical microbiology, 126

Chapter 7

The body as a whole, 160

Chapter 8

The skin, 177

Chapter 9

The skeletal system, 190

Chapter 10

The muscular system, 206

Chapter 11

The cardiovascular and lymphatic systems, 221

Chapter 12

The blood, 249

Chapter 13

The respiratory system, 264

Chapter 14

The digestive system, 286

Chapter 15

Metabolism, 308

Chapter 16

Nutrition, 320

Chapter 17

The urinary system, 328

Chapter 18

Inorganic metabolism, 337

Chapter 19

The nervous system, 348

Chapter 20

The eye, 388

Chapter 21

The ear, 400

Chapter 22

The endocrine system, 407

Chapter 23

Reproduction, 423

Chapter 24

Basic genetics, 444

General references, 451

Glossary, 453

INTEGRATED BASIC SCIENCE

STEWART M. BROOKS

Chapter 1

The history and nature of science

Science is an organized body of knowledge, especially that which seeks to establish general laws connecting a number of particular facts. Whereas theoretical or "pure" science is concerned solely with the discovery and formulation of new facts, laws, and theories, "applied" science is concerned with the application of such facts, laws, and theories to the matters of everyday living.

EVOLUTION OF SCIENCE

Science is as old as man, having evolved all the way from his first try at building a fire to landing on the moon. The true student has a keen interest in the history of science not only because the past serves as a guidepost to the future but also because the curious mind has an insatiable desire to learn about the great minds that have come and gone.

Prehistoric science. Man's first great scientific discovery was fire. In one stroke he was able to cook his meat, scare away vicious animals, and heat and light his cave. At about the same time he learned how to fashion tools and weapons from rough stone. Later these crude implements gave way to such refinements as whetstone edges equipped with handles. When the so-called New Stone Age gave way to the Age of Metals with the discovery of copper, bronze, and iron, man was well on the road to civilization. Indeed, by 5000 B.C. such items as dyes, vinegar, beer, wine, medicinals, soap, and objects of art were well known to those who inhabited the fertile valleys of the Middle East.

To those who think in terms of the modern laboratory, early man was certainly not "scientific." In a broad sense, though, he was. Early man had great curiosity—more perhaps than modern man—and curiosity is the essence of science.

Ancient science. From the earliest records of history to the fall of Rome there was unbelievable scientific progress. By 4200 B.C. the Egyptians had developed their knowledge of astronomy to such an extent that they were able to devise a calendar of 365 days. Other treasures of knowledge left by this first great civilization include the early concepts of astronomy, mathematics, chemistry, architecture, and engineering.

The reason for this breakthrough in scientific knowledge stems from the fact that the Egyptians had learned to write! The alphabet—perhaps the most significant contribution from the Nile—not only facilitated thinking but, just as important, enabled man to place his thoughts in history.

As the winds of civilization swept around the eastern end of the Great Sea, man's curiosity and thoughts began to soar to new heights. Genius flourished in Greece particularly. Pythagorus (2500 years ago!) taught that numerical relationships can be found in all nature. But the most shocking explosion of knowledge came when Leucippus (fourth century B.C.) and Democritus (fifth century B.C.) proposed that all matter is composed of indestructible particles called *atoms.* Other famous men of early Greece whose scientific curiosity played a role in shaping the world of thought include Aristotle, Euclid, Archimedes, Galen, Hippocrates, and Ptolemy.

The Roman scientist, in contrast to the Greek, was more interested in *applying* what seemed already known than in searching the mental protoplasm for new knowledge. Rome applied the scientific genius of ancient Greece and carried it to the farthest shores of the Mediterranean—to the "ends of the world."

One Roman scientist of note was Pliny the Elder (A.D. 23–A.D. 79). Although, paradoxically, his own scientific methods were questionable, he was the first to bring together the scientific knowledge of the past and present into one book. This immense work, called *Naturalis Historia,* covers geography, anthropology, botany, zoology, mineralogy, and applications of science to medicine and the fine arts.

Medieval science. When the Arabs came to power in the eighth century, they gathered together the scientific fruits of Rome and Greece. Although they paid little respect to the scientific method, they made outstanding contributions to mathematics, astronomy, chemistry, and medicine. As a matter of fact, had the Arabs not preserved the essence of Roman and Greek science, little would have survived from the ruins of the Roman Empire.

With the rediscovery of Aristotle's teachings in the thirteenth century and the translation of his complete works from Arabic and Greek, great scholars of the Church such as Albertus Magnus and Saint Thomas Aquinas sought to integrate these teachings with those of theology. Scientific inquiry virtually ceased during this period, and those who sought to challenge Aristotelian science (Galileo, for instance) were accused of heresy. This, of course, was no fault of Aristotle, for he could not foresee how his writings would be distorted centuries later.

It was in this stifled environment that alchemy, astrology, and the like came into their own. The alchemist had wild dreams of chemical magic and spent his dreary days toiling over smoldering cauldrons and retorts looking for the philosopher's stone, something that would change ordinary metals into gold.

In all fairness, though, it must be confessed that some alchemists made an honest attempt at experimentation. The most famous alchemist, and certainly one of the most colorful men of science, was the Swiss thinker Paracelsus (1493-1541). Although his work and writings were not infrequently tainted with the fantastic philosophies of his time, Paracelsus made some amazing discoveries and contributions. Among other things, he pointed out the fallacies in many current medical theories, taught the use of specific remedies instead of indiscriminate bleeding and purging, and introduced the medicinal use of opium, mercury, sulfur, iron, and arsenic.

The Middle Ages apparently produced only one great scientist—Roger Bacon (1214-1294). While other learned men of the time fell victim to the lethargy of unscientific thinking, Bacon proclaimed the "magic" of the scientific method. Indeed, this man anticipated the methods of modern science. "The end of all true philosophy," Bacon said, "is to arrive at a knowledge of the Creator through knowledge of the external world." It was he who first underscored the indispensability of mathematics and experimentation to science.

Renaissance science. The rebirth of scientific thinking in the fifteenth and sixteenth centuries is one of the marvels of man's existence on earth. Almost overnight, historically speaking, mental sparks appeared in the darkness of wayward thinking.

Nicolaus Copernicus, a priest (1473-1543), shocked the civilized world by his discovery that the sun, and not the earth, was the center of the universe. What disclosure could better herald a renaissance than such a revelation as this? A century later, Galileo Galilei confirmed the findings of Copernicus and struck out in bold fashion against medieval sorcery in general and the undue application of theology to science in particular. Other important scientists of the period were Kepler (astronomy), Boyle (physics), Vesalius (medicine), and Harvey (medicine).

By the end of the sixteenth century astronomy, mathematics, chemistry, physics, and medicine were well along the ever-widening path to scientific truth.

Seventeenth and eighteenth century science. During the seventeenth and eighteenth centuries modern science came into its own. Newton opened the door for Einstein; Huygens explored the nature of light; Franklin "solved" the mystery of electricity; Watt invented the steam engine; Lavoisier, Priestley, and Cavendish unlocked the basic laws of chemistry; and Desargues, Descartes, Fermat, and Pascal breathed new life into mathematical thinking.

Nineteenth century science. In the life sciences Darwin electrified this period with his theory of evolution. John Dalton revolutionized the concept of matter with his atomic theory, a piece of thinking so clear and simple we marvel that it was so long in coming. Faraday and Henry added to the findings of Franklin and laid the groundwork for our knowledge of electricity and magnetism. In 1838 Schleiden presented proof that all plant tissues were composed of cells, and in 1839 Schwann demonstrated that the cell is also the basis of animal tissue. These two pronouncements, together referred to as the *cell theory*, gave birth to modern biology.

The most phenomenal scientific happenings came at the turn of the century. Becquerel discovered radioactivity; the Curies isolated radium; Roentgen discovered x rays; Planck developed the quantum concept of light; Rutherford and Soddy probed the heart of the atom; and Einstein startled humanity with the theory of relativity.

HISTORY OF MEDICINE

Medicine, as an applied science, naturally bears close chronologic relation to the evolution of the natural sciences. However, the student will no doubt wish a more intimate picture than the one suggested in the foregoing section.

Ancient medicine. Prehistoric man had a keen interest in the preservation of health and instinctively searched his cave's environs for magical cures. Also, he probably learned something of "dentistry" and the care of broken limbs and infected wounds. It now appears, for instance, that antibiosis was a primitive art. At the dawn of written history, then, man had already amassed a considerable body of medical knowledge. Although it was obviously predicated upon the unknown, magic, and mysticism, the seeds of modern medicine had taken root.

The first great gifts to medicine came from the mind of the Greek genius Hippocrates (ca. 460 B.C.–370 B.C.). Since a good share of this man's teachings were 2000 years ahead of his time, he is, indeed, the father of medicine. Hippocrates rescued medicine from the clutches of superstition and placed it on the podium of scientific reasoning. His keen eye at the bedside and his nimble brain laid the foundation for modern clinical medicine. Equally significant is the fact that Hippocrates was a prolific writer and bent by nature to place all he knew in the written record. One of his best-known works is *Aphorisms,* a collection of concise statements relating to the practice of medicine.

Although Hippocrates was not the author of the so-called Hippocratic oath, he well deserves credit for the oath, for its message is the essence of his teachings.

Five centuries after Hippocrates, Greek medicine fell into the capable hands of Galen (ca. A.D. 130–A.D. 200). Galen founded an influential school of medicine whose teachings have survived the shifting sands of time. Though certain of his ideas were erroneous and seriously misleading, he did contribute significantly to the fields of surgery, anatomy, pathology, and particularly pharmacy. To this day, vegetable remedies are referred to among pharmacists as *galenicals.*

Another medical scientist of Greek birth, although he worked in Rome, was Asclepiades (ca. 124 B.C.–40 B.C.). He, too, was well ahead of his time and founded an influential school of medicine. Asclepiades recognized and stressed the importance of rest, massage, diet, and exercise.

Rome took its medical science from Greece and did little to improve upon its basic teachings. Indeed, Galen was the court physician to Marcus Aurelius and practiced surgery upon the Colosseum's mangled gladiators. The Arabs, in contrast, advanced medicine, particularly drug therapeutics, and left valuable records of medical knowledge.

Medieval medicine. Thanks to the Arabic world, medicine fared well during the strife-torn Middle Ages. This, the student will recall, was in stark contrast to the growth of the natural sciences. Famous schools of medicine were founded at Salerno, Padua, and other cities. All in all, medical knowledge was not only preserved but also advanced during the era.

Renaissance medicine. With the coming of the Renaissance, medicine was advanced tremendously at the hands of Vesalius (1514-1564). This brilliant Flemish investigator pioneered the dissection of the human body and probably contributed more to our knowledge of anatomy than any other man. His meticulous drawings, accurate to a hairbreadth, to this day are marvels of medicine and art.

Vesalius also practiced surgery. He operated on none other than Don Carlos of Aragon. He also performed several successful operations for removal of the breast. It was the findings and teachings of Vesalius that overthrew the misconceptions promulgated by Galen. Vesalius' *De Humani Corporis Fabrica* (1543) remains one of the great classics of medical science.

Other men of note in Renaissance medicine were Leonardo da Vinci (1452-1519) and Ambroise Paré (1510-1590). Da Vinci, "the genius of all sciences," added significantly to our knowledge of anatomy, and Paré contributed to the practice of medicine and surgery. The latter scientist, often the forgotten man in history, did much to advance bedside medicine. He reintroduced the ligature in amputations, promoted the use of artificial limbs, and introduced podalic version.

Modern medicine. William Harvey (1578-1657) is generally regarded as the father of modern medicine. He amplified and corrected the theories and practices of his predecessors and, most important, discovered the circulation of the blood. Although he lectured on the subject as early as 1616, the world was not generally apprised of his monumental findings until the publication of the now famous *Exercitatio Anatomica de Motu Cordis et Sanguinis* in 1628. With the exception of the capillary system, the complete circulation is described in this work.

In 1676 Antony van Leeuwenhoek, a draper's assistant from Amsterdam, struck out in a new direction and is credited with being one of the early discoverers of the microscope. He assembled over 250 microscopes and was the first to see bacteria, protozoa, and red blood cells. It is little wonder, then, that van Leeuwenhoek is commonly considered to be the father of bacteriology.

William Hunter (1718-1783), a Scottish physician, made notable contributions to anatomy and surgery. Equally significant were his talents as a lecturer and teacher, with which he did much to further the techniques of medical education. Hunter's priceless anatomic collections were bequeathed to the University of Glasgow.

Edward Jenner, a contemporary of Hunter, startled the world in 1796 by protecting a small boy (James Phipps) against a lethal dose of smallpox with a prior injection (vaccination) of cowpox virus. Thus, for the first time, man was given a weapon with which to ward off his invisible enemies. The magnitude of this discovery, together with the simplicity of the experiment and Jenner's status as a country doctor, teases the imagination and underscores the fact that great thoughts often stem from humble minds.

In the latter part of the nineteenth century Pasteur and Koch dominated the field of bacteriology. They firmly established the relationship between pathogenic organisms and disease and laid the foundations for modern microbiology. Pasteur, one of the greatest minds of all time, once and for all destroyed the concept of spontaneous generation. He discovered the staphylococcus and the pneumococcus, established the anthrax bacillus as the cause of anthrax, and devised the process that bears his name—pasteurization. Pasteur's brilliant career came to a climax in 1885 with his development of a treatment for rabies. The vaccine and the treatment employed today are essentially the same as those proposed by Pasteur.

Koch (1843-1910) of Germany stands as a close second to Pasteur. He discovered the anthrax bacillus, perfected the pure culture technique, and in 1882 demonstrated the causative agent of tuberculosis. Above all, he set forth the postulates relating to the germ theory of disease.

In America, surgery took its greatest step forward on October 16, 1846. On this day, before a gallery of skeptical spectators at the Massachusetts General Hospital, William T. G. Morton (a dentist) put Gilbert Abbott to sleep with ether. Dr. Bigelow, a surgeon attending the operation performed by Dr. J. C. Warren, explained, "I have seen something today that will go around the world."

In England, Lister (1827-1912) applied Pasteur's teachings to surgery with resounding success. The dramatic reduction of infectious complications in the postoperative patient soon established the concept of antiseptic surgery, a *sine qua non* of the operating room. This development, plus Morton's demonstration, finally placed surgery on a par with medicine.

Other milestones in surgery were the contributions of McDowell in America and Bergmann in Germany. In 1809 McDowell defied his time by performing the first ovariotomy. No less important was Bergmann's introduction of steam sterilization of surgical instruments.

The discovery of x rays by Roentgen in 1895, radioactivity by Becquerel in 1896, and radium by the Curies in 1898 brought new glory to medicine. Now man could not only stop the frenzied multiplication of cancerous tissue but could even look inside the body. Equally significant, in 1898 Sir Ronald Ross of England demonstrated the life history of the malarial parasite and proved its transmission by the bite of the female *Anopheles* mosquito.

The present century has seen medicine and surgery ascend to heights well beyond our wildest expectations. Ehrlich gave birth to the concept of chemotherapy, Fleming discovered penicillin, Domagk synthesized the first sulfonamide, and Banting and Best isolated insulin. In the last few years the heart and brain have yielded to routine surgery, and kidney and heart transplantations are everyday occurrences.

Perhaps the greatest achievements of the present, however, are often not appreciated by the public at large. This is paradoxical, for the chemist is now in the process of unraveling the workings of life itself. The general mechanism by which the cell synthesizes protein (the "backbone" of protoplasm) is now understood, and the genome (man's blueprint) is yielding its secrets. Above all, a virus—"life"—has actually been created in the test tube.

For more definitive information relating to the medical advancements of our century, the student should look over the Nobel Prizes awarded in medicine. From 1901, the first year in which the prize was awarded, through 1968 the laureates and their contributions are as follows:

1901 Emil von Behring (German*) *Diphtheria antitoxin.*

1902 Sir Ronald Ross (British) *Vector of malaria.*

1903 Niels R. Finsen (Danish) *Light therapy.*

1904 Ivan P. Pavlov (Russian) *Conditioned reflexes.*

1905 Robert Koch (German) *Discovery of tubercle bacillus.*

1906 C. Golgi (Italian) and S. Ramón y Cajal (Spanish) *Anatomy of nervous system.*

1907 Charles L. A. Laveran (French) *Discovery of parasite of malaria.*

1908 Paul Ehrlich (German) and E. Metchnikoff (French) *Studies on immunity.*

1909 Theodor Kocher (Swiss) *Physiology of the thyroid gland.*

1910 Albrecht Kossel (German) *Protein studies.*

1911 Allvar Gullstrand (Swedish) *Dioptrics of eye.*

1912 Alexis Carrel (American) *Organ transplants.*

1913 Charles Richet (French) *Anaphylaxis studies.*

*Nationality at the time the award was given.

1914 R. Bárány (Austrian) *Physiology of vestibular apparatus.*

1915 No prize awarded.

1916 No prize awarded.

1917 No prize awarded.

1918 No prize awarded.

1919 Jules Bordet (Belgian) *Immunity studies.*

1920 A. Krogh (Danish) *Capillary studies.*

1921 No prize awarded.

1922 A. V. Hill (British) and O. Meyerhof (German) *Muscle physiology.*

1923 F. G. Banting and J. J. R. Macleod (Canadian) *Discovery of insulin.*

1924 Willem Einthoven (Dutch) *Electrocardiograph.*

1925 No prize awarded.

1926 Johannes Fibiger (Danish) *Spiroptera carcinoma.*

1927 J. Wagner-Jauregg (Austrian) *Treatment of paresis.*

1928 Charles Nicolle (French) *Vector of typhus.*

1929 Sir F. G. Hopkins (British) and C. Eijkman (Danish) *Discovery of vitamin B_1.*

1930 Karl Landsteiner (American) *Discovery of human blood groups.*

1931 Otto Warburg (German) *Respiratory enzymes.*

1932 Sir C. S. Sherrington and E. D. Adrian (British) *Physiology of neuron.*

1933 T. H. Morgan (American) *Chromosome studies.*

1934 G. G. Whipple, G. R. Minot, and W. P. Murphy (American) *Liver therapy in pernicious anemia.*

1935 Hans Spemann (German) *Embryology.*

1936 Sir H. H. Dale (British) and O. Loewi (Austrian) *Neurohormones.*

1937 A. Szent-Györgyi (Hungarian) *Isolation of vitamin C.*

1938 C. Heymans (Belgian) *Physiology of carotid sinus.*

1939 Gerhard Domagk (German) *Sulfonamides.*

1940 No prize awarded.

1941 No prize awarded.

1942 No prize awarded.

1943 Edward Doisy (American) and Henrik Dam (Danish) *Discovery of vitamin K.*

1944 J. Erlanger and H. Gasser (American) *Nerve physiology.*

1945 Sir A. Fleming and Sir H. W. Florey (British) and E. B. Chain (German) *Penicillin.*

1946 H. J. Muller (American) *Radiation-induced mutation.*

1947 C. F. and G. T. Cori (American) and B. Houssay (Argentine) *Carbohydrate metabolism.*

1948 P. Mueller (Swiss) *Discovery of DDT.*

1949 W. R. Hess (Swiss) and A. Moniz (Portuguese) *Brain surgery.*

1950 P. S. Hench and E. C. Kendall (American) and T. Reichstein (Swiss) *Cortisone and ACTH.*

1951 Max Theiler (South African) *Yellow fever vaccine.*

1952 S. A. Waksman (American) *Discovery of streptomycin.*

1953 F. A. Lipmann (American) and H. Krebs (Belgian) *Cellular enzymes.*

1954 T. H. Weller, F. C. Robbins, and J. Enders (American) *Cultivation of poliovirus.*

1955 Hugo Theorell (Swedish) *Discovery of oxidative enzymes.*

1956 D. W. Richards, Jr., and A. F. Cournand (American) and W. Forssmann (German) *Cardiac catheterization.*

1957 D. Bovet (Italian) *Development of synthetic curare and antihistamines.*

1958 G. W. Beadle, E. L. Tatum, and J. Lederberg (American) *Genetics and heredity.*

1959 S. Ochoa and A. Kornberg (American) *Discovery of the enzymes that produce nucleic acid.*

1960 Sir M. Burnet (Australian) and P. B. Medawar (British) *Immunity studies.*

1961 Georg von Békésy (American) *Mechanism of hearing.*

1962 J. D. Watson and M. H. F. Wilkins (American) and F. H. C. Crick (British) *Determination of the structure of deoxyribonucleic acid (DNA).*

1963 A. L. Hodgkin and A. F. Huxley (British) and Sir J. C. Eccles (Australian) *Research on nerve cells.*

1964 K. E. Bloch (American) and F. Lynen (German) *Discoveries in cholesterol and fatty acid metabolism.*

1965 F. Jacob, A. Lwolff, and J. Monod (French) *Elucidation of regulatory activities of body cells.*

1966 C. B. Higgins and F. P. Rous (American) *Hormone treatment of cancer of prostate and discovery of tumor-producing viruses, respectively.*

1967 H. K. Hartline, G. Wald, and R. Granit (American) *Physiology of human eye.*

1968 R. W. Holley, H. G. Khorana, and M. W. Nirenberg (American) *Genetic code.*

BRANCHES OF SCIENCE

The almost endless varieties of science draw their sustenance from three prime disciplines of knowledge—*chemistry, physics,* and *mathematics.* This, however, is not a startling revelation if we recall that, dead or alive, the physical universe is composed of only two entities—*matter* and *energy.* Essentially, chemistry is concerned with the former and physics with the latter. Mathematics is an indispensable tool that serves both.

Specifically, physics is concerned with heat, light, electricity, sound, radiation, and the structure of matter. Chemistry, on the other hand, deals with the composition of matter and the changes that it undergoes. Mathematics is the science, if we may be so bold as to call it a science (some think of it as a form of philosophy), that deals with numbers and the measurement, properties, and relationship of quantities. Obviously, without mathematics there can be no science. As Lord Kelvin, the great English scientist, so aptly remarked, "When you can measure what you are seeking about and express it in numbers, you know something about it."

Medical science. The chief sciences relating to medicine include anatomy, physiology, microbiology, biochemistry, biophysics, pharmacology, and pathology. As indicated, these areas of knowledge are concerned, directly or indirectly, with the chemistry and physics (and mathematics) of living matter. Anatomy and physiology are the study of the structure and function, respectively, of the body. Microbiology deals with microscopic forms of life, particularly those which cause disease. Biochemistry and biophysics, respectively, are concerned with the application of chemical and physical principles to physiologic processes. Pharmacology is the study of drugs. Pathology, the study of disease, is, in a sense, medical science itself; among other sciences, it draws from the teachings of anatomy, physiology, biochemistry, histology, microbiology, and toxicology.

SCIENTIFIC METHOD

To say that science is knowledge is a slight understatement. Science is also the process by which knowledge is obtained, a process known as the scientific method.

The scientific method is concerned essentially with the *what's*, *how's*, and *why's*. Although no two scientists will set out in exactly the same way to answer these questions, there is a general technique that all men of science employ in the solution of a new problem. Basically, the scientific method is as follows.

Statement of problem. When the scientist sets out to solve a new problem, he must exercise extreme care in placing the problem on paper. In other words, the statement of the problem must be made in clear and concise language, free from the slightest ambiguity. It is the same idea as shooting at a target; unless one aims at the bull's-eye, the results are generally disappointing.

Searching literature. The next step, obviously, is to search the written record to obtain *all* the known facts that relate to the stated problem. In this way the scientist is availing himself of the fruits of previous research. Thus, he must have the best possible understanding of the literature pertaining to his field of work.

Experimentation. Experimentation is the phase of scientific method that identifies science to the man on the street. By discovering, collecting, and classifying facts, the scientist "builds up his case."

In carrying out an experiment, the scientist tries to find out what will happen (that is, the "effect") in a situation under meticulously controlled conditions when a single factor is varied. For instance, if he wished to study the effects of vitamin A deficiency in the rat, he would set up his experiment in such a way that the rat's diet contained all the known nutrients except vitamin A. Also, he would use not one rat but many rats of the same type, age, and weight to ensure against individual variation. The deficiency diet, of course, would be given to only half of the rats. Otherwise how would the scientist be able to see the difference? The rats on the normal diet constitute the *control* group. Any experiment, to be valid, must be run against some type of control.

Answer and explanation. From the foregoing data the scientist next attempts to answer the problem, and if an answer is found that fits all situations, then said answer becomes a *scientific law*. A law is not the end in itself, however, for what the scientist really wants to know is "Why?" In other words, he seeks an explanation of the law in the form of a hypothesis or theory. This requires great thinking, and here the scientist employs the laboratory of his highly developed brain.

Not infrequently, the terms *theory* and *hypothesis* are employed interchangeably. In ordinary usage the practice adds spice to the language, but that is not the case in scientific use. In science a hypothesis refers to a supposition or tentative theory that is provisionally adopted to explain certain facts and to guide in the investigation of others. As a matter of fact, the scientist commonly employs the expression *working hypothesis*. As students of science, therefore, we should understand that a hypothesis is an unverified theory or, put another way, a theory is a verified hypothesis.

Publishing results. Once the scientist has answered the problem, he publishes his findings in a reputable scientific journal. In days gone by this step was either slighted or completely neglected. History bears tragic testimony to important discoveries that were written on the sands of time rather than on paper. It is true that these findings were rediscovered, but only at the cost of precious time. Moreover, many a great scientist of the past could have avoided errors and made more outstanding contributions than he did if his predecessors had taken more to the written record.

Questions

1. Read several current newspaper articles of a scientific nature and identify the branch or branches of science discussed in each.
2. From your own personal experience cite some situation or problem that you solved and compare your method of approach with the scientific method discussed in the text.
3. Look up the latest Nobel Prizes awarded in chemistry, physics, and medicine and write a brief summary of the nature of the work and contribution in each area.

Chapter 2

Scientific measurement

The ability to measure is the keystone of the scientific method; without this ability, man's activities would soon grind to a halt. Obviously, therefore, the student of science at any level must have a command of the systems and units of measurement, particularly with respect to their magnitude and computation.

With the fall of the Roman Empire, progress in most areas of human endeavor was severely retarded by a lack of a precise and unified system of measurement. Although the Romans had contributed much toward unification by introducing their system into the conquered lands, each of the newly formed countries and nations went its own way in this regard. In practical terms this meant that an experiment performed in one country would not necessarily correspond with the same experiment performed in another. Things got so bad, not only in science but also in other areas of everyday life, that we might say that it took a revolution to straighten them out. Indeed, it was at the termination of the French Revolution in 1791 that the French Academy of Science urged adoption of international standards of measurement. It was not until 1872, however, that work was begun which led to adoption of the metric system. At that time the *International Commission on Weights and Measures* met in Paris and set about construction and distribution of prototypes of the standard meter and the standard kilogram.

The metric system is now used by scientists all over the world. Although many countries have also wisely adopted this system as the official system for trade and commerce, the United States and Great Britain continue to struggle along with the so-called English system. It is now widely appreciated that in relation to the metric system the English system is a highly cumbersome mode of measurement. Nonetheless, both systems are used, and the student of science is forced to understand both, or at least to know the equivalent values (Table 2-1) for the most commonly used units.

Basically, there are four characteristics of the physical world: *space, mass, energy,* and *time.* Although these entities are difficult to define, they become meaningful and manageable when viewed in the framework of magnitude. In brief, space, mass, energy, and time can be measured. Turned around, this means there are four fundamental categories of measurement: length, volume (both having to do with space), weight

Table 2-1. Metric system

Length	
1 micron (μ)	= 0.000001 meter
1 millimeter (mm.)	= 0.001 meter
1 centimeter (cm.)	= 0.01 meter
1 decimeter (dm.)	= 0.1 meter
Meter (m.)	= 1.0 meter
1 dekameter (dkm.)	= 10 meters
1 hectometer (hm.)	= 100 meters
1 kilometer (km.)	= 1000 meters
Weight	
1 microgram (μg)	= 0.000001 gram
1 milligram (mg.)	= 0.001 gram
1 centigram (cg.)	= 0.01 gram
1 decigram (dg.)	= 0.1 gram
Gram (gm.)	= 1.0 gram
1 dekagram (dkg.)	= 10 grams
1 hectogram (hg.)	= 100 grams
1 kilogram (kg.)	= 1000 grams
Volume	
1 microliter (μl)	= 0.000001 liter
1 milliliter (ml.)	= 0.001 liter
1 centiliter (cl.)	= 0.01 liter
1 deciliter (dl.)	= 0.1 liter
Liter (L.)	= 1.0 liter
1 dekaliter (dkl.)	= 10 liters
1 hectoliter (hl.)	= 100 liters
1 kiloliter (kl.)	= 1000 liters
Metric-English equivalents	
1 meter (m.)	= 39.37 inches
1 centimeter (cm.)	= 0.3937 inch
1 kilometer (km.)	= 0.62 mile
1 kilogram (kg.)	= 2.204 pounds
1 liter (l.)	= 1.057 quarts (liquid)
1 yard (yd.)	= 0.914 meter
1 foot (ft.)	= 30.48 centimeters
1 inch (in.)	= 2.54 centimeters
1 mile (mi.)	= 1.61 kilometers
1 ounce (oz.)	= 28.35 grams
1 pound (lb.)	= 453.6 grams
1 quart (qt.) (liquid)	= 0.956 liter
1 quart (dry)	= 1.101 liters

(mass), and time itself. These will now be discussed in relation to their respective metric units.

LENGTH

The meter is the standard unit of length, equal to exactly 39.37 inches. Formerly, it was defined as the distance between two marks on a platinum-iridium bar (kept in the International Bureau of Weights and Measures at Sèvres, France), but in 1960 a new standard was adopted. Now the meter is defined as 1,650,763.73 wavelengths of the orange-red light of krypton-86.

The meter, like the other basic units of the metric system, is divided and multiplied into series of tens to produce smaller and larger units, respectively. As shown in Table 2-1, these derived units carry the appropriate prefix followed by the suffix *-meter*. The major exception in the case of length units is the expression for 1 millionth of a meter. Instead of using the prefix *micro-* (millionth) and calling this unit a "micrometer," the term *micron* was coined. When one is dealing with dimensions too small to be seen with the unaided eye, this unit serves a highly useful purpose. In microbiology and histology (microscopic anatomy), for instance, the micron is the chief unit of length. The relationship between the centimeter and the inch is shown in Fig. 2-1.

Angstrom. When dealing with fantastically small distances (the diameter of the nucleus of an atom, for example), scientists use the angstrom (Å). This unit is equal to $\frac{1}{10}$ of a millimicron, or 10^{-8} cm.; in the English system this turns out to be $\frac{1}{254}$ millionths of an inch! The angstrom is the principal unit of length in atomic physics, particularly in the measurement of wavelength.

MASS AND WEIGHT

Mass, or *quantity* of matter, can be measured in several ways. The simplest pro-

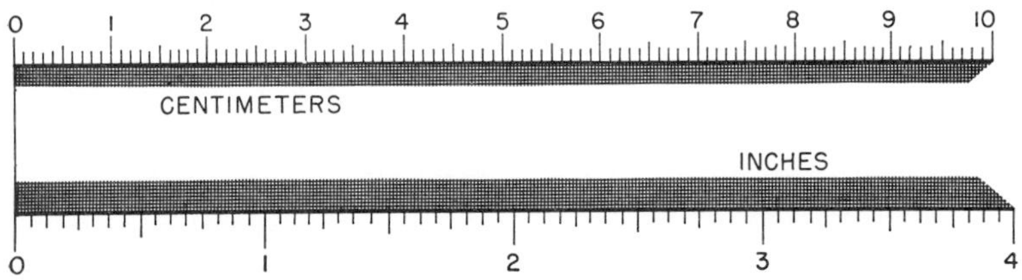

Fig. 2-1. Comparison of the inch and the centimeter.

cedure, however, is weighing. When we weigh an object, whether by stretching a spring or balancing the object against a standard mass, what we are really measuring is the pull of gravity, which we call *weight*. In the true sense, therefore, mass and weight are not the same. An object of a given mass on earth, for example, has the same mass anywhere else in the universe and vice versa. But this is not so in the case of weight. For example, on the moon, a much smaller body with much less gravity than the earth, a given mass weighs less than it does on earth. If the moon had an atmosphere, it might be an ideal home for "calorie counters."

The terms *mass* and *weight* are usually considered synonymous and are employed interchangeably in general chemistry and the applied sciences. The physicist, however, concerned as he is with gravity and other forces, must necessarily recognize the distinction between the two. In this text, mass and weight will be considered as one, and generally the more common expression *weight* will be used.

The metric unit of weight is the *kilogram* (kg.), which is equal to 2.2 pounds. The standard kilogram, a mass of an alloy of 90 percent platinum and 10 percent iridium, resides in the International Bureau of Weights and Measures at Sèvres, France.

VOLUME

The metric unit of volume is the *liter* (l.), which is the volume occupied by 1 kg. of water at its maximum density (4° C.). Although the *milliliter* (ml.) should equal the *cubic centimeter* (c.c.), the original standard kilogram (which is equal to 1000 ml.) turned out to occupy 1,000.028 c.c. instead of the intended 1000 c.c., making the milliliter a "tiny bit" larger than the cubic centimeter. However, for usual measurements the difference may be ignored.

DENSITY

In order to measure heaviness, the concept of density was introduced. Whether we realize it or not, what we really mean when we say that lead is heavier than cotton is that a given volume of the former weighs more than the same volume of the latter. Scientifically, we say that lead has a greater density than cotton. In precise terms, density (d) is equal to mass, or weight (w), divided by volume (v), or

$$d = \frac{w}{v}$$

In the metric system, density is expressed as grams per cubic centimeter. Gold, for instance, has a density of 19.3 gm. per cubic centimeter; that is, 19.3 gm. of this metal occupies a volume of 1 c.c. or, turned around, 1 c.c. weighs 19.3 gm. If we wish to compare the heaviness of gold to any other metal, all we need do is consult a reference work. Mercury, for example, is lighter than gold because its density is found to be 13.6 gm. per cubic centimeter (13.6 gm./c.c.).

Specific gravity. In order to compare the densities of different substances in a speedy yet accurate way, we use what is called the specific gravity. This is equal to the density of the substance in question divided by the density of water, or it may be de-

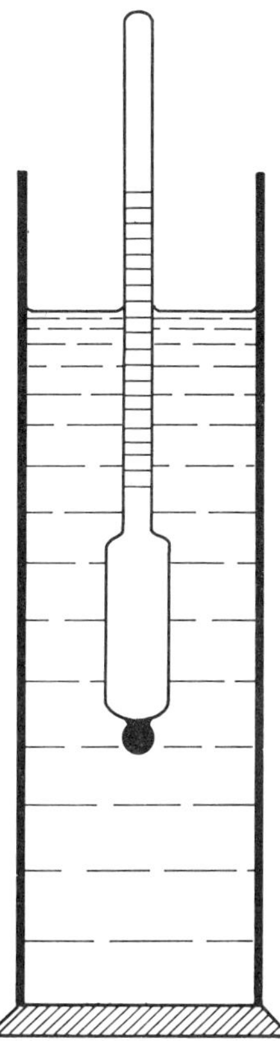

Fig. 2-2. Hydrometer. This instrument operates on the principle that an object floats "high" in a liquid of high specific gravity and "low" in a liquid of low specific gravity. The specific gravity is read where the surface of the liquid crosses the graduated scale.

fined as the weight of the substance divided by the weight of an equal volume of water. Thus,

$$\text{Specific gravity (SG)} = \frac{\text{Density of substance}}{\text{Density of water}} \quad \text{or}$$

$$\text{Specific gravity (SG)} = \frac{\text{Weight of substance}}{\text{Weight of an equal volume of water}}$$

The specific gravity of gold, for example, is computed by dividing 19.3, its density, by 1, the density of water:

$$\frac{\text{19.3 gm. per cubic centimeter}}{\text{1 gm. per cubic centimeter}} = 19.3$$

It should be noted especially that since the units cancel out the quotient (19.3) is merely a number without units. In other words, a specific gravity of 19.3 means that gold is 19.3 times heavier than water. Note, too, that a specific gravity of less than 1 means that a substance is lighter than water. The specific gravity of a liquid may be readily obtained by means of the *hydrometer* (Fig. 2-2).

ENERGY AND WORK

Energy is the ability to do work. This may sound like a rather strange definition, but we must remember that no one knows precisely what energy is. In short, we are forced to define energy in terms of what it can do—work. In practice there is nothing wrong with this definition, for work can be precisely measured, and as we know, measurement is the tool of scientific inquiry.

Erg. In science the term *work* is not used as casually as in everyday parlance. For instance, if we were to push in on a wall to prevent it from falling over, we would all agree that work was being done; scientifically, however, we would not be working. In the language of physics, work means a force moving through a distance, or

$$\text{Work } (w) = \text{Force } (f) \times \text{Distance } (d)$$

This, of course, introduces the term *force,* which for our present purposes we may think of as any "influence" that can change the position or motion of an object. Although force can be expressed in several ways, the simplest unit (and the one most suitable to delicate experimentation) is the *dyne,* a force that causes a mass of 1 gm. to accelerate 1 cm. per second. Now if we wish to measure work in the metric system, we multiply dynes times the distance in centimeters, which gives dyne centimeters of work, or ergs.

The erg, therefore, is the *metric unit of work.* It is defined as the work done (or the energy expended) in moving a body 1 cm. against a force of 1 dyne, or it is just as correct to say that an erg is the work performed when a force of 1 dyne moves through a distance of 1 cm. Since the erg is such an extremely small unit, equal to just about the muscular work expended in winking the eye, the much larger *joule* (a unit equal to 10 million ergs) is commonly used.

Foot-pound. In the United States the so-called foot-pound is the principal unit employed to measure mechanical work. This is the amount of work done when a force of 1 pound acts through the distance of 1 foot. It is computed simply by multiplying pounds by feet. For example, if a man lifts a 100-pound bag of grain 3 feet off the floor, he does 300 foot-pounds of work. By the same reasoning, a boy who pulls a 50-pound wagon a distance of 30 feet does about 1500 foot-pounds of work. The foot-pound is larger than the joule (1 joule is equal to 0.737 foot-pound).

Power. By power we mean the rate at which work is done; it is equal to work divided by time. One *horsepower* (hp), the usual unit of mechanical power, is equal to a rate of 550 foot-pounds per second. A machine, for example, that works at the rate of 5500 foot-pounds per second is designated as 10 horsepower.

Electrical power, on the other hand, is generally measured in watts or kilowatts. The watt is equal to 1 joule of work per second. One kilowatt, of course, would be equal to 1000 watts. It takes 746 watts of power to equal 1 horsepower.

TIME

Time, the fourth dimension, stands next to the Euclidean dimensions in describing the events of the cosmos. Even in everyday terms, how could we possibly mention an event on earth without reference to time? Thus, an examination is scheduled to take place not only at a given location but also at a given time. Without the latter dimension, the first part of the statement has no meaning. Thus, it is altogether possible that time was one of the first things man tried to measure. Since an ideal timepiece should be unchanging and readily available to all, it is not surprising that the "movement" of the sun and stars was selected as the mainspring of the fourth dimension.

For civil purposes the sun is the clock. The time from one *true noon* (the sun at its highest elevation) to the next true noon equals one *solar day*. However, because the solar day gradually changes in length throughout the year, the *mean solar day* is selected as the standard; this is equal to the average of all the solar days over a whole year. The mean solar day, as we well know, is divided into 24 hours, with each hour divided into 60 minutes and each minute into 60 seconds.

When high precision is required, the mean solar day is calculated from its relation to *sidereal time,* the latter being determined from observation of the meridian transits of stars. The mean sidereal day equals 23 hours 56 minutes 4.09 seconds of mean solar time.

GEOLOGIC TIME

As inhabitants of the earth, we are naturally interested and curious about the history of our planet and what it was like before man appeared. Here, particularly, we would like to know its relation to time—in short, its age and "what happened when."

On the basis of radioactive dating, the earth is now believed to be about 4 billion years old. The geologist divides this abysmal past into *eras,* which are delineated by the major changes that have occurred in the earth's crust (Table 2-2). The first, or Precambrian era, came to an end when the processes responsible for the oldest rocks came to a halt; the Paleozoic era marks the formation of the large land masses above sea level; the Mesozoic era

Table 2-2. The geologic timetable*

Era	Period	Dominant life forms	Years ago (in millions of years)
	(Primitive man)		2
Cenozoic	Quaternary	Mammals	17
	Tertiary		58
	Cretaceous	Dinosaurs	100
Mesozoic	Jurassic	Dinosaurs	150
	Triassic	Dinosaurs	210
	Permian	Reptiles	215
	Carboniferous	Amphibians	220
	Devonian	Fishes	255
Paleozoic	Silurian	Sea scorpions	310
	Ordovician	Nautiloids	350
	Cambrian	Trilobites	440
	Late	Soft-bodied invertebrates	600
Precambrian	(Black Hills, U. S. A.)		1600
	(Russian Karelia)	One-celled organisms	1800

*From Slabaugh, H. W., and Butler, A. B.: College physical science, Englewood Cliffs, N. J., 1958, Prentice-Hall, Inc.

started with the upheavals associated with the formation of the Appalachian Mountains in the United States and ended with the upthrusts of the Rocky Mountains; our present era, the Cenozoic, began with the last-mentioned event.

As shown in Table 2-2, the eras are subdivided into *periods,* each of which is generally associated with the appearance of certain flora and fauna. For example, fossil evidence indicates that fishes first appeared in the Devonian period, dinosaurs in the Triassic period, and last (but we hope certainly not least) man appeared in the Quaternary period. Most of what we know of the biology of these periods has been deduced from the order of succession of the sedimentary rocks and of their contained fossils.

Questions

1. A glass rod is 90 cm. long. What is its length in millimeters? In meters?
2. A boy is 5 feet 2 inches tall. What is his height in centimeters?
3. A golf ball weighs 46.2 gm. What is its weight in milligrams? In ounces?
4. If one tablet of morphine contains 10 mg., how many can be made from ½ ounce?
5. A table measures 3 × 2 m. What is its area in square inches?
6. How many liters of water does it take to fill a rectangular tank that is 75 cm. long, 60 cm. wide, and 70 cm. deep?
7. A cube of wood measuring 8 cm. on a side weighs 43 ounces. What is its density?
8. The specific gravity of urine gives a clue to the ability of the kidneys to excrete wastes. Explain.
9. At each heartbeat about 70 c.c. of blood is shot into the circulation. Using this figure, and taking the heart rate to be 70 beats per

minute, how many quarts of blood does the heart pump per minute?

10. A man weighs 154 pounds. What is his weight in kilograms?
11. An object that weighs 600 gm. in air weighs only 450 gm. when immersed in water. What is its volume?
12. What is the specific gravity of a substance that has a density of 12.5 gm. per cubic centimeter?
13. If a man lifts a stone weighing 15 pounds a distance of 3.5 feet off the ground, how much work does he do?
14. How many ergs of work are done when a force of 225 dynes acts through a distance of 6 inches?
15. What is the difference between power and work?
16. Assuming ideal conditions, how many kilowatts of electricity can be obtained from a generator run by a 2-horsepower engine?
17. What is the apothecaries' system of weights and measures?
18. A cylindrical vessel is 8 inches high and has a diameter of 3 inches. What is its volume in terms of milliliters?
19. Glycerin has a density of 1.25 gm. per cubic centimeter. What volume is used if a formula calls for 60 gm. of this liquid?
20. If 2 c.c. of mercury weighs 26 gm., what is its density?
21. Upon what physical principle does the hydrometer depend?
22. If a substance has a specific gravity of 2, what does this mean in practical terms?
23. In the metric system the specific gravity and density are numerically the same. Explain.
24. Whereas the density of a substance is understood to mean grams per milliliter (or grams per cubic centimeter), specific gravity is merely a number "without units." Using the formula specific gravity = gm. per c.c. divided by gm. per c.c., show why this is true.
25. What is the simplest way to demonstrate whether a solid has a specific gravity above or below 1?

the scale is pushing up with the same force. It sometimes happens that an object fails to develop certain reaction, with ineffectual results. For example, while a dry road resists the backward push of a car's wheels and pushes the latter forward, an icy road cannot react to the backward push, and the wheels merely spin.

The third law of motion, which makes it possible for man to explore outer space, can be easily demonstrated by blowing up a toy balloon and then letting it "fly away." The fiery gases streaking from the tail of a rocket develop sufficient forward thrust to overcome the pull of gravity.

Gravity. We are also indebted to Newton for the law of gravitation. Although no one seems to know exactly what this mysterious and cosmic force really is, it can be measured. The law asserts that every body, from an atom to a planet, attracts every other body with a force *directly proportional to their masses and indirectly proportional to the square of the distance between them.*

Though the gravitational force between objects of ordinary size is insignificant, it is far from insignificant in the case of massive objects the size of celestial bodies. The gravitational pull of the earth upon an object on its surface is called *weight;* that is, when a man and the earth are attracted by a force of 160 pounds, we say that the man weighs 160 pounds. It should be emphasized that gravity has no bearing upon an object's quantity of matter, or *mass.* This obviously will *not* depend upon location. For all *practical* purposes, however, we employ the terms *weight* and *mass* interchangeably.

Simple machines. Even the most complex machine can be analyzed in relation to certain basic parts called simple machines, namely, the lever, the pulley, the screw, and the inclined plane. Indeed, throughout daily life all of us use simple machines in the pure form. As a matter of fact, since our bodies contain an array of levers, how could we avoid the practice? The lever, the inclined plane, and the pulley are discussed here.

Lever. The lever is merely a rigid "bar" so arranged as to permit rotation about an axis called the *fulcrum.* In the operation of this machine a force (F) is applied at one point on the lever in order to move an object or load (L) located at some other point. The distance between the force and the fulcrum is called the *force arm* (Fa), and the distance between the load and the fulcrum is called the *load arm* (La). Now, the law of levers states that the *force times the force arm equals the load times the load arm,* or

$$F \times Fa = L \times La$$

Just a glance at this simple equation shows that if we wish to move or raise an object that could not be lifted, we could use some type of lever to multiply our strength. Herein lies the essence of the machine—to multiply force to do work. At the playground, for example, a small boy weighing 50 pounds can easily balance a 100-pound boy on the seesaw by sitting farther away from the fulcrum. As shown in Fig. 3-3, if the big boy sits 3 feet from the fulcrum, the distance the small boy must sit from the fulcrum is computed as follows:

$$\begin{aligned} F \times Fa &= L \times La \\ 50 \times Fa &= 100 \times 3 \\ 50\ Fa &= 300 \\ Fa &= 6 \text{ feet} \end{aligned}$$

The seesaw is an example of a first-class lever; that is, the fulcrum is between F and L. In the second-class lever, for example, a wheelbarrow (Fig. 3-3), L is between the fulcrum and F. In the third and last class of lever, for example, the elbow-forearm (Fig. 3-3), F is between the fulcrum and L.

Inclined plane. An inclined plane is a simple machine that permits a heavy load to be lifted by a relatively small force. A 300-pound barrel of beer, for example, can be easily loaded onto a platform 5 feet from the ground by the use of 15-foot planks. The exact force required to do the job can be calculated by the equation for the inclined plane:

$$\text{Force} \times \text{Force distance} = \text{Load} \times \text{Load distance}$$
$$\text{Force} \times 15 = 300 \times 5$$
$$\text{Force} \times 15 = 1500$$
$$\text{Force} = 100 \text{ pounds}$$

Thus, the inclined plane in this instance permits a force of 100 pounds to lift a weight of 300 pounds.

Pulley. A pulley consists of a wheel with a grooved rim to permit it to carry a rope or cable. In the simple fixed pulley (Fig. 3-4) the force (*F*) required to lift the load (*L*) would obviously have to be equal to the load. In contrast, in the movable single pulley (Fig. 3-4) the force needed to raise the load is only one-half the load, or put another way, a given force will lift a load twice as large. The reason for this advantage, of course, stems from the fact that the load is supported by two ropes or, more accurately, two forces—the rafter and the force applied. One never gets something for nothing, however, and in this instance the worker will have to pull the rope on the movable pulley twice the distance that he would pull the one on the single pulley to lift the load the same distance.

Combinations of pulleys are often used to move extremely heavy loads. One arrangement, the so-called *block and tackle,* is shown in Fig. 3-4. Since the load in this instance is supported by four ropes, we

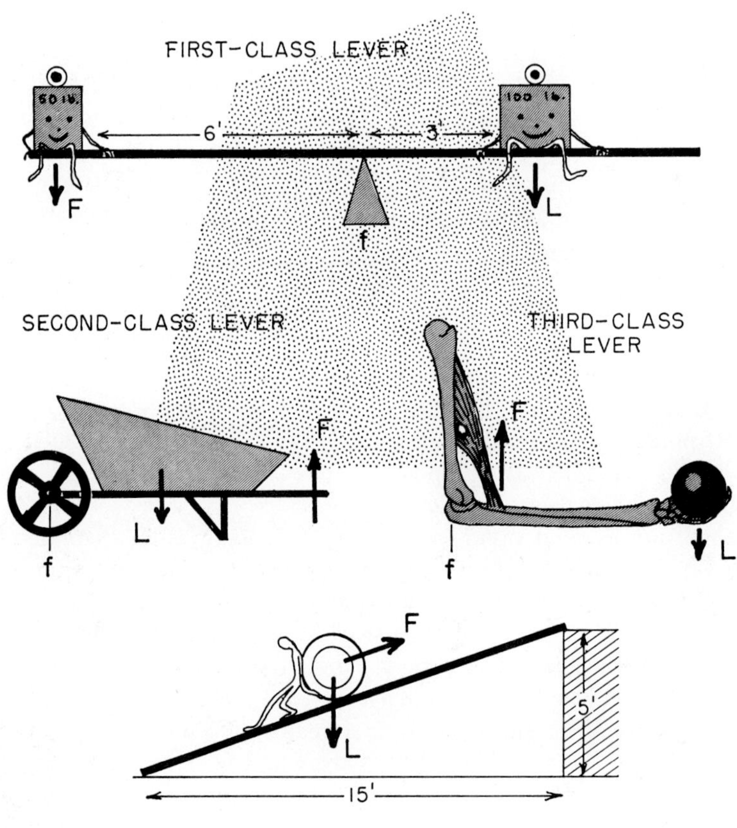

Fig. 3-3. The three classes of levers and the inclined plane.

see (neglecting friction and weight of the lower pulley) that the force applied to the free end need be only one-fourth the weight of the load. By the same token, the applied force will have to move four times farther than the load; that is, in order to raise 100 pounds 2 feet, one would have to pull the rope 8 feet with a force of 25 pounds. From the foregoing, then, we arrive at the equation for the pulley:

$$\text{Force} \times \text{Force distance} = \text{Load} \times \text{Load distance}$$

Thus, the equations for the lever, inclined plane, and the pulley are in essence the same; that is, the force needed to do the job times the distance through which it works equals the weight of the load times the distance the load moves. Since work equals force times distance (p. 13), we arrive at the basic law of the machine: *Work output equals work input.* Apparently, then, there is scientific truth to the old adage: "You never get more out than you put in."

Mechanical advantage. By mechanical advantage is meant the amount by which a given machine multiplies the force applied. In the pulley this is a simple matter; one merely counts the ropes supporting the load. For the block and tackle shown in Fig. 3-4, the mechanical advantage is 4. For example, an applied force of 25 pounds will lift a load weighing 100 pounds. The ideal mechanical advantage of any machine is given by the following formula:

$$\text{Mechanical advantage} = \frac{\text{Load}}{\text{Force}}$$

or

$$\text{Mechanical advantage} = \frac{\text{Force distance}}{\text{Load distance}}$$

Note that we say *ideal* mechanical advantage, for friction is not taken into consideration. If friction is taken into account, as it must be in actual practice, we speak of the *actual* mechanical advantage. Thus, in the case of the block and tackle having

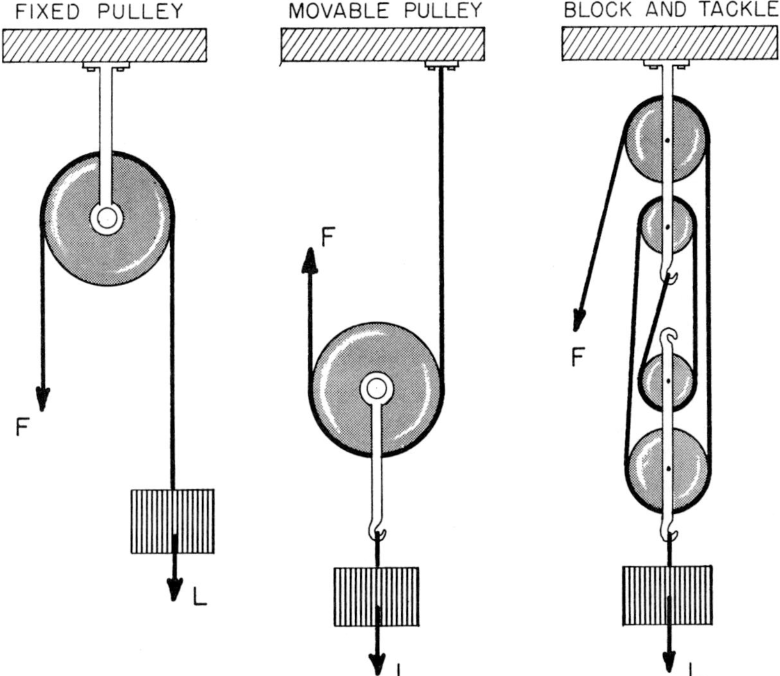

Fig. 3-4. Types of pulleys.

the ideal mechanical advantage of 4, its actual mechanical advantage would probably be in the vicinity of 3.5.

Efficiency. A machine's efficiency means just what it says—to wit, how well it utilizes work input. This is expressed mathematically as follows:

$$\text{Efficiency} = \frac{\text{Actual mechanical advantage}}{\text{Ideal mechanical advantage}} \times 100$$

Assuming an actual mechanical advantage of 3.5 for the block and tackle, the latter's efficiency would be

$$\frac{3.5}{4} \times 100, \text{ or } 87.5\%$$

As the student probably suspects, no machine has an efficiency of 100 percent, for it is impossible to annihilate friction completely.

Elasticity. When a substance is subjected to an external force, it may undergo a change in size or shape. If the substance returns to its original size and shape after the force is removed, it is said to be elastic. For quantitative purposes, the phenomenon is best described according to Hooke's law, which states that for an elastic body the ratio of the *stress* (the force which produces the distortion) to the *strain* (the ratio of the change in size or shape to the original size and shape) is a constant.

The usual types of stress are tension, compression, and bending. These forces are encountered not only in the construction of buildings and bridges but also throughout the body itself. The skeleton, for instance, represents top engineering, for where the stresses are the greatest the bones are the thickest and the cross bracing is the most extensive.

The liquid state. In this section certain features of the liquid state, one of the three states of matter, will be discussed.

Pressure. In the physics of fluids, pressure and force are not the same thing. Thus, in a tank of water the force against the bottom is equal to the weight of water, whereas the pressure against the bottom is equal to the force on a unit area, or

$$P = \frac{F}{A}$$

where P is the pressure, F the total force, and A the area. As an example, suppose that a fish tank 600 cm. long and 300 cm. wide is filled with water to a depth of 400

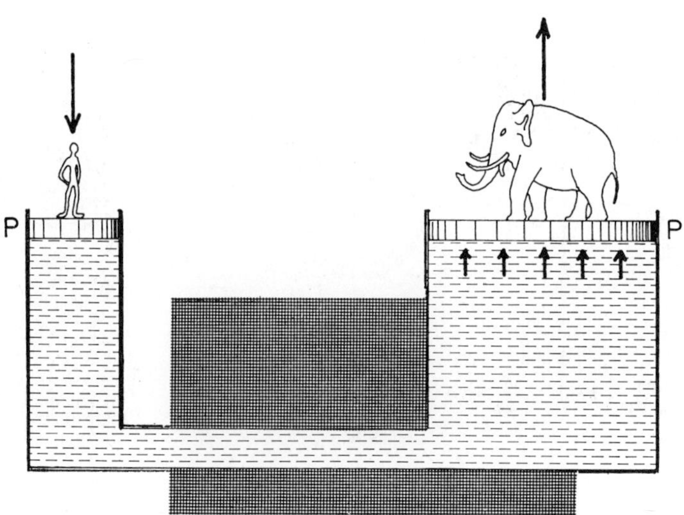

Fig. 3-5. Hydraulic press. **P**, Piston. (See text.)

cm. What would be the force and pressure on the bottom of the tank?

First, we compute the weight of the water:

Length × Width × Depth
or
600 × 300 × 400 cm.
or
72,000,000 c.c.

Since 1 c.c. of water weighs 1 gm., the weight, or force, of the water is 72,000,000 gm. Now, to find the pressure, we figure the area of the botton (600 × 300 cm., or 180,000 cm.²) and divide this into the force, as indicated by the formula

$$P = \frac{F}{A}$$

$$P = \frac{72{,}000{,}000}{180{,}000}$$

$$P = 400 \text{ gm. per square centimeter } (400 \text{ gm./cm.}^2)$$

Pascal's principle. Pascal's principle states that *whenever the pressure in a confined liquid is increased or diminished at any point the change in pressure is transmitted equally throughout the entire liquid.* There are many applications of the principle—the hydraulic press, hydraulic break, barber's chair, and operating table, to name but a few. In the hydraulic press (Fig. 3-5) the force applied to the small piston is multipled by the larger piston according to the proportion

$$\frac{\text{Force on large piston } (F)}{\text{Force on small piston } (f)} = \frac{\text{Area of large piston } (A)}{\text{Area of small piston } (a)}$$

Thus, with the proper design, a given force can be multiplied tremendously. In the hyperbolic illustration a 1-ton elephant standing on the 100-square foot piston can be lifted by a 200-pound man standing on the 10-square foot piston. This is in accordance with the foregoing formula. That is,

$$\frac{2000\ (F)}{200\ (f)} = \frac{100\ (A)}{10\ (a)}$$

Once again, however, we never get "something for nothing." In this instance the man will have to "drop" 10 feet down to lift the elephant 1 foot. And if you think that this is fair enough since all the man has to do is stand there, do not forget that the farther down he goes, the harder it will be for him to climb out.

Manometer. The manometer, a simple and useful device for measuring pressure, operates in accordance with Pascal's principle. The usual version consists essentially of a bent tube (with both arms vertical) partially filled with some liquid (generally water or mercury). One end is "open" and the other is connected to the system (liquid or gas) in which the pressure is to be measured. The device is so calibrated that the difference in the levels of the liquid in the arms indicates the pressure of the system being measured. For the mercury manometer the pressure is usually expressed as millimeters of mercury (mm. Hg).

Archimedes' principle. We are told that the great Greek scientist Archimedes was struck by the principle that bears his name while he was taking a bath, and well it could have been, for the observant bather notices two things when floating or submerged in water: (1) he feels lighter and (2) the water rises. On further investigation, Archimedes found that the *buoyant force on a floating or submerged object is equal to the weight of the fluid displaced.*

By way of illustration, if a cube of wood measuring 3 cm. on a side and weighing 50 gm. is submerged in water, it will be found to weigh 23 gm. This is because the cube has a volume of 27 c.c. (3 × 3 × 3) and thus displaces 27 c.c. of water; that is, the cube weighs 27 gm. less because the displaced water pushes it up with a force of 27 gm.

Liquids in motion. So far we have talked about fluids at rest. It is quite another matter when they are in motion. Here, we encounter a variety of factors, any one of which has a significant bearing on the overall motion. We should especially note that liquids seek their own level and that they gradually lose pressure as they move along through a tube or pipe. The latter effect is a result of fluid friction or viscosity and, naturally, varies with different liquids. As we know from experience, thick liquids such as molasses and blood have a higher viscosity than water or alcohol.

Another point of interest relating to liquids is the so-called *Bernoulli effect;* that is, when a fluid (liquid or gas) is forced to flow through a constriction in a tube (where its forward speed is increased), the pressure exerted sideways is decreased. This explains the operation of such devices as aspirators and atomizers.

Surface tension. At all surfaces liquids have a tendency to contract to the smallest possible area. This is vividly demonstrated when one tries to blow a soap bubble; that is, it takes energy to expand the soap film into a sphere. Moreover, when the pressure is released, the bubble contracts. This surface phenomenon, aptly referred to as surface tension, or surface energy, can be explained at the molecular level in a relatively simple way. In brief, while the molecules in the interior of a liquid are attracted equally on all sides by the surrounding molecules, those on the surface are pulled inward. In the laboratory, surface tension can be found accurately by the *tensiometer,* an instrument that measures the force necessary to detach a small circular ring from the surface of a liquid. Surface tension is expressed as ergs per square centimeter or dynes per centimeter.

Certain chemicals have the ability to lower surface tension. These so-called surface-active agents are extensively employed as wetting agents, emulsifiers, detergents, and antiseptics. Surface-active antiseptics (for instance, Zephiran and Cēpacol) owe a good part of their antimicrobial action to their ability to spread over the affected area and penetrate bacterial protoplasm.

Capillarity. If a capillary tube is held in water or any liquid that wets the tube, the liquid will rise to a certain level and remain there. The extent of the rise (h) depends upon the surface tension (T), the radius of the tube (r), the density of the liquid (d), and the acceleration of gravity (g), or

$$h = \frac{2T}{rdg}$$

In cases in which the liquid does not wet the tube (for example, mercury), there is capillary depression.

Osmosis. If pure water and an aqueous sugar solution are separated by a semipermeable membrane (for example, paper parchment or cellophane) that permits the passage of water molecules but retards the movement of sugar molecules, more water will diffuse into the sugar solution than out of it (Fig. 3-6). This is understandable

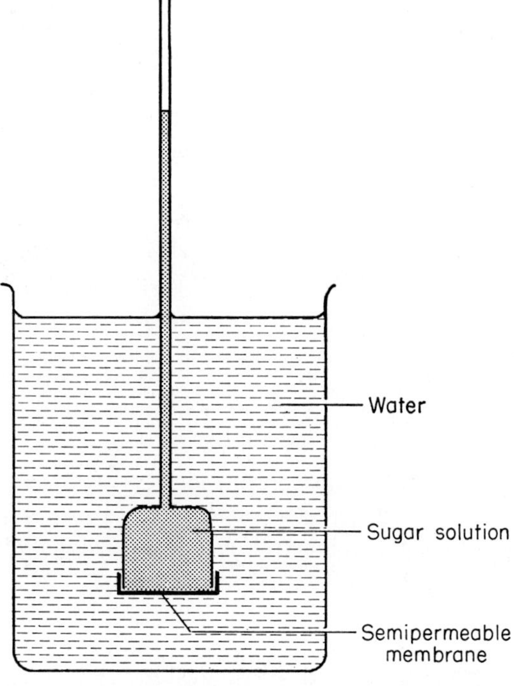

Fig. 3-6. Laboratory demonstration of osmosis.

when we consider that there is less water on the sugar side than on the pure water side. Such a flow always occurs when a semipermeable membrane separates aqueous solutions of unequal solute particle densities,* the principal flow being from the less dense solution (with the most water) to the more dense solution. This diffusion of water across the membrane is called osmosis.

As the apparatus shown in Fig. 3-6 clearly indicates, the flow of water from the less concentrated solution to the more concentrated one is evidenced by the rise of water in the tube. Moreover, the hydrostatic pressure excreted by this column of water is equal to the *osmotic pressure,* the magnitude of which depends upon the difference in the densities of the two solutions.

Because the cellular membrane of the plant and animal cell operates in a semipermeable fashion, the subject of osmosis is of vital interest to the biologist. For example, the passage of water through fruit skins and through the intestinal mucosa is effected largely by osmotic pressure.

The gaseous state. Regardless of chemical composition, all gases are similar in their physical behavior in response to changes in temperature (T) and pressure (P). In this section the mathematical laws governing these factors are discussed.

Boyle's law. In the seventeenth century the English scientist Boyle presented one of the most fundamental laws in physics. It is simple and may be stated as follows: *If the temperature remains constant, the volume of a gas varies inversely as the pressure on it.* If, for example, a given gas has a volume of 100 c.c. under a certain pressure, and the pressure is doubled (at a constant temperature), the new volume of the gas will be 50 c.c. If, on the other hand, the pressure is halved, the gas will expand to a volume of 200 c.c. The law may be stated mathematically as a simple inverse proportion:

$$\frac{\text{New volume}}{\text{Old volume}} = \frac{\text{Old pressure}}{\text{New pressure}} \text{ or } \frac{V^1}{V} = \frac{P}{P^1}$$

In scientific work, volume is usually expressed in cubic centimeters or liters and pressure is expressed in millimeters (mm.) of mercury; for example, the level of the mercury (in the mercurial barometer) at sea level stands at 760 mm.*

EXAMPLE: The volume of a gas measures 600 c.c. at 740 mm. pressure. Calculate the volume at 780 mm.

Since the pressure increases, the volume must decrease. The solution is as follows:

$$\frac{V^1}{V} = \frac{P}{P^1}$$

$$V^1 = \frac{VP}{P^1}$$

$$V^1 = \frac{600 \times 740}{780}$$

$$V^1 = 569 \text{ c.c.}$$

Charles' law. The exact relation between the volume of a gas and its temperature was first stated by the French chemist Charles. Like Boyle's law, Charles' law proved to be one of the building stones of modern physical science. Charles discovered that when a gas under constant pressure is heated 1° C. it expands 1/273 of its volume and that when cooled 1° C. it contracts 1/273 of its volume. Theoretically, then, at −273° C. a gas would have a volume of zero. It was Charles who designated the temperature of −273° C. as absolute zero. Charles' law is stated as follows: *If the pressure remains constant, the volume of a gas varies directly as the absolute*

*This is not necessarily the same as concentration in regard to solutions of different solutes; that is, two solutions may have the same percent concentration but not the same osmotic pressure by virtue of a difference in molecular weight and/or ability of solute to ionize.

*A pressure of 760 mm. Hg and a temperature of O° C. are referred to as *standard conditions.*

temperature. Mathematically, the law is stated as a direct proportion:

$$\frac{\text{New volume}}{\text{Old volume}} = \frac{\text{New temperature (absolute)}}{\text{Old temperature (absolute)}}$$

$$\text{or } \frac{V^1}{V} = \frac{A^1}{A}$$

In order for this proportion to be used, all centigrade temperature readings must be converted to absolute readings. This is done by merely adding degrees centigrade and 273° *algebraically.* A −10° C., for example, is 263° absolute and 10° C. is 283° A.

EXAMPLE: The volume of a gas measures 500 c.c. at 50° C. What will be its volume at 0 C.?

Since the temperature decreases, the volume will decrease. The solution is as follows:

$$\frac{V^1}{V} = \frac{A^1}{A}$$

$$V^1 = \frac{VA^1}{A}$$

$$V^1 = \frac{(0 + 273)(500)}{(50 + 273)}$$

$$V^1 = 423 \text{ c.c.}$$

General gas law. The formulas for Boyle's law and Charles' law may be combined into one formula. This formula enables us to find the new volume of a gas when there is both a temperature change and a pressure change, thus obviating the need for two calculations. The combined formula is as follows:

$$\frac{PV}{A} = \frac{P^1V^1}{A^1}$$

or

$$V^1 = \frac{PVA^1}{P^1A}$$

V^1 = New volume
P^1 = New pressure
A^1 = New absolute temperature
V = Old volume
P = Old pressure
A = Old absolute temperature

EXAMPLE: A gas has a volume of 100 c.c. at 70° C. and 760 mm. pressure. What will be its volume at 20° C. and 700 mm. pressure?

$$V^1 = \frac{PVA^1}{P^1A}$$

$$V^1 = \frac{(760)(100)(20 + 273)}{(700)(70 + 273)}$$

$$V^1 = \frac{(760)(100)(293)}{(700)(343)}$$

$$V^1 = 93 \text{ c.c.}$$

Dalton's law. Provided there is no chemical reaction involved, each gas in a mixture of gases behaves independently of the other gases present. Moreover, according to Dalton's law, the pressure of such a mixture *is the sum of the partial pressures of the constituent gases,* the partial pressure being defined as the pressure that the individual gas would exert if it occupied the same volume alone at the same temperature. Thus,

$$P = P_1 + P_2 + P_3 \ldots$$

where P equals total pressure, and P_1, P_2, P_3, and so forth, the partial pressures.

Graham's law. Graham found that when a gas distributes itself throughout a containing vessel or mixes with other gases (via diffusion), it does so according to the following expression:

$$\frac{D_1}{D_2} = \frac{\sqrt{d_2}}{\sqrt{d^1}}$$

This states that the *rates of diffusion* (D) *of gases are inversely proportional to the square roots of their densities.* Thus, a light gas such as hydrogen diffuses at a faster rate than a heavier gas such as oxygen—in this instance, four times as fast.

Henry's law. The solubility of a gas in a liquid bears a relationship to the pressure bearing upon the surface of the liquid. Specifically—according to Henry's law—though the *volume of a gas absorbed by a liquid remains constant, the weight of the absorbed gas rises and falls in proportion to the pressure.*

The atmosphere. Since air has weight, it

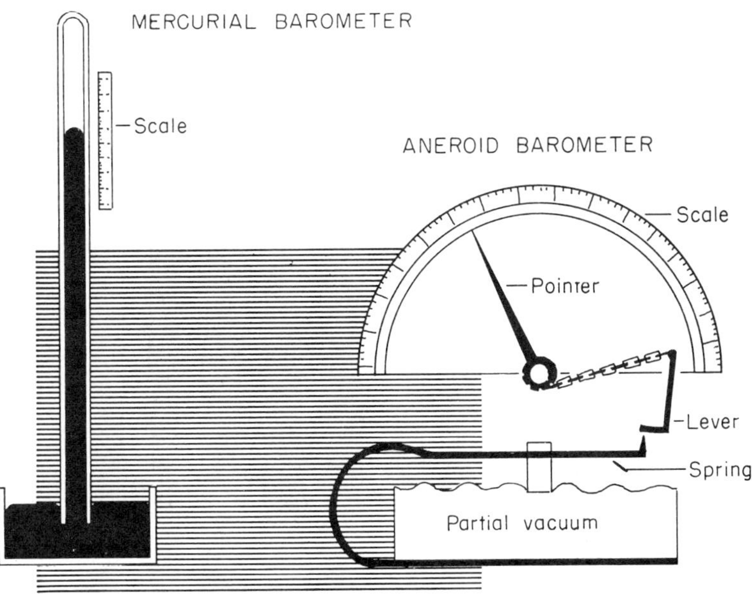

Fig. 3-7. Mercurial and aneroid barometers.

exerts a pressure upon the face of the earth. To register this pressure, we employ a simple but valuable device called a *barometer,* of which there are two types in general use; mercurial and aneroid. The *mercurial* barometer, the most accurate, is made by taking a glass tube about 3 feet long (closed at one end) and filling it with mercury. With the finger over the open end, the tube is inverted into an open dish of mercury and the finger is removed. As a result, the column of mercury drops slightly and comes to rest at a height of about 30 inches above the level of the mercury in the dish (Fig. 3-7). For scientific work, standard atmospheric pressure at sea level is defined as a column of mercury 76 cm. (760 mm.) high at 0° C. (this corresponds to 29.92 inches).

The *aneroid* barometer, a more convenient instrument, consists of a partially evacuated corrugated metal pillbox (Fig. 3-7). As can be seen easily from the illustration, any change in atmospheric pressure causes the pillbox surface to move up or down, thereby moving the pointer over the scale, which is measured off in inches of mercury. Naturally, the instrument must be calibrated by a standard mercurial barometer.

The barometer is one of the most important instruments for dealing with gases. Also, since the day-to-day change in atmospheric pressure gives a fairly accurate indication of the weather conditions 24 hours hence, it serves as the meteorologist's "right arm." Finally, when graduated to read in terms of distances above sea level, the barometer becomes an *altimeter.*

SOUND

Sound is a *wave disturbance* produced by a substance in vibration. This definition can be readily understood by considering a vibrating metal band. As the band vibrates back and forth, the air molecules adjacent to either surface are alternately *compressed* (*C*) and *rarefied* (*R*). The situation perpetuates itself forward, in all directions, and the air becomes filled with sound waves, which we hear. We hear the sound by virtue of the fact that the waves cause the eardrum to vibrate.

For convenience of study, sound waves

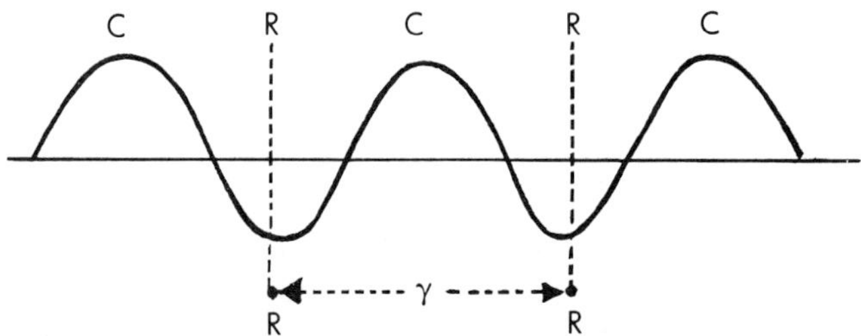

Fig. 3-8. Sound wave. **C,** Crest of the wave, representing the compression of air molecules; **R,** trough of the wave, representing rarefaction of air molecules. The distance between corresponding points is called the wavelength (λ).

are symbolized by the so-called sine wave shown in Fig. 3-8. This manner of representation is especially apropos because it reminds us of waves on the surface of water. Herein lies a singular analogy; that is, whether in air or in water, a "disturbance" is transmitted in all directions in wave formation. Indeed, it also underscores the fact that without a medium (air, water, steel, wood, or what have you) there can be no waves—and hence no sound.

Wavelength. Wavelength, the most basic feature of sound, is the distance between corresponding points on the sound wave. Obviously, different fundamental sounds will have different wavelengths, depending upon their frequency (number of vibrations per second) and velocity. Mathematically, this is expressed by the following formula:

$$\lambda = \frac{V}{f}$$

where λ (lambda) is the wavelength, V the velocity, and f the frequency. For example, a piano string with a frequency of 200 vibrations (or cycles) per second produces a sound with a wavelength of 5.5 feet, assuming a velocity* of 1100 feet per second. On the other hand, a string with a frequency of 100 cycles per second would produce a sound double this wavelength.

*In air at 0° C. the speed of sound is about 1087 feet per second, and for *each degree centigrade rise* in temperature it increases about 2 feet per second. Thus, at 20° C. the speed of sound is about 1127 feet per second.

Pitch. By pitch we mean the response of the brain to the frequency. For instance, if the tones of two tuning forks of different frequencies are compared, all normal ears will agree that the fork with the higher frequency emits the tone with higher pitch. Thus, pitch depends upon the frequency. However, it is interesting to note that the human ear cannot detect sounds beyond 20,000 cycles per second. This explains why sounds such as that emitted by the bat cannot be heard by human beings.

Loudness. In addition to pitch, a given tone has loudness, the auditory response to the intensity of the sound. Generally, this obeys *Fechner's law,* which states that the intensity of a sensation produced by a varying stimulus varies directly as the logarithm of that stimulus. For instance, the harder the drummer hits the drum, the louder will be the sound. Here, too, the symbolic sound wave proves useful, for we can nicely represent an increase in loudness by increasing the height of the crest (C) and the depth of the trough (R).

Quality. As we know from common experience, there is more to what we hear than pitch and loudness; there is also quality, or *timbre.* Indeed, what a monotonous world this would be if this were not true! In other words, a sound wave usually has a more subtle design than that shown in Fig. 3-8.

Let us illustrate this interesting point by performing a simple experiment with three tuning forks of different frequencies. If tuning forks A and B—with B having a frequency double that of A—are sounded together, the two notes combine to produce an overtone called the *first harmonic.* Now, if we repeat the experiment, this time using tuning fork C (with a frequency three times that of tuning fork A) instead of tuning fork B, a different overtone is produced—the so-called *second harmonic.* Although the two sounds are noted to have the same pitch and loudness, we can easily distinguish between them because they do not have the same quality or wave pattern.

And so it is with musical sounds in general; that is, there is always the fundamental note embellished by overtones and harmonics, the possible combinations of which are known only to the great masters and electronic calculators. What an astonishing thing it is that nature allows such a multitude of audible beauty through a mere disturbance of the molecules!

Beats. If two tuning forks of slightly different frequencies are sounded together, there appears a phenomenon known as beats, that is, a rise and fall of intensity. As a matter of fact, the number of beats is equal to the difference between the two frequencies. For instance, if one fork vibrates 256 times per second and the other 260 times per second, there will be 4 beats per second. Beats can be readily explained by the all-purpose symbolic wave; indeed, lest we put the cart before the horse, the beat phenomenon affords good evidence to support the wave theory.

Resonance. If we sound a tuning fork and hold it over a graduated cylinder into which water is being very gradually added, the intensity of the sound will vary, and for a certain column of air it will reach a maximum. When this occurs, the fork and the air are said to be in *resonance,* or *sympathetic vibration;* that is, the air column, having a frequency of vibration exactly equal to that of the fork, emits a sound wave in step with the wave emanating from the fork and thereby reinforces the latter and enhances the loudness.

Reflection. Just as ocean waves are reflected back when they hit the rocky coast, sound waves are reflected upon striking an obstruction. Out-of-doors we refer to this phenomenon as an *echo,* and indoors we call it a *reverberation.* Although generally looked upon as a nuisance, this feature of sound finds application in such devices as sonar (undersea radar) and clinical instruments used to detect foreign objects in the tissues.

HEAT

Heat is a form of energy and, like all forms of energy, leaves us in ignorance as to what it really is. However, we can measure it, control it, transform it, and use it. In this section we shall touch upon the highlights of its behavior and manifestations.

Temperature. Temperature is a word that all of us use in our work and daily conversation. The housewife sets the oven at 350° F. to bake a cake, and the man next door tells us, "The mercury today is going over 90." We all know that a flatiron is hotter than an ice cube, and that the refrigerator is colder than the radiator. But what are we really talking about? More to the point, what is the relationship between temperature and heat?

Temperature is the intensity of heat. In more precise language, and in accordance with the kinetic theory of heat, the temperature of a body is proportional to the average kinetic energy of its molecules (p. 18). In other words, a hot body has a higher temperature than a cold body because the molecules of the former are moving faster (or have more energy) than the molecules of the latter. What an exquisite explanation! Thus, as a cold body is gradually heated to higher and higher temperatures, we can, with little difficulty, visualize how the chilly, sluggish molecules begin to move faster and faster. Indeed, the body will expand!

Temperature scales. To measure the temperature, the scientist long ago devised the thermometer, an instrument familiar to one and all. On the Celsius or *centigrade* scale, water freezes at 0 degrees and boils at 100 degrees, and on the *Fahrenheit* scale it freezes at 32 degrees and boils at 212 degrees. Thus, there are 100 divisions between the two points on the centigrade scale, as opposed to 180 divisions on the Fahrenheit scale. One Fahrenheit division, therefore, equals $\frac{5}{9}$ centigrade division, or 1 centigrade division equals $\frac{9}{5}$ Fahrenheit divisions. Thus, to convert one reading into the other, we employ the following formulas:

$$\text{C.} = 5/9\ (\text{F.} - 32)$$

$$\text{F.} = 9/5\ \text{C.} + 32$$

The centigrade scale is used throughout the world in scientific work, and in many countries it is used for all purposes. In this country the Fahrenheit thermometer is, as we know, the household thermometer.

Another scale of scientific importance is the *absolute* or *Kelvin* scale on which absolute zero (the limit of coldness) is equal to −273° C. Although temperatures have been reduced to within a few thousandths of this reading, the figure itself is theoretically unobtainable, since it corresponds to the absence of all molecular motion. We use the absolute temperature scale in dealing with Charles' law, ". . . the volume of a gas varies directly to the absolute temperature. . . ." (See p. 27.)

Quantity of heat. We know from common experience that it takes longer to heat a large beaker of water than it does a small beaker of water. Quite logically, this means that the larger beaker of water "holds" more heat. After both beakers are boiling, however, their temperatures are the same (100° C.). Thus, we see that the quantity of heat and the temperature are

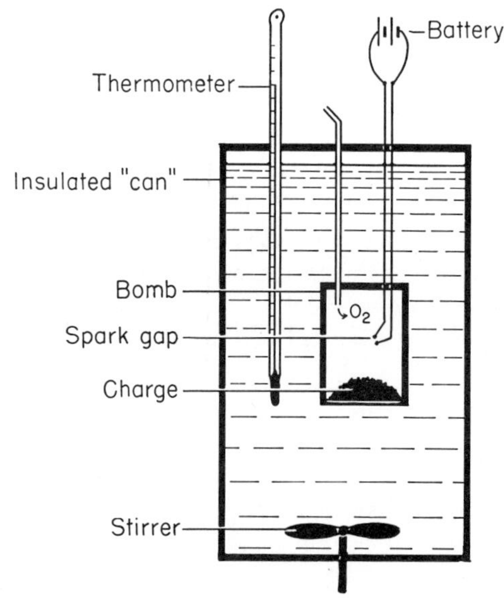

Fig. 3-9. Calorimeter.

not the same thing. For this reason, then, special units have been devised to measure heat quantitatively.

Calorie. The calorie (cal.), the heat unit employed in scientific work, is the quantity of heat required to raise the temperature of 1 gm. of water 1° C. (specifically, from 15° to 16° C.). This is not to be confused with the so-called *large calorie* (Cal.), or *kilocalorie,* which is equal to 1000 small calories. The large calorie is used by dieticians in stating the energy values of food.

The calorie content of foods and fuels is determined by the calorimeter (Fig. 3-9), a device in which an accurately measured sample is burned, and the heat released thereby is absorbed by water and measured. For example, if a slice of bread caused the temperature of 1000 gm. of water to rise 50° C., then 50 large calories were released during combustion.

British thermal unit. The British thermal unit (BTU) is the amount of heat required to raise the temperature of 1 pound of water 1° F. This unit is used in engineering and commercial work in the United States and England.

Specific heat. The specific heat of a substance is the number of calories of heat energy that 1 gm. of the substance must absorb in order to increase in temperature 1° C. The specific heat of water is obviously 1, for the calorie itself is defined in terms of water. Iron has a specific heat of 0.11, aluminum 0.22, and silver 0.056 cal. per gram per degree. The specific heats of most substances have been determined and tabulated.

Latent heat. As indicated in the discussion of the molecule, the three states of matter differ from one another in respect to molecular motion; that is, the molecules are most energetic in the gaseous state and least energetic in the solid state. In essence, then, the three states differ relative to their energy content. Since heat is a manifestation of molecular kinetic energy (p. 31), we can immediately appreciate the basic relationship between state and heat energy.

This relationship is underscored by the phenomenon of latent heat. When ice melts, the surrounding temperature starts to drop, as can be conclusively proved by squeezing an ice cube in the bare hand. Conversely, when water freezes, heat is liberated. This explains why the air warms up just prior to a snowfall and why autumn weather does not change suddenly into winter (nor winter into spring) in the vicinity of large bodies of water.

Heat of fusion. Even though heat is absorbed and liberated at the freezing and melting points, the temperature of a substance does not change during the transformation—hence, the adjective *latent.* The heat of fusion is a form of latent heat defined as the amount of heat required to melt 1 gm. of a substance without changing its temperature. For example, the heat of fusion of ice is 80 cal. per gram. In other words, for each gram of ice that melts, 80 cal. are taken from the environment. By the same token, for each gram of water that freezes, 80 cal. of heat are liberated.

Heat of vaporization. Just as heat is needed to "jump" the molecules of the solid state into the liquid state, latent heat is also needed to change a liquid into a gas or vapor. Called the heat of vaporization, this latent heat is defined as the amount of heat needed to vaporize a unit mass of a liquid without changing its temperature. For example, the heat of vaporization for water at its normal boiling point is 540 cal. per gram; that is for each gram of water converted into water vapor (or steam), 540 cal. are absorbed from the environment. Conversely, when water vapor or steam condenses, each gram liberates 540 cal. of heat. This explains why a steam burn is more serious than a hot water burn. It explains, too, why the temperature sometimes rises during a summer shower.

Evaporation. The cooling effect of evaporation is easily explained by the heat of vaporization; that is, when a liquid evaporates, it absorbs heat from the surrounding area. Nature puts this principle to work during vigorous exercise, as the evaporation of perspiration helps the body to maintain its normal temperature. Artificially, we apply the principle in the mechanical refrigerator in which a highly volatile gas such as ammonia is alternately vaporized and condensed.

Heat transmission. Heat is transmitted from one place to another in three ways —conduction, convection, and radiation. By *conduction* we mean the passage of heat from molecule to molecule, as through a metal. Silver and copper are the best of all conductors.

By *convection* we mean the manner in which heat is transferred through a gas or liquid. In the heating of a room, for example, the air in contact with the radiator is warmed, expanded, and driven upward by the cooler, heavier air. The circulation thereby set up carries the heat to all parts of the room.

Radiation, the third mode of heat transfer, requires no medium; that is, radiant heat passes straight through space in the form of electromagnetic waves at the speed of light (186,000 miles per second). This is the method by which we warm our hands by an open fire and by which the earth receives its heat from the sun.

MAGNETISM

There exists in nature a dark brown iron ore called *magnetite* that the Greek Thales discovered strongly attracted pieces of iron. Samples of the ore, called *loadstones,* soon became the "mystery of the day" and still fascinate the seasoned physicist as well as the youngster. Alas, magnetism, like other forms and manifestations of energy, teases the imagination.

Magnetic poles. If we take a loadstone and gently stroke it over a steel knitting needle from end to end, always in the same direction, we find that the needle becomes a magnet. It will attract iron filings, and if suspended at its center by a very fine thread to permit horizontal movement, it will always come to rest in a north-south direction. The latter phenomenon, observed by the Chinese long before Marco Polo's visit, serves to identify the magnetic poles. The north-pointing end is the north pole of the needle, and the south-pointing end is its south pole.

If the north pole of one magnet is brought near the north pole of another magnet, they repel one another, and the same action occurs if two south poles are brought near each other. The reverse is true of unlike poles. Thus, *like* magnetic poles repel and *unlike* magnetic poles attract each other. The force of this attrac-

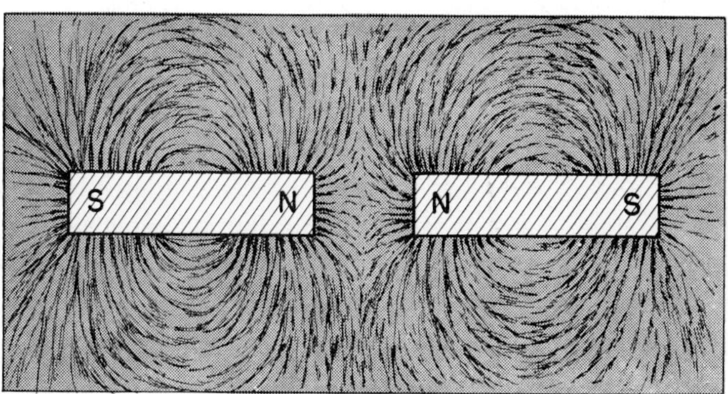

LIKE POLES REPEL

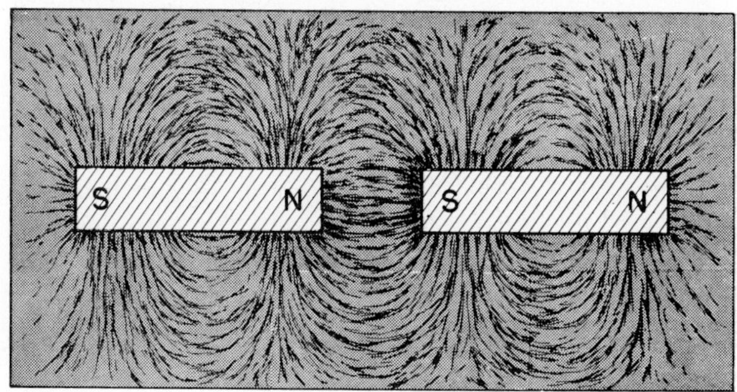

UNLIKE POLES ATTRACT

Fig. 3-10. Magnetic fields. **N,** North pole; **S,** south pole.

tion or repulsion is directly proportional to the magnetic pole strength and inversely proportional to the square of the distance between the poles (*Coulomb's law*).

Magnetic fields. The region in which magnetic forces exist is called a magnetic field. This can be dramatically demonstrated by sprinkling iron filings upon a piece of paper lying over a bar magnet, carefully tapping the paper a few times for best results (Fig. 3-10). As shown in the illustration, the filings arrange themselves along the lines of force that compose the magnetic field. In the same illustration, note that the lines of force "seek" an unlike pole but "resist" a like pole.

Theory of magnetism. Let us take a small bar of iron and proceed to magnetize it in the same way that we magnetized the knitting needle (p. 34). By testing its magnetism between strokes, we note a gradual increase in strength (up to a point, of course). If the fully magnetized iron bar is now strongly heated, it will become demagnetized. Hammering produces the same effect, though to a less degree.

These results can be readily understood if we assume the iron bar to be composed of "molecular magnets," which in the unmagnetized bar are pointing in every direction. Now, when we stroke the bar with the north pole of our magnet, all the molecular magnets will line up with their south poles facing the end toward which we stroked the magnet; thus, this end becomes the south pole and the opposite end the north pole. Demagnetizing, then, is the reverse situation; that is, the violence of molecular motion occasioned by heat and hammering throws the magnetic particles out of line.

The earth as a magnet. As indicated, the earth behaves as though a giant bar magnet were buried in its center along the axis. The magnetic poles of the earth, however, are several degrees from the *geographic* poles. In other words, the compass needle at most locations does not point exactly to *true* north. This offers no problem in navigation, however, since the appropriate "correction" has been found for all areas of the globe.

ELECTRICITY

Electricity is a form of energy, the effects of which were first observed centuries before the birth of Christ. The word *electricity* comes from the Greek word *electron,* which means "amber." (When amber is rubbed with wool, it becomes electrified.)

Electrostatics. Apparently, there are two forms of electricity: static (stationary electrical charges) and dynamic (moving electrical charges). Let us first consider static electricity, or *electrostatics.*

Two kinds of charges. The essence of static electricity resides in the fact that there are two electrical charges. This can be strikingly demonstrated by a very simple experiment. When a glass rod is rubbed with silk and placed in a freely rotating stirrup, it will be repelled by another silk-rubbed glass rod. If the experiment is repeated, this time using two ebonite rods that have been rubbed with fur, we witness the same result. But there is more to be learned. If the suspended charged ebonite rod is now approached by the charged glass rod, they attract each other. Moreover, the glass rod attracts the silk and the ebonite rod attracts the fur. The latter effect explains why the hair stands up when we comb it.

Benjamin Franklin, who considered electricity to be a "tenuous invisible weightless fluid," reasoned that a charged body had either too much or too little such fluid. Since he believed the charged glass rod had an excess, he said it carried a positive charge. The charge carried by the ebonite rod would therefore be negative. It is another monument to this great man that the designations positive (+) and negative (−) are still used today.

From the foregoing, then, we can derive these basic facts: First, there are two kinds of electrical charges (positive and negative). Second, *like* charges *repel* each other, and *unlike* charges *attract* each other. Third, positive and negative charges appear *simultaneously*.

Electron. Much has happened in the electrical laboratory since Franklin's time. Scientists now believe that the phenomenon of electrostatics resides in the electron, a negative particle of electricity that orbits about the nucleus of the atom (Chapter 4).

According to the present view, a negatively charged object has an *excess* and a positively charged particle has a *deficiency* of electrons. This simple theory accounts for all the findings just cited. For example, when the ebonite rod is rubbed with fur, it becomes negatively charged, for electrons are rubbed off the fur onto the surface of the rod, making the fur positively charged in the process. By the same token, electrons leave the glass rod and accumulate on the silk, making the former positively and the latter negatively charged.

Coulomb's law. Coulomb found that the same relationship exists between opposite electrostatic charges as between opposite magnetic poles; thus, the force exerted between two charges varies *directly* as the magnitude of the charges and *inversely* as the square of the distance between them.

Condenser. The electrical condenser is perhaps the most important electrical device having to do with electrostatics. Nature uses it to operate nervous tissue, and the engineer uses it to construct radios, radar, and television sets.

Essentially, the condenser consists of two conducting surfaces (plates) separated by a nonconductor. Its function is to accumulate charges of electricity. For example, if one plate is charged by either an electrostatic machine or a battery, an opposite charge will appear on the second plate. Since electrons cannot leak across the insulator (thereby neutralizing the charges), the condenser is said to "hold" the charge, the presence of which can be proved by touching a wire between the plates and producing a spark.

Electrostatics "in action." Electrostatics is of vital importance in nature and everyday experience. Recent work, for instance, strongly suggests that the movement of particles in and out through the cellular membrane is controlled in part by electrical charges; that is, positive pores in the membrane do not allow positive particles to pass but readily admit negative particles. By the same token, negative pores readily pass positive particles but not negative particles

Again, all of us are aware of the charge that builds up on the surface of the body, particularly in cold, dry weather. Sometimes the charge is of sufficient intensity to produce a sizable spark when a metal object is touched. Indeed, there is such a good possibility of igniting flammable gases and vapors by this means that all personnel in a hospital operating room must wear shoes fitted with a metal strap that touches the floor. As in the case of the lightning rod, the metal strap leads off ("grounds") the electrons, thereby preventing any buildup of charge.

As a final example, let us consider lightning. The water particles that compose rain clouds become electrified in their movement through the atmosphere, rendering the upper part of the cloud negative and the bottom part positive. When the intensity of the charge reaches the "breaking point," the electrons burst forth, producing a giant spark that we call lightning. The noise that we hear results from the explosive expansion of the air as the hot bolt darts through the molecules.

Dynamic electricity. Dynamic electricity deals with electrons in motion, or electric currents. The current produced by batteries and by certain types of generators is called *direct current* (DC), which means that the electrons flow in one direction. Conversely, certain generators produce an *alternating current* (AC), in which the electrons flow first one way in the conductor and then the other way. Since AC current can be easily and efficiently reduced or increased, it is the type usually generated in the United States.

Since an electric current can be made to do just about anything, from beating an egg to receiving a message from outer space, we can readily appreciate the endless variety of electrical devices. Not to be forgotten, too, is the fact that the body itself employs such currents to think and move and control its various parts. In the present section we shall review a few basic facts.

The battery. This is a device that transforms some other form of energy into an electric current. In the so-called *primary* or *voltaic* cell a strip of zinc (Zn) and a strip of copper (Cu) are immersed in a solution of dilute sulfuric acid. A chemical reaction ensues in which the zinc gradually dissolves, and electrons leave the zinc electrode and gather on the copper electrode. From our knowledge of electrostatics this makes the zinc strip the anode (positive electrode) and the copper strip the cathode (negative electrode). If a wire is now connected from each electrode to a sensitive voltmeter, we shall discover that a direct current is being generated at a pressure of 1.1 volts (v.). This may be visualized as a rush of electrons from the cathode to the anode via the external circuit.

The cell continues to function as long as the zinc strip remains. If, after the zinc has dissolved, the solution is removed from the cell and evaporated, crystals of zinc sulfate remain. Thus, in this particular cell an electric current is generated by the chemical reaction between zinc and sulfuric acid, producing zinc sulfate and hydrogen gas (the latter being released at the cathode). In short, chemical energy is transformed into electrical energy; indeed, this is the principle of the electric battery.

The generator. The generator produces most of the electrical energy used in the world. *Electromagnetic induction*, the principle upon which it operates, may be very simply demonstrated by the use of a bar magnet, a coil of wire, and a galvanometer (Fig. 3-11). When the magnet is moved in and out of the coil, the galvanometer needle moves, indicating an electric current. This is a real phenomenon and one that can be "explained" by saying that an electric current is generated as a consequence of magnetic lines of force cutting through a conductor, or vice versa.

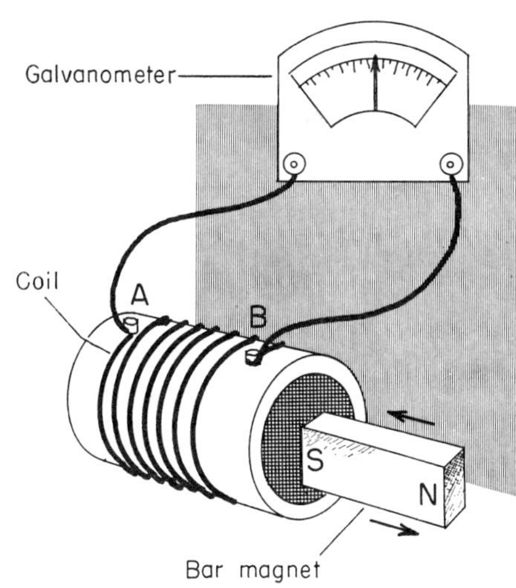

Fig. 3-11. Demonstration of electromagnetic induction.

In the actual generator the coil of wire, or *armature*, is made to rotate in a magnetic field supplied by a powerful magnet, the amount of current generated depending upon both the strength of the magnet and the speed at which the armature turns. If there is water power nearby, we let nature do the job for us. Otherwise we use steam, which in turn is "generated" by coal, oil, or nuclear energy. Thus, the electric generator serves as an excellent example of the convertibility of energy. Suppose we use coal to turn the generator. Coal (*potential* energy) becomes *heat* energy, heat energy becomes *mechanical* energy, and mechanical energy becomes *electrical* energy. Indeed, if we use such a generator to heat a kettle of water on an electric stove, the sequence is reversed!

Ohm's law. The basic features of current electricity are expressed by Ohm's law, one of the most important basic laws in science. This states that the *current (I) in a circuit varies directly as the electromotive force (E), and inversely as the resistance (R):*

$$I = \frac{E}{R}$$

To be of practical value, however, this formula must be expressed in the proper units. The *ampere* (amp.), the unit of current (measured by an ammeter), represents the passage of 1 coulomb of electricity (6.3×10^{18} electrons) per second. The *volt,* the unit of electromotive force (the force that "pushes" the electrons through the circuit), is defined as the electromotive force that will produce a current of 1 amp. in a circuit whose resistance is 1 ohm. By the same token, the *ohm* is that amount of resistance in a circuit that permits 1 v. to "develop" a current of 1 amp. Volts and ohms are measured by the voltmeter and the ohm-meter, respectively. Thus, the formula given in the preceding paragraph becomes

$$\text{Amperes} = \frac{\text{Volts}}{\text{Ohms}}$$

There is no circuit that does not offer at least some resistance. In sending current through a wire, it is obviously advantageous to use good conductors such as copper. Sometimes, however, we must use nonconductors to protect against short circuits ("shorts") and electric shocks. Such substances as glass, porcelain, rubber, and Bakelite are called insulators.

Aside from the basic nature of a given conductor, that is, whether it is a good one or poor one, resistance also depends upon its *length, diameter,* and *temperature.* Resistance, as we might guess, varies directly with the length and inversely with the diameter. This applies even to the nerves in the body, where the fastest impulses are carried by the fibers with the largest caliber. As for the temperature, resistance drops and rises with the mercury. Indeed, at extremely low temperatures, resistance essentially disappears, a phenomenon referred to as *superconductivity.*

Electric power. The amount of power supplied by a battery or generator, or the amount needed to do a certain job, is naturally of great practical concern. For electrical energy, power is measured in *watts (P),* the latter being equal to the voltage times the current *(I).* Thus, $P = VI$.

The transistor. In 1948 at the Bell Laboratories, Bardeen, Shockley, and Brattain invented the transistor, one of the most ingenious devices to emerge in the present century. Not much larger than a pea, the transistor can perform just about every function of the vacuum tube—heretofore the unchallenged heart and soul of electrical communications and electronic gadgetry—at an operating power only about one millionth of that required by the tube! Moreover, it is adaptable to areas where the bulky vacuum tube is worthless—hearing aids, miniature radios, computers, biophysical devices, and satellite communications, to name a few.

Basically, the transistor operates on the principle that certain "impure" crystals (for example, germanium or silicon) act as semiconductors. That is, when an infinitesimal electromagnetic signal (for example, a radio wave) is delivered to the crystal surface, a shower of electrons is set loose within, thereby amplifying the signal. In actual practice, however, it is far from being this simple, the production of transistors being a most exacting and sophisticated business.

The maser and the laser. Another major breakthrough in electronics was Charles Townes' invention of the so-called maser (1954). This device for "*m*icrowave *a*mplification by the *s*timulated *e*mission of *ra*diation" (the sobriquet formed by combining the letters shown in italics) operates on the principle that atoms or electrons, once excited by some suitable outside agency (such as an electric field or light beam), can be induced to fall back to their original energy level, in the process *intensifying* the input energy. The maser is the heart of the atomic clock and may, in the future, be used to transmit signals over great, even astronomical, distances. Moreover, when the maser principle is used to produce amplification of light—in the so-called *laser*—the possibilities are boundless. The laser light, the most powerful light known to man, can easily pass through steel. Already it is being used in delicate pinpoint surgery, and for the future the light holds great promise in communications systems.

LIGHT

Light is a form of energy that we perceive by its action upon the eye. Beyond this statement, anything that we say is likely to plunge the discussion into the depths of advanced physics. Nevertheless, it is possible, fortunately, to sharpen our understanding and appreciation through a review of certain basic and commonly observed phenomena.

First, however, we shall have to accept the premise that light is an electromagnetic (pp. 33-34) wave phenomenon that travels through empty space at about 186,000 miles per second—seven times around the earth at a single tick of the clock! Its speed in the atmosphere is only slightly less, but in certain media it is substantially reduced. Through glass, for example, light travels at about 125,000 miles per second. In just a moment we shall consider some visible proof of this medium-induced speed change.

Color. In the same way that the pitch of sound depends upon frequency and wavelength, the color of light depends upon the *frequency* and *length of the waves* of which it is composed. Light with a wavelength of 800 millimicrons ($m\mu$) produces a sensation of red, 650 $m\mu$ produces orange, 600 $m\mu$ produces yellow, 550 $m\mu$ produces green, 450 $m\mu$ produces blue, and 400 $m\mu$ produces violet. Indeed, this is the visual electromagnetic spectrum, for beyond the longest and shortest wavelengths there is darkness. Ultraviolet light and x rays, for instance, are too short to excite the retina.

White and black are physically as well as figuratively diametrically apart. White is a mixture of all the colors; black is the absence of all colors. The nature of white light can be demonstrated by both synthesis and analysis. A color wheel, for instance, containing equal segments of red, orange, yellow, green, blue, and violet looks white when spun at high speeds. Conversely, when a ray of sunlight passes through a glass prism, it forms a continuous spectrum of the six colors in the order just mentioned.

Colored objects. How do we explain the color of nonluminous bodies such as this page or the cover of this book? Provided that we understand the wave nature of light, this presents little difficulty. For instance, a red object is red because it *reflects* red light and *absorbs* the other colors of the spectrum. By the same reasoning, a white object reflects all colors and a black object absorbs all colors. What about colored glass? This can be answered by an example. A blue glass is blue because it transmits blue and absorbs all other colors.

Reflection and refraction. When a ray of light (represented by a straight line) strikes a reflecting surface obliquely, it is reflected obliquely; indeed, *the angle of reflection equals the angle of incidence* (Fig. 3-12). This is known as the *law of reflection.*

As indicated previously, the speed of light varies inversely with the density of the medium through which it passes. This explains the deviation, or refraction, of light in passing obliquely from one medium into another of a *different density* (Fig. 3-12). The only exception to the rule is when the original direction of the ray is exactly perpendicular to the surface of contact between the two bodies, in which case the ray passes through without refraction.

A look at Fig. 3-12 will demonstrate that a light ray is bent *toward* the normal when it enters a more dense medium. By the same token, a light ray is bent *away* from the normal when it enters a *less* dense medium.

Index of refraction. Referring once again to Fig. 3-12, we can readily define the so-called *relative index of refraction (n).* This is equal to the sine of the angle of incidence *(i)* divided by the sine of the angle of refraction *(r)*, or

$$n = \frac{\sin i}{\sin r}$$

The quotient is a *constant* that obviously depends on the density of the two media.

Optical instruments. The ability of glass to refract light is utilized in the operation of optical instruments, whether they be simple magnifying glasses or telescopes. The workings of the eye and eyeglasses are discussed in detail in Chapter 20.

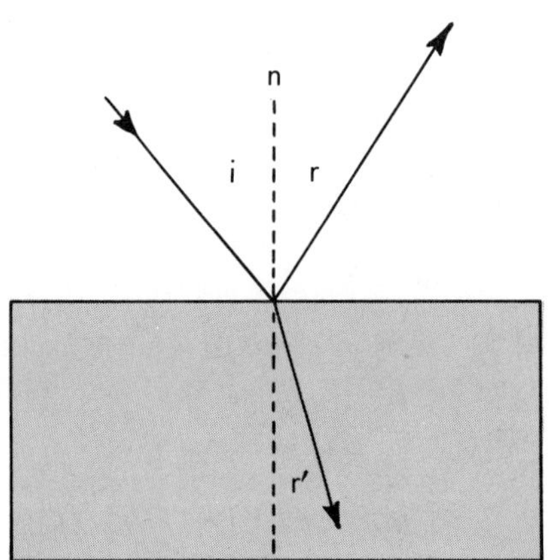

Fig. 3-12. Reflection and refraction. When a ray of light strikes the smooth surface of a glass plate, it is both reflected and refracted. Note that the angles of incidence, **i**, and reflection, **r**, are equal and that the angle of refraction, **r′**, is less than the angle of incidence. All three angles are measured from a perpendicular to the surface called the normal, **n**.

X RAYS

In 1895 Wilhelm Roentgen, a German physicist, discovered that mysterious rays were produced when a high voltage was placed across two electrodes housed in an evacuated glass tube. Such rays fogged photographic plates placed anywhere in the vicinity, even though the plates were wrapped in heavy dark paper. Not knowing the nature of this phenomenon, Roentgen quite aptly called the radiation *x rays.* Today we know that x rays are electromag-

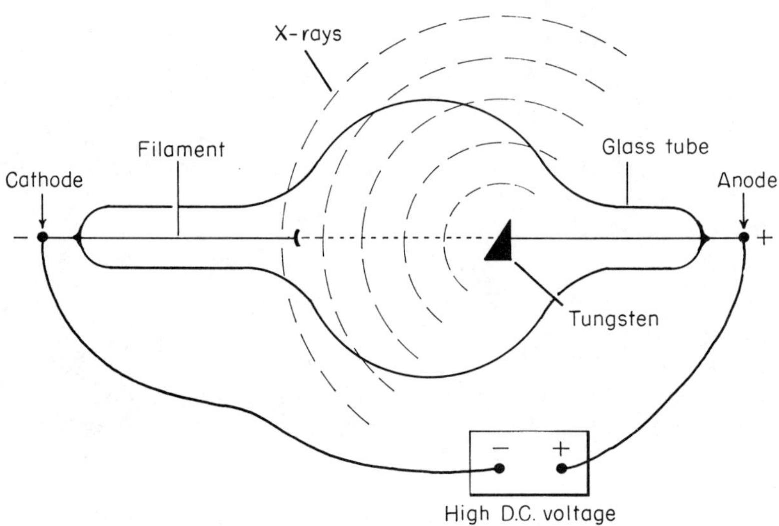

Fig. 3-13. Production of x rays.

netic waves that differ from other emanations such as light, ultraviolet light, and radio waves only in respect to their wavelength.

The essentials of x-ray production can be obtained from a study of the early type of tube shown in Fig. 3-13. The stream of electrons (*cathode rays*) emitted by the tungsten filament strike the tungsten anode and produce the rays. The abundance of rays increases rapidly with the temperature of the filament (and hence the amount of current supplied to the filament), and the penetrating power of the rays increases with the voltage supplied to the tube. By the use of such modern atomic devices as the *betatron* and the *electron synchrotron,* which whirl electrons at energies exceeding several billion electron volts, x rays powerful enough to pass through a foot or so of steel or concrete can be produced.

Ever since their discovery, x rays have played an important role in the investigation of matter in general and the atom in particular. As everyone knows, x rays are of incalculable value in diagnosis and therapeutics. In the well-known x-ray shadowgraph the "picture" depends upon the fact that x rays pass readily through flesh but not through bone or areas injected with x-ray contrast media. By absorbing x rays as bone does, contrast media (organic compounds of iodine) cast a shadow on the x-ray film. Such agents are employed for visualization of the gastrointestinal tract, gallbladder, bile ducts, urinary tract, and miscellaneous body cavities.

X rays have proved to be one of man's chief weapons in the treatment of cancer. Their use in this area depends upon the fortunate fact that rapidly dividing malignant cells are more easily inhibited and destroyed than those of healthy tissue. However, x rays may be dangerous, for they can destroy such rapidly dividing healthy structures as the bone marrow and gonads. For this reason, the physician and technician must pay strict attention to the dose to protect not only the patient but also themselves.

Roentgen. The roentgen (R) is the unit employed to measure the energy of x rays and gamma rays. One roentgen is the amount of radiation that will produce 2.08×10^9 ions in 1 c.c. of air under standard conditions. For the average population the federal Radiation Council has recommended that the yearly whole-body exposure not exceed 0.17 R and that the 30-year value be less than 5 R, exclusive of the dose due to natural background.

Rem and rad. The rem, which stands for "roentgen-equivalent-man," is a dose of radiation that when absorbed by man produces a biologic effect equivalent to the absorption of 1 R of x or gamma radiation. The rad, which stands for radiation dosage, corresponds to an energy transfer of 100 ergs per gram of irradiated object, including living tissue.

Questions

1. What is Avogadro's law?
2. What is the kinetic theory of matter?
3. What is meant by brownian movement? Cite two examples.
4. Distinguish between kinetic and potential energy.
5. Distinguish between adhesion and cohesion.
6. Distinguish between vector and scalar quantities.
7. If a force of 5 pounds and a force of 8 pounds act upon a point at an angle of 40 degrees, what is the resultant force?
8. Distinguish between resultant and equilibrant.
9. Cite several examples to illustrate Newton's first law of motion.
10. Distinguish between acceleration and velocity.
11. Distinguish between speed and velocity.
12. A crystal of dye dropped to the bottom of a glass of water will, in time, impart a uniform color. Explain how this occurs.
13. If a car travels 300 miles in 4½ hours, what is its average speed?
14. If a motorist is traveling at 50 mph, what distance will he cover in 4 hours?
15. What is momentum?
16. Cite several examples to illustrate Newton's third law.
17. What effect does size and distance have upon the force of gravity?

18. Distinguish between weight and mass.
19. What force must the flexor muscles (inserted 3 inches from the elbow) exert in order for the hand to hold an 8-pound ball? (Assume that the hand is 1½ feet from the elbow.)
20. When a block and tackle are used (with four ropes supporting the movable pulley), what force must be applied to lift a 700-pound safe? What is the mechanical advantage of this machine? How much work must be expended to lift the safe 30 feet?
21. Can a machine ever have an efficiency of 100 percent?
22. Distinguish between stress and strain.
23. What is the pressure on the bottom of a cylindrical vessel filled with water that has a diameter of 5 cm. and a height of 30 cm.?
24. Is steel elastic? Are bones elastic?
25. Cite several examples to illustrate Pascal's principle.
26. What force buoys up a 150-pound man floating in water?
27. Describe the manometer and how it operates.
28. A metal ball with a diameter of 6 cm. weighs 14 ounces. What will be its weight in water?
29. Examine the construction of an atomizer or hand spray and, on the basis of the Bernoulli effect, explain how it works.
30. A mouthwash containing a surface-active germicide is more effective than preparations that are not surface active. Explain.
31. When a drop of water and a drop of alcohol are placed on a glass plate, the latter spreads out more than the former. Which has the greater surface tension?
32. When blood cells are placed in distilled water, they swell and rupture. Explain.
33. During the process of inspiration the pressure within the lung falls to about 753 mm. Hg. In this instance, what amount of pressure forces atmospheric air into the lung?
34. Assuming no change in temperature, how much would 3 liters of nitrogen gas expand if the pressure were lowered from 750 to 700 mm. Hg?
35. Assuming no change in pressure, what would be the effect of heating 500 c.c. of helium gas from 70° to 78° F.?
36. A gas at 20° C. and 771 mm. Hg has a volume of 600 c.c. What will its volume be at standard conditions?
37. In reference to the pressure of gases, explain the meaning of the formula $P = P_1 + P_2 + P_3$.
38. Why does hydrogen pass through a porous surface more readily than helium?
39. Compare the mercurial and aneroid barometers.
40. Compare a sound wave and a water wave.
41. What is the wavelength of a sound that has a frequency of 400 vibrations per second and a velocity of 1100 feet per second.
42. Distinguish between pitch and loudness.
43. What is meant by the quality of a sound?
44. What is the relationship of a harmonic to the fundamental?
45. What is a beat?
46. Give an example of sympathetic vibration.
47. Distinguish between the degree and quantity of heat.
48. Convert 68° F. to centigrade.
49. Convert 17° C. to Fahrenheit.
50. Relative to the kinetic theory of heat, compare the three states of matter.
51. Compare the small calorie and the large calorie.
52. What is a BTU?
53. If 10 gm. of ice are added to 100 c.c. of water at 18° C., what will be the temperature after the ice melts?
54. If 30 gm. of steam condenses in 500 ml. of water at 22° C., what will be the resulting temperature?
55. Why is a steam burn more serious than a boiling water burn?
56. What is insensible perspiration?
57. Explain how sweating cools the body.
58. Compare conduction and radiation.
59. What is the theory of magnetism?
60. Compare Coulomb's laws for magnetism and electrostatics.
61. Current flows from negative to positive. Explain.
62. Describe the structure and function of the condenser.
63. Why is tungsten used in the electric light bulb?
64. Describe the components and operation of the electric generator.
65. What are the essentials of the electric battery?
66. A nerve impulse travels with greater speed over a large nerve than over a small one. Explain.
67. Why does nature provide a layer of fat beneath the skin?
68. What is the current in a circuit that has a resistance of 30 ohms and an electromotive force of 100 v.?
69. What is the basic difference among the six colors?
70. Compare reflection and refraction.
71. What effect does optical density have upon the index of refraction?
72. What are x rays? How are they produced?
73. Compare the effects of x rays upon healthy and tumorous tissue.
74. What are x-ray contrast media?
75. Compare the roentgen, rem, and rad.

Chapter 4

Basic inorganic chemistry

The distinction between chemistry and physics is essentially one of different points of view rather than of subject matter. Whereas the physicist is concerned with all forms of energy—its source, its measurement, and its changes from one form to another—the chemist is concerned with energy chiefly insofar as it relates to the properties and changes that occur in matter. Chemistry, then, is primarily the study of matter.

LAW OF CONSERVATION OF MATTER

The French scientist and father of chemistry Lavoisier experimentally established the first vital principle of chemistry—the law of conservation of matter. This law states that matter is neither created nor destroyed but may be changed from one form into another. The same wording also applies to the *law of conservation of energy.* These two great laws, however, must be slightly modified if we wish to be absolutely correct, for under extraordinary conditions they are not true. It is now possible to convert matter into energy and energy into matter in accordance with Einstein's famous equation $E = mc^2$ (pp. 80-81). Although, as indicated, the conservation laws are suitable for "everyday" science, strict accuracy calls for combining the two into a single statement; that is, *the total amount of matter and energy together in the universe is constant.*

CHANGES IN MATTER

Matter may undergo two types of change —*physical* and *chemical.* A physical change is one that does not alter the composition of a substance. The breaking of glass, the melting of ice, and the boiling of water are physical changes, because in each instance the internal constitution of the substance remains the same. Water is water, whether it is ice or steam, and glass is glass, whether it is in a window or smashed to pieces by a boy who should have been studying chemistry. In contrast, a chemical change alters the composition of a substance; indeed, in this type of change the original substance becomes transformed into one or more new substances. The explosion of gunpowder, the souring of milk, the rusting of iron, and the burning of paper are all common examples of the chemical change.

CHEMICAL AND PHYSICAL PROPERTIES

A given substance is known by its so-called physical and chemical properties. Physical properties are those characteristics of a substance as ascertained or observed without chemical action. Conversely, chemical properties are those characteristics that relate to action, or lack of action, with other substances. Oxygen, for example, is a colorless gas that is heavier than air and only slightly soluble in water; these are its physical properties. Its ability to support combustion and its reaction with certain elements to form oxides are its chemical properties. Any reference source in general chemistry such as a handbook always contains a detailed account of the physical and chemical properties of important compounds.

STATES OF MATTER

Matter may exist in three forms or states —*solid, liquid,* and *gaseous.* A solid is characterized by its definite shape and volume, a liquid by its definite volume and its readiness to assume the shape of the receptacle into which it is placed, and a gas by its indefinite shape and volume. Many substances, naturally, exist in two or all three states.

The change of state is a physical act. Specifically, and according to the kinetic theory (p. 18), the three states of matter are merely examples of an energy differential. In the solid state the molecules have the least energy and therefore the least motion. In the gaseous state, on the other hand, the molecules have the most energy and the most motion. The liquid state is merely an intermediate energy level. This energy differential can be readily appreciated if one compares the amount of energy needed to convert ice and water to steam. Since ice (the solid state) represents a lower energy level than water, it follows that more heat energy must be added to the former than to the latter to change it into steam.

The various physical characteristics of the three states, such as density, specific gravity, surface tension, and so on, have already been presented in the foregoing chapters.

KINDS OF MATTER

While the physicist is interested primarily in the states of matter, it is fair to state that the chemist concerns himself primarily with the kinds of matter. To be sure, there are three kinds of matter (or substances): elements, compounds and mixtures. Obviously, the student must have a clear understanding of these terms before progressing to more advanced ground.

Elements. The earth and its flora and

Table 4-1. Common elements

Element	Symbol	Atomic number	Atomic weight
Aluminum	Al	13	27
Barium	Ba	56	137.4
Boron	B	5	10.8
Bromine	Br	35	79.9
Calcium	Ca	20	40
Carbon	C	6	12
Chlorine	Cl	17	35.5
Chromium	Cr	24	52
Cobalt	Co	27	58.9
Copper	Cu	29	63.5
Fluorine	F	9	19
Gold	Au	79	197.2
Helium	He	2	4
Hydrogen	H	1	1
Iodine	I	53	126.9
Iron	Fe	26	55.9
Lead	Pb	82	207.2
Magnesium	Mg	12	24
Manganese	Mn	25	54.9
Mercury	Hg	80	200.6
Nickel	Ni	28	58.7
Nitrogen	N	7	14
Oxygen	O	8	16
Phosphorus	P	15	30.9
Platinum	Pt	78	195.2
Potassium	K	19	39.1
Silicon	Si	14	28.1
Silver	Ag	47	107.9
Sodium	Na	11	22.9
Sulfur	S	16	32.1
Tin	Sn	50	118.7
Uranium	U	92	238.1
Zinc	Zn	30	65.4

fauna are constituted of ninety-two elements in an astronomical number of combinations. Years ago an element was defined as a substance that cannot be decomposed into simpler material. However, since man now has the ability to take apart the atom, the "simplest" particle of matter, it is more accurate to define an element as a substance that cannot be decomposed into simpler material by ordinary chemical means.

For convenience in describing the constitution of matter, the chemist uses a system of chemical shorthand whereby each element is assigned a symbol. This consists of one or two letters of the English or Latin name, with the first letter capitalized. The more common and important elements and their symbols are presented in Table 4-1.

There is some convenience, for the beginning student, in classifying the elements as either *metals* or *nonmetals.* Metals are recognized by their luster, opacity, and high conductivity of heat and electricity. Such elements as iron, tin, lead, copper, silver, and gold are familiar to us as metals. Although the nonmetalic elements (oxygen, iodine, and sulfur, to name a few) are certainly common, we usually do not think of them as nonmetals, or as a group, because of their highly variable properties. Also, it is only fair to say that some elements which look like metals sometimes behave chemically like nonmetals, and vice versa. Arsenic, for example, resembles a metal but, chemically, acts as a nonmetal.

Compounds. A compound is a substance that consists of two or more elements chemically united, that is, combined in such a manner that each constituent has lost its individual characteristics. Each compound has its own static personality by virtue of another basic law of chemistry: the *law of definite proportions.* This law states that when two or more elements chemically combine, they always do so in a definite proportion by weight. Thus, when hydrogen and oxygen come together in Istanbul, they produce the same compound—*water* (H_2O)—as when the synthesis takes place in New York. Other common examples of compounds are sugar, salt, and aspirin.

Mixtures. Most substances in nature do not fit the definition of either an element or a compound. These are mixtures, which may be defined as two or more elements or compounds that are not chemically combined and that are put together in any proportion. Anything that is not a pure element or a pure compound, then, can be deduced to be a mixture. Air, soil, petroleum, candy, and blood are examples.

STRUCTURE AND BEHAVIOR OF MATTER

If we were to take a piece of matter—let us say a banana—and by some means proceed to break it up into an infinite number of pieces, what would the ultimate particle look like? More to the point: Is there a fundamental unit of matter? Though the Greeks answered the question in the affirmative and called the particle the atom, the discussion remained in the domain of philosophy until 1803, when a rather obscure English schoolteacher by the name of John Dalton presented to man the first unified idea concerning the true structure and behavior of matter. Borrowing the 2000-year-old word *atom,* and with due regard to the law of conservation of matter and the law of definite proportions, Dalton's assumptions (the atomic theory) ran as follows.

1. All matter is composed of very small particles called *atoms.*
2. All the atoms of the same element are alike in size, shape, and weight but differ from the atoms of every other element.
3. Atoms of most elements are able to unite with the atoms of other elements.
4. In all chemical changes atoms do not break up but act as individual units.

Dalton's statements are truly remarkable for their simplicity. Even more remarkable, they have essentially withstood the test of time. Although today we know that the atom cannot truthfully be called *the* particle, it nevertheless still serves as a practical unit of the universe.

Electron theory. The atomic theory sparked the great minds that followed Dalton to probe beyond the atom, and at the beginning of the present century these researches began to bear fruit. This probing and searching, however, have never ceased, for the end still remains out of sight. Indeed, as atomic science plods along, learning more and more about less and less, we cannot help but feel that matter becomes more and more involved. Regardless of these shortcomings, however, man has amassed sufficient knowledge, embodied in the electron theory, to explain the bulk of the chemical events associated with the workings of the elements and their compounds.

The electron theory holds that the atom is an arrangement of particles not unlike the arrangement of the solar system (Fig. 4-1). The basic ideas of the theory are as follows.

1. The atoms of all the elements are made up of a characteristic number of positively charged particles called *protons* and negatively charged particles called *electrons,* the proton being about 2000 times heavier than the electron.

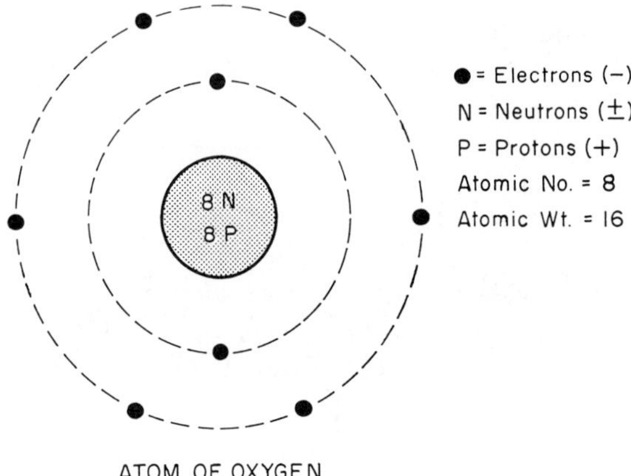

Fig. 4-1. The atom.

2. The atoms of each element contain the same number of protons as electrons and therefore are electrically neutral.

3. A dense central core, the *nucleus,* contains the protons and neutral particles, aptly called *neutrons;* the latter particle is believed to be the union of an electron and a proton.

4. About the nucleus revolve the electrons in rather definite orbits.

As will be shown, the chemical behavior of the atom is dictated by the number and spatial arrangement of these planetary electrons. In nuclear reactions, however, which are discussed at the end of the chapter, the protons, neutrons, and other nuclear particles too numerous to mention play the major roles.

Atomic number. As shown in Table 4-1, each element has a characteristic atomic number, which is defined as the number of planetary electrons about the nucleus of each of its atoms or preferably as the number of protons. The atomic number of oxygen, for example, is 8 (Fig. 4-1).

Mass number and atomic weight. The mass number, which stands next to the atomic number in significance, is equal to the sum of the neutrons and protons in the nucleus of each atom. The atomic weight of an element is the weight of its atoms compared to the weight of a carbon atom, to which has been assigned 12 atomic units.* Since for a single atom the atomic weight is equal to the mass number, we would expect all the elements to have integral atomic weights. However, a glance at Table 4-1 will disclose that most elements do not. This is because an element is usually composed of two or three varieties of atoms that differ in respect to their mass number. Thus, the atomic weight (35.5) of the gas chlorine represents the statistical average of its two kinds of atoms. One kind, with seventeen protons and eighteen neutrons and a mass number of 35, constitutes

*Formerly, the standard was oxygen 16.

75 percent of the gas; the other, with seventeen protons and twenty neutrons and a mass number of 37, constitutes 25 percent of the gas. Such atoms, that is, those which are alike save for the atomic weight, are called *isotopes*. Thus, chlorine has two isotopes: Cl^{35} and Cl^{37}. In summary, then, the atomic weight of an element is best defined as the average weight of its atoms compared to carbon.

Valence. Valence means the combining capacity of an atom or its behavior toward other atoms. Since chemistry is essentially the study of what happens when atoms meet and combine, the expression is obviously a keystone of the science.

The mechanism of valence resides among the palentary electrons. Substantial evidence indicates that the orbit, or shell, nearest the nucleus (the so-called k orbit) can contain no more than two electrons, and the second (l), third (m), and fourth (n) no more than 8, 18, and 32, respectively. But most interestingly, the *outermost* orbit of any atom has a maximum number of 8.

Using these rules, let us now consider the electronic pattern for the elements from hydrogen (atomic number of 1) to argon (atomic number of 18). All we need do is place two electrons in the first orbit, eight electrons in the second, and the remaining electrons in the third or last orbit. Once this is done, it will be noted that three of these elements—helium, neon, and argon—contain the maximum number of electrons in the outer orbit. Moreover—and here is the central idea—these are the *only* elements of the eighteen that under ordinary conditions are chemically inactive, or inert. From this interesting fact the chemist has

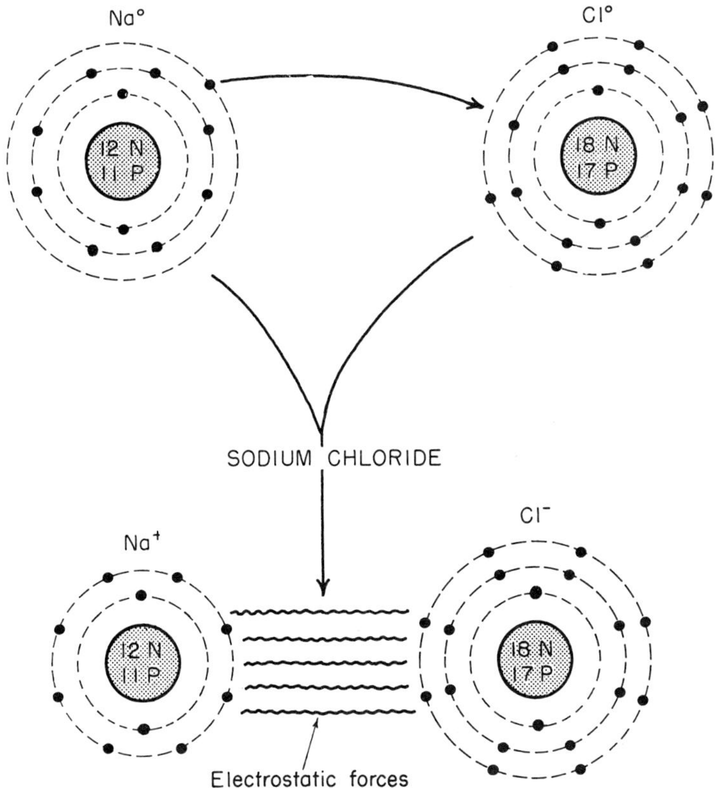

Fig. 4-2. Electrovalence. (From Brooks, S. M.: Basic facts of general chemistry, Philadelphia, 1956, W. B. Saunders Co.)

theorized that elements or, more to the point, their atoms react with one another to obtain an outer orbit with the maximum number of electrons—their "happiest" state. As we shall now see, this can be effected by either losing, gaining, or sharing electrons.

Electrovalence. When the elements sodium and chlorine are brought together, a violent reaction ensues, producing heat and, most important, the compound sodium chloride. As shown in Fig. 4-2, the reaction is one of electron transfer; that is, the one electron in the outer orbit of the sodium atom travels to the outer orbit of the chlorine atom, thereby establishing outer orbits containing the maximum number of electrons (eight) for both atoms. Of course, the same result could be achieved by a transfer of all seven electrons from the outer orbit of the chlorine atom to the sodium atom. This does not occur, however, for the simple reason that nature follows the most logical path, which in this instance is the easiest path—a transfer of one instead of seven.

This is not quite all, however, for, once the electron transfer has taken place, the atoms are no longer atoms; they are now charged particles called *ions.* The sodium atom that has lost one electron acquires a positive charge of one (Na^+) and the chlorine atom that has gained one electron acquires a negative charge of one (Cl^-). Now, since unlike charges attract, we may look upon a crystal of salt as a latticework of sodium and chlorine ions, in equal numbers, held together by *electrostatic forces.* That they are in equal numbers is of cardinal significance, for this means that the smallest possible particles of salt is composed of one sodium ion and one chlorine ion. This is expressed simply as NaCl.

This, then, is electrovalence, or the combining of elements by the loss and gain of electrons. Elements such as sodium that lose electrons are said to have a positive electrovalence; elements such as chlorine that gain electrons are said to have a negative electrovalence. Of general importance is the fact that metals are electropositive and nonmetals are electronegative. In brief, metals react with nomentals because the former are electron donors and the latter are electron recipients, a mutually satisfactory arrangement in obtaining the desired state of the maximum electron count in the outer orbit.

Just a little thought now will disclose some further enlightening ideas. First, the degree of electrovalence tells us the number of atoms needed to form a *molecule,* the smallest theoretical particle of a compound. In the instance of sodium chloride the one electron donated by each sodium atom required only one chlorine atom to accept it—hence, the formula NaCl. This formula tells us that in a crystal of salt there is one atom (strictly speaking, one ion) of sodium for every atom of chlorine. In other words, the electrovalence of sodium (+1) is equal to or balanced by the electrovalence of chlorine (−1). Similarly, the compound calcium chloride has the formula $CaCl_2$ for the simple reason that two negative chlorine ions are needed to balance the +2 charge of the calcium ions. Thus, with the electrovalences shown in Table 4-2, we can easily write the desired formula by the use of the appropriate subscript(s). By convention, the electropositive symbol precedes the electronegative symbol. Also, when there is only one atom of an element per molecule, no subscript is written; *one* is understood. Finally, and by convention, only the smallest possible subscripts are used; that is, although the formulas NaCl and Na_2Cl_2 are "balanced," the former is the accepted designation.

The student may wonder what to do about the formula of a compound such as aluminum sulfide, formed in the reaction between aluminum and sulfur. How does one balance the valence of aluminum (Al^{+++}) with the valence of sulfur ($S^{=}$)? It is quite easy: We merely use subscripts

Table 4-2. Valences of common elements and radicals

Electrovalent		
Metals		
Aluminum	3	(Al^{+++})
Barium	2	(Ba^{++})
Bismuth	3,5	(Bi^{+++}), (Bi^{+++++})
Calcium	2	(Ca^{++})
Copper	1,2	(Cu^{+}), (Cu^{++})
Hydrogen	1	(H^{+})
Iron	2,3	(Fe^{++}), (Fe^{+++})
Lead	2	(Pb^{++})
Magnesium	2	(Mg^{++})
Mercury	1,2	(Hg^{+}), (Hg^{++})
Nickel	2	(Ni^{++})
Potassium	1	(K^{+})
Silver	1	(Ag^{+})
Sodium	1	(Na^{+})
Tin	2,4	(Sn^{++}), (Sn^{++++})
Zinc	2	(Zn^{++})
Nonmetals		
Bromine	1	(Br^{-})
Chlorine	1	(Cl^{-})
Fluorine	1	(F^{-})
Iodine	1	(I^{-})
Oxygen	2	($O^{=}$)
Sulfur	2	($S^{=}$)
Radicals		
Ammonium	1	(NH_4^{+})
Bicarbonate	1	(HCO_3^{-})
Carbonate	2	($CO_3^{=}$)
Chlorate	1	(ClO_3^{-})
Hydroxyl	1	(OH^{-})
Nitrate	1	(NO_3^{-})
Nitrite	1	(NO_2^{-})
Phosphate	3	($PO_4^{\equiv}$)
Sulfate	2	($SO_4^{=}$)
Sulfite	2	($SO_3^{=}$)
Covalent		
Carbon	4	
Hydrogen	1	
Nitrogen	1,2,3,4,5	
Oxygen	2	
Phosphorus	3,5	
Sulfur	4,6	

in such a way that the subscript of aluminum times its valence equals the subscript of sulfur times its valence. We see immediately that the answer is Al_2S_3, that is, $2 \times 3 = 3 \times 2$. As we know, this means that a molecule of aluminum sulfide consists of two atoms of aluminum and three atoms of sulfur.

Covalence. While electrovalent compounds combine via the loss and gain of electrons, covalent elements do so by the *sharing* of electrons.* When oxygen reacts with hydrogen to form water, for example, one atom of oxygen combines with two atoms of hydrogen (H_2O). As shown in Fig. 4-3, the reason for this ratio lies in the fact that oxygen has six electrons in its outer orbit and hydrogen has one. Each atom of oxygen shares two pairs of electrons, and each atom of hydrogen one pair of electrons. Thus, we say that oxygen has a covalence of 2 and hydrogen a covalence of 1, covalence being defined as the number of electron pairs shared. Carbon, nitrogen, oxygen, phosphorus, and sulfur are other common elements that react or combine via covalence (Table 4-2). In the writing of chemical formulas, however, we employ the same rules that were discussed under electrovalence. For example, we write the formula for carbon dioxide as CO_2; that is, the subscript of C (1) times its valence (4) is equal to the subscript of O (2) times its valence (2), or $4 = 4$.

Several elements can combine by both mechanisms. Oxygen, for instance, sometimes gains two electrons, giving it an electrovalence of -2. Sulfur can have an electrovalence of -2 or a covalence of 4 or 6. To repeat, this does not alter the way in

*In some covalent compounds the electrons are not shared equally and this gives polarity to the molecule. In water, for example, oxygen has a greater affinity for electrons than does hydrogen, and this makes the oxygen portion of the molecule negative with respect to the hydrogen portion. Thus, water is a *polar* compound. *Nonpolar* compounds are those in which the electrons are shared *equally*.

which we write a formula, for all we need to use is the valence *number.*

Multiple valence. A glance at Table 4-2 will show that some elements have more than one valence. In other words, they are capable of losing, gaining, or sharing more than one set number of electrons. Iron (Fe), for example, depending upon external conditions, sometimes loses two electrons, becoming Fe^{++}, and sometimes three, becoming Fe^{+++}. Which of the two valences one uses in writing the chemical formula for the compounds of such elements depends upon the specified circumstances.

Radicals. A radical is defined as a combination of atoms that ordinarily acts as though it were a single atom; it exhibits a regular valence and possesses an electrical charge (Table 4-2). The atoms of a radical in most instances are held together by a special kind of covalence called *coordinate* valence. Whereas in ordinary covalence each atom involved contributes an electron to the pair that is shared between the two atoms, in coordinate valence both electrons are contributed by one of the two atoms. As a result, for reasons that we need not take up here, the radical acquires an overall charge.

In the formulas for compounds containing radicals the student handles the situation in exactly the same manner as already described, just remembering that a radical is a *unit.* For example, the formula for cal-

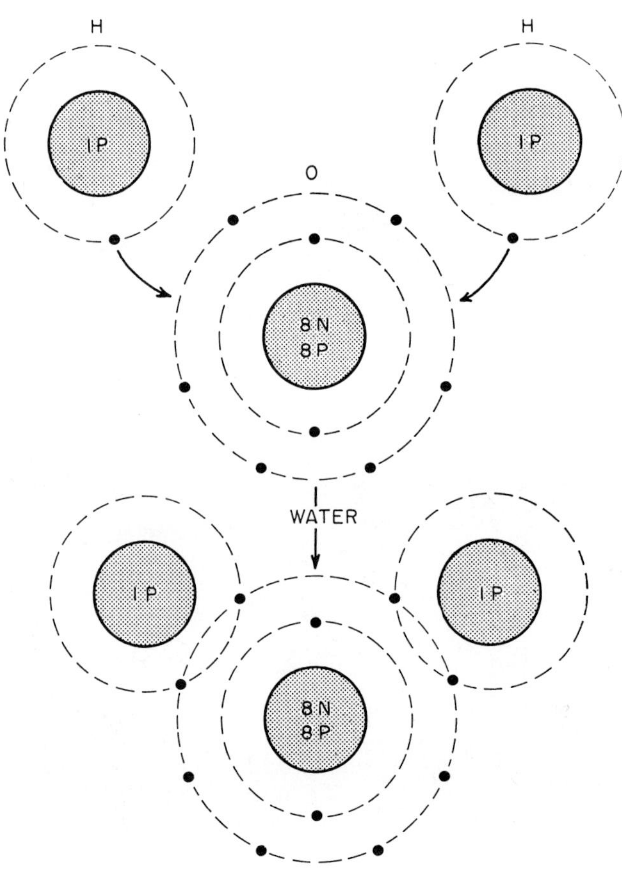

Fig. 4-3. Covalence. (From Brooks, S. M.: Basic facts of general chemistry, Philadelphia, 1956, W. B. Saunders Co.)

cium sulfate is simply $CaSO_4$; that is, the valence of Ca (+2) is balanced by the valence of SO_4 (−2). In the event subscripts are required, we must use parentheses about the radical because it is a unit. The formula for aluminum sulfate, for instance, is $Al_2(SO_4)_3$. As a further example, and one that should dismiss all difficulties at the elementary level, the formula for ammonium phosphate is $(NH_4)_3PO_4$.

Ions. The term *ion* is one of the smallest and yet biggest words in science. The chemist uses it over and over again in talking about matter in general and chemical reactions in particular. But this is not difficult to understand if we recall that ions are the charged particles that compose *electrovalent* compounds. Let us now return to these compounds and explore their properties more fully.

When electrovalent compounds are dissolved in water, the ions leave their electrostatic moorings of the solid state and diffuse throughout the solution, a phenomenon referred to as *dissociation* or more commonly, but less correctly, as *ionization*—less correctly because electrovalent compounds are ionized even in the solid state. The presence of these charged particles can be demonstrated by the simple apparatus shown in Fig. 4-4. Herein lies a fundamental principle: Whereas electrovalent compounds are conductors of electricity, covalent compounds may generally be regarded as nonconductors. The word *electrolyte* is used to describe a compound that, in solution, conducts a current; a *nonelectrolyte* is a compound that does not have this property.

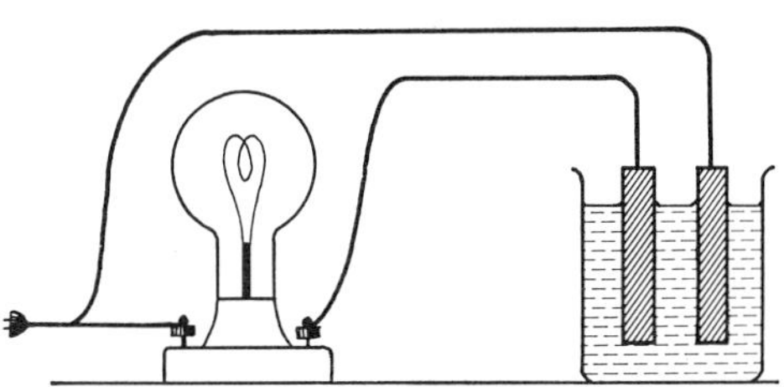

Fig. 4-4. Apparatus used to test the ability of a solution to conduct an electrical current. (From Brooks, S. M.: Basic facts of general chemistry, Philadelphia, 1956, W. B. Saunders Co.)

An electrolyte is always neutral. This is not because the number of positive ions equals the number of negative ions, as one might be prone to say, but because the number of positive charges equals the number of negative charges. For example, when aluminum chloride ($AlCl_3$) dissolves in water, three chlorine ions (Cl^-) are released for each aluminum ion (Al^{+++}). The resulting solution, therefore, will obviously contain the same number of negative charges as positive charges.

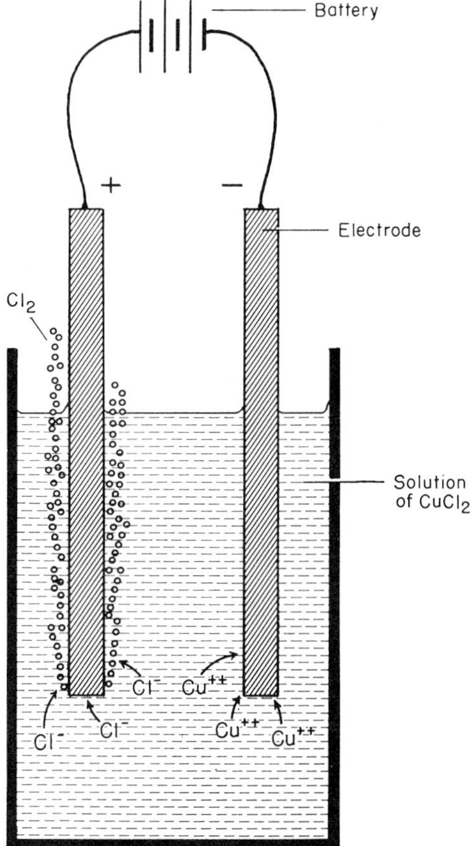

Fig. 4-5. Electrolysis of $CuCl_2$. (From Brooks, S. M.: Basic facts of general chemistry, Philadelphia, 1956, W. B. Saunders Co.)

Electrolysis. When a current of electricity passes through an electrolyte, the latter is decomposed into its constituent elements by a process known as electrolysis. A close study of the electrolytic events depicted in Fig. 4-5 is eminently instructive, for it will not only corroborate but also amplify the theory of ionization.

In the apparatus shown in Fig. 4-5, when the switch is thrown, copper ions (Cu^{++}) are drawn to the cathode (negative electrode) and the chlorine ions (Cl^{-}) are drawn to the anode (positive electrode). This, as we know, follows the law of electricity which states that like charges repel and unlike charges attract. Now, upon arriving at the cathode, the copper ions become copper atoms, as proved by the fact that the electrode becomes copper coated. Simultaneously, at the anode the chlorine ions become chlorine atoms, as attested by the appearance of gas bubbles at that electrode. If the current is kept on long enough, no copper chloride will remain in solution; that is, it will have been completely decomposed into copper (plated out on the cathode) and chlorine (released to the air).

These events can be explained and summarized by the equations that follow:

$$CuCl_2 \longrightarrow Cu^{++} + 2Cl^{-} \text{ (ionization)}$$
$$Cu^{++} + 2e \longrightarrow Cu^{\circ} \text{ (cathode)}$$
$$Cl - 1e \longrightarrow Cl^{\circ} \text{ (anode)}$$

Let us note especially that Cu^{++} *gains* two electrons (*e*) from the cathode (thereby becoming neutral, Cu°), and that Cl *loses* an electron (thereby becoming neutral, Cl°). Essentially, we can say that the chlorine electrons lost at the anode travel through the wire and neutralize the copper ion. Indeed, two chlorine ions are required to neutralize one copper ion.

In a practical sense the central theme in what we have just discussed is that *electrolysis is the reverse of synthesis,* or

$$Cu + Cl_2 \longrightarrow CuCl_2 \text{ (synthesis)}$$
$$CuCl_2 \longrightarrow Cu + Cl_2 \text{ (electrolysis)}$$

Theoretically, however, and this is our present concern, the events of electrolysis confirm the concept of electrovalence and ions.

Anions and cations. In talking about ions, it is customary to use the expressions *anions* and *cations.* An anion is simply a negative ion, so called because it travels to the anode during electrolysis. Conversely, a cation is a positive ion because it travels to the cathode.

Oxidation and reduction. Oxidation and reduction are very commonly used terms in chemistry. Unfortunately, the beginning student often seems to struggle a little whenever he encounters them, but this need not be. When the word *oxidation* is used in connection with ions, it means simply a loss of electrons; conversely, the word *reduction* means a gain of electrons. In the equations that follow note that copper is *reduced* and chlorine *oxidized:*

$$Cu^{++} + 2e \longrightarrow Cu^{\circ} \text{ (reduction; electrons gained)}$$
$$Cl - 1e \longrightarrow Cl^{\circ} \text{ (oxidation; electrons lost)}$$

With regard to the element oxygen, however, which must be mentioned although we are not concerned with it in this section, the term *oxidation* means the combining of oxygen with some other element. Conversely, reduction means the removal of oxygen.

The reaction. A chemical reaction is said to occur when two or more substances react with one another to produce new substances. Thus, the chemical changes mentioned earlier are now seen to be the result of a chemical reaction. Most reactions release energy in the form of heat; these are referred to as *exothermic* reactions. Sometimes energy is released in the form of light and electricity, but even in these instances some heat is formed. A chemical reaction may liberate energy gradually, as do most of the chemical reactions in our bodies, or with explosive violence, as when one pulls the trigger of a gun. There are reactions, however, that require energy in the form of heat, light, or electricity. In contradistinction to the first type, these are called *endothermic* reactions.

Equation. What happens in the test tube—the chemical reaction—is succinctly described and explained by the chemical equation. The following steps are taken in the writing of an equation.

1. The symbol or formula for each of the substances participating in the reaction is written to the left of an arrow.

2. In a similar manner the products formed are expressed on the right side of the arrow.

3. The equation is balanced by placing appropriate numbers (called *coefficients*) before the symbols or formulas in such a way that the number of atoms of each element is the same on both sides of the equation. *Above all, one must not change the subscripts!*

Let us now see how these rules apply to a specific reaction, for example, the reaction between magnesium and hydrochloric acid, forming magnesium chloride and hydrogen.

Step 1: $Mg + HCl \longrightarrow$
Step 2: $Mg + HCl \longrightarrow MgCl_2 + H_2$
Step 3: $Mg + 2HCl \longrightarrow MgCl_2 + H_2\uparrow$*

Our complete equation now reads: 1 atom of magnesium plus 2 molecules of hydrochloric acid yield 1 molecule of magnesium chloride plus 1 molecule of hydrogen. (Note that the absence of a coefficient is, by convention, understood as 1).

Finally, there are two points that the student must remember in addition to the mechanical steps just stated. During a chemical change a radical often remains intact and therefore should be treated as a chemical unit. For example, in the reaction between aluminum sulfate and ammonium hydroxide, which forms aluminum hydroxide and ammonium sulfate, the equation is written as follows:

$$Al_2(SO_4)_3 + 6NH_4OH \longrightarrow 3(NH_4)_2SO_4 + 2Al(OH)_3$$

*$\uparrow$ indicates gas.

Types of reaction. Now that we have some understanding of the chemical reaction and equation, it seems appropriate to make an important generalization; to wit, *countless chemical reactions can be grouped into four categories,* as follows:

1. Direct combination—a reaction in which two or more elements or compounds react to form a more complex substance (sometimes called *synthesis*)

$$C + O_2 \longrightarrow CO_2$$

2. Decomposition—a reaction in which a compound is broken up into its constituent elements or into simple compounds (sometimes called *analysis*)

$$2H_2O \longrightarrow 2H_2\uparrow + O_2\uparrow$$

3. Substitution—a reaction in which a free element replaces a combined element (sometimes called *single replacement*)

$$Zn + CuSO_4 \longrightarrow ZnSO_4 + Cu$$

4. Double replacement—a reaction in which the elements of the reacting compounds "change partners"

$$AgNO_3 + NaCl \longrightarrow NaNO_3 + AgCl\downarrow^*$$

Speed of reaction. The speed, or rate, at which a reaction takes place is obviously of great practical importance. Indeed, some chemicals refuse to react at all unless certain environmental factors are just right. The principal factors having a bearing upon the reaction are discussed in the paragraphs that follow.

Nature of the reacting substances. As we have learned from common experience, some chemicals react faster than others. For instance, it takes longer for a nail to rust than it does for a match to burn. At a more sophisticated level we note that the speed of reaction between electrovalent compounds generally exceeds the speed between convalent compounds.

Temperature. A rise in temperature greatly increases the speed of reaction.

*$\downarrow$ indicates precipitate.

Roughly speaking, a rise of 10° C. just about doubles the speed. Conversely, when the temperature is lowered, chemical activity is decreased. Refrigeration, for example, is nothing more than a method of retarding chemical reactions in food.

Catalysis. Catalysis is a subject of vital concern not only to the chemist but also to the biologist, for *enzymes*—the keystones of cellular activity—are catalysts. Catalysis is the altering of a chemical reaction via the influence of an agent (the catalyst) which, itself, remains unchanged. If two boys are fighting because of something said by a third boy, the latter is a bona fide catalyst.

To get back to the laboratory, there are many substances that react with difficulty, or not at all, unless a catalyst is present. In the preparation of oxygen by heating potassium chlorate, the reaction is extremely sluggish without a little manganese dioxide. On the other hand, to retard the decomposition of hydrogen peroxide, the manufacturer adds a pinch of acetanilid to the bottle. Thus, catalysts are employed to speed up or to slow down reactions. Just how the catalyst does its job is not completely understood, but much evidence points to some kind of intermediary role whereby the reacting substances are brought into more "intimate" atomic contact.

Concentration. The effect of concentration upon a given reaction is succinctly put forth by the *law of mass action,* which states that the speed of a chemical reaction is directly proportional to the concentration of the reacting substances. For example, if A and B react to form C, we can speed up the reaction by increasing the concentration of either A or B.

Chemical equilibrium. So far in our discussion of chemical reactions we have not considered the likelihood of the products "re-reacting" to form the original reactants; that is, if $A + B \rightarrow C + D$, might not $C + D \rightarrow A + B$? In short, are there reactions of the type $A + B \rightleftarrows C + D$? The answer is Yes. These are called *reversible* reactions in contradistinction to the *irreversible* type.

If we add a solution of potassium nitrate (KNO_3) to a solution of sodium chloride ($NaCl$), there is no manifestation of a reaction. Something is taking place, however, at the "ionic level," as follows:

$$KNO_3 + NaCl \leftrightarrows KCl + NaNO_3$$

In other words, this equation tells us that K^+ ions encounter Cl^- ions to form KCl, and Na^+ ions encounter NO_3^- ions to form $NaNO_3$. Once these ionic compounds are formed, there is, in this case, nothing to prevent them from dissociating and recombining with their former partners. Thus, there are two reactions going on, as indicated by the two arrows. Technically, this state of affairs is referred to as *dynamic equilibrium;* that is, chemical events take place in both directions simultaneously. Obviously, unless something is done to push the reaction to the right, the new products (KCl and $NaNO_3$) cannot be obtained.

From this the student can readily appreciate the importance of knowing whether a given reaction is reversible or irreversible. As far as ionic reactions are concerned, if one of the products is "nonionizable," insoluble, or a gas, the reaction will be irreversible. By the same token, other reactions will be reversible because the products, once formed, will not be removed from the "field of activity." The following are examples of irreversibility:

$NaOH + HCl \longrightarrow NaCl + H_2O$ (H_2O is only very slightly ionized)

$2KHCO_3 + H_2SO_4 \longrightarrow K_2SO_4 + 2H_2O + 2CO_2\uparrow$ (CO_2 escapes into the air)

$AgNO_3 + NaCl \longrightarrow NaNO_3 + AgCl\downarrow$ (AgCl is insoluble and settles out)

WATER

Now that we have an idea of the structure and behavior of matter, let us turn to some specific points of interest. In this

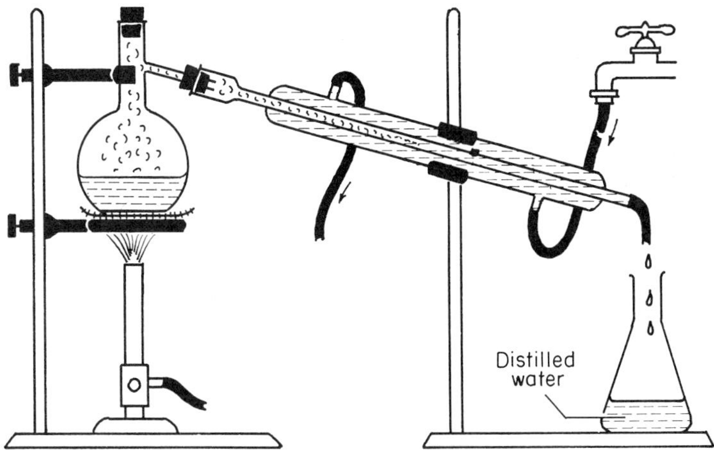

Fig. 4-6. Distillation apparatus. (From Brooks, S. M.: Basic facts of general chemistry, Philadelphia, 1956, W. B. Saunders Co.)

regard, one can do no better than start with water.

Water (H_2O) is our most familiar, most abundant, and most useful compound. It is especially interesting to the chemist because of its unique properties. It is tasteless, colorless, and odorless and at standard pressure freezes at 0° C. and boils at 100° C. At 4° C. it has its greatest density: 1 gm. per milliliter. Above or below this temperature 1 ml. of water weighs very slightly less than 1 gm. Although water displays extreme stability, even at high temperature, it does react with several substances, for example, the alkali metals (p. 71) and certain oxides.

Purification. Water for human consumption must be free of poisonous materials and harmful microbes (Chapter 6). For laboratory use, however, it must be free of *all* dissolved substances, particularly mineral matter. Mineral-free water is prepared by *distillation*, a process that consists of *evaporation* (conversion of the liquid to the gaseous state) and *condensation* (conversion from the gaseous to the liquid state). The basic apparatus for carrying out distillation is shown in Fig. 4-6.

Solutions. A true solution is a *homogeneous* mixture of two or more substances whose particles are of molecular or atomic size. The solute refers to the substance that goes into solution and the solvent (usually water) to the substance that dissolves the solute. When the solute and the solvent are both liquids and mix in all proportions, they are said to be *miscible* (for example, water and alcohol). Nonmiscible or immiscible liquids do not mix (for example, oil and water).

A common way to classify solutions is based on the proportion of solute to solvent. Later we shall learn more precise ways to express concentration.

Dilute solution. A dilute solution is one that contains a small amount of solute in relation to solvent.

Concentrated solution. A concentrated solution is a solution that contains a large amount of solute in relation to the solvent.

Unsaturated solution. An unsaturated solution is a solution that is capable of dissolving more solute under the same conditions of temperature and pressure.

Saturated solution. A saturated solution is a solution that contains all the solute it can normally dissolve at a given temperature and pressure.

Supersaturated solution. The supersaturated solution is of little practical importance but of some interest. It is one that contains more solute than it could ordinarily hold at a given temperature. The condition is extremely unstable, and all the excess solute over and above the saturation point will crystallize out of solution if a pinch of solute is added to the cooled solution. Other disturbances such as agitation or scratching the sides of the vessel may also initiate the "fallout."

Colligative properties. Solutions have certain properties that are related solely to the concentration of the solute rather than to the nature of the solute. These properties, namely, freezing point, boiling point, and osmotic pressure, are known as colligative properties. The freezing point of a solution is always lower than that of the solvent; the boiling point of a solution containing a nonvolatile solute is always higher than that of the solvent; and the osmotic pressure is proportional to the concentration of the solute (p. 27).

ACIDS, BASES, SALTS, AND OXIDES

Inorganic compounds fall into four major categories: acids, bases, salts, and oxides. The vast array of organic compounds (that is, compounds of carbon) will be discussed elsewhere.

Acids. According to the classic view and for ordinary purposes, an acid may be defined as a compound that furnishes hydrogen ions (H^+). Although in aqueous solutions the H^+ exists as the *hydronium* ion (H_3O^+), that is, $H_2O + H^+ \rightarrow H_3O^+$, no harm is really done in employing the symbol "H^+."*

Properties. Acids taste sour and cause certain dyes, or indicators, to undergo a color change. For example, they turn litmus from blue to red and methyl orange from orange to red. Acids react with certain metals to form hydrogen and salts and with all bases to form salts and water (neutralization):

$$\underset{\text{Metal}}{Zn} + \underset{\text{Acid}}{2HCl} \longrightarrow \underset{\text{Salt}}{ZnCl_2} + \underset{\text{Hydrogen}}{H_2\uparrow}$$

$$\underset{\text{Base}}{2NAOH} + \underset{\text{Acid}}{H_2SO_4} \longrightarrow \underset{\text{Salt}}{Na_2SO_4} + \underset{\text{Water}}{2H_2O\uparrow}$$

Acids differ greatly in strength, depending upon the degree of ionization. This can be easily demonstrated by the setup shown in Fig. 4-4. Whereas acetic acid (CH_3COOH), a weak acid, is a poor electrolyte (bulb lights dim), hydrochloric acid (HCl) is a good electrolyte (bulb lights bright). Using equations, this may be represented as follows:

$$HCl \longrightarrow H^+ + Cl^- \text{ (completely ionized)}$$
$$CH_3COOH \rightleftharpoons H^+ + CH_3COO^- \text{ (slightly ionized)}$$

Preparation. In the laboratory, acids may be prepared by the reaction between a nonmetallic oxide (acid anhydride) and water or by the reaction between sulfuric acid and the appropriate salt. The following are examples:

$$\underset{\text{Sulfur trioxide}}{SO_3} + H_2O \longrightarrow \underset{\text{Sulfuric acid}}{H_2SO_4}$$

$$\underset{\text{Sulfuric acid}}{H_2SO_4} + \underset{\text{Sodium nitrate}}{2NaNO_3} \longrightarrow \underset{\text{Sodium sulfate}}{Na_2SO_4} + \underset{\text{Nitric acid}}{2HNO_3}$$

Nomenclature. Binary acids (those composed of only two elements, that is, hydrogen and some nonmetal) are named by using the stem of the nonmetal with the prefix *hydro-* and suffix *-ic.* Ternary acids (hydrogen, oxygen, and another element) are named according to the amount of oxygen (Table 4-3).

Because acids represent one of the chief kinds of chemicals, the student should memorize the names and formulas for the ones most commonly used in general chemistry. These include hydrochloric acid

*Since the H^+ ion is really a proton (the hydrogen atom has one proton in the nucleus and one planetary electron), the Brönsted theory defines an acid as a *proton donor.* While the "hydrogen ion definition" applies to aqueous solutions, the Brönsted view is all-inclusive, applying to any solvent.

Table 4-3. Naming of acids

Acids of chlorine	Formulas	Acids of bromine	Formulas
Hydrochloric acid	HCl	Hydrobromic acid	HBr
Hypochlorous acid	$HClO$	Hypobromous acid	$HBrO$
Chlorous acid	$HClO_2$	Bromous acid	$HBrO_2$
Chloric acid	$HClO_3$	Bromic acid	$HBrO_3$
Perchloric acid	$HClO_4$	Perbromic acid	$HBrO_4$

Table 4-4. Naming of salts

Acid	Sodium salt
Hydrochloric acid (HCl)	Sodium chloride ($NaCl$)
Hypochlorous acid ($HClO$)	Sodium hypochlorite ($NaClO$)
Chlorous acid ($HClO_2$)	Sodium chlorite ($NaClO_2$)
Chloric acid ($HClO_3$)	Sodium chlorate ($NaClO_3$)
Perchloric acid ($HClO_4$)	Sodium perchlorate ($NaClO_4$)

(HCl), sulfuric acid (H_2SO_4), nitric acid (HNO_3), and acetic acid ($H \cdot C_2H_3O_2$).

Bases. According to the classic theory, a base is a compound of a metallic element with one or more hydroxyl (OH) groups; in aqueous solution, therefore, bases furnish OH^- ions.*

Properties. Bases have a bitter taste, and their action on indicators is opposite to that of acids; for example, bases turn litmus from red to blue and methyl orange from orange to yellow. Another important indicator is phenolphthalein, which turns red in a basic medium and remains colorless in an acid medium. Bases neutralize acids to form salts and water. As in the case of acids, the strength of a base depends upon the degree of ionization; for example, ammonium hydroxide (a weak base) and potassium hydroxide (a stronge base) may be depicted as follows:

$$NH_4OH \leftrightarrows NH_4^+ \; OH^-$$
$$KOH \longrightarrow K^+ \; OH^-$$

Stronge bases such as $NaOH$ and KOH are referred to as *alkalies.*

Preparation. Bases are prepared by reacting metallic oxides with water or by reacting salts with sodium hydroxide. Thus,

$$CaO + H_2O \longrightarrow Ca(OH)_2$$
$$MgCl_2 + 2NaOH \longrightarrow 2NaCl + Mg(OH)_2$$

Nomenclature. Bases are very easily named. The name of the metal is simply followed by the word *hydroxide*—for example, sodium hydroxide ($NaOH$), potassium hydroxide (KOH), ammonium hydroxide (NH_4OH), and calcium hydroxide ($Ca[OH]_2$).

Salts. A salt is a compound that results from the substitution of a metal for hydrogen in an acid, or it may be defined as

*According to the Brönsted theory, a base is defined as a proton acceptor. Therefore, many substances other than hydroxides can be technically considered bases.

a compound consisting of a metal combined with a nonmetal or acid radical. Ionically, a salt may be considered the product of the union of a cation of a base with the anion of an acid.

Preparation. Salts are prepared in a variety of ways, for example, neutralization, reacting a metal with an acid, and reacting a metallic oxide with an acid:

$$Mg(OH)_2 + 2HCl \longrightarrow MgCl_2 + 2H_2O$$
$$Mg + 2HCl \longrightarrow MgCl_2 + H_2\uparrow$$
$$MgO + 2HCl \longrightarrow MgCl_2 + H_2O$$

Nomenclature. Salts are named after the metal and the corresponding acid. Those derived from binary acids are named simply by affixing the suffix *-ide* to the stem. Those derived from a ternary acid carry the suffix *-ate* for acids ending in *-ic* and *-ite* for acids ending in *-ous.* If the ternary acid has the prefix *hypo-* or *per-*, this is made the prefix of the salt. These simple rules are illustrated by the acids and salts shown in Table 4-4.

Types. It is sometimes convenient to classify a salt as an "acid salt" or a "double salt." An acid salt is one in which all the hydrogen has not been replaced from the acid. For example, the sodium salts of phosphoric acid (H_3PO_4) include, in addition to Na_3PO_4, monosodium phosphate (NaH_2PO_4) and disodium phosphate (Na_2HPO_4). It is common practice to use the prefix *bi-* to name an acid salt of a dibasic acid such as H_2CO_3 and H_2SO_4. Thus, Na_2CO_3 is called sodium carbonate and $NaHCO_3$, sodium bicarbonate. A double salt is a compound containing two metals combined with one acid radical. Common alum, or potassium aluminum sulfate, is a good example. It has the formula $KAl(SO_4)_2$. A great many mineral substances are double salts.

Hydrolysis. From what has been said we would expect all salt solutions to be neutral. However, this is not the case; some are quite acidic and some are quite basic. The explanation resides in hydrolysis, which for all practical purposes may be considered a reversible reaction between water and the salt, producing an acid and a base. If the resulting acid and base are both strong, the solution is neutral; if the acid is stronger than the base, the solution is acidic; and if the base is stronger than the acid, the solution is basic. Further, if we remember that NaOH and KOH are common strong bases, and H_2SO_4, H_2SO_3, HNO_3, HCl, HI, and HBr are common strong acids, we can predict the character of a great many salts, relative to neutrality, by simply writing out the hydrolysis reaction. In the following equations note that water is expressed as HOH:

$$NaCl + HOH \rightleftharpoons \underset{\text{Strong}}{NaOH} + \underset{\text{Strong}}{HCl} \text{ (solution neutral)}$$

$$AlCl_3 + 3HOH \rightleftharpoons \underset{\text{Weak}}{Al(OH)_3} + \underset{\text{Strong}}{3HCl} \text{ (solution acidic)}$$

$$Na_2CO_3 + 2HOH \rightleftharpoons \underset{\text{Strong}}{2NaOH} + \underset{\text{Weak}}{H_2CO_3} \text{ (solution basic)}$$

pH. Now is the time to introduce the idea of hydrogen ion concentration, or pH—a convenient way to express the degree to which a solution is acidic or basic.

In a liter of pure water the hydrogen ions (H^+) weigh 0.0000001 gm., and since water is neutral, there are as many hydroxyl ions (OH^-) as there are hydrogen ions; that is, the OH^- concentration, too, is 0.0000001 gm. per liter. Thus, in any solution that is not neutral, the two concentrations will not be the same. By definition, pH is expressed as the common logarithm (log) of the reciprocal of the hydrogen ion concentration ($[H^+]$) per liter of solution, or

$$pH = \log\left(\frac{1}{[H^+]}\right)$$

In the case of pure water or a neutral solution this turns out to be as follows:

$$pH = \log\left(\frac{1}{0.0000001}\right)$$
$$pH = \log(10^7)$$
$$pH = 7$$

Let us try another example. What is the pH of a solution having a $[H^+]$ of 0.00001 gm. per liter? The calculation is as follows:

$$pH = \log \left(\frac{1}{[H^+]}\right)$$

$$pH = \log \left(\frac{1}{0.00001}\right)$$

$$pH = \log (10^5)$$

$$pH = 5$$

Note that as $[H^+]$ increases, the pH decreases; that is, the lower the pH, the greater will be the acidity. Conversely, on the other side of 7, the higher the pH, the greater will be the basicity. As shown in Fig. 4-7, the pH range extends from 0 ("pure" acid) to 14 ("pure" base).

Oxides. An oxide is a compound composed of oxygen and another element. A so-called basic anhydride is a metallic oxide that reacts with water to form a base (p. 57); an acid anhydride is a nonmetallic oxide that reacts with water to form an acid (p. 56).

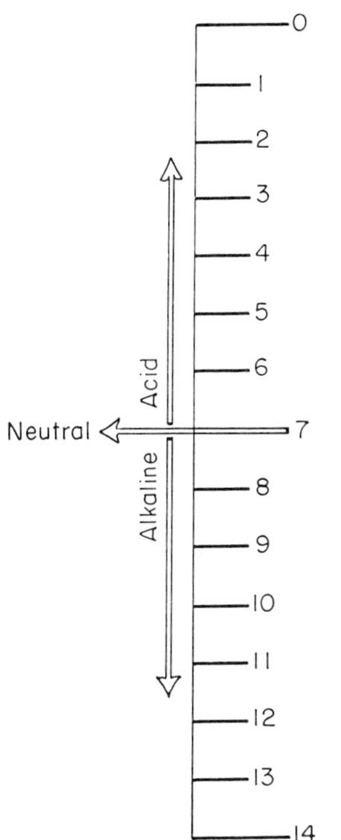

Fig. 4-7. The pH range. (From Brooks, S. M.: Basic facts of general chemistry, Philadelphia, 1956, W. B. Saunders Co.)

The name of an oxide is derived from the name of the element and the word *oxide*. In instances where an element has more than one valence and forms a series of oxides, they are distinguished from one another by the appropriate prefix: *mono-*, *di-*, *tri-*, *tetra-*, and so on. For example, calcium oxide is CaO, carbon monoxide CO, carbon dioxide CO_2, phosphorus trioxide P_2O_3, and phosphorus pentoxide (P_2O_5).

PERIODIC TABLE

In the latter half of the nineteenth century the Russian chemist Mendeléeff discovered that when the elements (omitting hydrogen) were arranged in order of their atomic weights there was a periodic recurrence of similar chemical properties. Now, if these "periods" were placed under one another in a table, the similar elements fell into vertical columns. Mendeléeff's table, however, later proved to have certain discrepancies, and in the latter part of the present century Moseley in England remedied the situation by arranging the elements according to their atomic number. Thus, according to the *periodic law*, the properties of the elements are periodic functions of their atomic numbers.

The "secret" of the table (a simple version of which appears in Table 4-5) is readily disclosed if we consider the electronic patterns. In short, elements of the same vertical column, or group, are similar because the outer orbits of their atoms have the same number of electrons and hence the same valence. Thus, the elements lithium, sodium, and potassium in Group I are alike because each has a valence of +1. Similarly, the elements of Group VII, with seven electrons in the outer orbit, have a valence of −1, and so on.

Table 4-5. Periodic table

Periods	Group 0 A B	Group I A	Group I B	Group II A	Group II B	Group III A	Group III B	Group IV A	Group IV B	Group V A	Group V B	Group VI A	Group VI B	Group VII A	Group VII B	Group VIII
1		1 H														
2	2 He	3 Li		4 Be		5 B			6 C		7 N		8 0		9 F	
3	10 Ne	11 Na		12 Mg		13 Al			14 Si		15 P		16 S		17 Cl	
4	18 A	19 K		20 Ca		21 Sc		22 Ti		23 V		24 Cr		25 Mn		26 27 28 Fe Co Ni
			29 Cu		30 Zn		31 Ga		32 Ge		33 As		34 Se		35 Br	
5	36 Kr	37 Rb		38 Sr		39 Y		40 Zr		41 Nb		42 Mo		43 Te		44 45 46 Ru Rh Pd
			47 Ag		48 Cd		49 In		50 Sn		51 Sb		52 Te		53 I	
6	54 Xe	55 Cs		56 Ba		57-71 Rare earths		72 Hf		73 Ta		74 W		75 Re		76 77 78 Os Ir Pt
			79 Au		80 Hg		81 Tl		82 Pb		83 Bi		84 Po	85 At		
7	86 Rn	87 Fr		88 Ra		89 Ac		90 Th		91 Pa		92* U				

*Eleven man-made elements lie beyond U-92. These so-called transuranium elements include Np-93, Pu-94, Am-95, Cm-96, Bk-97, Cf-98, E-99, Fm-100, Md-101, No-102, and Lw-103.

Group O is so designated because its elements have a "full" outer orbit and no valence; hence, under most conditions they are chemically inert. Also, the "true," or "chemically active," metals are located on the left side of the table, and the true nonmetals are located on the right side. Generally speaking, the elements occupying the central portion of the table are amphoteric; that is, they resemble both metals and nonmetals. With the exception of O and VIII, each group is divided into two families (A and B). The elements of a family are almost identical in this chemical behavior but often differ considerably from those in the other family of the group. Finally, the elements identified as the rare-earth metals (57-71) are so much alike that they occupy the same position in Group III.

From the student's standpoint the greatest value of the periodic table resides in its simplification and unification of inorganic chemistry. Specifically, if one is familiar with the chemical and physical properties of representative elements, he becomes familiar with the group as a whole and eventually with all the elements.

With this in mind, we shall now take up the more important elements from the various groups.

HALOGENS

The halogens (salt-formers)—fluorine, chlorine, bromine, and iodine—epitomize the chemical family. Since they belong to Group VII, they are nonmetals with seven electrons in the outer orbit (Fig. 4-8). Hence, all four have a valence of -1.

Fluorine. Being the most active of the halogens, fluorine occurs in the combined state, mostly as fluorspar (calcium fluoride) and cryolite. The free element is a pale yellow gas, a little heavier than air, with an extremely pungent odor. It is a powerful poison. With hydrogen it forms hydrogen fluoride (HF) which, in water solutions, becomes hydrofluoric acid (HF). Salts of this acid are called fluorides. Of considerable interest is the fact that the fluoride ion (F^-) plays a vital role in the chemistry of the teeth (Chapter 8).

Chlorine. Chlorine occurs chiefly as sodium chloride (salt) in the oceans and solid salt beds. The chloride ion (Cl^-) is an essential inorganic constituent of protoplasm. Chlorine, a greenish yellow gas with a powerful irritating odor, is about two and one-half times as dense as air and is fairly soluble in water. The gas is easily liquefied.

Commercially, chlorine is prepared by the electrolysis of brine (salt and water), the gas escaping from the anode:

$$2NaCl \longrightarrow 2Na + Cl_2\uparrow$$

In the laboratory the gas may be prepared by heating a mixture of manganese dioxide and concentrated hydrochloric acid (Fig. 4-9). The equation for the reaction is as follows:

$$MnO_2 + 4HCl \longrightarrow MnCl_2 + 2H_2O + Cl_2\uparrow$$

The foregoing is a good example of an oxidation-reduction or *redox* reaction. Chlorine becomes oxidized, and manganese is reduced:

$$Cl^- - 1e \longrightarrow Cl^\circ \text{ (oxidation)}$$
$$2Cl^- - 2e \longrightarrow Cl_2$$
$$Mn^{++++} + 2e \longrightarrow Mn^{++} \text{ (reduction)}$$

Also, a little thought will, with reference to this equation, substantiate the following rules:

1. An oxidizing agent (for example, MnO_2) brings about the oxidation of some other substance.

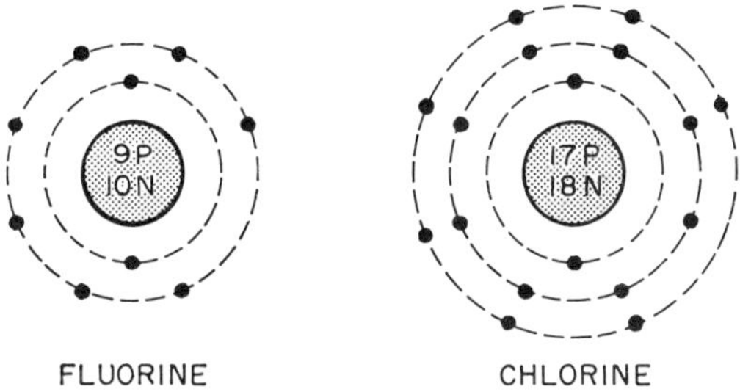

Fig. 4-8. Atoms of chlorine and fluorine. (From Brooks, S. M.: Basic facts of general chemistry, Philadelphia, 1956, W. B. Saunders Co.)

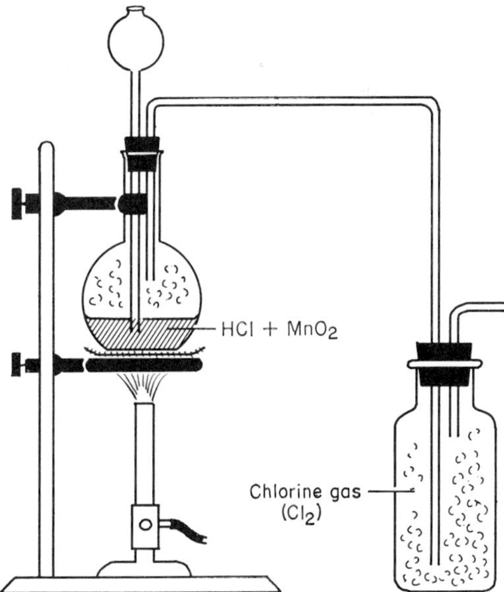

Fig. 4-9. Preparation of chlorine. (From Brooks, S. M.: Basic facts of general chemistry, Philadelphia, 1956, W. B. Saunders Co.)

2. A reducing agent (in this case HCl) brings about the reduction of some other substance.

3. An oxidizing agent *itself* undergoes reduction.

4. A reducing agent *itself* undergoes oxidation.

Chlorine gas is a useful bleach, an antiseptic, and a disinfectant. Its compounds, particularly sodium chloride, have endless applications in the laboratory and industry. Also, the chloride ion is vital to the processes of life (Chapter 18).

Test for chloride. When a solution of silver nitrate ($AgNO_3$) is added to a solution of a chloride (Cl^-), a dense white precipitate—silver chloride ($AgCl$)—forms immediately. The test is confirmed by the ability of ammonium hydroxide to redissolve the precipitate. The equation for the first reaction is as follows:

$$AgNO_3 + NaCl \longrightarrow NaNO_3 + AgCl\downarrow$$

Bromine. Bromine occurs in nature in the form of bromides. The free element, a volatile dark red liquid about twice as dense as water, has a disagreeable, pungent, and irritating odor. Commercially, bromine is prepared by the electrolysis of bromides; in the laboratory it is prepared by heating a bromide salt with manganese dioxide and sulfuric acid (Fig. 4-10):

$$2NaBr + 2H_2SO_4 + MnO_2 \longrightarrow Na_2SO_4 + MnSO_4 + 2H_2O + Br_2$$

Bromine compounds enjoy wide use in industry and in the laboratory, but the element itself has few uses outside the laboratory. Perhaps the most important compound is silver bromide ($AgBr$), which is used in the manufacture of photographic film.

Test for bromide. To test for the bromide ion (Br^-), chlorine water is added to the unknown solution in a test tube. If a yellow to brown color appears, a little carbon tetrachloride is added and the mixture vigorously shaken. The carbon tetrachloride, being immiscible, is allowed to settle and its color noted. A reddish brown color indicates a bromide. A purple color indicates an *iodide.* The test is based upon the fact that chlorine (Cl_2), being more active than bromine (or iodine), replaces the latter from their compounds The element thus released dissolves in the carbon tetrachloride. In the case of KBr and KI the reactions are as follows:

$$2KBr + Cl_2 \longrightarrow 2KCl + Br_2$$
$$2KI + Cl_2 \longrightarrow 2KCl + I_2$$

Iodine. Iodine occurs in nature as iodides in sea water and as iodates in Chile saltpeter deposits. In the body it is a constituent of thyroxine, the hormone of the

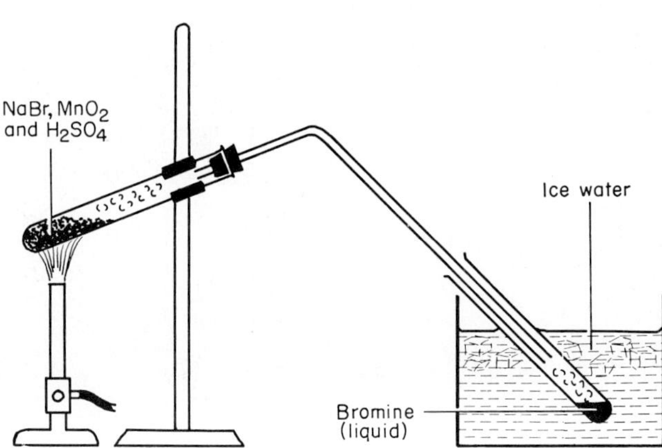

Fig. 4-10. Preparation of bromine. (From Brooks, S. M.: Basic facts of general chemistry, Philadelphia, 1956, W. B. Saunders Co.)

thyroid gland. Elemental iodine is a crystalline, steel-gray solid, which quickly turns to purplish black upon contact with air. The solid vaporizes into beautiful purplish red fumes that return directly to the solid state when cooled. This process of passing from the solid to the vapor and then back to the solid state is called *sublimation.*

Commercially, iodine is prepared from seaweed (kelp), ocean water, and Chile saltpeter. In the laboratory the element is prepared by heating an iodide with a mixture of manganese dioxide and sulfuric acid (Fig. 4-11). The equation for the reaction is balanced in the same fashion as that shown for the preparation of bromine (p. 62).

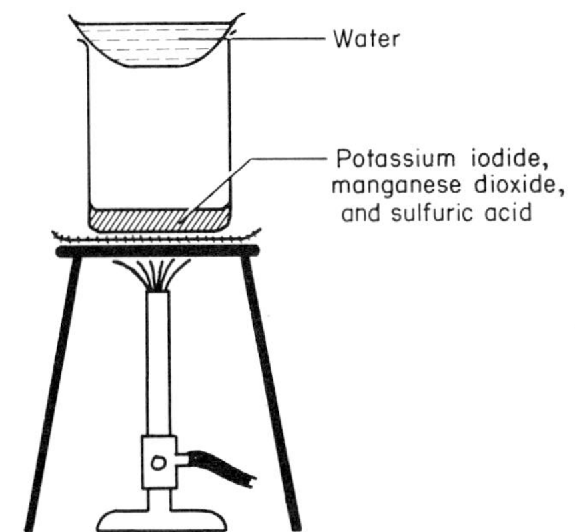

Fig. 4-11. Preparation of iodine. (From Brooks, S. M.: Basic facts of general chemistry, Philadelphia, 1956, W. B. Saunders Co.)

The principal commercial use for free iodine is in the production of tincture of iodine, a 2 percent solution of the element in alcohol. Sodium and potassium iodides are used in medicine in conjunction with other drugs in the treatment of thyroid dysfunctions. Other compounds of iodine, both organic and inorganic, enjoy a variety of uses in the laboratory, in medicine, and in industry.

Test for iodide. The test for an iodide (I^-) is performed according to the procedure described for the bromide test. Also, it is interesting to note that, whereas iodide and starch do not produce a color, *elemental* iodine and starch produce an intense purplish black coloration. The latter reaction is used to test for the presence of starch in foods.

OXYGEN

Oxygen, the most abundant element, occurs in the free state in the atmosphere at a concentration of about 21 percent, and in the combined state, namely water,

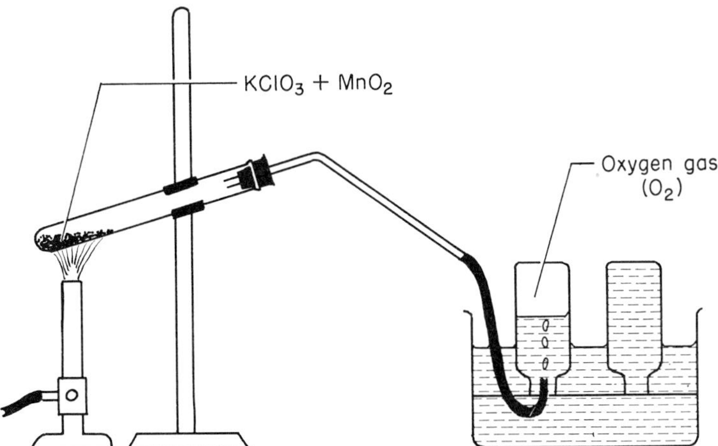

Fig. 4-12. Laboratory preparation of oxygen. (From Brooks, S. M.: Basic facts of general chemistry, Philadelphia, 1956, W. B. Saunders Co.)

quartz, clay, and limestone, constitutes 50 percent of the earth's crust. Priestley, the first to prepare oxygen (1774), made the gas by heating mercuric oxide (HgO)

$$2HgO \xrightarrow{\Delta} 2Hg + O_2\uparrow$$

Usually, however, the element is prepared in the laboratory by heating a mixture of potassium chlorate ($KClO_3$) and manganese dioxide (MnO_2), the latter serving as a catalyst (Fig. 4-12). The equation for the reaction is as follows:

$$2KClO_3 \xrightarrow{MnO_2} 2KCl + 3O_2\uparrow$$

Oxygen is generally prepared commercially by the electrolysis of water:

$$2H_2O \longrightarrow 2H_2 + O_2$$

Oxygen is a colorless, odorless, tasteless gas that is slightly soluble in water and slightly denser than air. Chemically, the gas combines with most other elements, forming oxides (oxidation). Iron and sulfur react with oxygen as follows:

$$4Fe + 3O_2 \longrightarrow 2Fe_2O_3$$
$$S + O_2 \longrightarrow SO_2$$

Oxidation is said to be *slow* or *rapid.* For example, when iron remains in contact with the atmosphere, it slowly forms ferric oxide (Fe_2O_3). In pure oxygen, on the other hand, it burns (still forming Fe_2O_3). In other words, burning, or combustion, is rapid oxidation. This brings to mind the so-called *kindling temperature,* which may be defined as the temperature to which a substance must be heated in order to burn. The more combustible the substance, the lower will be the kindling temperature.

Oxygen is marketed in steel cylinders. In medicine it is employed extensively in persons with poor respiration, and in industry it is used to provide high temperatures for welding and cutting. The oxyhydrogen torch and the oxyacetylene torch produce temperatures of 4000° C. and over.

Ozone. Oxygen and several other elements have the unique and interesting physical property of existing in two or more physical forms, a property referred to as *allotropism.* Ozone (O_3), the allotropic form of oxygen, is a colorless gas with a garliclike odor. Chemically, it is a much more powerful oxidizing agent than oxygen. The gas is readily prepared by passing a powerful spark through air or oxygen:

$$3O_2 \longrightarrow 2O_3$$

SULFUR

Since sulfur and oxygen are members of the same family of the periodic table, we should not be surprised to find striking similarities in their chemistry. Physically, sulfur is a golden yellow solid with little taste or odor. Of the five allotropic forms of the element, two are liquid and three are solid. The latter include two crystalline forms (rhombic and prismatic) and a noncrystalline variety called amorphous sulfur. Chemically, sulfur reacts with oxygen to form oxides and with metals to form sulfides:

$$S + O_2 \longrightarrow SO_2 \text{ (sulfur dioxide)}$$
$$2Ag + S \longrightarrow Ag_2S \text{ (silver sulfide)}$$

Commercially, sulfur is perhaps our most important element. There is scarcely a laboratory or industry that does not employ sulfur compounds in one form or another. For instance, it is an economic fact that the degree of civilization of a country bears a direct proportion to the consumption of sulfuric acid (H_2SO_4), the "King of Chemicals." To supply this great demand, sulfur is mined in prodigious amounts by the Frasch process (Fig. 4-13).

Hydrogen sulfide. Hydrogen sulfide (H_2S), a highly odoriferous gas with an odor resembling rotten eggs, is formed by decaying organic matter that contains sulfur. In the laboratory it is readily prepared by the action of dilute acid on a sulfide:

$$FeS + 2HCl \longrightarrow FeCl_2 + H_2S\uparrow$$

The principal use of the gas is in chemical

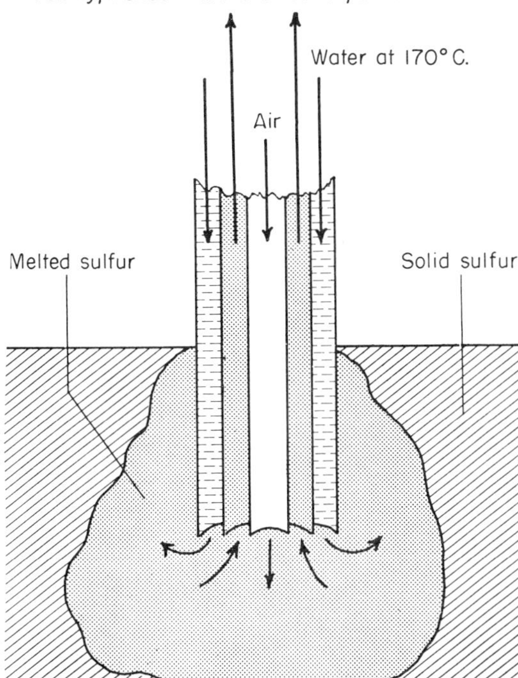

Fig. 4-13. Frasch process for mining sulfur. (From Brooks, S. M.: Basic facts of general chemistry, Philadelphia, 1956, W. B. Saunders Co.)

analysis to identify certain metals. Some illustrative equations follow:

$$ZnCl_2 + H_2S \longrightarrow 2HCl + \underset{\text{White}}{ZnS\uparrow}$$

$$CuSO_4 + H_2S \longrightarrow H_2SO_4 + \underset{\text{Black}}{CuS\downarrow}$$

$$2BiCl_3 + 3H_2S \longrightarrow 6HCl + \underset{\text{Brown}}{Bi_2S_3\downarrow}$$

$$2SbCl_3 + 3H_2S \longrightarrow 6HCl + \underset{\text{Orange}}{Sb_2S_3\downarrow}$$

Sulfur dioxide. Sulfur dioxide (SO_2), a heavy colorless gas with a strong pungent odor, is prepared by the action of dilute acid upon a sulfite ($SO_3^{=}$) or a bisulfite (HSO_3^{-}):

$$Na_2SO_3 + 2HCl \longrightarrow 2NaCl + H_2O + SO_2\uparrow$$

$$NaHSO_3 + HCl \longrightarrow NaCl + H_2O + SO_2\overrightarrow{}$$

Chemically, the gas is a stable compound that does not burn or support combustion. The most important property, however, concerns its reaction with water to form sulfurous acid (H_2SO_3):

$$H_2O + SO_2 \longrightarrow H_2SO_3$$

As we know, this acid reacts with bases to form salts called sulfites ($SO_3^{=}$) and bisulfites (HSO_3^{-}).

Test for sulfite. To test for a sulfite or a bisulfite, all we need do is add a little dilute acid to the unknown in a test tube and pass any gas that is formed through a purplish red solution of potassium permanganate. The acid causes the release of SO_2, and the latter decolorizes the solution.

Sulfur trioxide. Sulfur trioxide is a white solid made by reacting sulfur dioxide with oxygen in the presence of a hot platinum catalyst. Thus,

$$2SO_2 + O_2 \longrightarrow 2SO_3$$

The most important feature of this substance is the fact that it is the acid anhydride of sulfuric acid (H_2SO_4):

$$SO_3 + H_2O \longrightarrow H_2SO_4$$

Test for sulfate. To test for a sulfate ($SO_4^{=}$), a solution of barium chloride ($BaCl_2$) is added to a solution of the unknown. If a white precipitate forms (which is insoluble in concentrated hydrochloric acid), the test is positive. Magnesium sulfate, for example, reacts with $BaCl_2$ to form magnesium chloride ($MgCl_2$) and barium sulfate ($BaSO_4$). Thus,

$$MgSO_4 + BaCl_2 \longrightarrow MgCl_2 + BaSO_4\downarrow$$

NITROGEN

Nitrogen is the most abundant element of the atmosphere, constituting 78 percent of dry air by volume (Table 4-6). In the combined state it occurs in a vast number of both organic and inorganic compounds. The chief inorganic salt is sodium nitrate ($NaNO_3$), or Chile saltpeter. Since nitrogen is the key element of proteins, and since proteins are the backbone of protoplasm, the element is obviously as essential to life as oxygen.

Table 4-6. Average composition of dry air (percent by volume)

Gas	Percent
Nitrogen	78 %
Oxygen	21 %
Carbon dioxide	0.04%
Argon	0.94%
Neon	Traces
Helium	Traces
Krypton	Traces
Xenon	Traces
Hydrogen	Traces
Ozone	Traces

Physically, nitrogen is a colorless, tasteless, odorless gas, slightly lighter than air, and slightly soluble in water. Chemically, the element is rather inactive; it does not burn, support combustion, or readily react with other elements. Under certain conditions, however, it reacts with hydrogen to form ammonia and with oxygen to form a series of gaseous oxides. Nitrous oxide (N_2O), commonly called laughing gas, is extensively used in dentistry and medicine as an anesthetic.

Nitrogen cycle. As indicated, nitrogen is necessary for life, and a complex relationship exists between the plant and animal worlds relative to this element. Essentially, this is a reciprocal agreement whereby the plants feed the animals, and the animals, in turn, aid in maintaining the plants. Since *free* nitrogen is usable to but a very few plants, it must be converted into the proper compounds. The chemical events involving the free nitrogen of the air and its compounds in protoplasm and the earth's soil constitute the so-called nitrogen cycle.

Briefly, the cycle may be described as follows: Certain microorganisms in the soil bring about the decay or putrefaction of organic matter derived from dead plants and animals and animal wastes. As a result of this microbial action, ammonia is liberated. Another group of microorganisms, called nitrifying bacteria, convert this ammonia into soluble nitrate salts, for example, sodium nitrate. Plants absorb these nitrates into their roots and utilize them to manufacture proteins for protoplasm. In turn, herbivorous animals obtain their proteins by consuming plants. In time, plants and animals die and return their nitrogen to the soil in the manner just described.

This situation is somewhat complicated by the fact that another group of bacteria, called denitrifying bacteria, act upon soil nitrates to form nitrogen gas, which escapes into the air. If there were not some mechanism, therefore, whereby this lost nitrogen could be returned to the soil, the earth would become depleted of its nitrates—and of life. An interesting group of bacteria, called nitrogen-fixing bacteria, are able to convert atmospheric nitrogen directly into bacterial protein. Since these organisms live a symbiotic life on the roots of certain plants (for example, alfalfa and clover), they share their proteins with the plants. Thus, the return of nitrogen to the soil by the nitrogen-fixing bacteria completes the cycle. The nitrogen cycle is shown in Fig. 4-14.

Ammonia. Ammonia (NH_3), perhaps the most important compound of nitrogen, is a light colorless gas with a strong, pungent odor. It is extremely soluble in water, 1 volume of the latter dissolving 700 volumes of the gas. Ammonia burns in pure oxygen and reacts with water to form the important base, ammonium hydroxide:

$$NH_3 + H_2O \longrightarrow NH_4OH$$

Ammonium hydroxide reacts with acids to form ammonium (NH_4^+) salts. For instance,

$$NH_4OH + HNO_3 \longrightarrow NH_4NO_3 + H_2O$$

Commercially, ammonia is prepared mainly by the famous Haber process, an innovation that heralded the era of synthetic chemistry. In this process, nitrogen

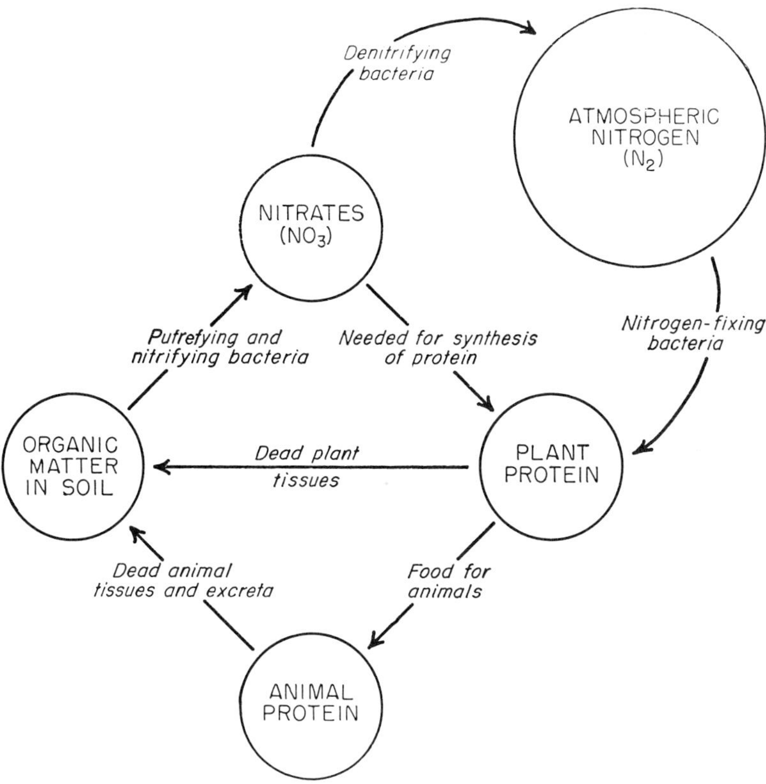

Fig. 4-14. Nitrogen cycle. (From Brooks, S. M.: Basic facts of general chemistry, Philadelphia, 1956, W. B. Saunders Co.)

(from liquid air) and hydrogen (from water) are made to unite under high temperatures and pressures according to the following equation:

$$N_2 + 3H_2 \longrightarrow 2NH_3$$

In the laboratory ammonia is prepared by heating a dry mixture of an ammonium salt and calcium hydyroxide (Fig. 4-15):

$$2NH_4Cl + Ca(OH)_2 \xrightarrow{\Delta} CaCl_2 + 2H_2O + 2NH_3\uparrow$$

Huge amounts of ammonia are used in the manufacture of ammonium hydroxide, nitric acid, and ammonium sulfate. The latter compound is a common ingredient of fertilizers.

Test for ammonia and NH_4 radical. Ammonia gas will turn red litmus blue, provided that water is present. To test for an ammonium salt, the unknown is heated

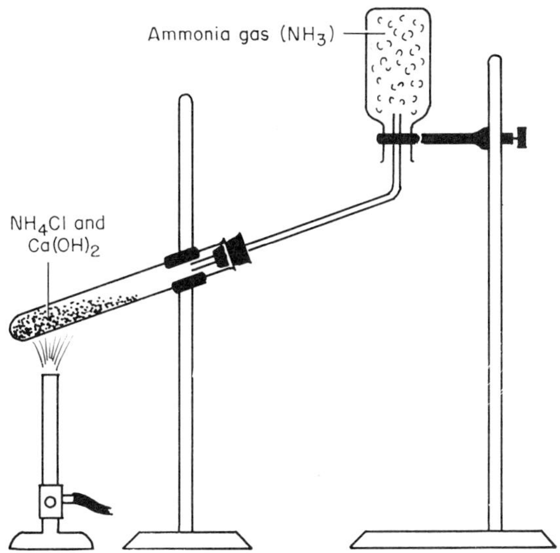

Fig. 4-15. Laboratory preparation of ammonia. (From Brooks, S. M.: Basic facts of general chemistry, Philadelphia, 1956, W. B. Saunders Co.)

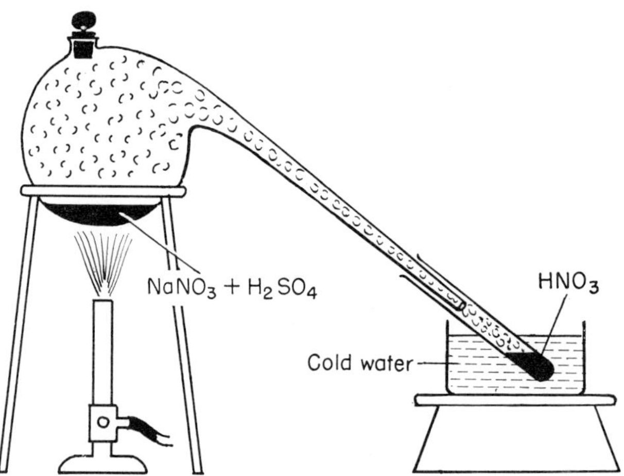

Fig. 4-16. Preparation of nitric acid. (From Brooks, S. M.: Basic facts of general chemistry, Philadelphia, 1956, W. B. Saunders Co.)

with sodium hydroxide and the issuing vapors are tested for the presence of ammonia. The equation for the reaction is as follows:

$$NH_4Cl + NaOH \xrightarrow{\Delta} NaCl + H_2O + NH_3\uparrow$$

Nitric acid. Nitric acid (HNO_3) is a strong acid and an extremely powerful oxidizing agent. It is prepared commercially by dissolving nitrogen peroxide (NO_2) in water, and in the laboratory it is prepared by heating a mixture of sodium nitrate and sulfuric acid (Fig. 4-16):

$$2NaNO_3 + H_2SO_4 \longrightarrow Na_2SO_4 + 2HNO_3$$

In addition to its many uses in the laboratory, nitric acid is employed in the manufacture of nitroglycerin, nitrocellulose, dyes, and nitrates.

Test for nitrate. To identify a nitrate, the following test is performed: A freshly prepared solution of ferrous sulfate ($FeSO_4$) is added to a solution of the substance being tested. Concentrated sulfuric acid is then allowed to run slowly down the side of the test tube and to collect at the bottom. The formation of a brown ring at the junction of the two liquids indicates the presence of nitric acid or a nitrate. The sulfuric acid reacts with the nitrate to produce nitric acid which, in turn, reacts with the ferrous sulfate to form a brown-colored compound.

CARBON

In the natural free state, carbon occurs in three allotropic forms: coal, graphite, and diamonds. In the combined state it serves as the key element of all organic substances (Chapter 5). Coke, charcoal, boneblack, and lampblack are amorphous forms of the element produced industrially.

Carbon dioxide. Carbon dioxide, a vital constituent of the atmosphere (pp. 28-29), is a colorless gas with a very slight taste and odor. It is about one and one-half times as dense as air and is moderately soluble in water. Soda water and other carbonated beverages contain relatively large quantities of the gas held in solution under pressure. Solid carbon dioxide ("snow") is formed by the sudden evaporation of the liquefied gas. The useful refrigerant dry ice is made by pressing the carbon dioxide snow into cakes.

Chemically, carbon dioxide is a stable and rather inactive gas that does not burn or support combustion. It reacts with water

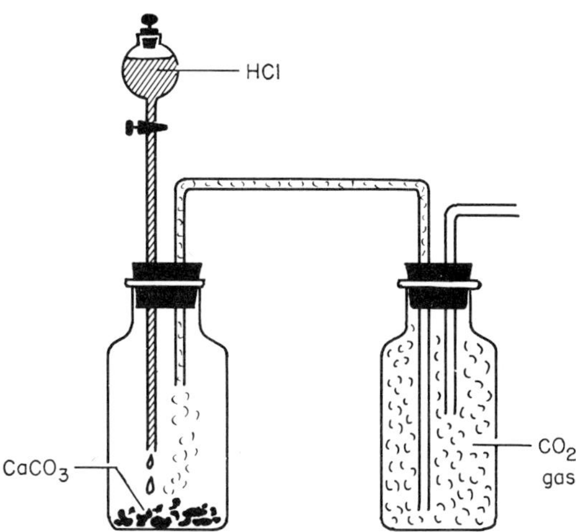

Fig. 4-17. Laboratory preparation of carbon dioxide. (From Brooks, S. M.: Basic facts of general chemistry, Philadelphia, 1956, W. B. Saunders Co.)

to form the weak and unstable carbonic acid:

$$H_2O + CO_2 \rightleftharpoons H_2CO_3$$

In the laboratory the gas may be readily prepared by reacting a carbonate or bicarbonate with dilute acid (Fig. 4-17):

$$CaCO_3 + 2HCl \longrightarrow CaCl_2 + H_2O + CO_2\uparrow$$
$$NaHCO_3 + HCl \longrightarrow NaCl + H_2O + CO_2\uparrow$$

Commercially, carbon dioxide is made by burning carbon (usually coke) or by heating limestone:

$$C + O_2 \longrightarrow CO_2$$
$$CaCO_3 \xrightarrow{\Delta} CaO + CO_2\uparrow$$

Test for carbonate. To test for a carbonate or a bicarbonate, all we need do is add a little acid to the unknown and pass any gas formed through a solution of limewater ($Ca[OH]_2$). If the limewater turns milky (as a result of the formation of $CaCO_3$), the test is positive. The reaction is as follows:

$$Ca(OH)_2 + CO_2 \longrightarrow CaCO_3 + H_2O$$

Uses. Carbon dioxide is one of the most important gases in industry and commerce.

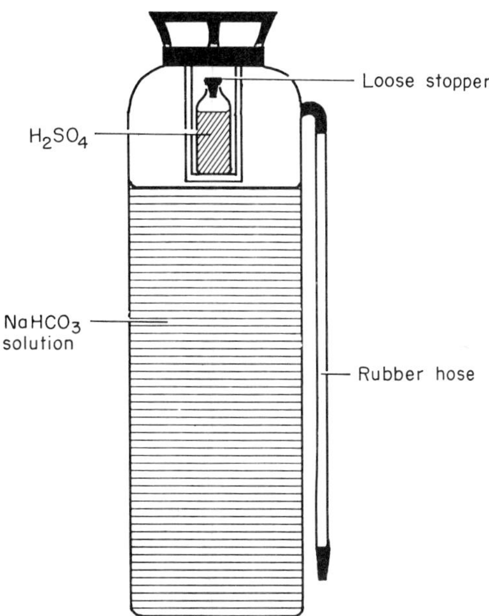

Fig. 4-18. Soda-acid fire extinguisher. When the extinguisher is inverted, the acid and the soda solution react violently, forming CO_2, which forces the solution out of the nozzle with great pressure. (From Brooks, S. M.: Basic facts of general chemistry, Philadelphia, 1956, W. B. Saunders Co.)

Huge quantities of the gas are employed in the making of carbonated beverages and carbon dioxide fire extinguishers. It also serves as the active principle in baking powder (when water is added) and in the soda-acid fire extinguisher (Fig. 4-18).

Photosynthesis. Photosynthesis, a chemical process vital to the survival of life on our planet, is made possible by the presence of carbon dioxide, water, chlorophyll, and sunlight. Although the details of the complex events that lead to the synthesis of carbohydrates (for example, glucose) are only now beginning to be really understood, the overall picture may be *summarized* as follows:

$$6CO_2 + 6H_2O \xrightarrow[\text{Chlorophyll}]{\text{Sunlight}} \underset{\text{Glucose}}{C_6H_{12}O_6} + 6O_2$$

In this reaction, chlorophyll (the green pigment of the leaf) "traps" the light energy and makes it available for the various reactions. The plant stores the glucose as starch (largely in the roots), and the oxygen is released to the air. Thus, the energy of the sun first becomes locked in the sugars and starches and then is released in the processes of respiration and burning. Relative to the latter, let us not forget that wood, coal, and oil ultimately derive from decayed plant life.

Carbon dioxide–oxygen cycle. The so-called carbon dioxide–oxygen cycle refers to the mutually sustaining processes of photosynthesis and oxidation; that is, carbon dioxide is constantly being added to the atmosphere as a consequence of respiration and burning and constantly being withdrawn as a consequence of photosynthesis—and the oxygen produced as a by-product in the latter process makes oxidation possible. The balanced aquarium (Fig. 4-19) microcosmically demonstrates this life-and-death relationship.

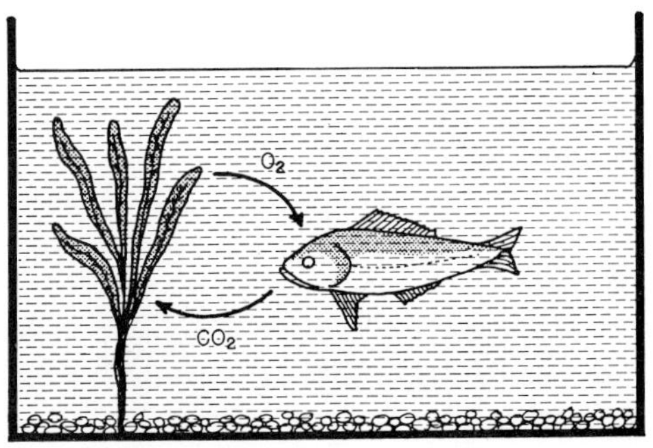

Fig. 4-19. Balanced aquarium. (From Brooks, S. M.: Basic facts of general chemistry, Philadelphia, 1956, W. B. Saunders Co.)

Carbon monoxide. Carbon monoxide (CO) is formed when carbon or some compound containing carbon burns in an insufficient supply of air:

$$2C + O_2 \longrightarrow 2CO$$

Carbon monoxide is a colorless, odorless, and tasteless gas, somewhat lighter than air and only slightly soluble in water. In contrast to the dioxide, it burns readily:

$$2CO + O_2 \longrightarrow 2CO_2$$

Toxicity. Carbon monoxide causes more deaths than all other poisons combined. This is due to its omnipresence (in engine exhausts), its insidious physical characteristics, and its affinity for the hemoglobin molecule in the red cell. Since the gas combines with hemoglobin to form carboxyhemoglobin, a compound unable to carry oxygen, the injury to the body stems from anoxia, or lack of oxygen. A concentration of as little of 0.1 percent in the air is dangerous and may cause death.

The treatment of carbon monoxide poisoning is successful, even in severe cases, if instituted early. Indeed, the victim of mild intoxication is generally out of danger if removed to the out-of-doors. Severe intoxication, however, demands oxygen and artificial respiration.

METALS

Of the ninety-two natural elements that constitute the earth, some seventy or more are metals. Of this number, the great majority are so rare and of such limited commercial value that they are seldom mentioned, even among chemists. Only about fifteen metals are commonly encountered in everyday life. Indeed, such an unbelievably complex substance as protoplasm contains no more than ten metallic elements. In this section we shall touch upon the highlights of the more important metals.

Hydrogen. Although hydrogen has the physical properties of a nonmetal, it possesses the chemical properties of a metal—hence, its inclusion in the present section. Hydrogen, the chief element of the stars, is contained in all living things. In essence it is the primordial element.

Hydrogen is a colorless, odorless, tasteless gas that is only very slightly soluble in water. Its outstanding physical property, however, is that it is the *lightest gas known.* Chemically, it combines with other elements at high temperatures. For instance,

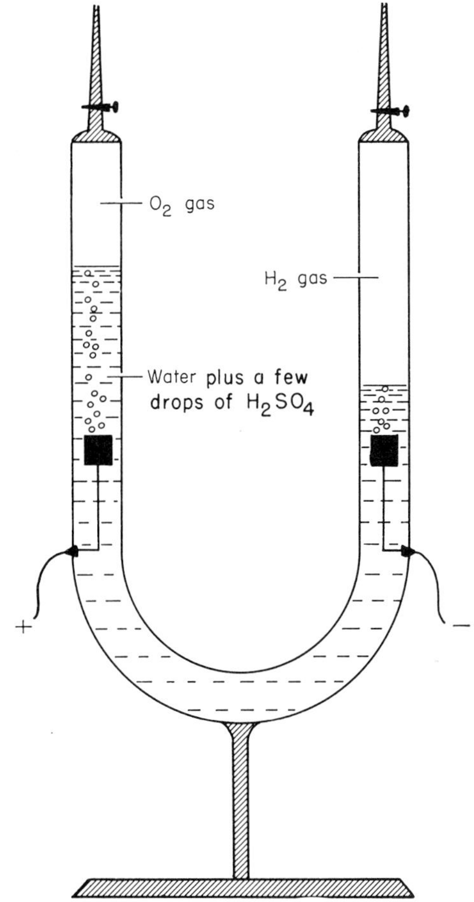

Fig. 4-20. Electrolysis of water. (From Brooks, S. M.: Basic facts of general chemistry, Philadelphia, 1956, W. B. Saunders Co.)

$$2H_2 + O_2 \longrightarrow 2H_2O$$
$$H_2 + Cl_2 \longrightarrow 2HCl$$
$$3H_2 + N_2 \longrightarrow 2NH_3$$

As we know, hydrogen is the characteristic element of acids, being released in solution as the hydrogen ion:

$$H_2SO_4 \longrightarrow 2H^+ + SO_4^=$$

Hydrogen is prepared commercially by the electrolysis of water, hydrogen being liberated at the cathode and oxygen at the anode (Fig. 4-20). In the laboratory the gas is best prepared by reacting certain metals with dilute hydrochloric or sulfuric acid:

$$Zn + 2HCl \longrightarrow ZnCl_2 + H_2\uparrow$$

As indicated, not all metals replace hydrogen from acids. In the following so-called replacement or electromotive series all the metals above hydrogen release the gas from acids, whereas those below it do not:

Potassium (most active)
Sodium
Calcium
Magnesium
Aluminum
Zinc
Iron
Nickel
Tin
Lead
HYDROGEN
Copper
Mercury
Silver
Platinum
Gold (least active)

The location of an element in the series is also indicative of its chemical activity. In other words, a metal will replace from their salts all metals below it but will, itself, be replaced by all metals above it. For example, copper does not replace iron, but iron does replace copper. Thus,

$$Cu + FeSO_4 \longrightarrow \text{No reaction}$$
$$Fe + CuSO_4 \longrightarrow FeSO_4 + Cu^\circ$$

In the laboratory, hydrogen is used as a reducing agent. Commercially, huge quantities of the gas go into the synthesis of ammonia (p. 66). Since the tragic explosion of the *Hindenburg* in 1937, hydrogen has been replaced by helium (nonflammable) for use in dirigibles and balloons.

Alkali metals. The elements of Family A, Group I, are referred to as the alkali metals because their hydroxides are all strong bases. Since sodium and potassium are by far the most important members, we shall confine our specific remarks to these two elements.

Because of their extreme activity, sodium

and potassium are never found in the free state. Their principal natural compounds include sodium chloride (common table salt), sodium nitrate (Chile saltpeter), sodium tetraborate (borax), potassium chloride (potash), and potassium aluminum silicate (feldspar). The free metals are very similar in appearance and soft enough to be cut with a knife, the bright, freshly cut surfaces soon darkening upon exposure to air.

Like the other alkali metals, sodium and potassium react vigorously with other substances. With water, for example, they liberate sufficient heat to ignite the hydrogen gas that is formed:

$$2Na + 2H_2O \longrightarrow 2NaOH + H_2\uparrow$$
$$2K + 2H_2O \longrightarrow 2KOH + H_2\uparrow$$

Although the free elements are not widely used commercially, their compounds are of extreme importance. Among many others, these include sodium chloride (common salt), sodium bicarbonate (baking soda), sodium hydroxide (caustic of soda), potassium hydroxide (caustic of potash), potassium chloride, and potassium chlorate.

Flame test. When sodium and potassium or their compounds are heated in the Bunsen flame, they produce a yellow and a violet color, respectively. Other metals that color the flame include lithium (crimson), calcium (orange-red), barium (green), and strontium (bright red). These flame colorations are the basis of *spectroscopy*, an important tool of analytical chemistry.

Calcium. Calcium is the principal member of the alkaline-earth metals (Family A, Group II). Next to aluminum and iron, it is the most abundant metal of the earth's crust. Its most common salts include calcium carbonate, calcium sulfate, calcium fluoride, and calcium phosphate, the latter substance being the chief constituent of bones and teeth.

Calcium is a light silver-white metal that tarnishes rapidly in moist air. It reacts with oxygen to form calcium oxide and with water to form calcium hydroxide and hydrogen:

$$2Ca + O_2 \longrightarrow 2CaO$$
$$Ca + 2H_2O \longrightarrow Ca(OH)_2 + H_2\uparrow$$

Elemental calcium has few uses. Its compounds, however, are of vast importance in the laboratory, in industry, and in medicine. Calcium carbonate, the most abundant calcium compound, occurs as marble, limestone, chalk, and calcite, the latter being a crystalline substance. Marble and limestone have served the building needs of man since antiquity. Powdered calcium carbonate (precipitated chalk) is employed in the making of tooth powder, toothpaste, polishes, and stomach remedies. Other important compounds include calcium hydroxide (slaked lime), calcium sulfate (gypsum), and calcium phosphate. The latter material is used as a fertilizer to supply phosphorus.

Hard water. Water that reacts with soap to produce a scum and an anemic suds is referred to as "hard water." This is due principally to the presence of the salts of calcium, magnesium, and iron. A typical reaction is as follows:

$$CaSO_4 + \underset{\text{Soap}}{2NaC_{17}H_{35}CO_2} \longrightarrow Ca(C_{17}H_{35}CO_2)_2\downarrow + Na_2SO$$

In contrast to sodium stearate ("regular" soap), calcium stearate is a worthless precipitate. To circumvent this annoying and costly situation, we employ agents (water softeners) which, in one way or another, remove the interfering ions. Also, the so-called detergents (which are not conventional soaps) do not react with mineral matter.

Iron. Iron, the second most abundant metal of the earth's crust, occurs chiefly in the from of *oxides*. For example, hematite—an important iron ore—has the formula Fe_2O_3. In the biologic world, iron (in the form of hemoglobin) is found in the blood of nearly all animals. As we know, the metal is of vast importance. In the form of steel it has revolutionized our civilization. In addition, its compounds serve hundreds of diversified uses in the laboratory, in commerce, and in industry.

Because the blast furnace is almost synonymous with the industrial age, we should say at least a word or two concerning its operation. Into this huge firebrick device (Fig. 4-21) are placed iron ore (Fe_2O_3), coke (a porous form of carbon), and limestone ($CaCO_3$). The mixture is ignited, and hot air is blown up through the bottom to intensify the tremendous heat. In brief, the coke at the bottom forms carbon dioxide (CO_2) which, in passing up through the furnace, is reduced to carbon monoxide (CO) by the hot coke above. The carbon monoxide now reduces the ore to molten iron, which collects at the bottom of the furnace. The purpose of the limestone is to combine with the impurities (namely, SiO_2), terminating as molten *slag* above

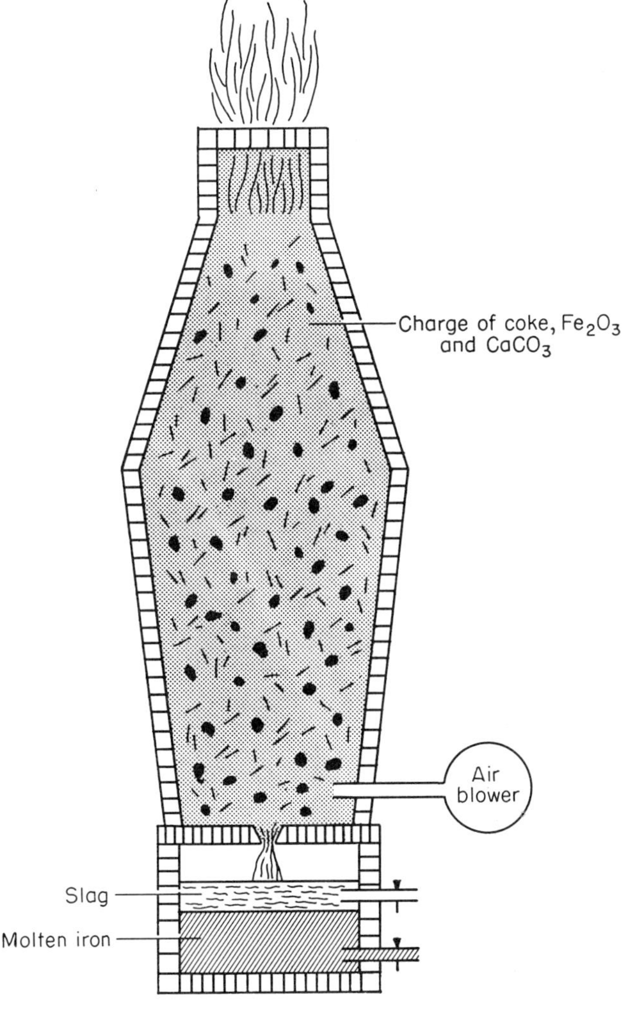

Fig. 4-21. Blast furnace. (From Brooks, S. M.: Basic facts of general chemistry, Philadelphia, 1956, W. B. Saunders Co.)

the iron. The iron and slag are finally run off from the notches at the bottom of the furnace.

Ferrous and ferric compounds. Depending upon the prevailing conditions, iron has a valence of +2 (ferrous) or +3 (ferric). For example, the formulas for ferrous and ferric sulfates are $FeSO_4$ and $Fe_2(SO_4)_3$, respectively. Ferrous compounds are generally quite unstable and, upon exposure to air, gradually change to the ferric variety.

To distinguish between the two types of compounds, the chemist employs potassium ferricyanide ($K_3Fe[CN]_6$) and potassium ferrocyanide ($K_4Fe[CN]_6$) as test reagents. This may be illustrated as follows:

$FeCl_2 + K_4Fe(CN)_6 \longrightarrow$ White precipitate
$FeCl_2 + K_3Fe(CN)_6 \longrightarrow$ Turnbull's blue
$FeCl_3 + K_3Fe(CN)_6 \longrightarrow$ No reaction
$FeCl_3 + K_4Fe(CN)_6 \longrightarrow$ Prussian blue

Aluminum. Aluminum is the most abundant metal, making up approximately 7 percent of the earth's crust. Never found free because of its high degree of chemical activity, aluminum occurs in the combined state in such compounds as clay, feldspar, mica, cryolite, and bauxite, the latter being the principal ore. Prior to development of the Hall process for extracting aluminum, the metal was about as rare as gold. In this ingenious process, bauxite (Al_2O_3) is dissolved in molten cryolite, and a powerful direct current is then passed through the mixture (Fig. 4-22). The aluminum ions (Al^{+++}) are attracted to the negative walls of the box and the oxygen ions ($O^{=}$) to the graphite anodes. Because of the high temperatures generated, molten aluminum runs to the bottom, where it is drawn off.

Aluminum is silver-white in color and the lightest of the common metals. It possesses great tensile strength and is highly malleable, ductile, and a good conductor of heat and electricity. Chemically, it reacts with metals to form salts and hydrogen gas and with strong bases to form *aluminates.* The reaction between aluminum and sulfuric acid is as follows:

$$2Al + 3H_2SO_4 \longrightarrow Al_2(SO_4)_3 + 3H_2\uparrow$$

Aluminum is employed in huge quantities in the manufacture of airplanes, kitchen utensils, and aluminum foil. When used for construction purposes, its alloys, for example, aluminum bronze (Al, Cu), are preferred to the plain metal. Its principal compounds of commercial value in-

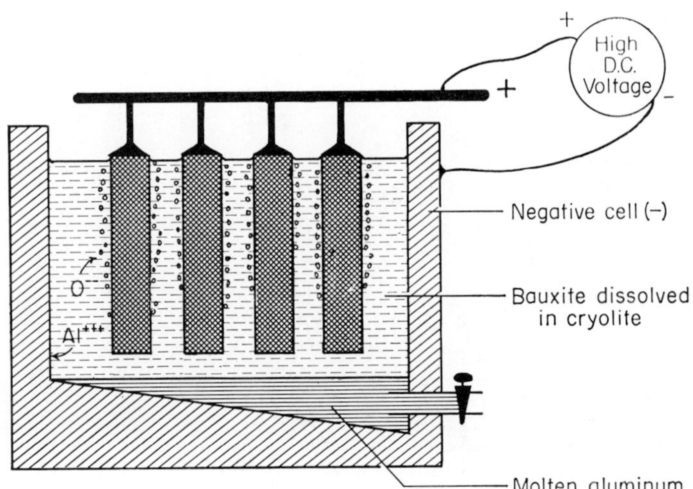

Fig. 4-22. Hall process for the extraction of aluminum. (From Brooks, S. M.: Basic facts of general chemistry, Philadelphia, 1956, W. B. Saunders Co.)

clude clay, alum, aluminum hydroxide, and aluminum oxide. The latter compound exists in several forms in nature, namely, bauxite, corundum, emery, rubies, and sapphires. The ruby and sapphire are precious stones that owe their characteristic beauty to minute impurities.

Magnesium. Magnesium, a light, silver-white metal, burns with a brilliant white light, and reacts with acids to form hydrogen:

$$2Mg + O_2 \longrightarrow 2MgO$$
$$Mg + 2HCl \longrightarrow MgCl_2 + H_2\uparrow$$

The metal is used chiefly in the production of light alloys (for example, Duralumin), and several of its compounds are used widely in the laboratory, in commerce, and in medicine. Magnesium hydroxide ($Mg[OH]_2$) is used to make milk of magnesia, and magnesium sulfate ($MgSO_4$) is none other than Epsom salt.

Mercury. Mercury is uniquely distinguished in that it is the only liquid metal. Chemically, it displays a valence of +1 (mercurous) or +2 (mercuric). For example, the formula for mercurous oxide is Hg_2O, and that for mecuric oxide HgO.

Mercury is particularly well adapted for use in thermometers, barometers, and electrical devices. Mercury alloys, or amalgams, are also useful. Silver amalgam, for example, is used by the dentist to fill tooth cavities. Certain compounds of mercury are extensively employed in the laboratory and in medicine. Mercuhydrin, a complex organic compound containing the metal, is a powerful diuretic, and mercuric oxide is commonly used (as an ointment) in certain eye inflammations.

Copper. Because copper occurs abundantly in the free state, it was the first metal that primitive man learned to use as a material for tools and weapons. The passing of time has certainly not diminished the importance of this reddish metal; indeed, the centuries have enhanced the utility of copper. Of all its many roles, however, this metal finds its greatest use in the making of electrical wire. As a conductor of electricity, it is surpassed only by silver.

Copper reacts with strong concentrated acids and certain elements to form two

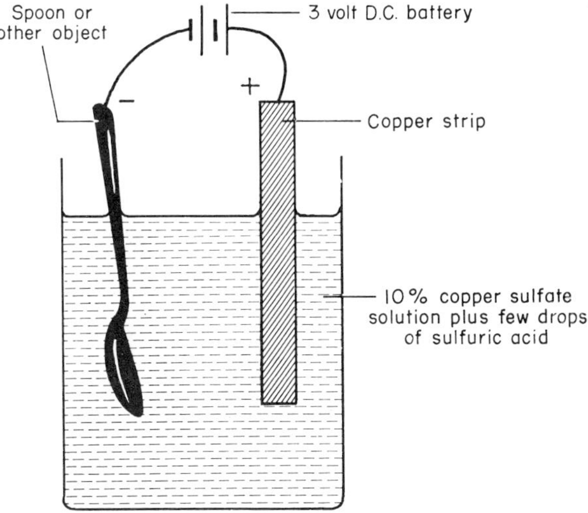

Fig. 4-23. Electroplating of copper. Copper ions (Cu^{++}) in solution are attracted to the negative object, where each ion receives two electrons and becomes a copper atom (Cu°). To replenish the ions removed from solution, copper atoms from the anode enter the solution. (From Brooks, S. M.: Basic facts of general chemistry, Philadelphia, 1956, W. B. Saunders Co.)

types of compounds—*cuprous* (Cu^{+}) and *cupric* (Cu^{++}). For instance, cuprous oxide, a red powder, has the formula Cu_2O; cupric oxide, a black powder, has the formula CuO. By far the most important compound of copper is copper sulfate. The hydrous form, $CuSO_4 \cdot 5H_2O$, is composed of beautiful deep blue crystals that turn to a white powder ($CuSO_4$) when the water of crystallization is driven off by heat. Copper sulfate (more correctly called cupric sulfate) is used in wet batteries, dyeing, Benedict's solution (Chapter 5), and electroplating (Fig. 4-23). In medicine the compound is employed as an anti-infective, as an emetic, and as an antidote in cases of phosphorus poisoning.

Silver. Silver, the most precious of the common metals, occurs in both free and combined states. A soft, whitish element having a high luster, silver stands next to gold as the most ductile and malleable metal. Of interest, too, is the fact that silver surpasses all metals as a conductor of electricity. Silver is inert toward oxygen but readily reacts with sulfur to form silver sulfide (Ag_2S), a black compound known unpleasantly to housewives and pleasantly to the manufacturers of silver polish. With concentrated acids, the metal readily forms the corresponding salts.

Silver is used in coins and jewelry and as a coating on silver-plated ware. So-called solid silver contains a certain percentage of copper to increase its hardness. Silver coins containing 90 percent silver and 10 percent copper are said to be "900 fine," that is, 900 parts silver per 1000 parts alloy. Sterling silver is 925 fine. The main compounds of silver are silver nitrate ($AgNO_3$) and silver bromide (AgBr). Silver nitrate, sometimes called *lunar caustic,* has been used in medicine for years as a caustic and antiseptic (Chapter 23). The bromide, the most important compound, is the backbone of the photographic arts and sciences. Over 200 tons of silver annually goes into the manufacture of film. When a photographic film is exposed by opening the shutter of the camera, the grains of AgBr that are struck by light become sensitized in such a way as to make them easily reduced by the developer, the degree of reduction at any point depending upon the intensity of light. Thus, the film becomes a "chemical picture" of the object photographed.

Lead. Lead, the heaviest of the common metals, is unusually soft and malleable. The bright luster that it has when freshly cut soon dulls because of the formation of a protective coating of oxide. Though the metal does not react with hydrochloric or sulfuric acids, it is readily attacked by nitric and acetic acids. Lead finds extensive use in the making of water pipes, sheeting, storage batteries, alloys, and white lead for paints. The latter substance, the most important compound of lead, has the somewhat cumbersome formula $Pb(OH)_2 \cdot 2PbCO_3$.

Lead is the leading industrial poison. Lead poisoning, or plumbism, is almost always chronic and occurs among persons who work with the metal or its compounds. The signs and symptoms are insidious because of their gradual onset and their similarity to other abnormalities. Treatment of the condition is largely symptomatic.

Zinc. Zinc is a bluish white metal that readily reacts with most dilute acids, forming zinc salts and liberating hydrogen gas. The metal is used for roofing, lining tanks, coating iron to prevent rusting (galvanizing), and making alloys (namely, brass, bronze, and German silver). Its most important compounds are zinc sulfate ($ZnSO_4$), zinc oxide (ZnO), and zinc chloride ($ZnCl_2$).

Tin. Tin is a silver-white metal that is practically inert to air and ordinary corrosive agents. For this reason, the metal finds its widest use as a protective material for other metals. The common "tin can," for instance, is not pure tin but merely tin coated. Among the many important alloys of tin are bronze, pewter, solder, type metal, and Babbit metal. Tin salts are of limited value.

Manganese. Manganese, a hard, steel-like metal, is used extensively in the making of iron alloys and manganese steel. Probably its two most important compounds are manganese dioxide (MnO_2) and postossium permanganate ($KMnO_4$), both employed as oxidizing agents in the laboratory. In addition, the permanganate is used in medicine as an antiseptic and fungistatic agent.

Nickel. Nickel, a hard, silver-white metal, is commonly coated on other metals (by electroplating) to fight corrosion. The element is also extensively used in producing such valuable alloys as German silver, nickel coin, invar, nickel steel, and nichrome.

Chromium. Like manganese, chromium is a hard metal used in making special steel alloys. It also is commonly electroplated on other metals to prevent corrosion.

Gold. Gold, a metal that has appealed to the eye since time immemorial, occurs almost exclusively in the free state in dust, nuggets, and gold-bearing quartz. This heavy, bright-yellow element is not only astonishingly soft, but it is also the most malleable and ductile of all the metals. Although generally inert to most chemical agents, it readily dissolves in aqua regia (a mixture of concentrated HCl and HNO_3), forming chlorauric acid ($HAuCl_4$). As we know, of course, the free metal is the "element of economics" and the backbone of the jewelry store.

Platinum. Platinum, a white lustrous metal, is harder, heavier, and more expensive than gold. It has an extremely high melting point and is resistant to all common chemical reagents. Because of these qualities, the metal is used to make resistant ware for the laboratory. Industrially, powdered platinum serves as a valuable catalyst.

Radioactive metals. Radium, uranium, and other radioactive metals are discussed in the section that follows.

NUCLEAR CHEMISTRY

At the turn of the last century certain discoveries shifted the chemist's spotlight from the planetary electrons to the nucleus, the kernel of the universe. In the present section an attempt will be made to acquaint the student with the major findings in this area and their application to our everyday activities.

Radioactivity. The discovery of x rays (p. 5) by Roentgen in 1895 stimulated other scientists to look for similar mysterious radiations. Becquerel found that uranium compounds emitted penetrating rays, and in 1903 Marie and Pierre Curie isolated radium, an element two million times more "potent" than uranium. Radium, uranium, and other elements that emit energy rays are said to be radioactive.

By the use of photographic plates and a powerful magnetic field, Rutherford and associates demonstrated that radium (and

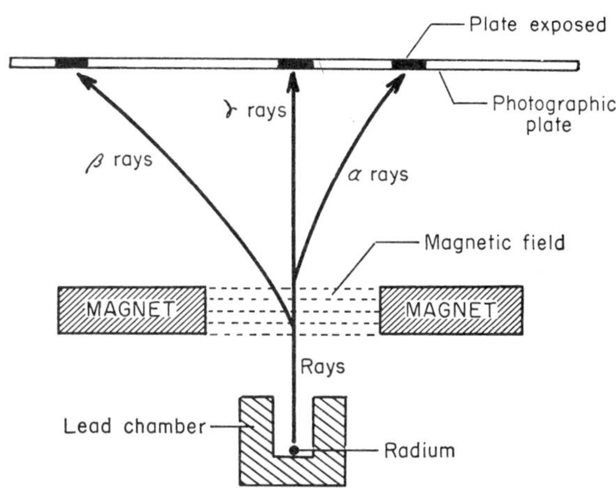

Fig. 4-24. Effect of a magnetic field upon the rays emitted by a radioactive substance. The magnetic field is perpendicular to the plane of the paper and directed into the paper.

other radioactive elements) emit three types of rays: alpha, beta, and gamma (Fig. 4-24). Alpha and beta rays are particulate; that is, they consist of helium nuclei (two protons and two neutrons) and electrons, respectively. The latter, it is now known, come from the disintegration of neutrons. Gamma rays, nonparticulate electromagnetic waves of energy, are similar to x rays but are more penetrating. Indeed, the gamma emanations are the most powerful of the three forms of radiation.

Why should some elements behave in this radioactive fashion, while others do not? Briefly, it is a matter of stability. Apparently, radioactive atoms are unhappy about their allotment of protons and neutrons and do something about it by emitting "undesirable" particles. This will continue until all the nuclei have attained the desired combination.

Curie. The quantitative unit that we use to measure radioactivity is called the curie. One curie represents the disintegration of 3.7×10^{10} atoms of radioactive substance per second, which is approximately equal to the radioactivity of 1 gm. of radium. Because of the relative largeness of the curie, the millicurie (0.001 curie) is the more useful unit in medical work.

Half-life. Since the disintegration, or decay, of radioactive nuclei is spontaneous

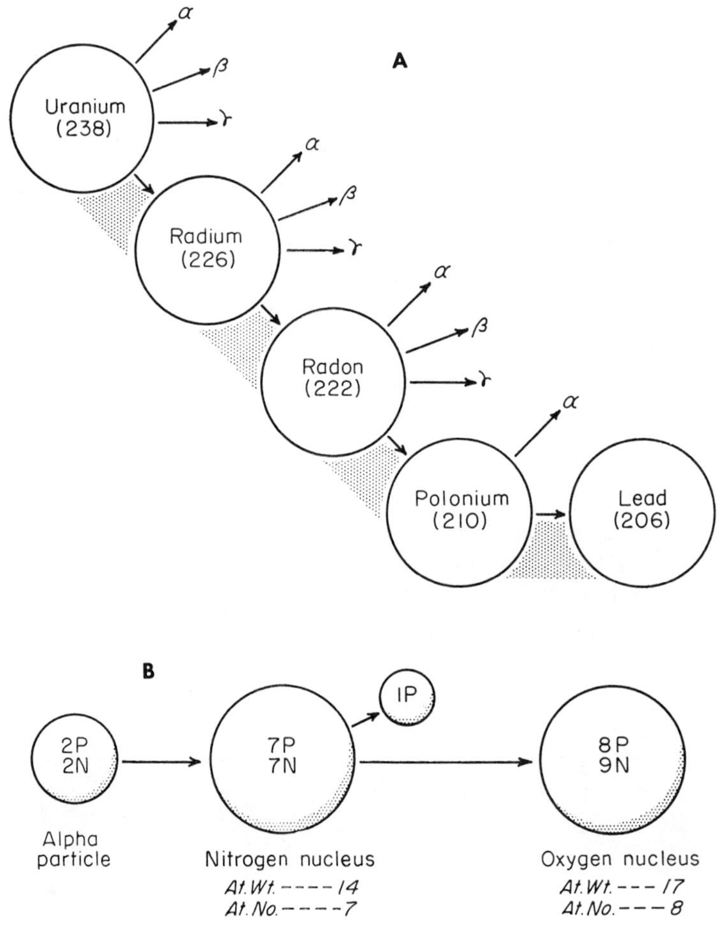

Fig. 4-25. Natural, **A**, and artificial, **B**, transmutation. (See text.)

and not changed by outside forces, each radioactive element acts as an atomic timepiece. To express this time, we employ the term *half-life,* which is defined as the length of time it takes one-half of the atoms in any given sample of radioactive material to decay. Interestingly, this period varies fantastically among the elements. For example, while polonium has a half-life of less than a millionth of a second, uranium has a half-life of almost 5 billion years!

Transmutation. Because each atom has a characteristic atomic number, it follows that a radioactive atom will change into a new atom subsequent to its emission of nuclear particles. In other words, chemical analysis of a radioactive element will disclose the presence of other elements. In time the original element will disappear and a new *stable* element will remain; the earth's lead, for instance, resulted from the radioactive decay of radium, which in turn resulted from the decay of uranium (Fig. 4-25). We call this natural phenomenon of one element changing into another element *transmutation.*

The discovery of transmutation served as a most powerful stimulus for atomic research. It raised the question: If nature can effect transmutation, why can't man? The great work of Rutherford demonstrated that artificial transmutation was indeed possible. Using alpha particles (supplied by radium) as "atomic bullets," he succeeded in knocking protons out of nitrogen nuclei, converting the latter element into oxygen (Fig. 4-25). Since Rutherford's time, a great many other transformations have been achieved, yielding new elements and radioactive isotopes.

Detection of radioactivity. Since radiation cannot be detected by the eye or measured by usual procedures, the chemist and physicist have devised special techniques. In addition to photographic methods (Fig. 4-24), the atomic scientist employs such pieces of equipment as the Wilson cloud chamber, the scintillator, and the Geiger-Müller counter. The latter, in one modification or another, is used in all establishments that employ radioactive elements and isotopes. As indicated by its name, this device not only detects radiation but, equally important, also determines the intensity of radiation.

Radioactive isotopes. Radioactive isotopes have been employed in innumerable ways in just about every branch of science. As indicated, their usefulness depends upon the emission of telltale energy rays.

In the biologic sciences, radioactive isotopes are used to tag compounds in order to trace their metabolic fate within plant and animal bodies. Carbon dioxide, for instance, prepared from ${}_6C^{14}$ (Fig. 4-26), has enabled the researcher to learn a great deal more about the process of photosynthesis. In general, this so-called tracer technique has brought forth information that otherwise could never have been elicited by conventional methods.

Radiation has a profound influence upon living material. In excessive amounts it not only denatures protoplasm but also alters the genes in such a way as to pass the injury on to future generations. Indeed, herein lies one of the great questions of our time. On the positive side, however, radiation has proved to be our principal weapon against cancer. Although x rays and radium have been employed in this capacity

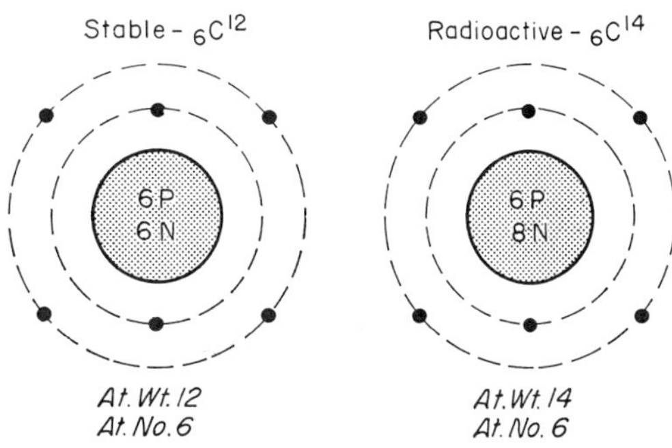

Fig. 4-26. Isotopes of carbon.

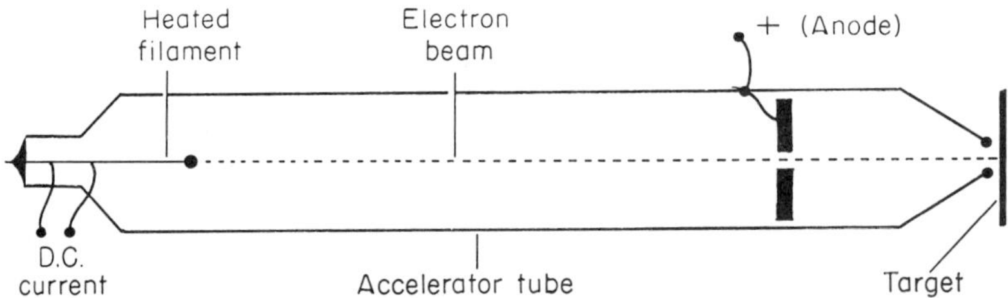

Fig. 4-27. Electron accelerator atom smasher. Electrons, emitted by the heated filament and accelerated by the high charge on the anode, pass through the small opening in the latter electrode and strike the target. (See text.)

for the greater part of the century, they are being supplemented and often replaced by radioactive isotopes. Moreover, certain isotopes offer special advantages. For example, radioactive iodine has proved to be highly effective against cancer of the thyroid. Since the element accumulates in the gland, a powerful dose of radiation is delivered at the exact spot where it is needed. Other radioactive isotopes used in medicine include carbon-14 ($_{6}C^{14}$), sodium-24 ($_{11}Na^{24}$), phosphorus-32 ($_{15}P^{32}$), cobalt-60 ($_{27}Co^{60}$), gold-198 ($_{79}Au^{198}$), strontium-90 ($_{38}Sr^{90}$), iron-59 ($_{26}Fe^{59}$), and hydrogen-3, or tritium ($_{1}H^{3}$).

Nuclear fission. A cataclysmic experiment in 1942 disclosed that man had learned to tap the enormous energy trapped within the atom. Using an atomic pile charged with uranium-235, Enrico Fermi demonstrated the first controlled *chain reaction,* a phenomenon destined to change the course of history.

It had long been appreciated that the nucleus of an atom was heavily dosed with energy to hold it together, for how else could the protons, with their strong force to repel one another, be held together? It was further realized that if the nucleus could be "split," this energy could be released. The atom smasher (Fig. 4-27) sustained both hypotheses. However, the amount of energy released was so infinitesimally small compared to the astronomic amounts of energy needed to run the machine that the scientist looked in other directions. The breakthrough came with the isolation of U-235, the natural radioactive isotope of uranium. (The bulk of uranium is made up of U-238.) Not only did the U-235 atom undergo fission ("splitting"), but in the process it also shot out two neutrons that triggered the fission of two other atoms, which in turn set off four others, which in turn set off sixteen others, and so on (Fig. 4-28). If the student considers the trillions upon trillions of atoms in a piece of matter the size of a pea, he can readily appreciate the fantastic quantity of energy released in the process. Indeed, unless the rate of fission is *controlled,* a certain mass of fissionable material explodes with a violence known only to the survivors of Hiroshima and Nagasaki.

Fermi's apparatus, then, housed a controlled reaction. Aptly called an atomic pile because of its shape, a charge of "enriched uranium" in graphite was interlaced with cadmium-boron rods to capture a certain proportion of the neutrons released during fission. Thus, by pushing the rods in and out of the pile, the rate at which the chain reaction was proceeding along could be kept below the critical value. Since projects such as this were carried out on the fringes of the unknown, early nuclear scientists were not only brilliant but brave. History records, for example, that on one occasion the first atomic pile "went critical."

Einstein's formula. Perhaps we can better

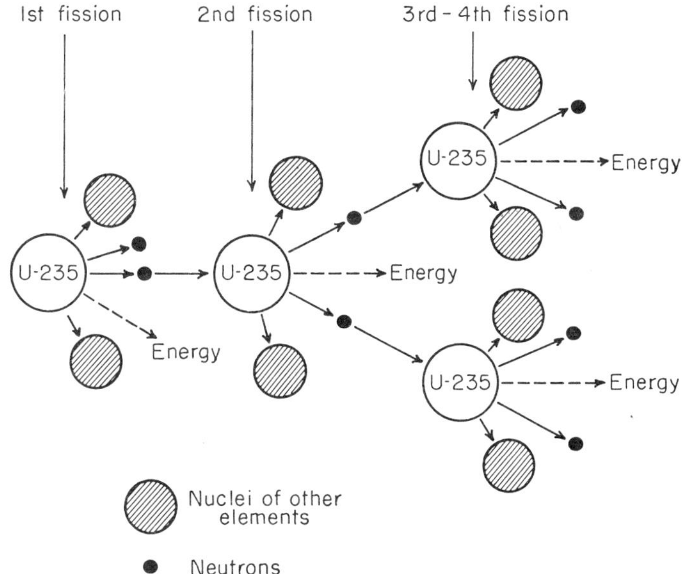

Fig. 4-28. Diagram illustrating nuclear fission and the chain reaction. (From Brooks, S. M.: Basic facts of general chemistry, Philadelphia, 1956, W. B. Saunders Co.)

appreciate the energy of the atom if we consider the now famous Einstein formula ($E = mc^2$), which states that energy equals mass times the speed of light squared. Since the fission products of U-235 weigh *less* than the original atom, matter has disappeared as energy in accordance with the formula. Note that even though the vanished mass is unbelievably small, it is multiplied by the speed of light squared, a fantastic figure. Moreover, this, in turn, is multiplied by the atronomical number of atoms present.

Atomic blast. The early work with fission was prompted by the last Great War when President Truman directed that an atomic bomb be made and dropped before the know-how was acquired by the enemy. The making of the bomb was the most complex and expensive project that man had ever undertaken. The chief obstacle centered about the herculean task of separating U-235 from uranium ore, the former constituting less than 1 percent of a given quantity of the element. Progress was greatly accelerated, however, when it was discovered that another element—plutonium—also possessed fissionable powers. This element can be produced from the relatively abundant U-238.

The bomb itself consists of two charges—a small mass of U-235 separated from a larger mass of plutonium. As long as the two masses are kept apart, no explosion occurs. When brought together, however, the combination "goes critical" (Fig. 4-29). The two bombs used against Japan unleashed an energy equivalent to about 20,000 tons of TNT.

Atomic reactor. The knowledge gained as a result of working with the bomb was readily channeled into peaceful uses following the war. Atomic power is now a giant reality. The trip of the atomic submarine *Nautilus* over the North Pole and the first atomic electric plant at Calder Hall, England, are already history.

Atomic power is obtained by placing a charge of fissionable material in a reactor, a special heat-resistant device that permits a controlled chain reaction. The tremendous heat evolved is carried away by an "exchange fluid" (for example, liquid sodium) that circulates between the reactor core and water, the latter being converted to steam in the process. The steam is then used to generate electricity. Some comparison of this mode of power with conventional means can be gained by the fact that the *Nautilus* made its trip around the world on a charge of uranium no larger than a golf ball!

Nuclear fusion. The swift pace of present-day developments has, in a sense, made fission itself a thing of the past, for the atomic scientist has discovered that it is not fission but *fusion* that yields the last word in energy. The principle, however, is the same; that is, mass is converted into energy in accordance with Einstein's formula of $E = mc^2$.

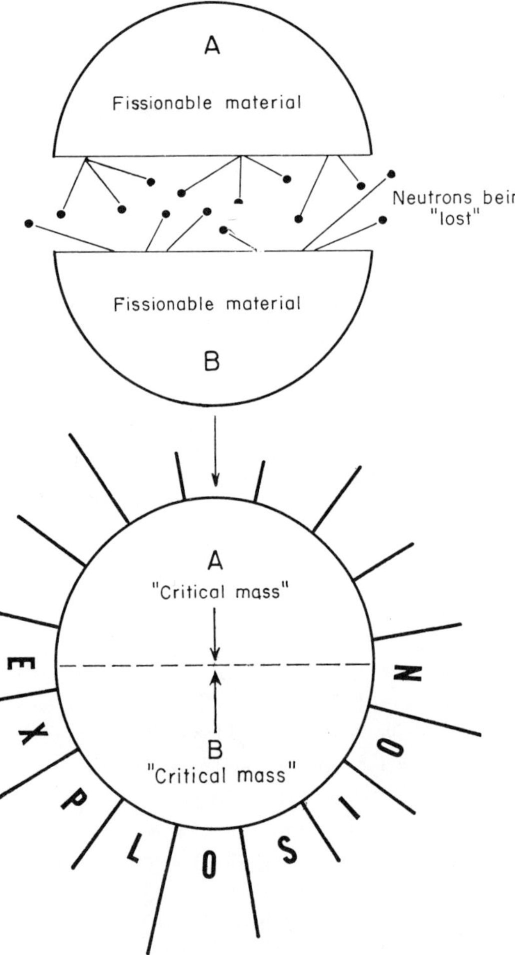

Fig. 4-29. The atomic bomb is set off by bringing together two masses of fissionable material to form the critical mass. When kept apart, the two masses (each "subcritical") lose sufficient neutrons to the air to prevent an uncontrolled chain reaction.

Science first suspected fusion in the sun and stars, and postulated that hydrogen atoms fuse into helium atoms, with a *loss* of mass and the release of tremendous energy. Thus, energywise, the cradle of life resides in a hydrogen furnace 93 million miles away A man-made fusion reaction has already been achieved in the form of the hydrogen bomb. Although the details of this thermonuclear device are not publicly known, the reaction probably entails the fusion of tritium ($_1H^3$) and deuterium ($_1H^2$), iostopes of hydrogen. The initiation of such a reaction requires a temperature of 100 million degrees or so and necessitates the use of the atom bomb as a detonator.

At present, nuclear laboratories throughout the world are feverishly searching for a means to effect a *controlled* fusion reaction for peaceful purposes. Even though the obstacles are formidable, progress has already been made in this country and abroad. Once controlled fusion becomes a reality, man will never want for energy, for the ocean and seas serve as fathomless sources of deuterium and tritium.

COLLOIDS

A colloid, or a colloidal system, may be defined as a solid, liquid, or gas dispersed (or subdivided) to such a degree that the size of the particles becomes an important factor in determining its properties.* Since most substances in nature are usually in the colloidal state, the subject demands a few special remarks.

Types of colloids. The dispersed phase

*A colloidal particle usually measures somewhere between 10^{-7} and 10^{-5} cm.

Table 4-7. Examples of colloidal systems

Dispersed phase	Dispersing phase	Example
Solid	Solid	Colored glass
Solid	Liquid	Glue
Solid	Gas	Smoke
Liquid	Solid	Cheese
Liquid	Liquid	Milk
Liquid	Gas	Fog
Gas	Solid	Pumice
Gas	Liquid	Whipped cream
Gas	Gas	—

of a colloidal system may be a solid, liquid, or gas. Likewise, the dispersing phase may be a solid, liquid, or gas. Although theoretically there are nine possible systems (Table 4-7), actually there are only eight because gases always form true solutions.

Colloidal systems are named according to the states of the dispersed and dispersing phases. If the dispersed phase is a solid and the dispersing phase a liquid, the system is called a *sol;* if both phases are liquid, the system is called an *emulsion.* Colloidal systems in which the dispersing medium is a semisolid are called *gels.* Common and important examples of the various

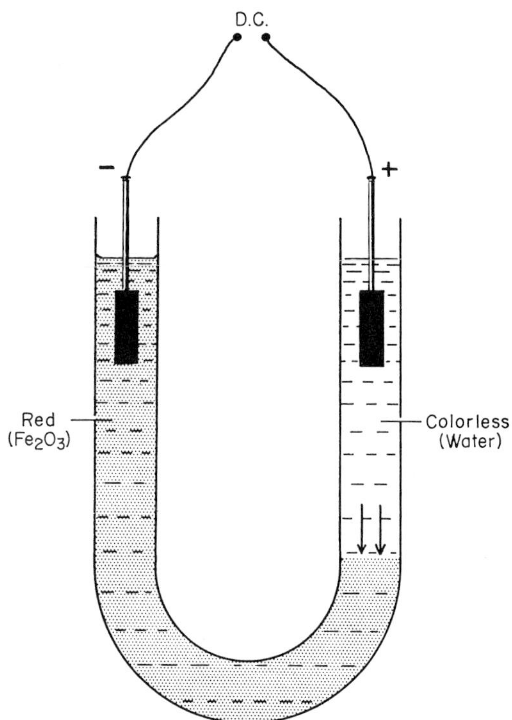

Fig. 4-30. Demonstration of electrophoresis. As the current passes through the solution, the colloidal particles of ferric oxide (Fe_2O_3) migrate toward the cathode. This proves that all the particles carry the same (positive) charge. (From Brooks, S. M.: Basic facts of general chemistry, Philadelphia, 1956, W. B. Saunders Co.)

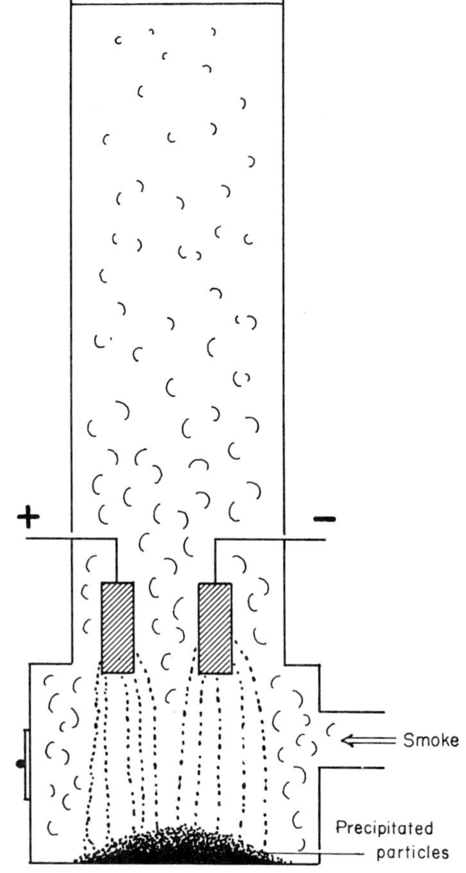

Fig. 4-31. "Smokeless chimney." Its operation depends upon the fact that the charged particles in the smoke are neutralized by the electrodes.

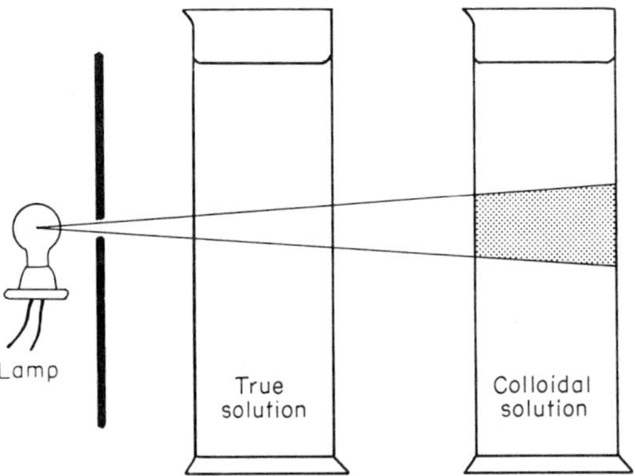

Fig. 4-32. Demonstration of the Tyndall effect.

colloidal systems are presented in Table 4-7.

Colloidal properties. A colloidal system is a two-phase heterogeneous mixture in which, characteristically, the suspended or dispersed phase does not settle out from the dispersing phase. The particles of the dispersed phase remain suspended in part because they all carry the same electrical charge (Fig. 4-30). In other words, since they repel one another, they do not coalesce and thereby exceed colloidal dimensions. As a matter of fact, a colloidal system can be readily destroyed by neutralizing this charge. Advantage is taken of this fact in the so-called smokeless chimney (Fig. 4-31).

Tyndall effect. One of the more striking features of a colloidal system is the Tyndall effect. While a true solution does not show the path of light, a colloid outlines the path in clear detail (Fig. 4-32). Common examples of the Tyndall effect are a searchlight probing the night sky and a ray of sunshine passing through a darkened room.

Brownian movement. When colloidal particles are microscopically observed against a dark background, they appear as bright specks of light in rapid zigzag, or *brownian movement* (p. 18). This phenomenon is now known to be a consequence of the collision of high-speed molecules of the dispersing medium with the colloidal particles.

Adsorption. By adsorption we mean the adherence of molecules or ions to the surface of a solid. Because of the immense surface area of colloidal particles, colloids adsorb substances to a very high degree. For example, a cube having a length of 1 cm. on a side has a total surface area of 6 sq. cm. However, if this cube were to be divided into cubes measuring 0.001 mm. on an edge ("colloidal size"), the total surface area would be 600,000 sq. cm.! The use of charcoal and bone black to remove coloring matter and gases is a practical application of colloidal adsorption.

Color. Many colloidal systems are highly colored. Colloidal color is explained by the fact that the minute particles absorb certain wavelengths of light and reflect others. The specific color, however, depends primarily upon the size of the particle rather than upon its nature. For this reason, the color gives little clue as to what substance is present. Thus, colloidal gold may be red, blue, green, or violet, according to the size and uniformity of the particles.

It takes only a very small amount of colloidal substance to impart an intense color. Just a few milligrams of gold, for example, will color a liter of water. Red glass is manufactured by adding just a trace of selenium to ordinary glass. The blue of the sky and the ocean is explained on the basis of colloidal dust in the air and water. It is thought that the blue of the eyes is due not to pigment but to the presence in the iris of colloidal particles that scatter blue light and transmit red. The brilliant colors of some of the feathers of birds are due to the presence of colloidal air bubbles.

Dialysis. From a standpoint of size there are two types of solutions—those whose solute particles pass through a semipermeable membrane (such as parchment or cellophane) and those whose particles do

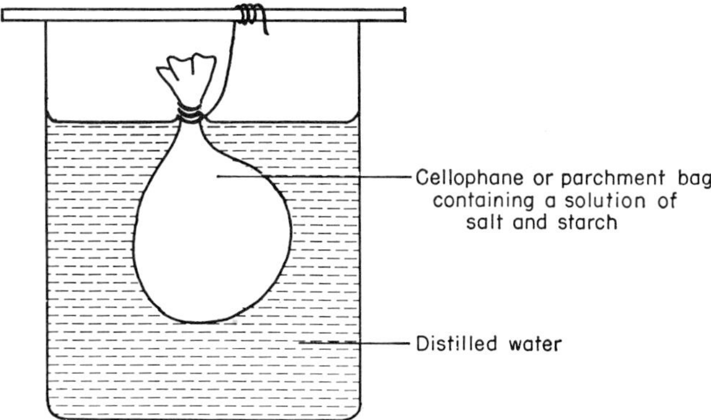

Fig. 4-33. Demonstration of dialysis. In this particular experiment a mixture of boiled starch and salt is placed in a cellophane bag, and the latter is immersed in a jar of water. When allowed to remain in this position, the salt (a crystalloid) diffuses through the bag, but the starch (a colloid) does not. This can be proved by adding a little $AgNO_3$ (to test for salt) and iodine (to test for starch) to the water. (From Brooks, S. M.: Basic facts of general chemistry, Philadelphia, 1956, W. B. Saunders Co.)

not pass through. The former constitutes a true solution and the latter a colloidal system called a *sol.* We take advantage of this feature in dialysis, a process whereby a crystalloid (a substance that forms a true solution) is separated from a colloid by means of a semipermeable membrane (Fig. 4-33).

The membrane that surrounds the living cell has selective properties; for example, it prevents the loss of protoplasm (a colloid) but permits the passage of nutritional and waste crystalloids.

Preparation of colloids. The various methods used to prepare colloidal systems may be placed in one of two categories: dispersion and condensation. Dispersion is the subdividing of a substance into particles of colloidal size. The grinding of solids and the agitation of liquids are common examples of dispersion. At the commercial level a device called a colloid mill is used to reduce a substance to the colloidal state by forcing a suspension between two revolving surfaces about 0.002 inch apart. The mill is used to make paints, inks, ointments, and emulsions. Colloidal systems of metals in liquids may be prepared by the unique dispersion method diagrammed in Fig. 4-34.

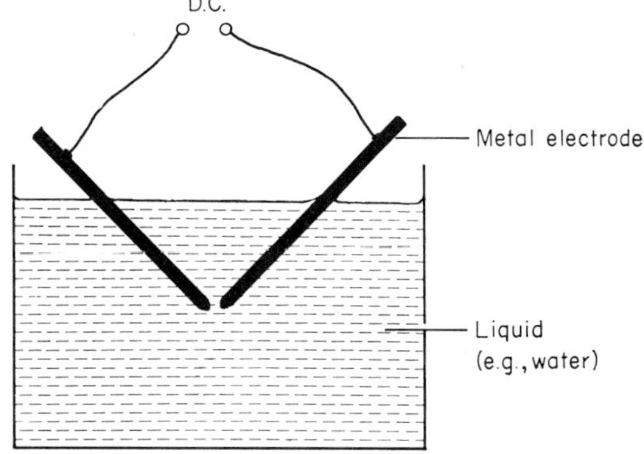

Fig. 4-34. Preparation of a colloid by producing an electric arc beneath the surface of water. The arc causes colloidal particles to be stripped away from the electrodes.

Condensation is the building up of colloidal particles from those of crystalloid dimensions. Usually this is done by forming a colloidal precipitate via chemical action between two solutions. When a few drops of acid are added to a dilute solution of sodium thiosulfate, for example, sulfur is released, producing a suspensoid of sulfur in water.

CHEMICAL ARITHMETIC

Now that we have explored some of the fundamentals of chemistry, let us take up a few practical situations that deal with chemical arithmetic.

The molecular weight. The molecular weight, or the formula weight, of a substance is the sum of the atomic weights of the constituent atoms as indicated by the formula.

EXAMPLE: The molecular weight of sulfuric acid (98) is computed as follows:

Element	*Atomic weight*		*Subscript*		
H	1	×	2	=	2
S	32	×	1	=	32
O	16	×	4	=	64
					98

Formula: H_2SO_4

Percentage composition. If one knows the molecular weight of a compound, it is a simple matter to compute the percentage composition of any of its constituent elements by use of the following formula:

$$\text{Percentage} = \frac{\text{Atomic weight} \times \text{Subscript}}{\text{Molecular weight}} \times 100$$

EXAMPLE: The percentage composition of hydrogen in water (11.1 percent) is calculated as follows:

Formula: H_2O
Molecular weight: 18

$$\text{Percentage} = \frac{1 \times 2}{18} \times 100 = 11.1\%$$

Computing the formula. To write the formula of an unknown substance, the chemist first determines the percentage composition for each of its constituent elements and then divides each percentage by the atomic weight of the element. The resulting quotients (the nearest whole number is used) indicate the subscripts.

EXAMPLE: A pure compound was found, upon chemical analysis, to be composed of 2 percent hydrogen, 33 percent sulfur, and 65 percent oxygen. Its formula was computed as follows:

Element	*Percent composition*	*Atomic weight*	*Subscript*
Hydrogen	2	1	2
Sulfur	33	32	1
Oxygen	65	16	4

Formula: H_2SO_4

Quantitative reactions. Since chemical compounds react in a definite way, it is very easy to compute the products or reactants if we know one quantity. The next example illustrates the so-called *weight-weight* problem, and it is followed by an example of the *volume-volume* problem.

EXAMPLE 1: What quantity of sulfuric acid is needed to neutralize 10 gm. of sodium hydroxide?

First step—Balance equation:

$$2NaOH + H_2SO_4 \longrightarrow Na_2SO_4 + 2H_2O$$

Second step—Write known and unknown *(X)* quantities above appropriate compound:

$$\overset{10}{2NaOH} + \overset{X}{H_2SO_4} \longrightarrow Na_2SO_4 + 2H_2O$$

Third step—Write in molecular weight times coefficient below appropriate compound:

$$\underset{2 \times 40}{\overset{10}{2NaOH}} + \underset{98}{\overset{X}{H_2SO_4}} \longrightarrow Na_2SO_4 + 2H_2O$$

Fourth step—Form proportion and solve for *X*:

$$\frac{10}{80} = \frac{X}{98}$$

$$80X = 980$$

$$X = 12.3 \text{ gm. of } H_2SO_4 \text{ needed}$$

EXAMPLE 2: How many liters of ammonia gas are formed when 10 liters of nitrogen react with sufficient hydrogen?

First step

$$N_2 + 3H_2 \longrightarrow 2NH_3$$

Second step

$$\overset{10}{N_2} + 3H_2 \longrightarrow \overset{X}{2NH_3}$$

Third step—Write *coefficients* below respective gases:

$$\underset{1}{\overset{10}{N_2}} + 3H_2 \longrightarrow \underset{2}{\overset{X}{2NH_3}}$$

$$\frac{10}{1} = \frac{X}{2}$$

$$1X = 20$$
$$X = 20 \text{ liters}$$

Solutions. In the laboratory the most common type of situation demanding arithmetic is the making of solutions. Indeed, a sound knowledge of the fundamentals presented here is of practical value out of the laboratory as well as in it.

Percentage solutions. Expressing the concentration of a solution via percentage is the method most commonly employed in commerce, pharmacy, and medicine. Unless otherwise specified, a solid dissolved in a liquid is computed *weight to volume,* and a liquid dissolved in a liquid is computed *volume to volume.*

EXAMPLE 1: Two grams of salt were dissolved in water contained in a graduated cylinder. If the resulting volume was 10 ml., what was the percentage concentration?

First step

$$\frac{\text{Grams of salt}}{\text{Volume of solution}} \times 100 = \%\ \text{Salt}$$

Second step

$$\frac{2}{10} \times 100 = 20\%$$

EXAMPLE 2: A solution is prepared from 700 ml. of alcohol, 100 ml. of glycerol, and 200 ml. of water. What is the percentage of alcohol?

First step

$$\frac{\text{Volume of alcohol}}{\text{Volume of solution}} \times 100 = \%\ \text{Alcohol}$$

Second step

$$\frac{700}{1000} \times 100 = 70\%\ \text{by volume}$$

Molar solutions. Molar solutions are commonly used in the chemical laboratory. A 1 molar solution is a solution that contains 1 *gram-molecular weight* of a chemical per liter of solution. A gram-molecular weight, or *mole,* of a compound is the molecular weight expressed in grams.

EXAMPLE: Prepare 500 ml. of 2 molar (2M) sulfuric acid (H_2SO_4).

(1) Molecular weight = 98
(2) 1 mole = 98 gm.
(3) Moles needed = 1 (2M for 1 liter, hence, 1M for 0.5 liter)

Thus, the solution is prepared by adding 98 gm. of H_2SO_4 to sufficient water to make a total volume of 500 ml.

The mole and colligative properties. One mole of any nonvolatile nonelectrolyte in 1000 gm. of water raises the boiling point to 100.52° C. and lowers the freezing point to − 1.86° C. In regard to electrolytes, the effect upon the boiling and freezing points depends upon the degree of dissociation. For electrolytes that yield two ions per molecule, such as NaCl, 1 mole in 1000 gm. of water raises the boiling point to 101.04° C. and lowers the freezing point to −3.72° C.—just *double* the effect of 1 mole of any nonelectrolyte. This, of course, relates to the fact that 1 mole of NaCl yields twice as many solute particles as does 1 mole of any nonelectrolyte, for instance, sugar.

Advantage is taken of the aforementioned colligative properties in the experimental determination of molecular weight.

EXAMPLE: If 120 gm. of some nonelectrolyte in 1000 gm. of water produced a boiling point of 100.26° C., what is its molecular weight?

(1) One mole of any nonelectrolyte produces a boiling point of 100.52° C.
(2) Therefore, since 120 gm. of the substance produced only one-half this effect, its molecular weight would be twice 120, or 240.

Normal solutions. Normality is perhaps the most useful mode of expressing concentration in chemistry. In a moment we shall see why.

A 1 normal (1N) solution contains 1 gm. of hydrogen ion—or its equivalent—per liter of solution, an equivalent being defined as 1 gram-atomic weight of any ion divided by the valence. Thus, 36.5 gm. HCl (that is, 1 gram-molecular weight of HCl) and 58.5 gm. NaCl (that is, 1 gram-molecular weight of NaCl) are chemically equivalent because this amount of HCl furnishes 1 gm. of H^+ ion, and this amount of NaCl furnishes 23 gm. of Na^+, or *one* equivalent of that ion. To prepare a 1N solution of HCl and a 1N solution of NaCl, therefore, we simply dissolve these amounts in sufficient water to make 1 liter.

To prepare a 1N solution of an acid that contains more than one atom of hydrogen per molecule, we must take the appropriate fraction of the gram-molecular weight: for dibasic acids one-half and for tribasic acids one-third. Thus, to prepare a 1N solution of H_2SO_4, we take one half of 98, or 49 gm. of acid, and sufficient water to make 1 liter. The same reasoning applies to salts and bases with cations having a valence greater than 1. Thus, to prepare a 1N solution of $MgCl_2$, we take one half of 95.3, or 47.7 gm., and sufficient water to make 1 liter.

Of course, normal solutions of any desired strength may be prepared—0.5N, 3N, 5N, and so on. This is done simply by calculating the amount needed to prepare a 1N solution and then multiplying by the appropriate fraction or whole number.

EXAMPLE 1: Prepare 2 liters of a 1N solution of HCl.

(1) Grams of HCl needed to make 1 liter of 1N = 36.5
(2) Grams of HCl needed to make 2 liters of 1N = 2 × 36.5, or 73 gm.
(3) The solution is made by adding the acid to about a liter of water contained in a graduate and then finally adding just enough water to bring the volume to the 2000 ml. or 2-liter mark.

EXAMPLE 2: Prepare 2 liters of 2N $AlCl_3$.

(1) Grams of $AlCl_3$ needed for 1 liter of 1N = ⅓ of 133.5, or 44.5 gm.
(2) Grams of $AlCl_3$ needed for 1 liter of 2N = 2 × 44.5, or 89 gm.
(3) Grams of $AlCl_3$ needed for 2 liters of 2N = 2 × 89, or 178 gm.
(4) The solution is made by dissolving 178 gm. of $AlCl_3$ in 500 ml. or so of water and then adding sufficient water to bring the volume to *exactly* 2 liters.

Titration. The value of normality resides in the fact that solutions of the same normal concentration react with one another, volume for volume. For example, 20 ml. of 1N HCl will exactly neutralize 20 ml. of 1N NaOH, and vice versa. By the same token, 20 ml. of 0.5N HCl reacts exactly with 10 ml. of 1N NaOH. Thus, normality follows a relationship that can be expressed arithmetically:

$$\underset{\text{(Solution A)}}{N \times \text{ml.}} = \underset{\text{(Solution B)}}{N \times \text{ml.}}$$

As an example of how the normal solution is used in quantitative analysis, let us suppose that a chemist is asked to determine the concentration of acetic acid in

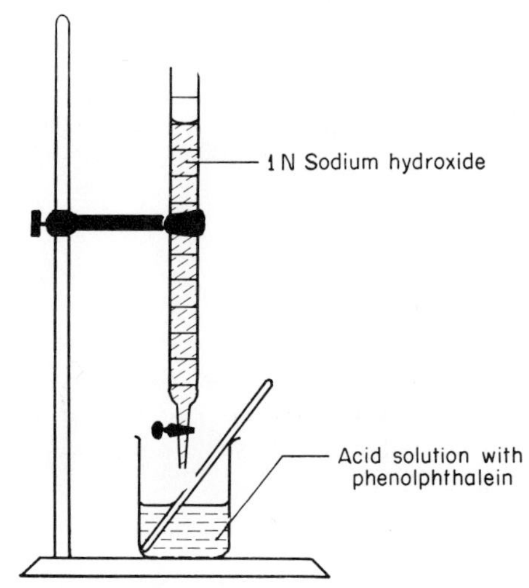

Fig. 4-35. Titration. (See text.)

a sample of vinegar, a very practical situation. Using a pipet, he would first put an *exact* volume of vinegar in a clean beaker and a drop or two of indicator to signal the "end point." Then he would place the beaker below a buret (Fig. 4-35) and into the vinegar would titrate (that is, add drop by drop) a base (for example, NaOH) of *known normality*. When the indicator turns color (the end point of neutralization), titration is stopped and the volume of base added is carefully noted on the buret. The normality of the vinegar is now simply calculated by substituting the three known values in the foregoing formula and solving for the unknown *N*. Thus,

$$\underset{\text{Vinegar}}{N \times \text{ml.}} = \underset{\text{Base}}{N \times \text{ml.}}$$

$$N\ (\text{vinegar}) = \frac{N \times \text{ml. (base)}}{\text{ml. (vinegar)}}$$

Milliequivalent. As the science of chemistry has more and more infiltrated the realm of physiology, the biochemist has become a physiologist and the physiologist has become a biochemist. This is epitomized by the very important expression *milliequivalent*, a term now as common in the hospital as in the chemical laboratory.

In the discussion of normality we learned that the concept of equivalency was of great practical value because it permitted us to compare chemicals arithmetically. In other words, *one* equivalent weight of one ion exactly replaces or combines with *one* equivalent weight of some other ion. Unquestionably, this is the most logical way to compare substances chemically. By the same reasoning, it is also the most logical way to talk about ions physiologically; therefore, the physiologist and the physician have adopted the expression in dealing with the electrolytes of the body (Chapter 18).

As stated, the equivalent weight or "equivalent" of an ion is its gram-atomic weight divided by its valence. For example, the equivalent weight of Na^{+} is 23 ÷ 1, or 23 gm., and the equivalent weight of Ca^{++} is 40 ÷ 2, or 20 gm. Because of the very low ionic concentrations encountered in the body fluids, however, the equivalent proves too large a unit—hence, the use of the much smaller milliequivalent (mEq.), which is equal to an ion's equivalent weight divided by 1000. Thus, the milliequivalent weights of Na^{+} and Ca^{++} are 0.023 and 0.020 gm., respectively.

It is often of practical importance to translate milliequivalents into milligrams or vice versa. For example, on the basis of milliequivalents, the concentration of potassium in the blood serum is 4 mEq. per liter. In terms of milligrams this is equal to 4 × 0.039 gm. (the milliequivalent weight of K), or 156 mg. per liter. Further, it is common practice to express concentration in *milligrams percent* (mg.%), meaning the number of milligrams per 100 ml. Thus, in the example just cited, this would be 15.6 mg.%.

Questions

1. Matter is neither created nor destroyed. Discuss this statement.
2. On the basis of the kinetic theory, describe the three states of matter.
3. Potassium has an atomic number of 19 and an atomic weight of 39. Sketch an atom of the element according to the electron theory.
4. What are isotopes?
5. Illustrate the theory of electrovalence by diagramming the "atomic reaction" between magnesium and chlorine (forming magnesium chloride).
6. What is meant by covalence?
7. Write formulas for the following compounds: aluminum floride, zinc phosphate, calcium carbonate, cupric nitrate, ammonium chlorate, lead nitrite, silver nitrate, mercuric oxide, ferrous sulfate, ammonium bicarbonate, dipotassium phosphate, sodium bisulfite, and magnesium hydroxide.
8. Describe the chemical events that occur when a direct electric current is passed through a solution of potassium iodide.
9. Distinguish between the expressions *oxidation* and *reduction*.
10. Write equations for the following reactions:
    Zinc + Dilute sulfuric acid →
    Aluminum hydroxide + Hydrochloric acid →

Reduction of nickel ion →
Burning of sulfur →
Potassium sulfate + Barium chloride →
Calcium bicarbonate + Sulfuric acid →
Lithium sulfite + Hydrochloric acid →
Oxidation of ferrous ion to ferric ion →
Hydrolysis of sodium carbonate →
Magnesium + Dilute nitric acid →
Ammonium chloride + Silver nitrate →

11. Discuss three factors that influence the speed of a reaction.
12. A solution may be saturated and still be dilute. Explain.
13. What is meant by a supersaturated solution?
14. What are immiscible liquids?
15. Describe the process of distillation.
16. What are colligative properties?
17. What is the hydronium ion?
18. If a solution has a $[H^+]$ of 0.004, what is its pH?
19. Discuss the Brönsted theory of acids and bases.
20. What is the $[H^+]$ of a solution with a pH of 8?
21. What is meant by a strong acid? Strong base? (Illustrate with equations.)
22. Why do neutralization reactions go to completion?
23. Name four binary acids and four ternary acids.
24. What is an acid salt? Give examples.
25. What would be the reaction of an ammonium chloride solution toward litmus? Explain your answer.
26. Why do elements in the same group in the periodic table have similar chemical properties?
27. When a solution of $AgNO_3$ is added to gastric juice, a white precipitate forms. Explain.
28. Describe a test that you could perform to distinguish between KI and KBr.
29. When an acid was added to a white powder contained in a test tube, a gas was liberated that decolorized a solution of potassimu permanganate. Explain.
30. Describe a test that you could perform to distinguish between NH_4Cl and $CaCl_2$.
31. Explain why there is belching subsequent to taking a "dose" of sodium bicarbonate.
32. Starch paste is an excellent antidote for iodine. Explain.
33. Salt water is an excellent antidote for silver salts. Explain.
34. Why is hydrogen peroxide marketed in brown bottles?
35. Compare oxygen and ozone.
36. Explain the tarnishing of silver.
37. How could you tell sodium bircarbonate from potassium nitrate?
38. Explain why a laboratory painted with a white lead paint darkens prematurely.
39. Discuss the composition of the atmosphere.
40. In agriculture what is the principal reason for growing alfalfa?
41. Discuss the Haber process.
42. How could you distinguish between KCl and NaCl?
43. What happens when chlorine water is added to a solution of sodium bromide?
44. How could you distinguish between KNO_3 and K_2SO_4?
45. Name five metals that are found in protoplasm.
46. What is spectroscopy?
47. Distinguish between cations and anions.
48. Write the equation for the reaction between calcium oxide and phosphoric acid.
49. What are the three chief elements of bone?
50. Briefly describe the extraction of iron from its ore.
51. Why does distilled water produce a better suds than regular water?
52. Following a "blood check" of the patient, the doctor prescribed ferrous sulfate. Explain.
53. How could you distinguish between $FeSO_4$ and $Fe_2(SO_4)_3$?
54. The layman is usually surprised to learn that aluminum is the most abundant metal. Why?
55. What is milk of magnesia?
56. What is the chief use of copper metal?
57. What is the chief copper compound?
58. Discuss the medical use of $AgNO_3$ in the prevention of *ophthalmia neonatorum.*
59. What is plumbism?
60. Why is gold ideally suited for the making of jewelry?
61. What is meant by radioactivity?
62. What is a radioactive isotope?
63. Explain the meaning of half-life.
64. Discuss natural and artificial transmutation.
65. Distinguish between fission and fusion.
66. Discuss the formula $E = mc^2$.
67. Briefly describe the construction of an atomic reactor.
68. Discuss the relationship of radioactivity to health and disease.
69. Distinguish between a solution and a sol.
70. What is an emulsion?
71. How could you distinguish between a true solution and a colloidal system?
72. What is brownian movement?
73. Charcoal and kaolin (a highly purified clay) are highly effective in preventing the absorption of poisons from the gastrointestinal tract. Explain.

74. A solution containing starch, sugar, and salt was poured into a cellophane bag, and the latter was immersed in a large beaker of water. What was the fate of the solutes?
75. Compute the molecular weight of $CuSO_4 \cdot 5H_2O$.
76. Explain how you would prepare 5 ounces of a 1 percent solution of silver nitrate.
77. If 1 liter of 5 percent glucose solution is given intravenously, how much glucose does the patient receive?
78. How many liters of 70 percent alcohol can be prepared from 10 liters of absolute (100 percent) alcohol?
79. How would you prepare 500 ml. of a 2M solution of HNO_3?
80. How many grams of $NaHCO_3$ does it take to neutralize 20 gm. of HCl?
81. How would you prepare 3 liters of 1N HCl?
82. How many liters of hydrogen are needed to yield 60 liters of ammonia via the Haber process?
83. If a solution has a $[K^+]$ of 7 mEq. per liter, what would this be in milligrams percent?
84. How many milliliters of 2N acetic acid does it take to neutralize 25 ml. of 0.5N ammonium hydroxide?
85. How would you prepare 2 ounces of 2 percent tincture of iodine?

Chapter 5

Basic organic chemistry

Although it is certainly not correct to consider one area of chemistry as being independent of other areas, we shall, for pedagogic reasons, follow standard procedure and devote a very special section to organic chemistry.

Organic chemistry is the study of *carbon compounds.* Whereas noncarbon or inorganic compounds number in the vicinity of seventy thousand, there are more than one million known compounds of carbon derived from synthetic and natural sources. This huge number of substances is explained by the fact that carbon atoms have the unique ability to combine with one another in an endless number of ways. Further, in many instances simple organic molecules may combine with each other to form highly complex molecules—a process called *polymerization.* For these reasons, that is, "number and complexity," the study of organic chemistry demands, at the elementary level at least, special concern with classification. This is the principal objective of the present chapter.

STRUCTURAL FORMULA AND ISOMERISM

The properties of an organic compound depend upon the arrangement of its atoms as well as upon their number and kind. This is epitomized by *isomerism,* the interesting situation in which two or more compounds have the same empirical formula but different properties. The organic chemist accounts for this phenomenon by means of the structural formula, a graphic representation showing the manner in which the atoms are apparently hooked together. This is exquisitely illustrated by the two isomers that have the empirical formula C_2H_6O. Their structural formulas are drawn as follows:

```
    H  H              H     H
    |  |              |     |
 H—C—C—O—H         H—C—O—C—H
    |  |              |     |
    H  H              H     H
```

The writing of structural formulas, then, is something that everyone must be able to do when dealing with organic compounds. For the present, when referring to the structures just given, the student should understand two basic facts: (1) carbon has a covalence of 4 (that is, it must be written with four valence bonds) and (2) the number of bonds about any one atom must be equal to its valence. In this regard it should be noted that each hydrogen atom has one bond, each oxygen atom two bonds, and each carbon atom four bonds.

To save time and space, the structural formula is often abbreviated. This procedure is acceptable, provided that there is no ambiguity. To illustrate, the structure for C_3H_7Cl may be condensed as follows:

```
    H  H  H
    |  |  |
 H—C——C——C—H
    |  |  |
    H  Cl H
```

or

$CH_3—CHCl—CH_3$

Optical isomerism. A peculiar type of isomerism is shown by many organic substances. Lactic acid will serve as a typical example. All three varieties of this acid possess the same physical and chemical properties but differ with respect to their effect upon polarized light; hence, they are said to be optically active. When polarized light is passed through each of the three acids, the following happens: One kind turns the plane of polarized light to the right and is called *dextro* or *d*-lactic acid, another turns the plane of light to the left and is called *levo* or *l*-lactic acid, and the third has no effect upon polarized light and is called *racemic* or *dl*-lactic acid. (The lat-

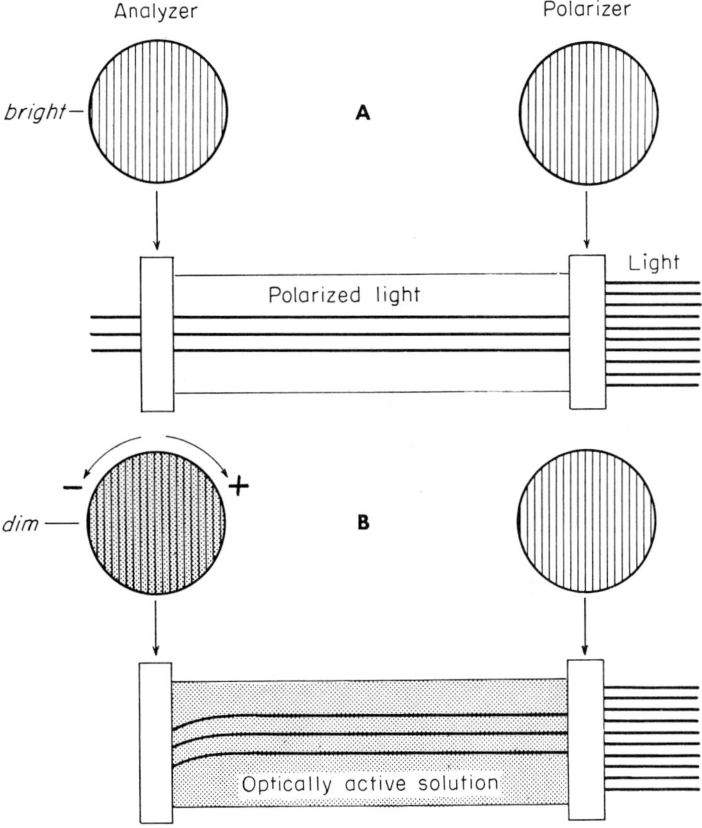

Fig. 5-1. Operation of the polarimeter. **A,** The "analyzer" Polaroid glass is first adjusted for maximum light transfer. **B,** An optically active compound in solution has been added to the glass tube. Since the compound causes polarized light "to turn," the light will not pass completely through the analyzer; hence, the latter becomes dim. Now by rotating the analyzer to the left or right, depending upon whether the compound is levorotatory or dextrorotatory, the brightness can be restored. The number of degrees through which the analyzer must be turned is then noted on a calibrated scale. (From Brooks, S. M.: Basic facts of general chemistry, Philadelphia, 1956, W. B. Saunders Co.)

ter is actually a mixture of equal parts of the *d*- and *l*- forms.) The polarimeter, the apparatus used to measure optical activity, is shown in Fig. 5-1.

Optical isomers, particularly optically active drugs, differ a great deal physiologically. *Dexedrine,* for example, which is chemically *d*-amphetamine, is considerably more stimulating to the cerebral cortex than *Benzedrine* or *dl*-amphetamine. Therefore, when a new synthetic drug turns out to be optically active, all three forms must be isolated and tested separately.

HYDROCARBONS

Hydrocarbons are composed of only two elements—carbon and hydrogen—and theoretically may be considered the "starting point" of all other organic compounds. They range in complexity from a few atoms per molecule to compounds with a hundred or more atoms per molecule. Hydrocarbons occur naturally in petroleum and coal tar (Fig. 5-2).

There are two major categories of hydrocarbons: those whose carbon atoms are joined in open chains (*aliphatic* hydrocarbons) and those whose atoms are joined in closed chains (*cyclic* hydrocarbons). The latter category, in turn, is divided into the so-called *aromatic* and *alicylic* hydrocarbons.

The aliphatic hydrocarbons fall into various classes, or series, depending upon their chemical structure. The most important are the *methane, ethylene,* and *acetylene* series.

Methane series. The hydrocarbons of the methane series are often termed *paraffins.*

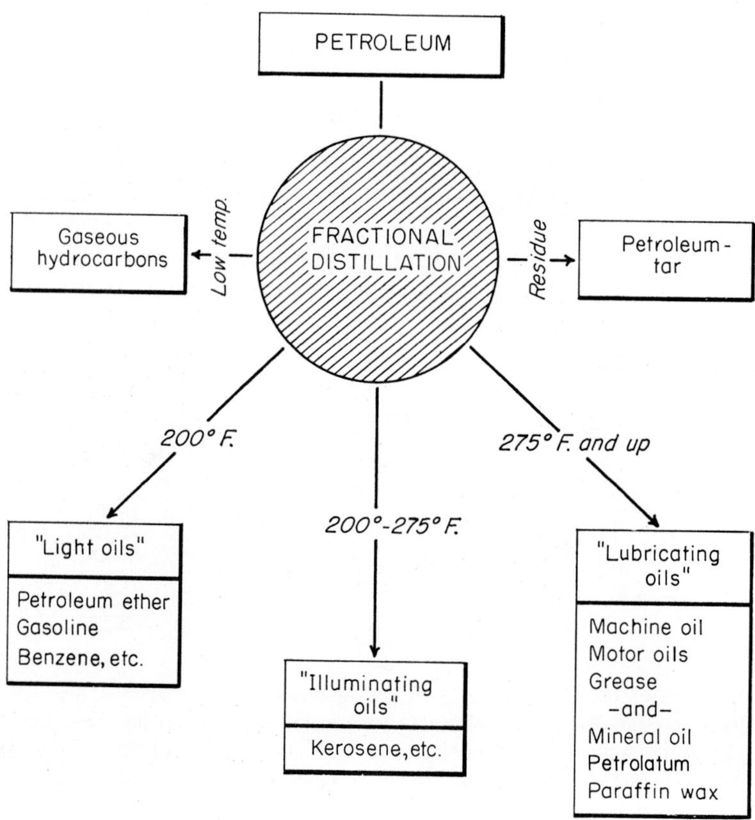

Fig. 5-2. Products of petroleum. (From Brooks, S. M.: Basic facts of general chemistry, Philadelphia, 1956, W. B. Saunders Co.)

Table 5-1. Methane series

	Formula	Boiling point (° C.)
Methane	CH_4	−161.5
Ethane	C_2H_6	− 88.3
Propane	C_3H_8	− 44.5
Butane	C_4H_{10}	− 0.45
Pentane	C_5H_{12}	36.2
Hexane	C_6H_{14}	68.9
Heptane	C_7H_{16}	98.5
Octane	C_8H_{18}	125.8
Nonane	C_9H_{20}	150.7
Decane	$C_{10}H_{22}$	174

(Paraffin is a mixture of solid hydrocarbons of this series.) The names, formulas, and boiling points of the first ten members are given in Table 5-1. Others are known as far up as twenty-eight carbon atoms; the first ten, however, are the most important.

A glance at the table will disclose the singular fact that each member of the series differs from the one preceding it by the group of atoms CH_2. Such a series of hydrocarbons is called a homologous series. Further, the formula for any member of the series is given by the general formula C_nH_{2n+2}, where n represents the number of carbon atoms. In general, the members of a homologous series are similar in their chemical characteristics. Their physical properties show a fairly regular gradation; for example, their physical state (gas, liquid, or solid) is a function of their molecular weight.

The methane hydrocarbons are all colorless compounds. The first four members—methane, ethane, propane, and butane—are gases, those containing five to sixteen carbon atoms are liquids, and those containing more than sixteen carbon atoms are solids. *All members of this series are insoluble in water. Chemically, they are rather inert; strong acids and bases have little or no effect upon them. All of them burn, however, to form carbon dioxide and water.*

Table 5-2. Ethylene series

	Formula	Boiling point (° C.)
Ethylene (ethene)	C_2H_4	−104
Propylene (propene)	C_3H_6	− 47
Butylene (butene)	C_4H_8	− 1.4
Amylene (pentene)	C_5H_{10}	40
Hexylene (hexene)	C_6H_{12}	64
Heptylene (heptene)	C_7H_{14}	95

Ethylene series. Ethylene is a hydrocarbon that has the formula C_2H_4. If we attempt to write a structural formula for this compound, we find that the laws of valence seem to be violated. Thus,

```
  H  H
  |  |
H—C—C—H
```

In this structural formula each carbon atom is surrounded by *three* bonds instead of *four*. Therefore, how can there be a compound with the empirical formula C_2H_4? The answer resides in the fact that there is a *double bond* between the two carbons. Thus,

```
  H  H
  |  |
H—C═C—H
```

Ethylene is the first member of the ethylene series of hydrocarbons (Table 5-2). Each member, like ethylene, is characterized by the presence of a double bond. The general formula for hydrocarbons of this series is C_nH_{2n}.

As in the methane series, the lower members are gases and the higher members are liquids or solids. Chemically, however, there is an important difference between the two series. In contrast to the paraffins, members of the ethylene series are relatively active. This can be explained only on a basis of the double bond. It appears that when given the opportunity the carbon atoms that share a double bond prefer to dissolve this relationship; that is, a double bond imparts an unstable nature to a molecule. The halogens, for example, swiftly break the bond and add onto the molecule. Bromine reacts with ethylene as follows:

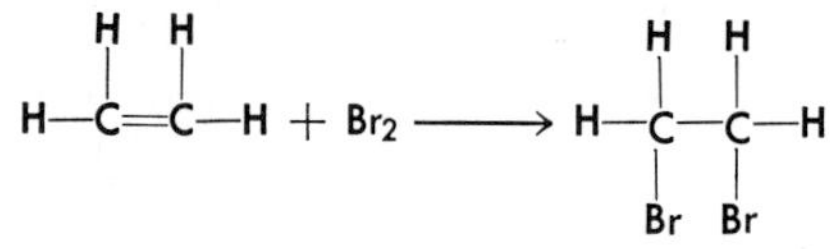

$$\mathrm{H{-}\overset{\displaystyle H}{\overset{|}{C}}{=}\overset{\displaystyle H}{\overset{|}{C}}{-}H + Br_2 \longrightarrow H{-}\underset{\displaystyle Br}{\underset{|}{\overset{\displaystyle H}{\overset{|}{C}}}}{-}\underset{\displaystyle Br}{\underset{|}{\overset{\displaystyle H}{\overset{|}{C}}}}{-}H}$$

A hydrocarbon or any other organic compound with *carbon* double bonds is said to be *unsaturated;* that is, it is capable of adding on atoms. The compound formed as a result of the *addition* is termed an addition product. Conversely, compounds that do not contain such bonds are said to be *saturated.* Saturated compounds react by *substitution;* that is, atoms are exchanged for hydrogen. Bromine reacts with methane in the presence of ultraviolet or other higher-frequency light as follows:

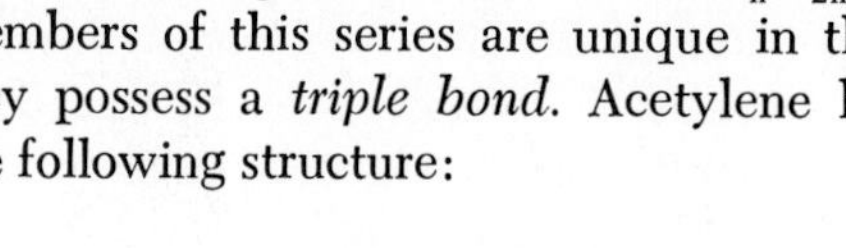

$$\mathrm{H{-}\underset{\displaystyle H}{\underset{|}{\overset{\displaystyle H}{\overset{|}{C}}}}{-}H + Br_2 \longrightarrow H{-}\underset{\displaystyle H}{\underset{|}{\overset{\displaystyle H}{\overset{|}{C}}}}{-}Br + HBr}$$

Acetylene series. Acetylene gas (C_2H_2) is by far the most important member of a series whose general formula is C_nH_{2n-2}. Members of this series are unique in that they possess a *triple bond.* Acetylene has the following structure:

$$\mathrm{H{-}C{\equiv}C{-}H}$$

The first three members of the series are as follows:

Ethyne (acetylene)	C_2H_2
Propyne	C_3H_4
Butyne	C_4H_6

The properties of acetylene are illustrative of its homologues. Physically, acetylene is colorless, possesses a garliclike odor, and is sparingly soluble in water. Chemically, it is marked by extreme activity. For example, it combines readily with chlorine, forming an addition compound having the formula, $C_2H_2Cl_4$.

The reaction is as follows:

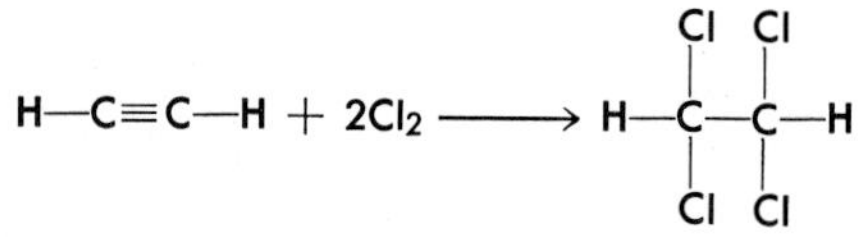

$$\mathrm{H{-}C{\equiv}C{-}H + 2Cl_2 \longrightarrow H{-}\underset{\displaystyle Cl}{\underset{|}{\overset{\displaystyle Cl}{\overset{|}{C}}}}{-}\underset{\displaystyle Cl}{\underset{|}{\overset{\displaystyle Cl}{\overset{|}{C}}}}{-}H}$$

Since it takes four atoms of chlorine to saturate one molecule, we are presented with good evidence that acetylene has a triple bond.

Naming aliphatics. The ability to name an organic compound is a *sine qua non* in organic chemistry. Although time and space obviously do not allow a study of the details here, we must not, however, stray from the fundamental ideas. Anyway, for our purposes, the latter will suffice.

Methane series. The name for any member of the methane series has the suffix *-ane* (Table 5-1). With the exception of the first four members, the first part of the name indicates the number of carbon atoms in the molecule. When a hydrogen atom is removed from any member of the methane series, the resulting group is called an *alkyl radical;* the radical is named by changing the final syllable of the hydrocarbon name from *-ane* to *-yl.*

In order to name paraffin isomers, we must modify our rule. There are, for example, three pentanes. In order to have a different name for each of the three structures, the following convention is followed: First, structural formulas are written for the possible arrangements; second, the longest chain is numbered in such a manner that the side radicals are attached to the carbons of the lowest possible numbers; third, we base the name for each compound on the longest chain. The naming of the three pentanes is done as follows:

$CH_3—CH_2—CH_2—CH_2—CH_3$
5 carbons in a straight chain
Name: *n*-Pentane*

```
1       2       3       4
CH3—CH—CH2—CH3
        |
        CH3
```
2-Methylbutane

```
CH3—CH2—CH2—CH2—CH2—CH3
    |       |
    CH3     CH3
```
2,3-Dimethylhexane

Ethylene series. The hydrocarbons of the ethylene series are named by replacing the suffix *-ane* of the paraffin hydrocarbon having the same number of carbon atoms with the suffix *-ylene* or *-ene.* Isomerism in this series is due not only to branching in the carbon chains but also to changes in the position of the double bond. Isomeric members and derivatives are therefore named by numbering the compound in such a way that the smallest possible numbers are assigned to the unsaturated carbon atoms. Thus,

```
                            CH3
                            |
CH3—CH═CH—CH2—CH—CH3
1       2       3       4       5       6
```
5-Methyl-2-hexene

Acetylene series. The name of any homologue of the acetylene series is derived from that of the methane hydrocarbon that contains the same number of carbon atoms by replacing the suffix *-ane* with *-yne.* Thus, C_2H_2 (acetylene) is called *ethyne,* and $CH_3C \equiv CH$ is called *propyne,* and so on. The triple bond is located in the manner used for the olefins.

Aromatic hydrocarbons. Use of the term *aromatic* has its origin in the fact that certain aromatic substances (for example, oil of bitter almonds, vanilla, and oil of wintergreen) are cyclic compounds. The possession of an odor is not characteristic, however, of all aromatic substances.

It is, indeed, a difficult task to find an adjective that embraces the significance of the chemistry of aromatic hydrocarbons and their derivatives. It is certainly an exact statement of truth to say that our lives have been revolutionized by discoveries in this area of organic chemistry. Miracle drugs, modern insecticides (for example, DDT), dyes, plastics, and explosives are but a small part of the complete picture.

Table 5-3. Benzene series

Benzene	C_6H_6
Toluene	C_7H_8
Xylene	C_8H_{10}
Mesitylene	C_9H_{12}
Cymene	$C_{10}H_{14}$

Benzene series. Benzene (C_6H_6) is the most important member of the so-called benzene series, whose general formula is C_nH_{2n-6}. The principal homologues are shown in Table 5-3.

Benzene, together with some of the other members of the series, is a product of the destructive distillation of bituminous coal; that is, the coal is heated in the absence of air. First, combustible gases escape; then a viscous black liquid distills out, leaving a residue of coke in the retort. This black liquid, called *coal tar,* is one of the most valuable raw materials of the chemical industry. When subjected to fractional distillation, it yields a conglomeration of aromatic substances; of these, benzene, toluene, naphthalene, anthracene, phenol, and cresol are the most important. Each of these substances serves as the source material from which thousands of other useful compounds are prepared (Fig. 5-3). Such compounds, whether obtained directly or indirectly, are commonly referred to as coal-tar derivatives.

The general properties of the series are reflected by those of benzene. Benzene

**n* means "normal" or straight chain.

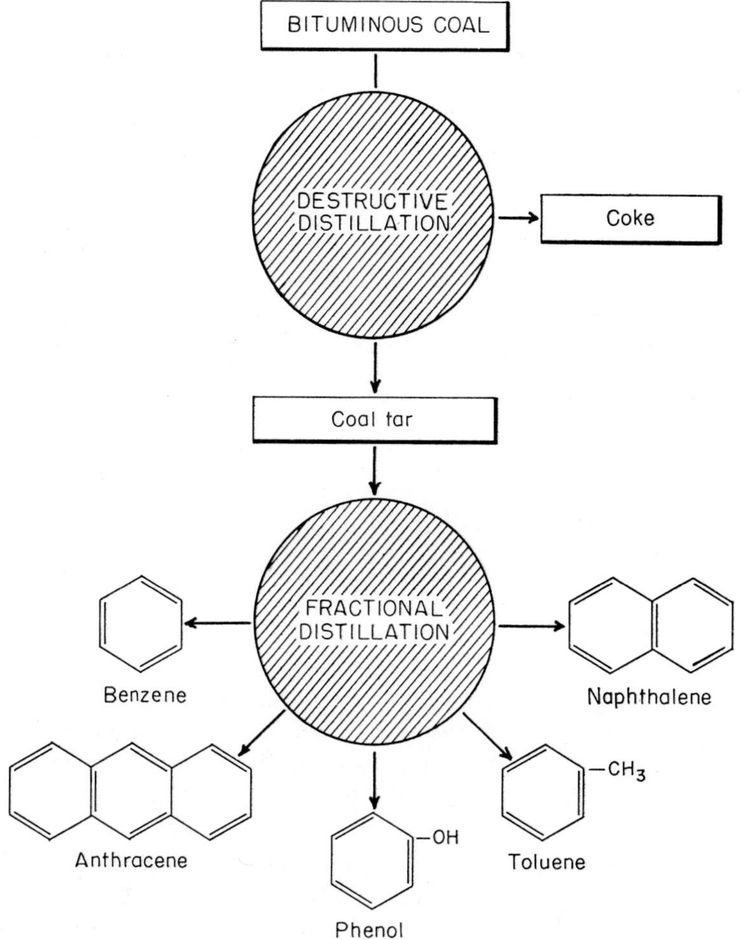

Fig. 5-3. Coal-tar derivatives. (From Brooks, S. M.: Basic facts of general chemistry, Philadelphia, 1956, W. B. Saunders Co.)

is a colorless liquid that boils at 80° C. It has a peculiar, pleasant odor. Several of the other homologues have a similar odor. Benzene is insoluble in water but soluble in alcohol and chloroform. It burns with a bright, luminous, smoky flame. The ring structure of the benzene molecule is well established:

H
C
HC CH
HC CH
C
H

For the sake of convenience, however, the organic chemist usually abbreviates the structure as follows:

Toluene, with the empirical formula C_7H_8, has the following structure:

CH_3

In contrast to the aliphatic hydrocarbons, benzene and its homologues react with a variety of common laboratory chemicals to form many highly useful substituted derivatives. With nitric acid, for example, benzene readily forms nitrobenzene—a source material from which several dyes and drugs are prepared:

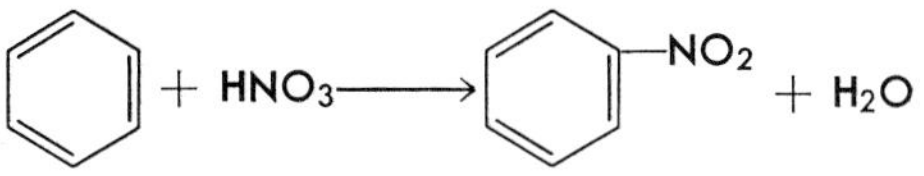

$$C_6H_6 + HNO_3 \longrightarrow C_6H_5NO_2 + H_2O$$

NOMENCLATURE. The first few members of the benzene series have common names ending in *-ene.* In order to name a more complex member, however, it is most convenient to consider the member as a derivative of benzene. For example, $C_{12}H_{18}$ is best named hexamethylbenzene:

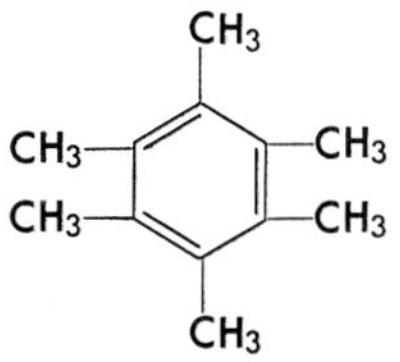

There are no isomers of benzene or toluene. Since all six carbon atoms of the benzene ring are "equivalent," it makes no difference at which position *one* group is attached. Xylene, however, presents a different situation. For reasons that are quite obvious (namely, the distance between the attached groups), the following structures are *not* the same:

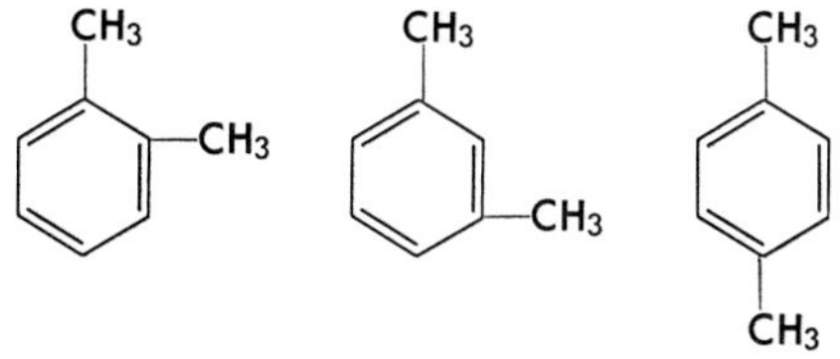

A B C

Formula A shows the two methyl groups on neighboring carbon atoms, formula B has one carbon atom separating the groups, and formula C has two carbon atoms between the groups. Isomer A is called *ortho-* or *o-xylene;* isomer B, *meta-* or *m-xylene;* and isomer C, *para-* or *p-xylene.* The prefixes *ortho-*, *meta-*, and *para-* are employed also for naming other derivatives of benzene. For example, *p*-dichlorobenzene is the name for the following structure:

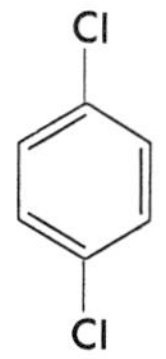

When more than two groups are attached to the benzene ring, we must employ numbers to locate their positions. The ring is numbered as follows:

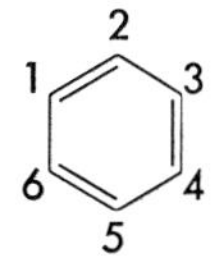

For example, 1,2,3,-tribromobenzene is the name for the following structure:

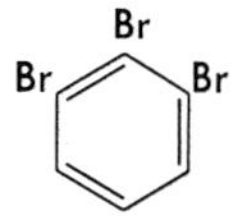

When a hydrogen atom is removed (that is, substituted by another atom or group) from a member of the benzene series, the residue is called an *aryl radical;* C_6H_5- is called *phenyl,* C_7H_7- is called *tolyl,* C_8H_9- is called *xylyl,* and so on. The phenyl radical is the most common of the aromatic substances. It will be recalled that important radicals *(alkyl radicals)* are also derived from the methane series (for example, methyl, ethyl, propyl, and the like). A knowledge of radicals is useful in the naming of organic compounds; we shall have frequent occasion to use them.

Naphthalene. Naphthalene ($C_{10}H_8$) is present to the extent of about 6 percent in coal tar, from which it is obtained in large quantities. Naphthalene is a white, volatile solid with a characteristic penetrating odor (mothballs are almost pure naphthalene). It is soluble in hot alcohol and ether.

The relation of naphthalene to benzene has been discovered through a careful study of its chemical conduct. Its structural formula is as follows:

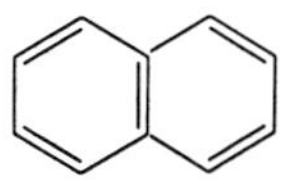

Naphthalene resembles benzene closely in its behavior with chemical reagents. Thus, derivatives are formed when it is treated with chlorine, bromine, nitric acid, or sulfuric acid. These derivatives are valuable source materials from which important dyes and drugs are manufactured.

Because of the presence of two rings, the opportunities for isomerism are great. Higher members of the class and their derivatives are named by numbering the carbon atoms as follows:

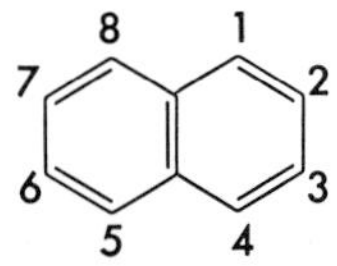

8 1 7 2 6 3 5 4

Monosubstitution products exist in two forms. The carbon atoms numbered 1, 4, 5, and 8 bear the same relation to the molecule. Compounds with an atom or radical in these positions are called *alpha* (α) compounds. Compounds with an atom in position 2, 3, 6, or 7 are called *beta* (β) compounds. For example, α-chloronaphthalene and β-chloronaphthalene are the names for the following structures:

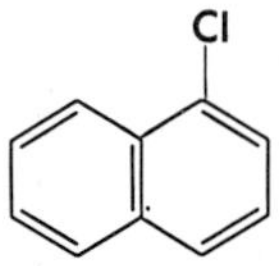

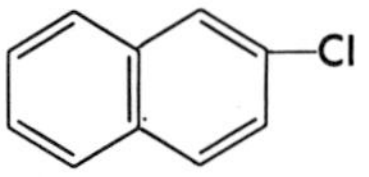

Cl Cl

α-Chloronaphthalene **β-Chloronaphthalene**

When two or more groups are present, however, numbers must be employed. For example, *2-ethyl-3-methyl-naphthalene* is the name for the following structure:

C_2H_5 CH_3

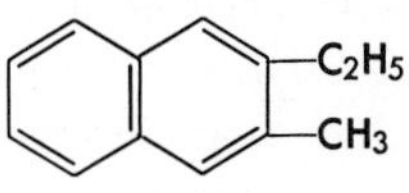

Anthracene. Anthracene ($C_{14}H_{10}$) is obtained from coal tar, in which it is present to the extent of less than 0.5 percent. When pure, it forms colorless monoclinic (needle-like) plates, showing a beautiful blue fluorescence. The structure of anthracene is of singular interest. The following structure is arrived at as a result of a number of syntheses of the hydrocarbon:

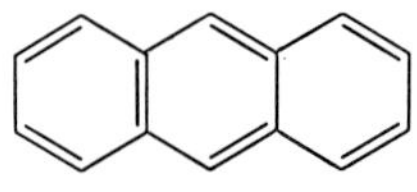

For the purpose of naming derivatives, the anthracene molecule is numbered as shown below:

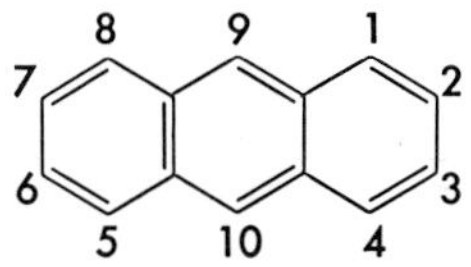

8 9 1 7 2 6 3 5 10 4

Monosubstitution products exist in three forms. The carbon atoms numbered 1, 4, 5, and 8 bear the same relation to the molecule. Compounds with a group in these positions are called *alpha* (α) compounds. Compounds with a group in position 2, 3, 6, or 7 are called *beta* (β) compounds. Positions 9 and 10 are called *gamma* (γ). For example, β-bromoanthracene has the following structure:

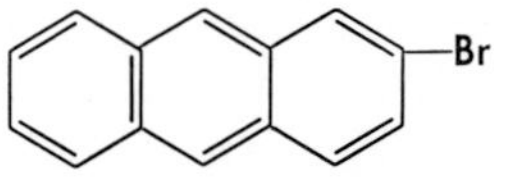

Br

When two or more groups are present, the numbers must be used. Thus, 1,2,9-tribromoanthracene is the name for the following structure:

Br Br Br

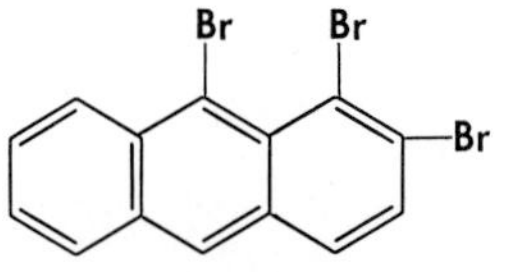

Phenanthrene. Phenanthrene ($C_{14}H_{10}$) is isomeric with anthracene. Its mode of synthesis indicates that its structure is as follows:

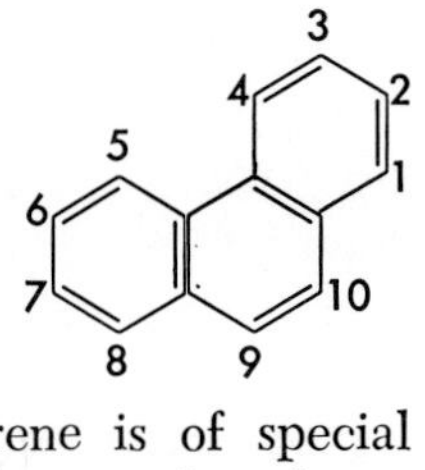

3 4 2 5 1 6 7 10 8 9

Phenanthrene is of special interest because morphine and codeine are phenanthrene derivatives. The structures for morphine and codeine are as follows:

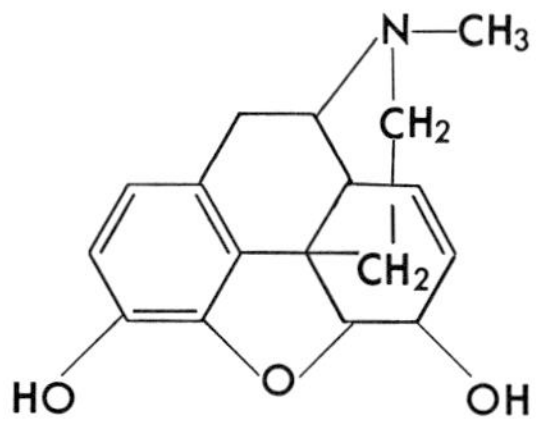

Morphine

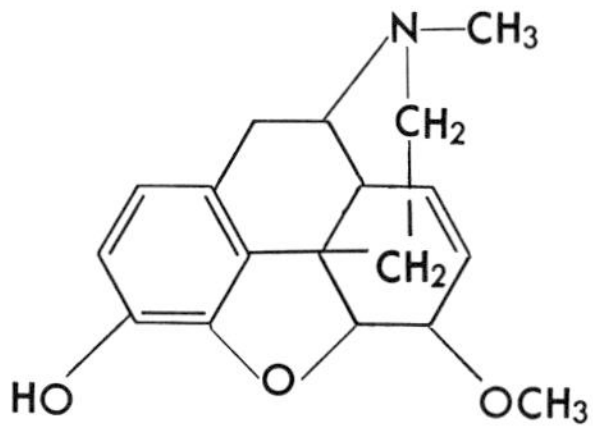

Codeine

Cyclopentanoperhydrophenanthrene. This unwieldy hydrocarbon, a relative of phenanthrene, and its derivatives are often referred to as steroids. For purposes of nomenclature, the structural formula is numbered as follows:

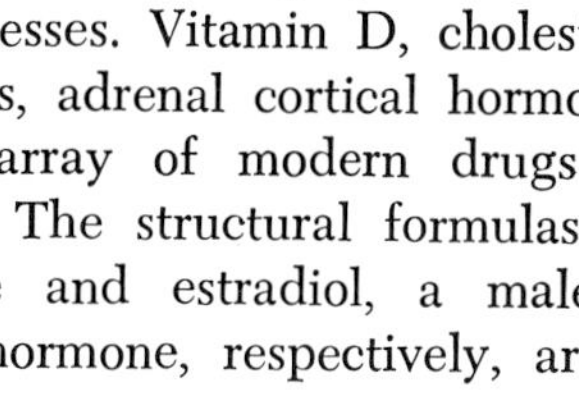

Steroid substances play a vital role in the life processes. Vitamin D, cholesterol, sex hormones, adrenal cortical hormones, and a vast array of modern drugs are all steroids. The structural formulas for testosterone and estradiol, a male and a female hormone, respectively, are as follows:

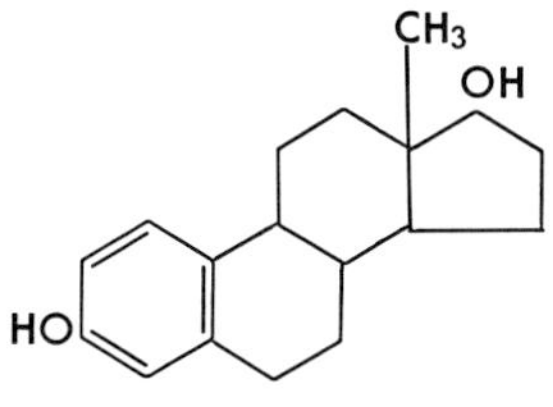

Estradiol

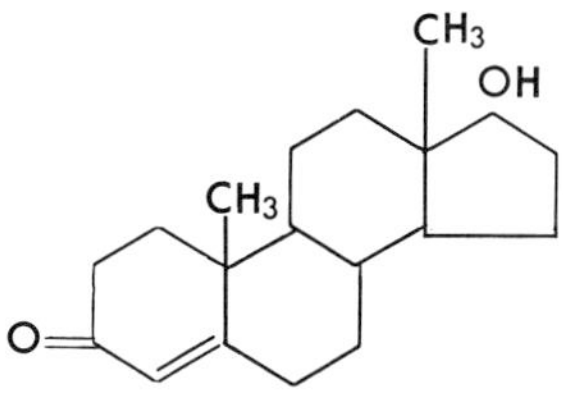

Testosterone

Just a glance at these structures lends some credence to the old saying that "the only difference between a male and female is a methyl group."

Alicyclic hydrocarbons. Alicyclic hydrocarbons are cyclic compounds that resemble both aliphatic and aromatic hydrocarbons, particularly the former. A compound of this class is named by adding the prefix *cyclo-* to the name of the aliphatic hydrocarbon that contains the same number of carbon atoms. Thus, cyclopropane and cyclohexane have the following structures:

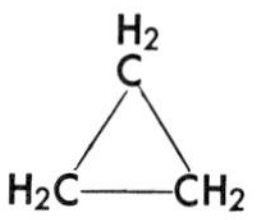

Cyclopropane

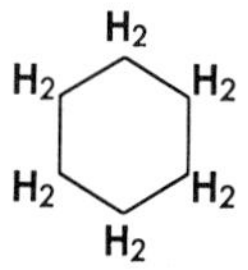

Cyclohexane

When using abbreviated ring symbols, we should make certain that we do not confuse the alicyclics with the aromatics. Benzene and cyclohexane, for example, should always be written as follows:

Benzene

Cyclohexane

Although many substances that occur in nature are alicyclics (for example, the terpenes, camphors, and naphthenes), the class at present is of lesser importance than the aromatics.

Cyclopropane. Cyclopropane ($[CH_2]_3$) deserves special mention because it is the simplest alicylic hydrocarbon. Moreover, it is steadily gaining in popularity as a potent anesthetic gas. As an anesthetic, however, it suffers a grave disadvantage in that it is extremely explosive.

HALOGEN DERIVATIVES

A large number of compounds may be formed from the hydrocarbons by the substitution of halogen elements (for example, fluorine, chlorine, bromine, and iodine) for hydrogen atoms. In the case of unsaturated hydrocarbons, addition takes place. Although it is possible to form such compounds through direct action of the halogen and the hydrocarbon, it is usually a much simpler matter to do this by other methods.

Chloromethanes. When chlorine reacts with methane (in the presence of sunlight) there are four possible derivatives, depending upon the conditions under which the reaction is carried out. The reactions are as follows:

$$(1)\quad \begin{array}{c} H \\ | \\ H{-}C{-}H \\ | \\ H \end{array} + Cl_2 \longrightarrow \begin{array}{c} H \\ | \\ H{-}C{-}Cl \\ | \\ H \end{array} + HCl$$

$$(2)\quad \begin{array}{c} H \\ | \\ H{-}C{-}H \\ | \\ H \end{array} + 2Cl_2 \longrightarrow \begin{array}{c} Cl \\ | \\ H{-}C{-}Cl \\ | \\ H \end{array} + 2HCl$$

$$(3)\quad \begin{array}{c} H \\ | \\ H{-}C{-}H \\ | \\ H \end{array} + 3Cl_2 \longrightarrow \begin{array}{c} Cl \\ | \\ H{-}C{-}Cl \\ | \\ Cl \end{array} + 3HCl$$

$$(4)\quad \begin{array}{c} H \\ | \\ H{-}C{-}H \\ | \\ H \end{array} + 4Cl_2 \longrightarrow \begin{array}{c} Cl \\ | \\ Cl{-}C{-}Cl \\ | \\ Cl \end{array} + 4HCl$$

These compounds and all other halogen derivatives are named on the basis of the hydrocarbon from which they were derived. Thus,

(1) CH_3Cl–monochloromethane (methyl chloride)
(2) CH_2Cl_2–dichloromethane
(3) $CHCl_3$–trichloromethane (chloroform)
(4) CCl_4–tetrachloromethane (carbon tetrachloride)

Compounds of extensive value such as trichloromethane and tetrachloromethane are usually known under a more popular name (in this instance, *chloroform* and *carbon tetrachloride*, respectively).

Chloroform. Chloroform ($CHCl_3$) is a heavy, colorless, sweet-smelling, nonflammable liquid with potent anesthetic properties. Because of its toxic effects upon the heart and liver (p. 113), however, it is seldom used as an anesthetic. Chloroform is an excellent solvent for fats, oils, and resins.

Carbon tetrachloride. Carbon tetrachloride (CCl_4) is a nonflammable, colorless liquid with a low boiling point. Because the liquid (and its vapor) has proved so highly toxic, it is no longer recommended for use as a fire extinguisher or cleaning fluid. It is an excellent organic solvent.

Iodomethanes. The most important iodine derivative of methane is triiodomethane, commonly known as iodoform (CHI_3). This is a yellow powder with an extremely characteristic odor (perhaps best described as medicinal). Iodoform still enjoys some use as an antiseptic dusting powder. It is readily prepared by the action of iodine and sodium hydroxide on ethyl alcohol. This reaction is often used as a test for ethyl alcohol.

Chlorobenzenes. Just about any halogen derivative desired can be prepared from the aromatic hydrocarbons. The reaction of benzene with chlorine will serve as an example. Of the chlorobenzene derivatives, *p*-dichlorobenzene is of commercial importance. This compound has the following structure:

Cl

Cl

From our previous work with isomerism we know that there are two other di-chlorobenzenes—ortho (*o*-) and meta (*m*-). Only the para form, however, possesses insecticidal properties.

Test for saturation. Bromine and iodine are frequently employed in the laboratory to determine whether a compound is saturated or unsaturated. It will be recalled that unsaturated compounds are much more reactive than are saturated compounds. When, for example, a solution of bromine is added to an unsaturated compound, the reddish brown color of the solution quickly disappears; that is, an "addition" product is formed. Saturated substances react at a much slower rate, and sometimes not at all. Ethylene reacts with bromine as follows:

$$H_2C{=}CH_2 + Br_2 \longrightarrow H_2C(Br){-}CH_2(Br)$$

Dibromoethane

Identification. Halogenated organic compounds may be identified in a rather crude but fairly accurate fashion. A copper wire is dipped into the compound and is then held in the flame of a Bunsen burner. A positive reaction is indicated by a green flame.

Generic formula. Throughout our work with the various classes of organic compounds, we shall find it convenient to employ a general or so-called generic formula. The generic formula for halogenated derivatives may be given by RX, where *R* stands for an alkyl or aryl group and *X* stands for the halogen element.

ALCOHOLS

Alcohols, a large and important class of organic compounds, are hydroxyl derivatives of hydrocarbons. There are three classes of alcohols: primary, secondary, and tertiary. A primary alcohol is one in which the hydroxyl group is attached to a carbon atom which, in turn, is attached to not more than *one* other carbon atom; a secondary alcohol is one in which the hydroxyl group is attached to a carbon atom which, in turn, is connected to *two* carbon atoms; and a tertiary alcohol is one in which the carbon atom is attached to *three* other carbon atoms. Therefore, there are three generic formula:

$$R{-}C(H)(H){-}OH \qquad (RCH_2OH)$$

Primary alcohol

$$R{-}C(H)(OH){-}R \qquad (R_2CHOH)$$

Secondary alcohol

$$R{-}C(R)(OH){-}R \qquad (R_3COH)$$

Tertiary alcohol

Although all alcohols share common properties, the behavior of any one alcohol depends to some degree upon whether it is primary, secondary, or tertiary. Those which contain two, three, four, five, or six hydroxyl groups are referred to as polyhydroxy alcohols.

The alcohols discussed here are the most important of the entire class, and they are illustrative of the general behavior of this large group of compounds.

Methyl alcohol. Methyl alcohol (CH_3OH), also known as methanol or wood alcohol, the simplest alcohol possible, is one of the volatile products formed when wood is subjected to destructive distillation. Under proper conditions, carbon monoxide and hydrogen unite and form methyl alcohol:

$$CO + 2H_2 \longrightarrow H{-}C(H)(H){-}OH$$

Methyl alcohol, a colorless liquid that boils at 65° C., mixes with water in all proportions and is an excellent solvent. Many substances that are insoluble in other liquids are soluble in methyl alcohol. The alcohol burns with a pale blue flame that does not deposit soot. The equation is as follows:

$$2CH_3OH + 3O_2 \longrightarrow 2CO_2 + 4H_2O$$

Chemically, methyl alcohol reacts with several substances. It reacts with acids, for example, to form an important group of compounds called *esters*. (Esters will be discussed in a subsequent section.)

Commercially, methyl alcohol is used extensively as a solvent and in the preparation of dyes and formaldehyde. In addition, it is a valuable solvent and reagent in the laboratory. Methyl alcohol is sometimes used in the biology laboratory as a preservative for specimens.

Of vital toxicologic interest is the fact that methyl alcohol is a potent poison, with small doses causing partial or complete blindness. Its inherent toxicity, coupled with its availability, makes methyl alcohol a dangerous article in the laboratory, in industry, and in the household. There are numerous poisonings among persons who ingest methyl alcohol as a substitute for "alcohol" (that is, grain alcohol). Each year about 150 deaths result from ingestion of this substance.

Methyl alcohol is not as depressant to the central nervous system as grain alcohol. It differs from ordinary grain alcohol also in that it is not completely oxidized in the body to carbon dioxide and water. As a result, intermediate products (formaldehyde and formic acid) are produced. At one time it was thought that these products were the cause of the blindness mentioned in the preceding paragraph.

Ethyl alcohol. Ethyl alcohol (C_2H_5OH), also known as ethanol, grain alcohol, or "alcohol," is unquestionably the most "famous and infamous" compound known to man. There seems to be no other substance that has enlisted as much comment from the sages of chemistry, biology, and philosophy—past and present. Alcohol (or at least its properties) has been known since time immemorial. The ancient Egyptians, for example, were well aware of its spirituous and preservative properties. Ethyl alcohol is a primary alcohol with the following structure:

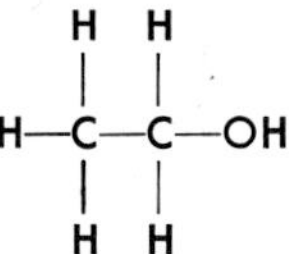

Ethyl alcohol is produced by the oldest chemical process known to man—*fermentation*, which may be defined as the degradation of carbohydrates (that is, sugars and starches) by organic catalysts called enzymes. (The subject of carbohydrates and enzymes is treated in some detail in Chapter 14.) For the present, let us just say that enzymes are complex chemical substances (of a protein nature) produced by living cells. Alcoholic fermentation is brought about by the addition of yeast to a warm solution of glucose ($C_6H_{12}O_6$). The yeast cells produce a variety of enzymes that collectively (as "zymase") bring about the following reaction:

$$\underset{\text{Glucose}}{C_6H_{12}O_6} \xrightarrow{\text{Zymase}} \underset{\text{Alcohol}}{2C_2H_5OH} + 2CO_2\uparrow$$

Cane sugar ($C_{12}H_{22}O_{11}$) is also fermented by yeast. Since zymase can act only upon simple sugars, the yeast must contain some other enzyme. This enzyme is called *invertase*. The fermentation of cane sugar is as follows:

$$C_{12}H_{22}O_{11} + H_2O \xrightarrow{\text{Invertase}} 2C_6H_{12}O_6$$

$$C_6H_{12}O_6 \xrightarrow{\text{Zymase}} 2C_2H_5OH + 2CO_2\uparrow$$

Starch, however, is the cheapest source material for producing ethyl alcohol and spirituous beverages. In this process, malt (which is made from sprouting barley) is added to a mixture of grain (source of starch) and water. An enzyme in the malt called *diastase* converts starch into maltose, an isomer of sucrose. Yeast is then added. The yeast acts upon the maltose in the manner described for sucrose, and alcohol is obtained from the mixture by fractional distillation. By distillation, however, it is possible to obtain only 95 percent alcohol.* When 100 percent alcohol *(absolute alcohol)* is desired, the 95 percent must be treated with a dehydrating agent such as lime. In recent years a totally synthetic process of producing ethyl alcohol has been adopted in some areas. The synthetic process starts with ethylene and sulfuric acid.

Pure ethyl alcohol has a peculiar, pleasant odor and boils at 78° C. It burns with a nonluminous flame that does not leave a deposit of soot. The effects of alcohol upon the body are a result of its depressant action upon the central nervous system. When taken in large doses, it may cause death. Chemically, ethyl alcohol reacts with a number of different chemical reagents, yielding a number of important ethyl esters.

Millions of gallons of alcohol are used annually in various types of industry. As a solvent, ethyl alcohol stands next to water. Numerous pharmaceutical preparations (for example, tinctures, spirits, and elixirs) contain medicaments dissolved in alcohol. Of course, all spirituous beverages contain ethyl alcohol as the "active" constituent. In order to provide alcohol for industrial use at low cost (that is, tax-free), the United States government permits the sale of *denatured* alcohol. Alcohol is denatured by adding substances such as methyl alcohol or pyridine, which render it unfit for human consumption.

Alcohols of propane. The alcohols of propane will serve to illustrate other facts about alcohols.

*Alcoholic beverages are commonly rated by "proof," which is equal to twice the percentage reading. For example, 80 proof means 40 percent alcohol.

Propyl alcohols. There are two alcohols with the empirical formula C_3H_7OH:

```
    H  H  H              H  H  H
    |  |  |              |  |  |
 H—C—C—C—OH          H—C—C—C—H
    |  |  |              |  |  |
    H  H  H              H  OH H
      (A)                  (B)
```

Compound A is called propyl alcohol and compound B is called isopropyl alcohol.* These alcohols have slightly different physical and chemical properties; for example, propyl alcohol boils at 98° C. and isopropyl boils at 82° C. It is to be noted that propyl alcohol is a primary alcohol, whereas isopropyl is a secondary alcohol. Derivatives of propyl and isopropyl alcohol contain the propyl (C_3H_7) and isopropyl radicals, respectively. The structures for these radicals are as follows:

```
    H  H  H              H  H  H
    |  |  |              |  |  |
 H—C—C—C—            H—C—C—C—H
    |  |  |              |     |
    H  H  H              H     H
    Propyl              Isopropyl
```

Glycerol. Glycerol ($C_3H_5[OH]_3$), also known as glycerin, is a trihydroxy derivative of propane. It has the following structure:

```
    H  H  H
    |  |  |
 H—C—C—C—H
    |  |  |
    OH OH OH
```

Glycerol is a heavy, sweet-tasting colorless liquid that is soluble in water. (A sweet taste is characteristic of polyhydroxy alcohols.) A by-product of the soap industry, it is employed in the manufacture of nitroglycerin and in the preparation of plastics, toilet articles, and pharmaceuticals. Since glycerol is a constituent of practically

*The prefix *iso-* is frequently employed when there are two isomers of a given empirical formula. Thus, there are two butanes: normal butane and isobutane. When there are more than two isomers, however, numbers are used.

all animal and vegetable fats and oils, it is obviously of biologic importance.

Nomenclature. Simple alcohols are named in the manner indicated previously (for example, methyl alcohol, ethyl alcohol, and so on). A more systematic and accurate method is to name the alcohol by replacing the final *-e* in the name of the hydrocarbon to which the alcohol is akin with the ending *-ol* (for example, methyl alcohol is methanol and ethyl alcohol is ethanol). When necessary, the name of the alcohol carries a number that indicates the position of the hydroxyl group of the chain. Alcohols that contain two or more hydroxyl groups are named in a similar way. And, too, the number of hydroxyl groups is indicated by prefixing the syllables *di, tri,* and so on to the suffix *-ol.* Alcohols with *one* hydroxl group at the end, that is, at the number 1 position, are often referred to as *normal.* The following are illustrative examples:

$CH_3—CH_2—CH_2—CH_2OH$

Butanol-1

$CH_3—CH_2—CHOH—CH_3$

Butanol-2

$CH_3—CH(CH_3)—CH_2—CH_2OH$

3-Methylbutanol-1

$CH_3—CHOH—CH_2OH$

Propanediol-1,2

$CH_2OH—CH_2—CH_2OH$

Propanediol-1,3
(isomeric with propanediol-1,2)

PHENOLS

The hydroxyl derivatives of the aromatic hydrocarbons are of two distinct classes: (1) those in which the hydroxyl group is situated in a side chain and (2) those in which the hydroxyl group is linked *directly* to the ring. The former class closely resembles the aliphatic alcohols, whereas members of the latter class, the phenols, possess acidic properties. Benzyl alcohol, for example, is a "regular" alcohol because the hydroxyl group is linked to the side chain. Its structure is as follows:

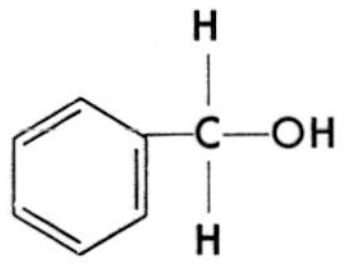

$C_6H_5—CH_2—OH$ $(C_6H_5—CH_2OH)$

Actually, this alcohol may be considered a substitution product of methyl alcohol, formed as the result of the replacement of one hydrogen atom by a phenyl radical.

Phenol. Phenol (C_6H_5OH), commonly known as carbolic acid, occurs in coal tar. It is a colorless substance that crystallizes in long needles that melt at 41° C. Phenol possesses a strong characteristic odor, described as phenolic.

Several of its derivatives, for example, picric acid and salicylic acid, are of commercial value. Phenol reacts with formaldehyde to form Bakelite and similar plastics. Although inferior to other antiseptics available at the present time, phenol continues to enjoy some use as a disinfectant and germicide. Of historic importance is the fact that phenol was the antiseptic used by Lister to herald "antiseptic surgery."

Cresol. Whereas phenol is derived from benzene, cresol is derived from toluene. There are three isomeric cresols:

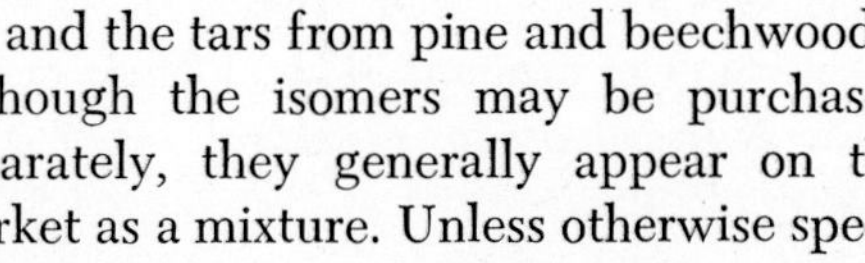

o-Cresol (CH3, OH)   *m*-Cresol (CH3, OH)   *p*-Cresol (HO, CH3)

These are all found along with other phenols in creosote. (Creosote is a mixture of chemical compounds contained in coal tar and the tars from pine and beechwood.) Although the isomers may be purchased separately, they generally appear on the market as a mixture. Unless otherwise specified, the term *cresol* refers to the mixture. Cresol closely resembles phenol and finds its most important use as a disinfectant and germicide. In this capacity it is superior to phenol.

ALDEHYDES

Aldehydes may be derived from primary alcohols by partial oxidation or, commercially, by catalytic dehydrogenation. This is of great theoretical and practical importance. Thus, from a given alcohol we can prepare the corresponding aldehyde. Aldehydes have the following generic formula:

$$\mathrm{R{-}C{\overset{\displaystyle H}{\diagup}}{\underset{\displaystyle O}{\diagdown\!\!\diagdown}}} \qquad (RCHO)$$

Formaldehyde. In the laboratory, formaldehyde (H • CHO) is obtained through the oxidation of methyl alcohol. When methyl alcohol vapor and air are passed over a hot copper gauze, formaldehyde gas and water are formed:

$$CH_3OH + [O] \longrightarrow HCHO + H_2O$$

Formaldehyde, the simplest aldehyde, is a water-soluble gas with a powerful, irritating odor. It is readily oxidized to formic acid and carbon dioxide; it is readily reduced by nascent hydrogen to methyl alcohol. Thus,

$$H{-}CHO + H_2 \longrightarrow CH_3OH$$

Formaldehyde appears on the market as formalin, a 37 percent aqueous solution of formaldehyde gas. The terms *formaldehyde* and *formalin* often are used synonymously, although at present *formaldehyde* seems to be the more popular term. Large quantities of formaldehyde are used in the manufacture of certain dyes, plastics (for example, Bakelite and Formica), and photographic films. In the biology laboratory it is used extensively as a preservative for anatomic specimens, and in the hospital it still enjoys some use as a disinfectant. Although formaldehyde was employed formerly as a food preservative, this practice now is prohibited by law.

Acetaldehyde. The liquid acetaldehyde ($CH_3 \cdot CHO$) is prepared by the oxidation of ethyl alcohol. The oxidation is effected by a mixture of sulfuric acid and potassium dichromate:

$$C_2H_5OH + [O] \longrightarrow H{-}\overset{\displaystyle H}{\underset{\displaystyle H}{\overset{|}{\underset{|}{C}}}}{-}\overset{\displaystyle H}{\overset{|}{C}}{=}O + H_2O$$

Acetaldehyde, commonly called acetic aldehyde or simply "aldehyde," is a colorless liquid that boils at 21° C. It mixes with water and alcohol in all proportions. From the chemical point of view the most characteristic property of aldehyde is its power to unite directly with other substances. Indeed, if left to itself, it changes readily into polymeric modifications, of which *paraldehyde* is the most important. The paraldehyde molecule is formed by the union of three aldehyde molecules; its formula is $(CH_3CHO)_3$. Paraldehyde has been used for years as a hypnotic.

Another interesting compound of acetaldehyde is chloral, which is formed by substitution of the three hydrogens of the methyl group with three chlorine atoms:

$$Cl{-}\overset{\displaystyle Cl}{\underset{\displaystyle Cl}{\overset{|}{\underset{|}{C}}}}{-}\overset{\displaystyle H}{\overset{|}{C}}{=}O$$

When chloral and water are brought together, they unite to form a crystallized compound called *chloral hydrate,* a valuable sedative and hypnotic.

Nomenclature. The simple aldehydes are usually named from the acids that they yield on oxidation; thus, H • CHO is *formic aldehyde,* or *formaldehyde,* and CH_3CHO is *acetic aldehyde,* or *acetaldehyde.* In the more systematic method the name of an aldehyde is formed by adding the suffix *-al* to the name of the hydrocarbon that contains the same number of carbon atoms. Accordingly, acetaldehyde is *ethanal.*

Identification. The ability of aldehydes to reduce other substances (that is, they are reducing agents) is of analytical significance. When an aldehyde or a compound containing an aldehyde group is added to an alkaline solution of a cupric salt (for example, Benedict's solution), a red precipitate of cuprous oxide (Cu_2O) is formed. The reactions may be summarized as follows:

$$Cu^{++} \xrightarrow{\text{Reducing agent}} Cu^{+}$$

$$2Cu^{+} + O^{=} \rightarrow Cu_2O\downarrow$$

KETONES

Ketones are closely allied to aldehydes. Whereas aldehydes are derived from *primary* alcohols by oxidation, ketones are derived from *secondary* alcohols by oxidation. The generic formula for ketones is as follows:

$$R{-}\underset{\underset{O}{\|}}{C}{-}R' \quad (RCOR')$$

The characteristic —C=O group is commonly referred to as the *carbonyl* group.

Although similar in structure, aldehydes and ketones differ in a few of their chemical properties. For example, aldehydes are reducing agents and ketones are not. This alone is of practical importance. The general properties of ketones are well illustrated by acetone.

Acetone. Acetone ($[CH_3]_2CO$) is the first member of the class and by far the most important. The formation of acetone as the result of the oxidation of isopropyl alcohol substantiates the generic formula for the group:

$$CH_3{-}\underset{\underset{OH}{|}}{\overset{\overset{H}{|}}{C}}{-}CH_3 + [O] \rightarrow CH_3{-}\underset{\underset{O}{\|}}{C}{-}CH_3 + H_2O$$

Acetone is a flammable liquid with a characteristic odor and a peppermint-like taste; it is miscible with water in all proportions and boils at 56.1° C. Acetone finds its greatest use as a solvent in a wide variety of industries. As a source material, it is used in the manufacture of chloroform, iodoform, and various resins and plastics.

Nomenclature. Ketones can be named in accordance with the groups represented by R:

$$CH_3{-}\underset{\underset{O}{\|}}{C}{-}CH_3$$

Dimethyl ketone

$$C_2H_5{-}\underset{\underset{O}{\|}}{C}{-}CH_3$$

Methyl ethyl ketone

When both R's are the same, we have a *simple ketone* (for example, acetone); when the R's are different, we have a *mixed ketone* (for example, methyl ethyl ketone). To name complex ketones, it is preferable to change the *-e* ending of the hydrocarbon with the same number of carbon atoms to *-one* and indicate the position of the carbonyl group, when necessary, by numbering the longest chain. Thus,

$$CH_3{-}\underset{\underset{O}{\|}}{C}{-}CH_3$$

Propanone

$$CH_3{-}CH_2{-}\underset{\underset{O}{\|}}{C}{-}CH_3$$

Butanone

$$CH_3{-}CH_2{-}\underset{\underset{O}{\|}}{C}{-}CH_2{-}CH_3$$

Pentanone-3

Identification. In contrast to aldehydes, ketones do not reduce Fehling's or Benedict's solution. They do, however, on standing produce a color with Schiff's reagent (aldehydes produce an immediate color). To establish the identity of a specific ketone, a derivative (an oxime or phenylhydrazone) is usually prepared from it.

Quinones. Quinones are aromatic compounds in which the carbonyl group (—CO) is a part of the ring. Several substances of this character are of considerable interest. Vitamin K, for example, is a

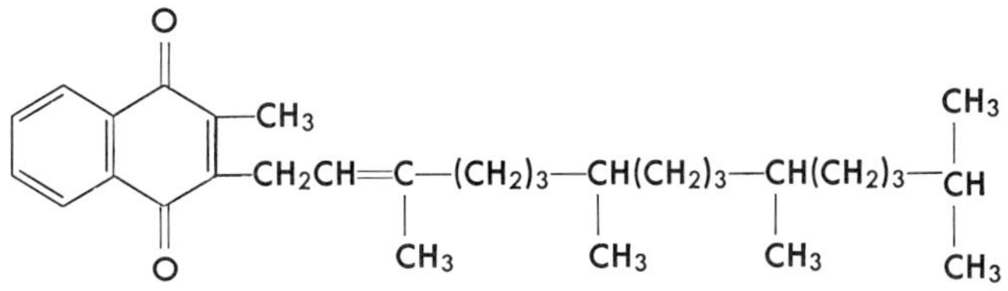

$$\text{1,4-naphthoquinone ring (C=O at 1 and 4)} \text{—}CH_3;\ \text{—}CH_2CH{=}\underset{\displaystyle CH_3}{C}\text{—}(CH_2)_3\text{—}\underset{\displaystyle CH_3}{CH}(CH_2)_3\text{—}\underset{\displaystyle CH_3}{CH}(CH_2)_3\text{—}\underset{\displaystyle CH_3}{\overset{\displaystyle CH_3}{CH}}$$

derivative of 1,4-naphthoquinone with the structure shown above.

ACIDS

When primary and secondary alcohols are *partially* oxidized, aldehydes and ketones, respectively, are produced. Aldehydes and ketones, however, are capable of being further oxidized to form products called *carboxylic* acids. The latter, therefore, result from the complete oxidation of alcohols. The generic formula for an organic acid is as follows:

$$R\text{—}\overset{\displaystyle O}{\overset{\|}{C}}\text{—}OH \quad (RCOOH)$$

The —COOH group is called the carboxyl radical.

The relationship of alcohols, aldehydes, ketones, and acids is shown at the bottom of the page.

When tertiary alcohols are oxidized, a mixture of acids and ketones is obtained.

Organic acids undergo a slight degree of ionization when placed in solution. Thus, solutions of organic acids are weak electrolytes. The ionization of organic acids may be represented as follows:

$$RCOOH \rightleftharpoons RCOO^- + H^+$$

The presence of hydrogen ions, then, endows such compounds with acidic properties. For example, organic acids neutralize bases to form salts and water:

$$RCOOH + NaOH \longrightarrow RCOONa + H_2O$$

In a similar fashion, organic acids react with alcohols to form organic salts called esters. There are numerous esters of importance.

Fatty acid series. Organic acids are present in the tissues of certain organisms or products derived from them. They occur in the form of either the free acid or some derivative (for example, ester) of the acid. Like the hydrocarbons, they can be arranged in series.

Of these, the so-called fatty acid series is perhaps the most important. The term *fatty acid* has its origin in the fact that most fats are derivatives of acids belonging to this series; in turn, all members of the fatty acid series may be derived from hydrocarbons of the paraffin series. Some of the more important acids of this series are given in Table 5-4. These acids are monobasic; that is, they contain only one carboxyl group.

Formic acid. Formic acid (HCOOH) is the simplest organic acid. It occurs in red ants, in stinging nettles, in the shoots of some varieties of pine, and elsewhere. Formic acid is a colorless liquid that boils at 99° C. and has an extremely penetrating

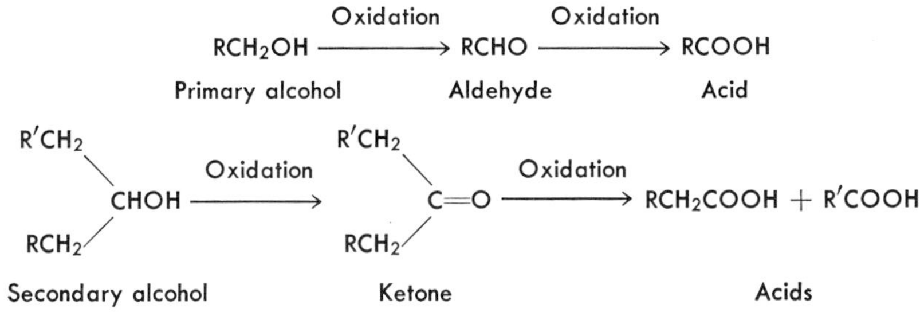

$$\underset{\text{Primary alcohol}}{RCH_2OH} \xrightarrow{\text{Oxidation}} \underset{\text{Aldehyde}}{RCHO} \xrightarrow{\text{Oxidation}} \underset{\text{Acid}}{RCOOH}$$

$$\underset{\text{Secondary alcohol}}{(R'CH_2)(RCH_2)CHOH} \xrightarrow{\text{Oxidation}} \underset{\text{Ketone}}{(R'CH_2)(RCH_2)C{=}O} \xrightarrow{\text{Oxidation}} \underset{\text{Acids}}{RCH_2COOH + R'COOH}$$

Table 5-4. Important fatty acids

Formic acid	HCOOH
Acetic acid	CH_3COOH
Butyric acid	C_3H_7COOH
Palmitic acid	$C_{15}H_{31}COOH$
Stearic acid	$C_{17}H_{35}COOH$

odor. Chemically, it is a fairly strong acid, forming salts and esters called formates.

Acetic acid. Acetic acid (CH_3COOH) is one of our most important acids in commerce and in the laboratory. Once prepared commercially by the distillation of wood, it is now produced in huge quantities by a synthetic process. In this process, acetylene reacts with water (via the catalytic action of mercuric sulfate) to form acetaldehyde. The aldehyde is then easily oxidized to acetic acid. The equations are as follows:

$$C_2H_2 + H_2O \xrightarrow{HgSO_4} CH_3CHO$$
$$CH_3CHO + [O] \longrightarrow CH_3COOH$$

Acetic acid is a clear, colorless liquid that boils at 118° C. It has a very penetrating, pleasant, acrid odor and a sharp, acid taste. The pure acid, solid at temperatures below 16° C., is known as glacial acetic acid. Chemically, acetic acid yields a large number of derivatives. Many of its salts and esters (acetates) are widely used in the laboratory, in industry, in pharmacy, and in medicine.

A discussion of acetic acid would not be complete without a word about vinegar, an aqueous solution containing 3 to 6 percent of the acid, a little alcohol, and other substances in small quantities. It is made by the fermentation of fruit juices such as cider. The sugar is first converted to ethyl alcohol (by yeast), and the latter is oxidized to acetic acid by bacteria *(Bacterium aceti)* present in the juice.

The reactions are summarized thus:

$$\underset{\text{Sugar}}{C_6H_{12}O_6} \xrightarrow{\text{Yeast}} \underset{\text{Alcohol}}{C_2H_5OH} \xrightarrow{\text{Bacteria}} \underset{\text{Acid}}{CH_3COOH}$$

Palmitic and stearic acids. Palmitic ($C_{15}H_{31}COOH$) and stearic ($C_{17}H_{35}COOH$) acids are of special interest because they are present as glyceryl esters (that is, esters of glycerol) in the fats and oils of most animals and plants. These esters will be discussed in detail in a later section.

Nomenclature. The names of several of the acids of this series are derived from their origin (for example, formic from formica, butyric from butter, and so on). These acids may also be named by changing the ending *-e* of the hydrocarbon containing the same number of carbon atoms to *-oic.* Thus, H • COOH is methanoic acid, CH_3COOH is ethanoic acid, and so on.

Lactic acid. Lactic acid (CH_3CHOH-$COOH$) has the following structure:

```
         H
         |
   CH3—C—COOH
         |
        OH
```

The souring of milk is due to the formation of this acid by the action of certain bacteria (which produce enzymes) on milk sugar, or lactose. In the body, lactic acid is found in muscle tissue during exercise.

Earlier in this chapter lactic acid was cited as an example of an optical isomer (*l*-lactic acid, *d*-lactic acid, and *dl*-lactic acid). The three forms, like all optically active compounds, are about identical in their chemical and physical properties except in regard to polarized light.

Benzoic acid. Benzoic acid, the simplest aromatic acid, may be prepared in the laboratory by the oxidation of benzyl alcohol:

```
          H                           O
          |                           ||
  C6H5 —C—OH   --Oxidation-->   C6H5 —C—OH
          |
          H
  Benzyl alcohol              Benzoic acid
```

It occurs as the free acid or ester in gum benzoin, resins, balsam of Tolu, berries, and other natural products. The acid itself finds application as an antiseptic in medicine and in the manufacture of dyes; its salts also enjoy wide use. Sodium benzoate, for example, is a common and safe food preservative; benzyl benzoate is used in medicine.

Salicylic acid. Salicylic acid, the simplest aromatic hydroxy acid, has the following structure:

```
        O
        ||
  ⬡—C—OH
  |
  OH
```

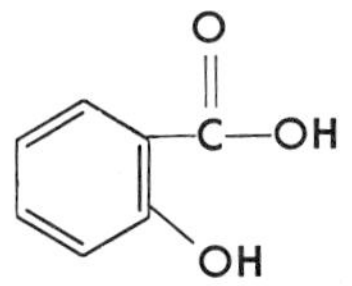

From our previous discussion we can see that this acid may also be named *o*-hydroxybenzoic acid. Salicylic acid is found in the form of its methyl ester (methyl salicylate) in oil of wintergreen, and it is prepared synthetically from phenol.

Salicylic acid and its salts and esters are some of our most common medicinal agents. Free salicylic acid is used widely as an antiseptic and fungistatic agent. Its most important derivative—aspirin—is unquestionably the most popular drug in medicine. Aspirin has the following structure:

```
           O
           ||
  ⬡—O—C—CH3
  |
  C—OH
  ||
  O
```

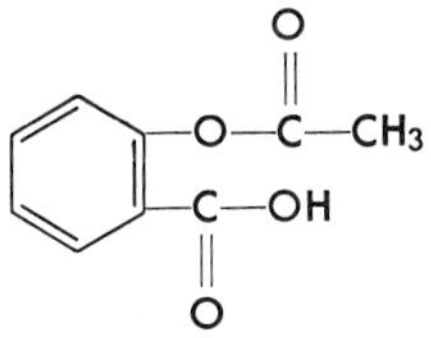

Chemically, aspirin is called acetylsalicylic acid. Other salicylates used in medicine include phenyl salicylate (salol) and methyl salicylate. Salicylates are also used in the manufacture of dyes.

Penicillin. Of interest and practical importance is the fact that penicillin is an organic acid. It has the following structure:

```
                              S     CH3
                            /   \  /
⬡—CH2—CO—NH—CH—CH     C
                  |       |       |  \
                  |       |       |   CH3
                 OC——N——CH—COOH
```

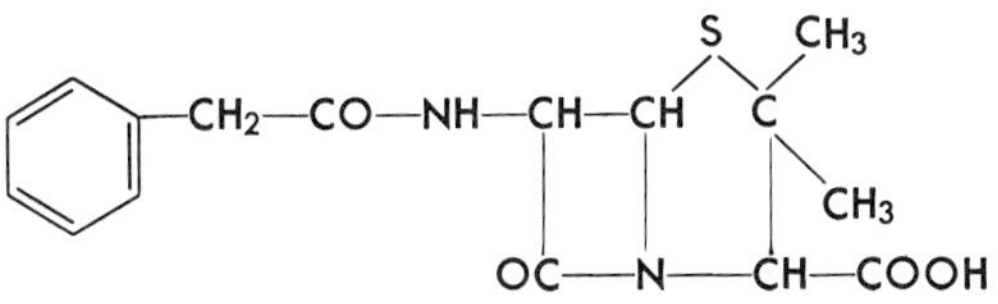

Penicillin is insoluble in water. Its alkali salts, which are very soluble, are employed when penicillin is to be administered by the intravenous route. Certain other salts, especially procaine penicillin, are highly insoluble and are employed for intramuscular injection to prolong absorption and thereby increase the duration of action.

ESTERS

Esters are prepared by the interaction of an alcohol and an acid (esterification). This is analogous to neutralization in inorganic chemistry. Esterification may be represented by the following generic equation:

$$R'OH + RCOOH \longrightarrow RCOOR' + H_2O$$

There are a large number of natural and synthetic esters. In nature these esters are responsible for the characteristic odor of many fruits and flowers. In general, they are neutral compounds that hydrolyze upon heating with a dilute acid or base.

A great many esters are of commercial value. Although several are used as flavoring materials and in perfumes, the majority are employed for a variety of uses in industry, in pharmacy, and in medicine. Some esters that are of special interest will be discussed here.

Glyceryl trinitrate. Glyceryl trinitrate, commonly called nitroglycerin, is prepared by the action of nitric acid on glycerin. In this reaction, and in other esterification reactions, H_2SO_4 is used as a dehydrating agent to hasten the speed of reaction:

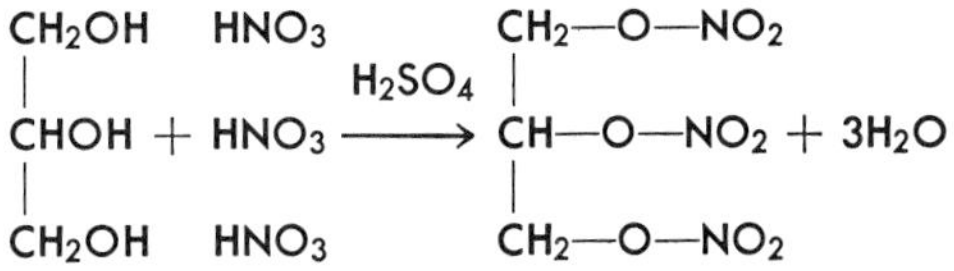

```
CH2OH    HNO3              CH2—O—NO2
|                   H2SO4  |
CHOH  +  HNO3  ———————→    CH—O—NO2 + 3H2O
|                          |
CH2OH    HNO3              CH2—O—NO2
```

Glyceryl trinitrate

Nitroglycerin is used in medicine as a vasodilator (especially in the treatment of angina pectoris) and is the active constituent of dynamite.

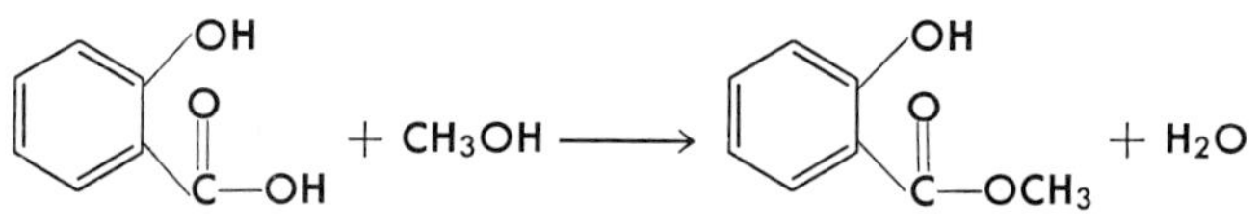

$$\text{Salicylic acid } (C_6H_4(OH)COOH) + CH_3OH \longrightarrow \text{Methyl salicylate } (C_6H_4(OH)COOCH_3) + H_2O$$

Salicylic acid — Methyl salicylate

Ethyl acetate. Ethyl acetate is prepared by reacting ethyl alcohol with acetic acid:

$$C_2H_5OH + CH_3COOH \longrightarrow \underset{\text{Ethyl acetate}}{CH_3COOC_2H_5} + H_2O$$

Ethyl acetate is one of the most important industrial solvents. In this capacity it is used in the manufacture of nitrocellulose, photographic films, resins, and essences.

Methyl salicylate. When methyl alcohol is heated with salicylic acid, methyl salicylate is formed, as indicated by its structural formula. (See above.)

Methyl salicylate is the chief constituent of oil of wintergreen and oil of birch. It is used in medicine as a rubefacient (in liniments and ointments) and as a substitute for the natural oil of wintergreen.

ETHERS

Ethers may be considered alcohols in which the H of ROH is replaced by an R group. Thus, they are organic oxides:

$$R—O—R$$

If the two R's represent the same group, the ether is referred to as a simple ether. If the two R's represent different groups, we have a so-called mixed ether. Thus, we have two generic formulas:

$$R—O—R \text{ (simple ether)}$$
$$R'—O—R \text{ (mixed ether)}$$

Ethers of low molecular weight are colorless, neutral liquids that are extremely volatile and flammable (especially the lower members). Since they are highly inactive, they are used extensively as solvents for other organic substances. Ethers of particular importance are discussed here.

Diethyl ether. Diethyl ether, also known as ether, sulfuric ether, and ethyl oxide, is the most important member of the class. It has the following structure:

$$C_2H_5—O—C_2H_5$$

Ether is prepared in great quantities by the reaction between sulfuric acid and ethyl alcohol:

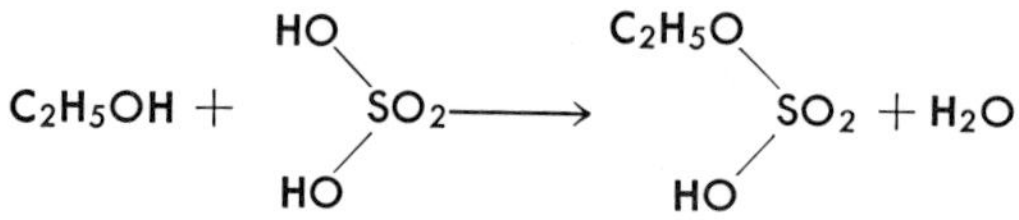

$$C_2H_5OH + \underset{\text{(first step)}}{(HO)_2SO_2} \longrightarrow \underset{\text{Ethyl sulfuric acid}}{(C_2H_5O)(HO)SO_2} + H_2O$$

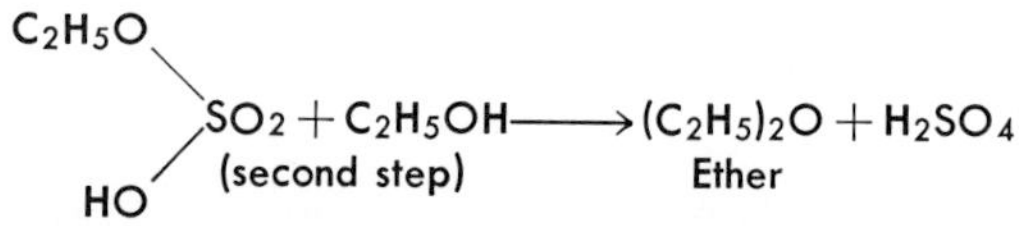

$$(C_2H_5O)(HO)SO_2 + C_2H_5OH \xrightarrow{\text{(second step)}} \underset{\text{Ether}}{(C_2H_5)_2O} + H_2SO_4$$

The laboratory setup for the preparation of ether is shown in Fig. 5-4.

Diethyl ether is a colorless, volatile liquid with a characteristic odor. It is highly flammable and explosive when mixed with air and ignited. Industrially, ether is unsurpassed as a solvent for a large number of organic substances, and in this capacity it is used in the manufacture of guncotton, collodion solutions, and certain plastics.

Of special interest is the fact that ether is one of our most important anesthetic agents (Fig. 5-5). Although other agents have appeared on the scene, ether is still considered a standard anesthetic. For this purpose, it must be highly purified.

AMINES

Amines are organic compounds that may be looked upon as derivatives of ammonia. Since ammonia has three replaceable hydrogens, there are three classes of amines—primary, secondary, and tertiary. These may be summarized as follows:

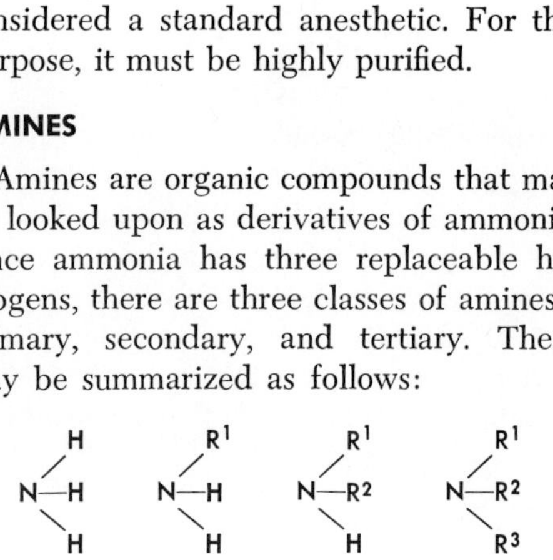

Ammonia	Primary amine	Secondary amine	Tertiary amine
$N(H)(H)(H)$	$N(R^1)(H)(H)$	$N(R^1)(R^2)(H)$	$N(R^1)(R^2)(R^3)$

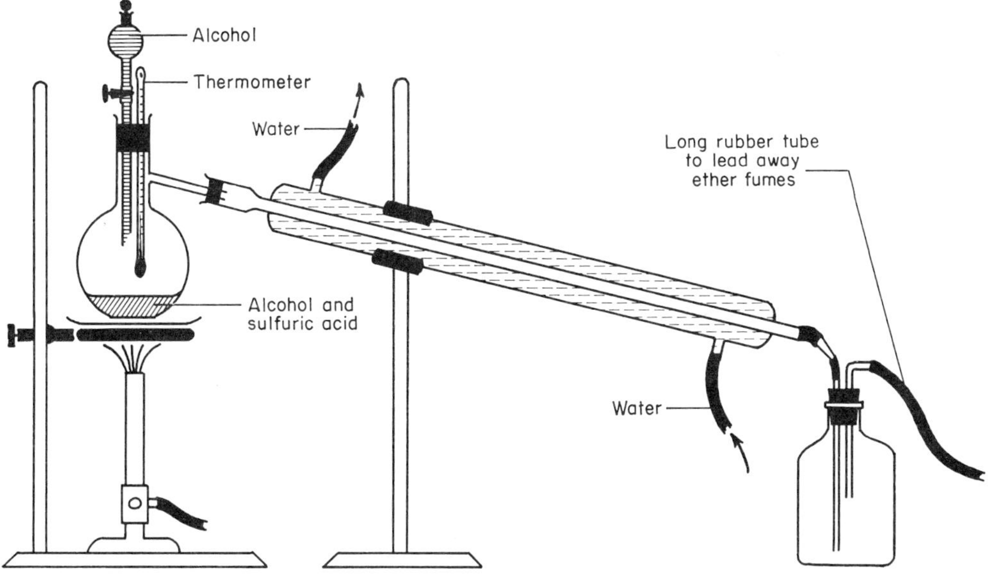

Fig. 5-4. Laboratory preparation of ether. (From Brooks, S. M.: Selected experiments in general chemistry, Philadelphia, 1956, W. B. Saunders Co.)

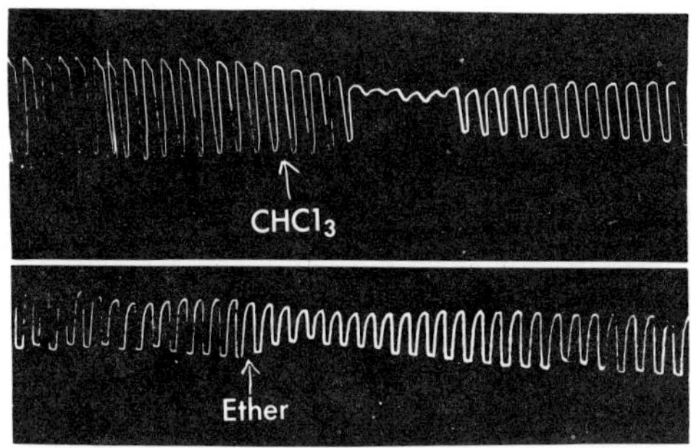

Fig. 5-5. Effects of chloroform ($CHCl_3$) and ether upon the frog heart. One drop of each was used. Note that chloroform almost stopped the heart. (From Brooks, S. M.: Basic facts of pharmacology, ed. 2, Philadelphia, 1963, W. B. Saunders Co.)

In primary amines, "$—NH_2$" is called an *amino* group; in secondary amines, "—NH" is called an *imino* group. The following examples will serve to illustrate the manner in which amines are named:

CH_3	CH_3	CH_3
N—H	N—C_2H_5	N—CH_3
H	H	C_2H_5
Methylamine	Methyl ethylamine	Dimethyl ethylamine

The most outstanding chemical characteristic of amines is their basic properties; indeed, they are more basic than ammonium hydroxide. By virtue of this property, amines combine with acids to form ammonium salts. Trimethylamine, for example, reacts with hydrochloric acid to form trimethylammonium chloride:

$$(CH_3)_3N + HCl \longrightarrow (CH_3)_3NHCl$$

Being a true salt, it is composed of ions, and for this reason its structural formula is best written as follows:

$$\left[\begin{array}{c} CH_3 \\ | \\ CH_3—N—CH_3 \\ | \\ H \end{array}\right]^{+} Cl^{-}$$

Aniline. Aniline (chemically, phenylamine), our most important amine, is the source material for a large number of our most popular dyes and drugs. It is prepared from benzene (obtained from coal tar) by the following reactions:

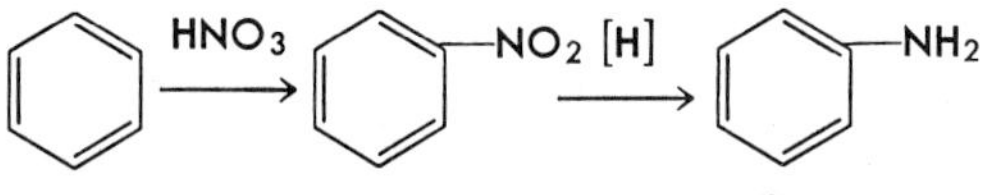

$$C_6H_6 \xrightarrow{HNO_3} C_6H_5\text{—}NO_2 \xrightarrow{[H]} C_6H_5\text{—}NH_2$$

Benzene Nitrobenzene Aniline

Aniline, a liquid with a characteristic odor, boils at 184° C. It is colorless when freshly distilled but darkens on standing.

The value of aniline was first appreciated in 1856 when Perkin found that aniline could be oxidized with chromic acid to yield a violet dye, to which was given the name *mauve*. This was the first *coal-tar dye* to be produced. Since then, about 3000 coal-tar dyes have been synthesized.

Physiologic amines. The amines discussed below are but a few of those employed in medicine. They clearly illustrate, however, how the organic chemist has revolutionized the practice of medicine.

Epinephrine. Epinephrine (commercial preparations are called Adrenalin) is a hormone of the adrenal glands with the following structure:

$$(HO)_2C_6H_3\text{—}CHOH \cdot CH_2 \cdot NH \cdot CH_3$$

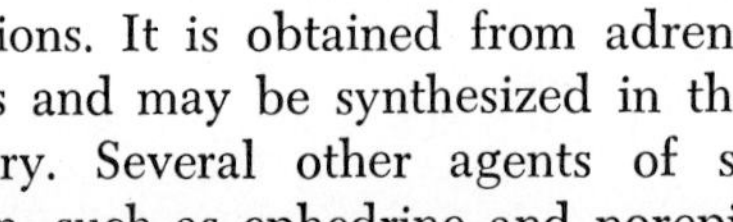

Epinephrine (secondary amine)

Although epinephrine acts on many tissues in the body, it is used mostly to relieve attacks of acute asthma and to stem allergic reactions. It is obtained from adrenal extracts and may be synthesized in the laboratory. Several other agents of similar action, such as ephedrine and norepinephrine, have similar structures.

Sulfonamides. The efficacy of the sulfonamides, or "sulfa drugs," in the treatment of infectious diseases is familiar to all. Sulfanilamide (chemically, *p*-aminobenzenesulfonamide), one of the first sulfonamides used in medicine, has the following structure:

$$H_2N\text{—}SO_2\text{—}C_6H_4\text{—}NH_2$$

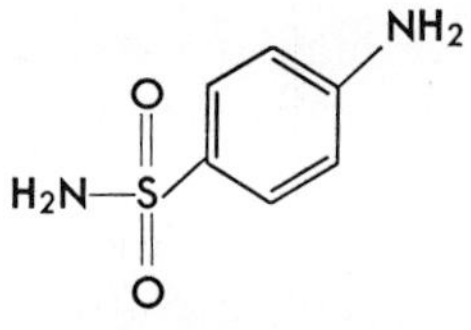

Sulfanilamide (primary amine)

Since sulfanilamide proved to be quite toxic to the kidneys and blood, the chemist synthesized an array of related agents. Most derivatives are prepared by replacing a hydrogen of the $—SONH_2$ group with some organic group (R):

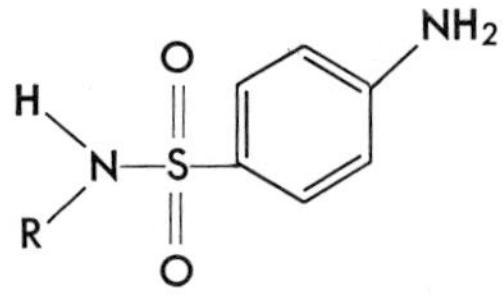

$$(H)(R)N\text{—}SO_2\text{—}C_6H_4\text{—}NH_2$$

Sulfadiazine, for example, a much less toxic agent than sulfanilamide, has the following structure:

$$NH_2\text{—}C_6H_4\text{—}SO_2\text{—}NH\text{—}C_4H_3N_2$$

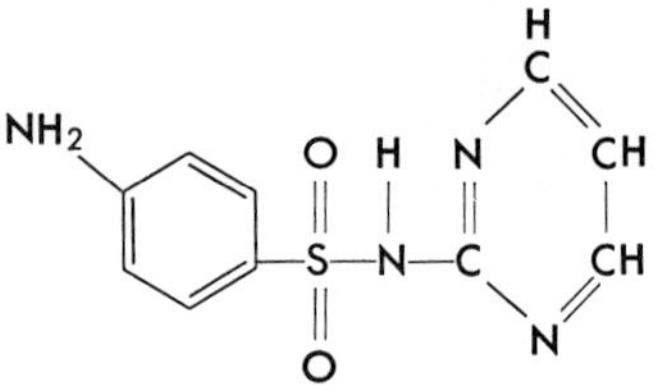

Sulfadiazine

Procaine. Procaine (Novocain) is also a familiar compound. Although hundreds of other local anesthetics have been synthesized, it is still a standard of its class. Procaine has the following structure:

$$NH_2\text{—}C_6H_4\text{—}COO\text{—}CH_2\text{—}CH_2\text{—}N(C_2H_5)_2$$

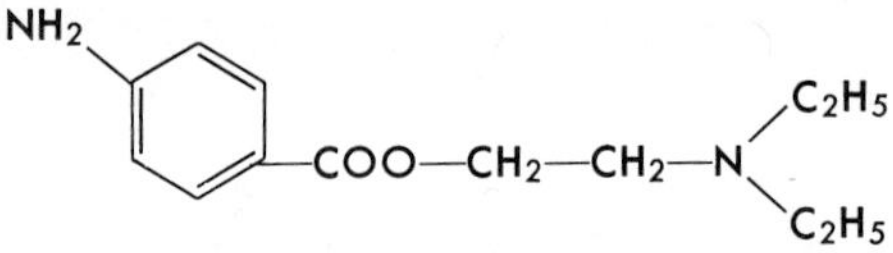

Procaine

Several other important local anesthetics have a similar structure.

Quaternary antiseptics. Several quaternary salts are highly useful as antiseptics, being more potent and much less toxic and irritating than such antiseptics as iodine and related agents. Their generic formula may be represented as follows:

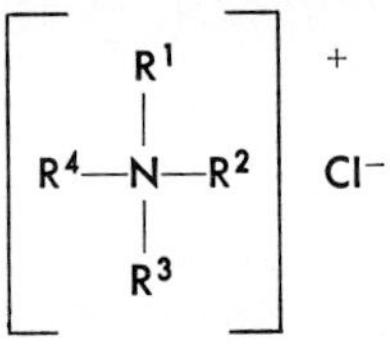

$$\left[R^4\text{—}N(R^1)(R^3)\text{—}R^2 \right]^+ Cl^-$$

One popular agent of this class, Zephiran, has the following structure:

$$\left[C_6H_5\text{—}CH_2\text{—}\overset{\displaystyle CH_3}{\underset{\displaystyle CH_3}{N}}\text{—}R \right]^+ Cl^-$$

Antihistamines. It has been postulated that in the allergic person an agent known as histamine (present within the cells of the body) is released in response to certain foreign proteinaceous substances called allergens. This has led to the synthesis of a large number of so-called antihistamines. Although not a cure, these drugs have brought dramatic relief to patients with a variety of allergic conditions. One popular agent of this class, *Pyribenzamine,* has the following structure:

$$C_6H_5\text{—}CH_2\text{—}N(C_5H_4N)\text{—}CH_2\text{—}CH_2\text{—}N(CH_3)_2$$

Acetylcholine. Acetylcholine is of special importance to the physiologist, for it is liberated at the endings of parasympathetic and voluntary nerves. Acetylcholine is a quaternary base, the structure of which is shown below.

$$\left[(CH_3)_3N\text{—}CH_2\text{—}CH_2\text{—}O\text{—}\overset{\displaystyle O}{\overset{\|}{C}}\text{—}CH_3 \right]^+ OH^-$$

The discovery of acetylcholine gave impetus to research concerning the relationship between quaternary compounds and nerve physiology. As a result, a large number of quaternary compounds have been introduced into medical therapeutics. Some of these agents augment the action of acetylcholine, and some inhibit acetylcholine. *Mecholyl, Doryl,* and *Urecholine,* for example, act like acetylcholine; *tubocurarine,* obtained from an extract called curare, is an inhibitor and produces paralysis of voluntary (skeletal) muscle.

HETEROCYCLIC COMPOUNDS

Some organic compounds are unique in that they are composed of rings in which elements in addition to carbon are present. Such compounds are referred to as heterocyclic; in contrast, aromatic and alicyclic compounds are referred to as carbocyclic. Many heterocyclic substances are derivatives of the following basic structures:

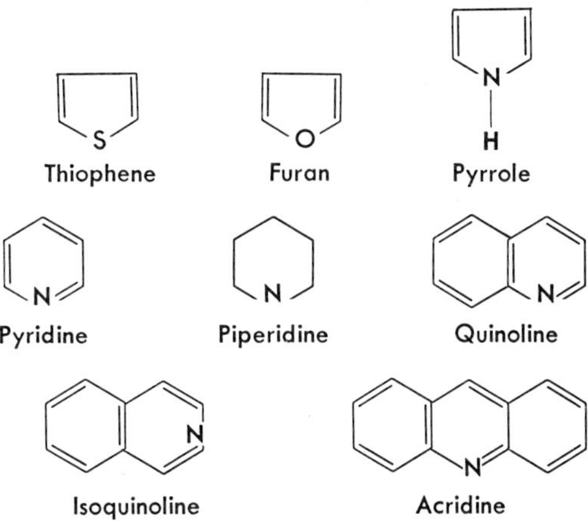

From these structures nature and the organic chemist have created a variety of highly useful flavors, dyes, drugs, and vitamins. Of special interest are the drugs of plant origin.

Alkaloids. Alkaloids are complex heterocyclic nitrogenous compounds of plant origin characterized by powerful physiologic activity. Physically, they are white crystalline solids that are insoluble in water but soluble in alcohol, ether, and chloroform. Alkaloids are optically active, and, interestingly enough, it is usually the levorotatory isomer that is physiologically active. Chemically, alkaloids are characterized by their basic nature; that is, they react with acids to form quaternary salts that are *soluble* in water. For this reason, they are usually used in the form of their salts. In addition to morphine and codeine

(p. 100), a few examples are presented herewith.

Cocaine. Cocaine, present is coca leaves, was the first agent to be used widely as a local anesthetic. It has the following structure:

```
         H
         |
H2C------C--------CH·COO·CH3
 |       |         |
 |  CH3--N        CH--O--C------(C6H5)
 |       |         |     ||
H2C------C--------CH2    O
         |
         H
```

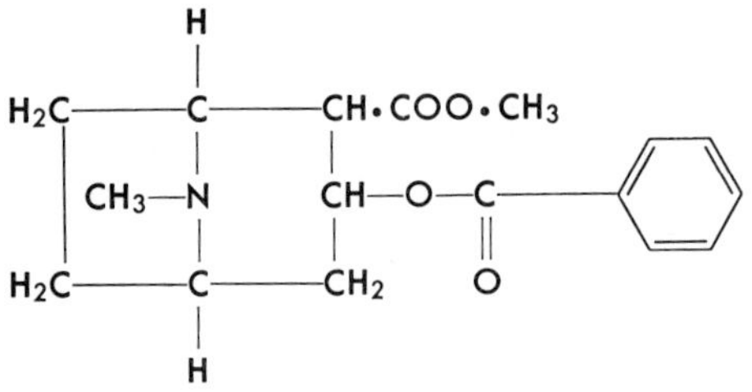

Atropine. Atropine, the active constituent of belladonna (deadly nightshade), is used in medicine as an antispasmodic to relax muscle and as a mydriatic to dilate the pupil. It has the following structure:

```
         H
         |
H2C------C--------CH2   O  CH2·OH
 |       |         | H  ||  |
 |       N--CH3    C/--O--C--C------(C6H5)
 |       |         |         |
H2C------C--------CH2        H
         |
         H
```

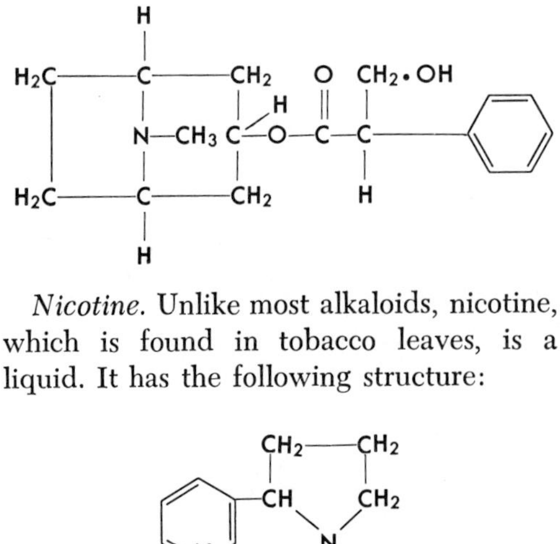

Nicotine. Unlike most alkaloids, nicotine, which is found in tobacco leaves, is a liquid. It has the following structure:

```
              CH2-----CH2
               |       |
(C5H4N)-------CH      CH2
                \     /
                  N
                  |
                 CH3
```

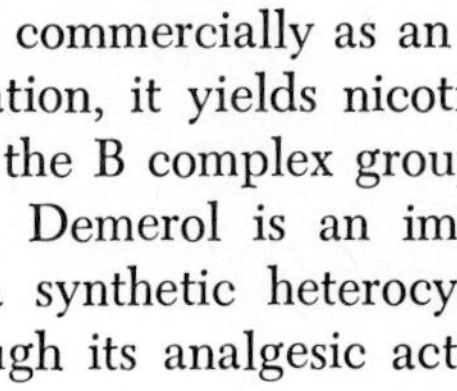

Nicotine is a highly poisonous substance that is used commercially as an insecticide. Upon oxidation, it yields nicotinic acid, a member of the B complex group.

Demerol. Demerol is an important example of a synthetic heterocyclic medicinal. Although its analgesic action is close to that of morphine, its toxicity is much lower. It has the following chemical structure:

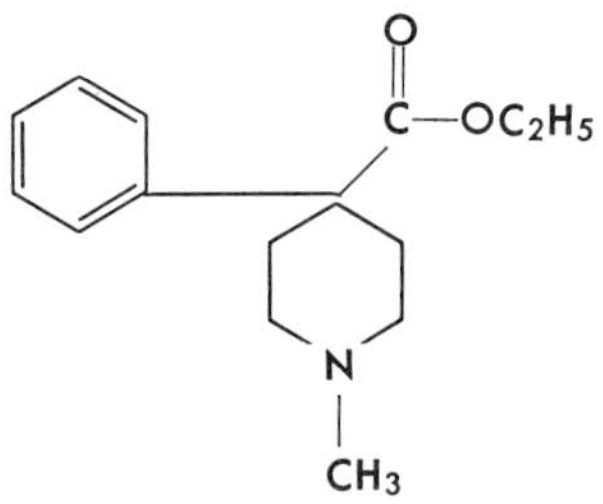

```
                    O
                    ||
                    C--OC2H5
                   /
(C6H5)------------C4 (piperidine ring)
                  |
                  N
                  |
                 CH3
```

ORGANOMETALLIC COMPOUNDS

Organometallic compounds contain one or more atoms of some metal per molecule. Important examples of naturally occurring compounds of this character are hemoglobin (iron) and chlorophyll (magnesium). An example of a synthetic organometallic compound is the mercurial antiseptic Merthiolate, which has the structure:

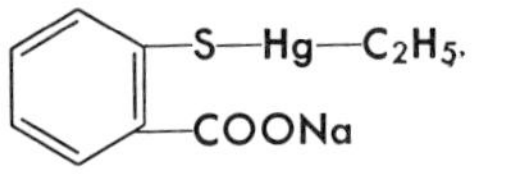

```
(C6H4)--S--Hg--C2H5.
   \
    COONa
```

CARBOHYDRATES

Carbohydrates constitute a very large class of organic compounds whose members contain carbon, hydrogen, and oxygen, the latter two elements being in the ratio of 2:1, respectively. Of chief interest is the fact that carbohydrates represent one of the three great classes of foodstuffs. In addition to their ability to sustain life, carbohydrates serve as essential raw materials in many industries.

In broad terms, carbohydrates may be placed into one of two categories of compounds: (1) those that are crystalline and sweet (sugars) and (2) those that are tasteless and noncrystalline, such as the starches, celluloses (woody substances), and similar substances. Sugars are subdivided into monosaccharides and disaccharides; starches and celluloses are classed as polysaccharides.

Monosaccharides. Monosaccharides, or simple sugars, are carbohydrates that cannot be further hydrolyzed, that is, broken down into simpler substances with dilute acids. They are constituted by molecules

Table 5-5. Monosaccharides

Trioses*	$C_3H_6O_3$
Tetroses	$C_4H_8O_4$
Pentoses	$C_5H_{10}O_5$
Hexoses	$C_6H_{12}O_6$

*The ending *-ose* refers to carbohydrates in general and to sugars in particular.

containing aldehyde or ketone groups linked directly to carbons which, in turn, are attached to hydroxyl groups. Monosaccharides are classified, as shown in Table 5-5, according to the number of carbon atoms.

Of the classes shown in Table 5-5, the hexoses are by far the most important—particularly glucose, fructose, and galactose. These three hexoses, like all hexoses, have the same empirical formula and are therefore isomeric. Their structural formulas are shown on p. 118.

Glucose. Glucose (also called dextrose or grape sugar) is one of the most important carbohydrates; physiologically, it is the most important. Present in the juice of many sweet fruits and in the blood of all animals, it is prepared commercially by the hydrolysis* of disaccharides and polysaccharides.

Physically, glucose is a sweet, white crystalline solid that is soluble in water. Glucose is optically active, *d*-glucose being the common form. Its chemical behavior is attributable mostly to the presence of the aldehyde or CHO group. For example, glucose produces a positive test with Fehling's or Benedict's solution. (At the present time, Benedict's solution is used commonly to test for the presence of glucose in urine.) As pointed out earlier, the enzyme "zymase," present in yeast, converts glucose into alcohol and carbon dioxide (alcoholic fermentation):

$$C_6H_{12}O_6 \xrightarrow{\text{Zymase}} 2C_2H_5OH + 2CO_2$$

In plant tissues, glucose reacts with a number of diverse substances to form a valuable class of compounds called glucosides. Similar compounds of any monosaccharide are generally called glycosides. Many glucosides (for example, digitoxin) and glycosides possess physiologic activity.

Glucose is used extensively in making candy, jellies, preserves, syrups, alcoholic beverages, and similar items. Its physiologic importance will be discussed later. For the time being, let us say that glucose is the principal end product of carbohydrate digestion.

Galactose. Galactose is obtained by the hydrolysis of lactose, or milk sugar. It reduces Fehling's solution and is slowly fermented by yeast. Galactose is of concern primarily because it is one of the end products of digestion; that is, it is absorbed into the blood along with glucose and fructose.

Fructose. Fructose, commonly called levulose, occurs naturally in honey; it is about 50 percent sweeter than sucrose. It may be obtained by the hydrolysis of cane sugar, or sucrose, and like other hexoses, it reduces Fehling's solution. Chemically and physiologically, fructose is much like glucose.

Disaccharides. Disaccharides are isomeric sugars that are synthesized in the tissues of plants from monosaccharide molecules. The most important (those formed from glucose, fructose, and galactose) are sucrose, lactose, and maltose.

Sucrose. Sucrose ($C_{12}H_{22}O_{11}$), or cane sugar, is in all respects the most important disaccharide. When an aqueous solution of sucrose is heated with dilute acid (hydrolyzed), it yields a mixture of glucose and fructose (invert sugar). The enzyme sucrase, which is present in the intestinal

*The term *hydrolysis* is applied to any reaction in which water takes part.

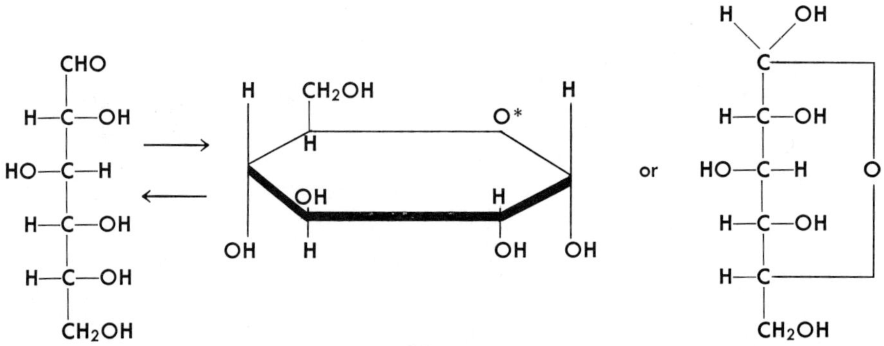

Glucose

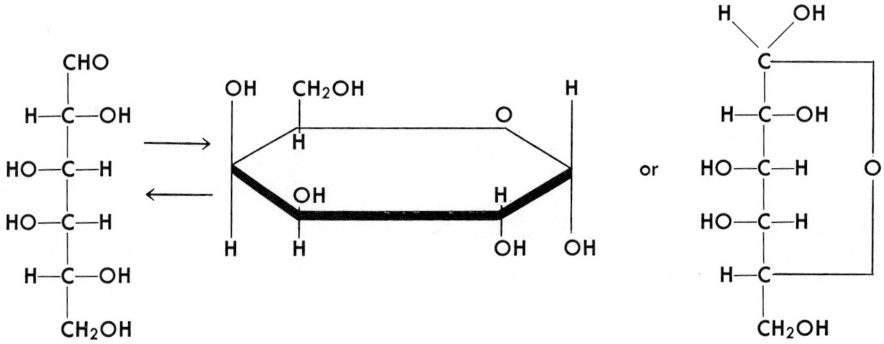

Galactose

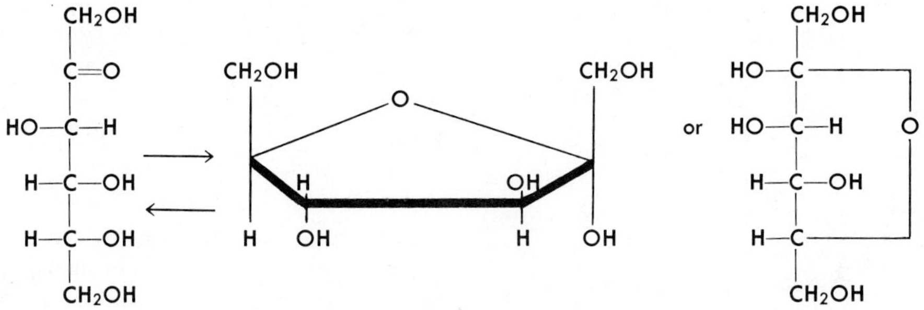

Fructose

*The ring is perpendicular to the plane of the paper, with the heavy lines facing out. The groups attached to the ring are perpendicular to the plane of the ring. The structure at the right is the "older" type of ring.

juice, brings about the same reaction. Unlike the other common sugars—glucose, fructose, galactose, maltose, and lactose—sucrose does not reduce Fehling's solution. From this information the chemist has suggested the following structure:

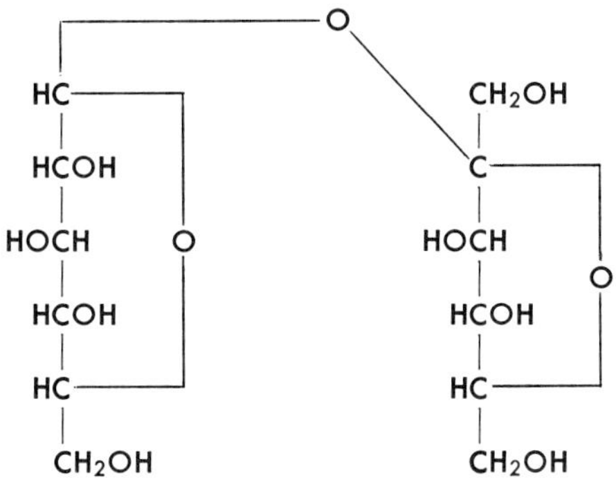

Sucrose

Sucrose is obtained from sugar cane and sugar beets. Essentially, the extraction process is carried out as follows: The juice is pressed from the cane or beets and separated from the insoluble fiber. Next, the albuminous impurities in the juice are precipitated and filtered off. The filtrate is then evaporated at low temperatures under vacuum, causing the sugar to crystallize out. The thick brown "mother liquor" remaining above the crystallized sugar is known as molasses. Molasses, which contains about 50 percent sucrose, is used in making alcohol, table syrup, and rum. When sucrose is heated above its melting point, a brown substance called caramel is formed. Caramel is commonly used as a food coloring.

Lactose. Lactose ($C_{12}H_{22}O_{11}$), or milk sugar, is present in milk to the extent of about 4 percent. Upon acid or enzyme (lactase) hydrolysis, one molecule yields one molecule of glucose and one molecule of galactose. The souring of milk is due to the conversion of lactose to lactic acid by the action of certain enzymes released by bacteria in the milk.

Maltose. Maltose ($C_{12}H_{22}O_{11}$), or malt sugar, is found in malt, the sprouting grain of barley. When a solution of maltose is hydrolyzed by acids or by maltase (present in the small intestine), one molecule yields two molecules of glucose. Maltose is a reducing sugar.

Polysaccharides. Polysaccharides are polymers of monosaccharides. This is proved by the fact that they can be hydrolyzed by acids and enzymes into monosaccharides. As stated previously, polysaccharides are noncrystalline, insoluble, tasteless substances; those with the formula $(C_6H_{10}O_5)_n$ are the most important. (This formula means that these substances are formed from an indefinite number of hexose, usually glucose, molecules that have undergone polymerization.)

Starch. Starch, a general name applied to a variety of similar polymers of glucose (for example, cornstarch, potato starch, and the like), has the empirical formula $(C_6H_{10}O_5)_n$ and the structure shown at the bottom of the page.

Upon hydrolysis by acids or enzymes, starch yields glucose as the final product. It is interesting to note, however, that several intermediate products are also formed in the process. The most important steps of the hydrolysis may be represented as follows:

Starch → Soluble starch → Erythrodextrin →
Achrodextrin → Maltose → Glucose

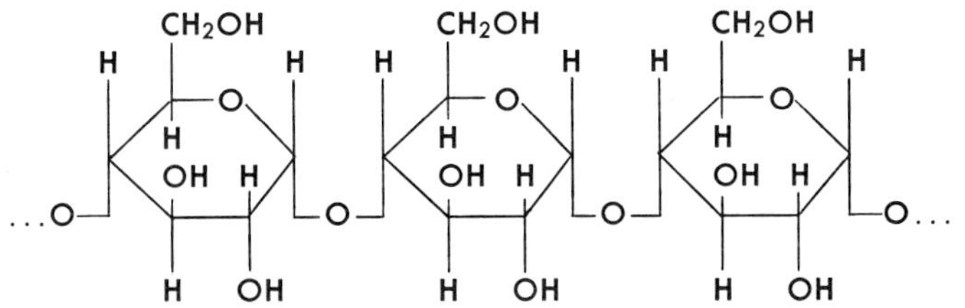

When boiled in water, starch granules swell and burst, forming a colloidal sol known as starch paste. The intense blue color that starch gives with iodine is highly characteristic and of analytical value.

Starches are widely distributed in the vegetable kingdom, being biosynthesized from the glucose formed in the process of photosynthesis. They are the principal carbohydrate food of plants and animals. Before starches can be converted into energy, however, they must be reconverted into glucose. Starch, therefore, represents stored carbohydrate, or energy.

Dextrin. Dextrin ($[C_6H_{10}O_5]_n$) is the name applied to a variety of polymers obtained in the course of the hydrolysis of starch by enzymes; these polymers are therefore less complex than starches. Dextrins that give a reddish brown color with iodine are called erythrodextrins; those which do not give a color are called achrodextrins.

Glycogen. Glycogen ($[C_6H_{10}O_5]_n$), sometimes called *animal starch,* is found in animal tissues, especially the muscles and liver. Like the starches and dextrins, it is a polymer of glucose because it yields glucose upon hydrolysis. When excess carbohydrate is taken into the body, a part is stored as glycogen. These physiologic events may be represented as follows:

$$\text{Carbohydrate} \longrightarrow \text{Glucose} \rightleftarrows \text{Glycogen}$$

Glycogen gives a red color with iodine.

Cellulose. All plant cells, in contrast to animal cells, contain a polysaccharide called cellulose ($[C_6H_{10}O_5]_n$), which is the chief constituent of the cell wall. (Cotton fiber is almost pure cellulose.) When hydrolyzed by acids, cellulose yields glucose. In general, however, cellulose is highly inert and is not acted upon by digestive enzymes.

Cellulose is of enormous industrial value, perhaps being the most important single raw material available at the present time. In the form of cotton and wood it is used in the manufacture of more than fifty different kinds of products; rayon, lacquers, plastics, food, chemicals, explosives, and paper are but a few examples (Fig. 5-6).

Other polysaccharides. Other polysaccharides of practical and theoretical im-

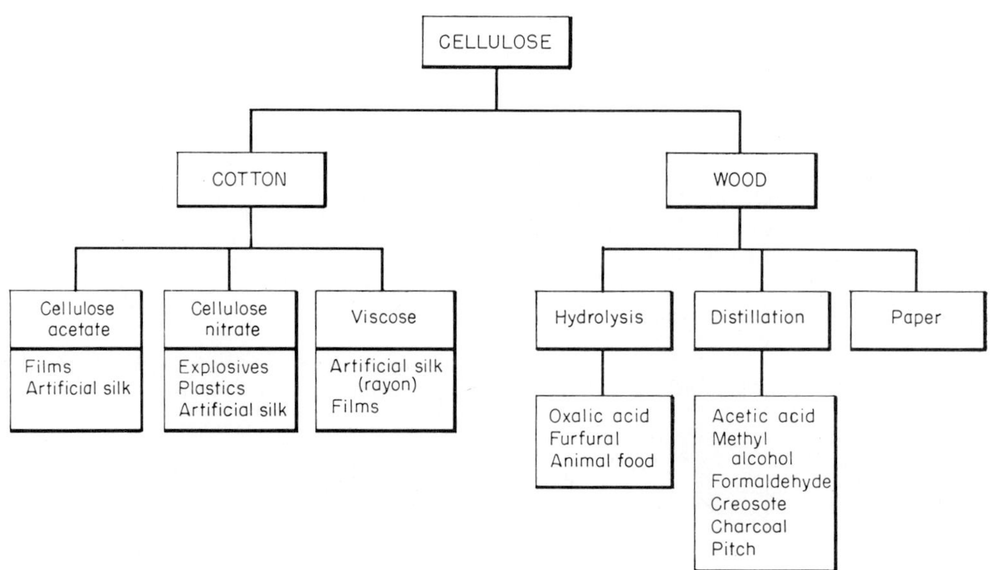

Fig. 5-6. Derivatives and products of cellulose. (From Brooks, S. M.: Basic facts of general chemistry, Philadelphia, 1956, W. B. Saunders Co.)

portance include gums, pectins, and mucilages. Gums (for example, gum arabic and gum tragacanth) are carbohydrates combined with acids; mucilages are substances that form viscous liquids; and pectins are polysaccharides present in fruit. The gelatinization of fruit extracts is due to the action of pectin. Dextran, a synthetic polysaccharide, is used (as a 6 percent aqueous solution) to raise the blood pressure in the emergency treatment of shock.

Molisch test. Most carbohydrates give a positive reaction to the Molisch test. This is a simple and valuable test performed by treating the substance under investigation with α-naphthol and concentrated H_2SO_4. If the substance is a carbohydrate or contains a carbohydrate, a violet color is produced.

LIPIDS

Lipids include fats, oils, waxes, sterols, and a variety of other substances of plant and animal origin that exhibit fatlike properties.

Fats and oils. Fats, in the main, are glyceryl esters of saturated fatty acids, whereas oils are glyceryl esters of unsaturated fatty acids. This "slight" chemical difference accounts for their physical difference; that is, fats are solid at room temperature, and oils are liquid at room temperature.

The glyceryl esters of stearic ($C_{17}H_{35}COOH$), palmitic ($C_{15}H_{31}COOH$), and oleic ($C_{17}H_{33}COOH$) acids constitute the bulk of the fats in vegetable and animal tissues.* The biosynthesis of glyceryl tristearate (commonly called stearin)—a typical fat—and glyceryl trioleate (olein)—a typical oil—may be summarized as shown at the bottom of the page.

Saponification. The hydrolysis of any ester employing alkali (that is, NaOH or KOH) may be called saponification. Usually, however, the term is applied to the reaction between an alkali and a fat or oil. In the latter reaction the sodium or potassium salt of a fatty acid—called a soap—and glycerin are formed. An example is shown at the top of page 122.

The kind of soap produced depends upon the type of fat or oil and upon whether sodium or potassium hydroxide is used. Glycerin is a by-product of the process. Fats are hydrolyzed in the body in a similar manner by the enzyme lipase. This is discussed in Chapter 14, in which the digestive system is considered.

Hydrogenation. Vegetable oils may be changed to solid fats by means of hydrogen and nickel (which act as catalysts), a process called hydrogenation. In this reaction the unsaturated glyceryl ester is converted into a saturated ester. For example, olein (glyceryl trioleate), a liquid,

*In nature, fats and oils are almost always mixtures of fatty compounds; for example, human fat contains the glyceryl esters of stearic, palmitic, oleic, butyric, and other acids.

$$\begin{array}{l} C_{17}H_{35}COO\boxed{H + HO-}-CH_2 \\ C_{17}H_{35}COO\boxed{H + HO-}-CH \\ C_{17}H_{35}COO\boxed{H + HO-}-CH_2 \end{array} \longrightarrow \begin{array}{l} C_{17}H_{35}COO-CH_2 \\ C_{17}H_{35}COO-CH \\ C_{17}H_{35}COO-CH_2 \end{array} \text{ or } C_3H_5(C_{17}H_{35}COO)_3 + 3H_2O$$

Stearic acid — Glycerol — Glyceryl tristearate (stearin)

$$\begin{array}{l} CH_3(CH_2)_7CH{=}CH(CH_2)_7COO\boxed{H + HO-}-CH_2 \\ CH_3(CH_2)_7CH{=}CH(CH_2)_7COO\boxed{H + HO-}-CH \\ CH_3(CH_2)_7CH{=}CH(CH_2)_7COO\boxed{H + HO-}-CH_2 \end{array} \longrightarrow \begin{array}{l} CH_3(CH_2)_7CH{=}CH(CH_2)_7COO-CH_2 \\ CH_3(CH_2)_7CH{=}CH(CH_2)_7COO-CH \\ CH_3(CH_2)_7CH{=}CH(CH_2)_7COO-CH_2 \end{array} + 3H_2O$$

Oleic acid — Glycerol — Glyceryl trioleate (olein)

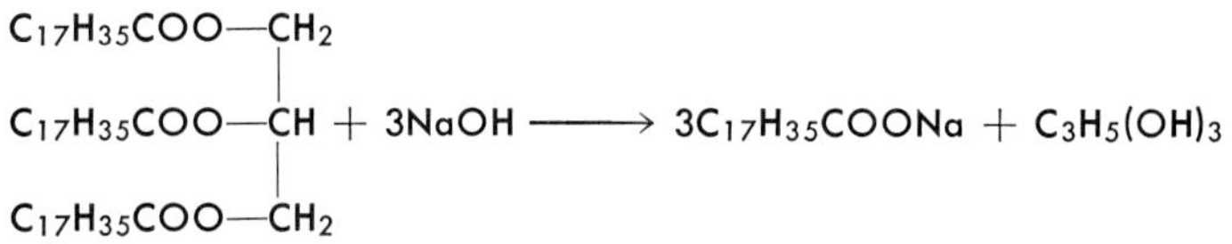

$$\begin{array}{l} C_{17}H_{35}COO-CH_2 \\ \qquad\qquad\quad | \\ C_{17}H_{35}COO-CH + 3NaOH \longrightarrow 3C_{17}H_{35}COONa + C_3H_5(OH)_3 \\ \qquad\qquad\quad | \\ C_{17}H_{35}COO-CH_2 \end{array}$$

Glyceryl tristearate — Sodium stearate (a soap) — Glycerol

becomes stearin (glyceryl tristearate), a solid:

$$C_3H_5(C_{17}H_{33}COO)_3 + 3H_2 \xrightarrow{Ni} C_3H_5(C_{17}H_{35}COO)_3$$

Olein — Stearin

Shortenings (for example, Crisco and Spry) are prepared by hydrogenation of cottonseed, peanut, and other edible oils.

Acrolein test. When fats and oils are heated with $KHSO_4$, a strong and penetrating odor is produced as a result of the formation of a compound called acrolein. Acrolein is derived from the glyceryl portion of the fat molecule. This reaction is used as a test for fats, oils, and glycerol.

Another test, which is crude but of some practical value, is to place a little fat or oil on a piece of paper; when held against a source of light, the spot is noted to be of exceptional translucence.

PROTEINS

Proteins, the organic backbone of protoplasm, are condensation polymers of amino acids. They are the most complex substances known to chemistry, with molecular weights in some instances in excess of 1,000,000,000. In one of the most brilliant pieces of work in the annals of science, Frederick Sanger and associates (1958) deciphered the chemical structure of insulin, a protein molecule composed of 777 atoms. This has proved a major breakthrough, because Sanger's techniques sparked an all-out attack on the "molecule of molecules." The student should well appreciate that the more we know about proteins, the more we know about the processes of life and disease.

An amino acid is a carboxylic acid containing one or more amino ($-NH_2$) groups. Glycine (aminoacetic acid), the simplest amino acid, has the following structure:

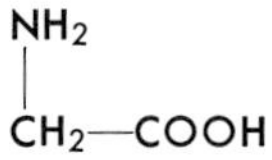

$$\begin{array}{l} NH_2 \\ | \\ CH_2-COOH \end{array}$$

The simplest possible protein, therefore, is glycylglycine, which is formed by the condensation of two molecules of glycine. Thus,

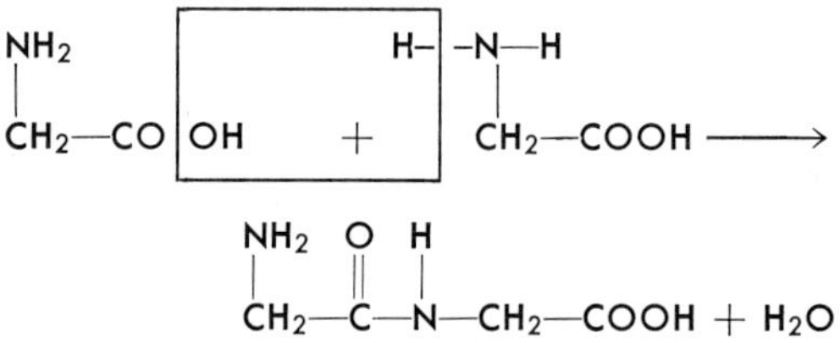

$$\begin{array}{l} NH_2 \qquad\qquad\qquad\qquad H-N-H \\ | \qquad\qquad\qquad\qquad\qquad\quad | \\ CH_2-CO\boxed{OH \quad + \quad H}-CH_2-COOH \longrightarrow \end{array}$$

$$\begin{array}{l} NH_2 \;\; O \;\; H \\ | \quad\;\; \| \quad | \\ CH_2-C-N-CH_2-COOH + H_2O \end{array}$$

Glycylglycine

Glycylglycine, in turn, can combine with another molecule of glycine to form diglycylglycine, and so on:

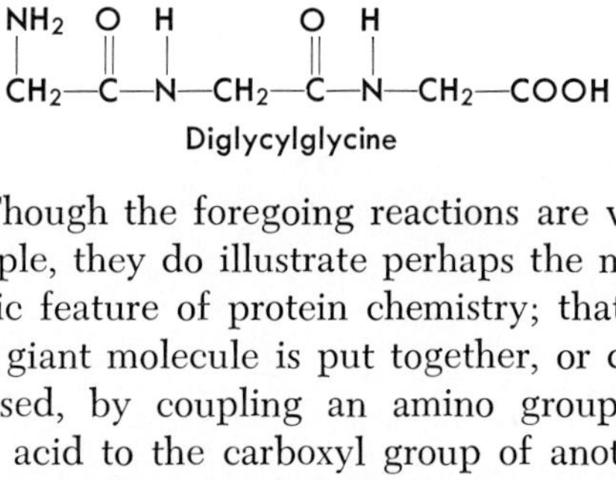

$$\begin{array}{l} NH_2 \;\; O \;\; H \qquad\quad O \;\; H \\ | \quad\;\; \| \quad | \qquad\qquad \| \quad | \\ CH_2-C-N-CH_2-C-N-CH_2-COOH \end{array}$$

Diglycylglycine

Though the foregoing reactions are very simple, they do illustrate perhaps the most basic feature of protein chemistry; that is, the giant molecule is put together, or condensed, by coupling an amino group of one acid to the carboxyl group of another via the splitting out of water.

A protein molecule, then, is a chain of amino acids. Now, is this a straight chain, a bent chain, or a twisted chain? And, moreover, does it make any difference? X-ray studies show that the chain is usually bent or twisted in the most cunning fashion. Indeed, one of nature's prize patterns consists of two coils wrapped about each other very much like a couple of interlocked spiral staircases. In this connection it is of singular interest to take a look at the amino acid cysteine:

$$\begin{array}{l} CH_2—S—H \\ | \\ CH_2NH_2 \\ | \\ COOH \end{array}$$

It has been shown that the sulfur atom of this acid in one chain cross-links with a sulfur atom of the acid in the other chain, giving a disulfide (—S—S—) bond.

The manner in which the molecular chains are bent, twisted, folded, or coiled does, indeed, have a key bearing upon protein behavior. As a matter of fact, enzymes (the protein catalysts of cells) owe their specificity to the way in which the substrate (the substance acted upon) dovetails into the chain. In other words, unless the substrate "fits," it cannot be acted upon.

Classification. Proteins are generally divided into three main classes: simple, conjugated, and derived. Simple proteins are those that yield only amino acids or their derivatives on hydrolysis. These include such substances as albumins, globulins, histones, and protamines. Conjugated proteins are those composed of a protein united to some other molecule, or *prosthetic* group. Important examples include nucleoproteins, glycoproteins, phosphoproteins, lipoproteins, and chromoproteins (for example, hemoglobin). Derived proteins include those obtained via the enzymatic or chemical hydrolysis of the other two classes. These include metaproteins, proteoses, peptones, and peptides.

Polypeptides. Polypeptides are compounds containing two or more amino acids. In a strict sense, then, polypeptides are simple proteins. In practice, however, the term is reserved for short amino acid chains, that is, dipeptides, tripeptides, tetrapeptides, and so on.

Properties. Physically, proteins are characterized by the fact that they are destroyed or denatured by heat. This is usually manifested by a change of color and solubility. For example, egg white, which is colorless and soluble in water, is changed to a white insoluble mass. Anyone who has ever fried an egg has observed this phenomenon. Heat kills cells because the proteins of the protoplasm are denatured.

Proteins are not soluble in strong alcohol or in solutions of salts such as ammonium sulfate. Chemists often take advantage of this fact when they desire to separate a protein from other substances. Alkaloidal reagents (for example, tannic acid, picric acid, and the like) and the salts of heavy metals (lead, mercury, silver, and copper) react with proteins to form precipitates. This action of heavy metals is thought to account for their antiseptic and disinfecting properties; that is, they react with and denature the protoplasm of the bacterial cell.

Color tests. A number of color tests are used as an aid in the identification of protein substances. Of these, probably the biuret and the xanthoproteic tests are the best known. The *biuret* test is performed by adding a strong solution of potassium hydroxide and a few drops of dilute copper sulfate to the unknown. A pinkish violet color signals a positive reaction. In the *xanthoproteic* test a few drops of concentrated nitric acid are added to the unknown; a yellow color that becomes an orange-yellow upon addition of a base signals a positive test.

NUCLEIC ACIDS

Nucleic acids are the chemical core of life. This is more than just a figure of speech when we consider that their twisted helical molecules direct and effect the synthesis of the proteins of cells. Whereas not a great many years ago the gene was looked upon as the "last word" in heredity and life, we now know that this honor belongs to *deoxyribonucleic acid* (DNA) because it is the stuff of which genes are made.

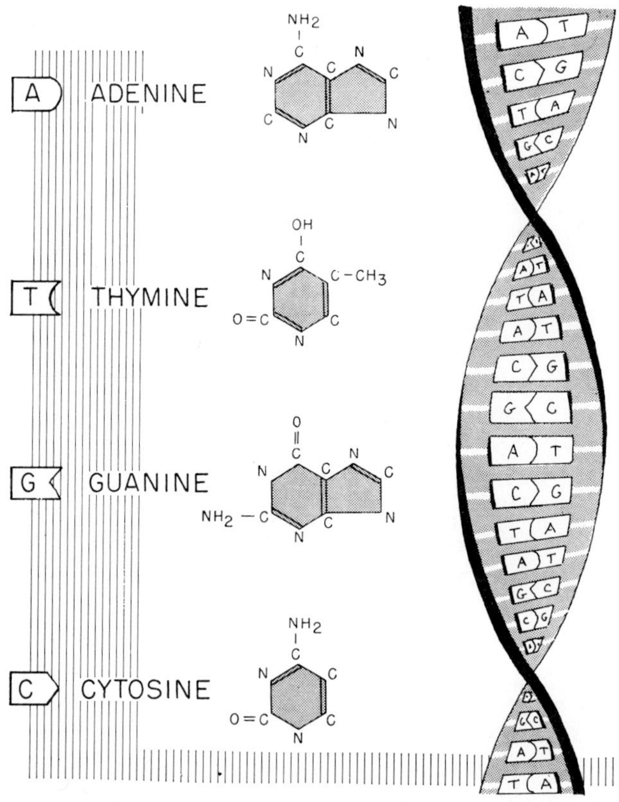

Fig. 5-7. Basic concept of the DNA molecule. The bases (**A, T, G,** and **C**) are attached to a "backbone" (broad dark lines) of phosphate and the sugar deoxyribose. (Modified from Medical News, May 11, 1960. Courtesy Ciba Pharmaceutical Co.)

Working hand in hand with DNA is a closely related substance called *ribonucleic acid* (RNA). Essentially, DNA directs the synthesis of *messenger* RNA, and the latter, with the help of *transfer* RNA, effects the condensation of amino acids into protein.

Structure of DNA and RNA. Both nucleic acids consist of long chains of phosphate and sugar residues, with nitrogenous bases attached to the sugars (Fig. 5-7). The sugar in RNA is *ribose,* and the sugar in DNA is *deoxyribose.* The bases include *adenine, guanine, cytosine, thymine,* and *uracil.* Both DNA and RNA contain the first three, but in the case of DNA the fourth base is thymine, whereas in RNA it is uracil.

According to x-ray analysis, DNA is actually a "double molecule," with one chain twined around the other in a *helical* fashion, the bases of one chain bonded neatly onto the bases of the other. In order to fit—and this we must deeply appreciate—a given base on one chain must be opposite a particular one on the other; specifically, guanine pairs only with cytosine and adenine only with thymine. *Thus, the sequence of bases on one chain determines the sequence on the other.* This means that if a piece of DNA wishes to duplicate or *replicate* itself, all it need do is untwine and have each chain line up the appropriate bases for a new partner chain. Thus, the chemical offspring are identical to the parent molecule, meaning that when a cell divides, the genes of the daughter cells are identical to those of the parent cell.

Questions

1. How could you distinguish between an organic and an inorganic compound?
2. Write the structural formulas for the three isomers of monobromopentane.
3. Account for the difference in pharmacologic potency between *dl*-amphetamine (Benzedrine) and dextroamphetamine (Dexedrine).
4. Compare the hydrocarbons of the methane and ethylene series.
5. Write the structural formula for pentylene.
6. How could you chemically distinguish between ethane and ethylene?
7. Using structural formulas, write the equation for the reaction between propylene and bromine.
8. Using structural formulas, illustrate "addition" and "substitution."
9. Write the structural formula for pentyne.
10. Write the structural formula for 2-iodo-5-methylheptane.
11. Name the following structure:

```
                 C2H5    CH3
                  |       |
CH3—CH2—CH2—C—CH2—CH—CH2—CH3
                  |
                 CH3
```

12. Distinguish between polymerization and condensation.
13. Write the structure for 1,3,5-triiodobenzene.
14. Write the structure for *p*-diiodobenzene.
15. Discuss the biologic significance of cyclopentanoperhydrophenanthrene.
16. Diabetic urine reduces Benedict's solution. Explain the mechanism of the reaction.
17. How could you chemically distinguish between acetone and acetaldehyde?
18. Write the structural formula for triiodomethane.
19. When grape juice is heated, it fails to ferment. Explain.
20. Using structural formulas, write the equation for the reaction between glyceryl trioleate and potassium hydroxide.
21. When iodine is added to olive oil, its color slowly disappears. Explain.
22. Explain how lye dissolves grease.
23. An ampule of penicillin reads "Penicillin Sodium." Explain.
24. What happens when a few drops of HCl are added to a solution of sucrose and the resulting mixture is boiled? Can you prove it?
25. Write the structure for methyl propyl ether.
26. Write the structure for methyl ethyl ketone.
27. Discuss the physiologic and pharmacologic significance of the amines.
28. Although strychnine is highly insoluble in water, a drop or two of HCl readily causes it to go into solution. Explain.
29. When a few drops of $AgNO_3$ are added to an aqueous solution of egg white, a precipitate is formed. Explain.
30. Using structural formulas, show what happens when a molecule of glycine condenses with a molecule of lysine.
31. A nitric acid burn turns the skin yellow. Explain.
32. What characteristics of egg white classify it as an albumin?
33. Name two important chromoproteins.
34. Following the complete enzymatic digestion of proteins, the latter fail to give a positive biuret test. Explain.
35. Explain the penetrating stench of burning fat.
36. Discuss the role of the nucleic acids in the life process.
37. Using methane, chlorine, silver hydroxide, and an oxidizing agent, tell how you could prepare formaldehyde. (*Hint:* First react the methane with chlorine.)
38. The end products of carbohydrate digestion are glucose, fructose, and galactose. Account for this fact.
39. Starting with starch, explain how ethyl alcohol can be manufactured.
40. Toluene is *carbocyclic* and pyridine *heterocyclic.* Explain.
41. Why are proteins said to be the most complex chemical substances?
42. Sweet cider changes into "hard" cider, and the latter changes into vinegar. Exactly what happens?
43. When water reacts with calcium carbide (CaC_2), calcium hydroxide and acetylene are produced. Write a balanced equation for the reaction.
44. It is said most dyes and drugs "come from coal tar." Explain.
45. Write the structural formula for benezene hexachloride.
46. Write a balanced equation for the burning of ethyl alcohol.
47. What is meant by denatured alcohol?
48. Distinguish between an alcohol and a phenol.
49. Write the equation for the reaction between formic acid and normal propyl alcohol.
50. Differentiate between esterification and saponification.

Chapter 6

Basic medical microbiology

Microbiology is the study of organisms too small to be studied without the aid of the microscope. Contrary to the consensus, these microorganisms, or *microbes,* are generally beneficial; indeed, through the processes of decay and putrefaction, they help to make our planet inhabitable. Also, microbes aid man in the manufacture of a great many useful products, ranging from vinegar to antibiotics. Here, however, our chief interest in the subject concerns those species that cause disease. To develop this interest, we shall discuss the basic ideas in the present chapter and reserve the details of the many infections until we arrive at the appropriate body system.

HISTORICAL DEVELOPMENT

The first concrete milestone in the history of microbiology was the discovery in 1675 by Antony van Leeuwenhoek that microbes do indeed exist. Using microscopes of his own design and construction, Leeuwenhoek described accurately the different shapes of bacteria and even pictured their arrangement in infected material. In view of this he is often referred to as the "father of bacteriology."

For many years it was generally believed that living organisms could arise from *non*-living organic matter, a belief called *spontaneous generation* or *abiogenesis.* Specifically, there was great controversy over the origin of bacteria that appeared in decomposing organic matter. Early experiments that seemed to support the theory of spontaneous generation were challenged by a number of investigators throughout the seventeenth century. However, it was not until 1861 that Louis Pasteur demonstrated beyond any reasonable doubt that living organisms have their origin only in other living organisms *(biogenesis).* That is to say, bacteria beget bacteria, protozoa beget protozoa, and so on.

The basic discovery in the field of immunity, or resistance to disease, was made as early as 1796 when Edward Jenner demonstrated that smallpox could be prevented by vaccination with the virus of cowpox. Interestingly, the discovery came at a time when other ideas about germs and disease were in a most primitive state.

In a very real sense the development of modern bacteriology began with the work of Pasteur. In 1865 he proved that "disease of wine" could be prevented (without altering the flavor of the wine) by the use of moderate heat *(pasteurization)*; and in 1881 and 1885 he developed vaccines against anthrax and rabies, respectively. Pasteur also discovered the staphylococcus and pneumococcus and was co-discoverer of the pathogen of gas gangrene.

Based on Pasteur's work, Lord Lister concluded that wound infections were caused by microorganisms. To test his theory, he started (1867) using dressings treated with carbolic acid (phenol) and spraying the air of the operating room with the substance *(antiseptic surgery)*. This practice drastically reduced the mortality rate and probably did more to advance surgery than any other single discovery or practice. Twenty years later Ernest von Bergmann reduced the rate still further through the use of steam sterilization of surgical instruments *(aseptic surgery)*.

In 1876 Robert Koch, considered by many to be second only to Pasteur, isolated the anthrax bacillus in pure culture and 6 years later discovered the tubercle bacillus. Koch was the first to stain bacterial smears on glass slides and also the first to work out methods for the isolation of bacteria in pure culture. In 1884 he proposed his famous principles *(Koch's postulates)* that established the relationship between an infectious disease and the causative microorganism. Thus, by this year the *germ theory of disease* was firmly established.

Medical microbiology now moved along rather swiftly. In 1880 Alphonse Laveran discovered the parasite of malaria, the most important infectious disease of man, and 3 years later Sir Ronald Ross proved that the parasite was transmitted by the *Anopheles* mosquito; in 1884 Elie Metchnikoff announced his discovery of phagocytosis (the ingestion and destruction of microbes by white cells) and proposed the phagocytic theory of immunity; in 1889 Shibasaburo Kitasato isolated the pathogen of tetanus; in 1890 he and Emil von Behring demonstrated the presence of an antitoxic substance *(antitoxin)* in the blood serum of infected animals that rendered the tetanus toxin harmless; and the very same year von Behring announced the discovery of an antitoxin against diphtheria.

In 1892 Dmitri Iwanowski demonstrated that tobacco mosaic disease was caused by an extremely small infectious agent—small enough to pass through a porcelain filter—and 6 years later Martinus Beijerinck proved that it was not a "tiny bacterium," as Iwanowski had supposed, but actually a new kind of microbe, known to us today as a *virus*. In 1909 Howard Ricketts discovered still another kind of microbe—the *rickettsia* (named in his honor).

The "closing of the ring" against microbes and infection came in 1909 when Paul Erhlich introduced the arsenical Salvarsan ("606") in the treatment of syphilis, thus creating the branch of medicine we call chemotherapy. In 1928 Alexander Fleming discovered penicillin; in 1935 Gerhard Domagk demonstrated the antimicrobial powers of Prontosil, the forerunner of the sulfa drugs; and in 1943 Selman Waksman and co-workers isolated streptomycin.

Perhaps the chief event in medical microbiology over the past quarter century was the development of successful vaccines against poliomyelitis and measles. This was largely an outgrowth of tissue culture methods perfected by John Enders and associates. And for microbiology as a whole, the most startling developments have been in the area of microbial genetics and biochemistry. Lo and behold, in 1967 Arthur Kornberg and co-workers actually succeeded in creating a virus in the test tube. Assuming that a virus is indeed a living thing, this is essentially *spontaneous generation!*

CLASSIFICATION

Six categories. Microorganisms fall into six general categories—protozoa, algae, fungi, bacteria, rickettsiae, and viruses

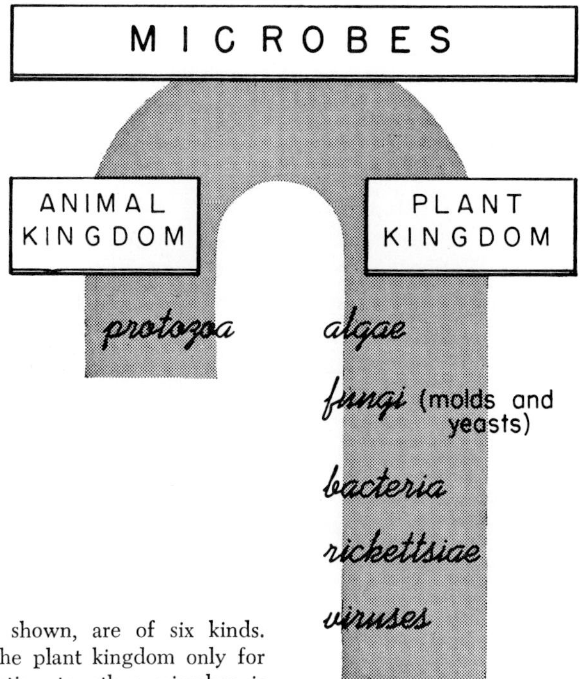

Fig. 6-1. Microbes, as shown, are of six kinds. Viruses are placed in the plant kingdom only for convenience. Their relation to other microbes is not presently understood. (From Brooks, S. M.: A programmed introduction to microbiology, St. Louis, 1968, The C. V. Mosby Co.)

(Fig. 6-1). Their salient features are as follows:

Protozoa are unicellular animals that are predominantly motile. Relative to other microorganisms, they have a complex internal structure. *Algae* are simple plants that show great variation in size and shape. The most primitive are unicellular, but others have a complex body structure with cell types designed for specific functions. Like all higher plant forms, algae contain chlorophyll and carry on photosynthesis. *Fungi* are simple plant forms *without* chlorophyll and therefore do not carry on photosynthesis. They range in size from microscopic forms such as yeasts to multicellular forms such as molds and mushrooms. *Bacteria* are unicellular plantlike microorganisms, the great majority of which do not contain chlorophyll. They are responsible for most infectious diseases of man and animals. *Rickettsiae* are unicellular *obligate* parasites present in various insects, the latter serving as vectors in the transmission of rickettsial infections to man. They are generally regarded as occupying a position intermediate between bacteria and viruses. *Viruses* are the smallest of the microbes and the great majority cannot be seen with the ordinary light microscope. They are *obligate* parasites that attack plants, animals, and bacteria. Based on present knowledge, viruses seem to inhabit the twilight zone between the living and the nonliving.

Basic units. The basic units used in the classification of living organisms are *kingdom, phylum, class, order, family, genus,* and *species.* Organisms that reproduce only their exact kind constitute a species; closely related species are grouped into genera; related genera constitute a family; and so on. In the *binomial system of nomenclature* each organism is known by two names: (1) the *genus* to which it belongs (always written with the initial letter *cap-*

italized) and (2) the name of the *species* (its initial letter never capitalized). By convention, both names are placed in *italics*. For example, the bacterium *Bacillus subtilis* belongs to the genus *Bacillus* and species *subtilis*.

Systems. The classification of microorganisms has proved a difficult task and there is considerable disagreement among authors (and textbooks) as to the best system. The trouble is not so much in regard to what we mean by "protozoa," "algae," "fungi," "rickettsiae," and "viruses," but rather where these groups belong in the general scheme of things—most particularly their relation to each other.

Most authors in microbiology (but not biology) subscribe to the scheme of classification set forth in the 1957 edition of *Bergey's Manual of Determinative Bacteriology,* a standard taxonomic work in the United States. According to this system, the plant kingdom (kingdom *Plantae*) is divided into five phyla (or divisions), two of which are of microbiologic concern—*Thallophyta* and *Protophyta.* To the former belong the algae and fungi, and to the latter belong the bacteria, rickettsiae, and viruses. (Protozoa belong to the animal kingdom—phylum *Protozoa.*)

Over the past decade the foregoing classification among most biologists (and some microbiologists) has given way to a system that gives phylum status to bacteria, fungi, and each of the various types of algae. In regard to viruses, there is a tendency among biologists and microbiologists alike to consider them an unknown entity in relation to other forms of life.

Some biologists and microbiologists take the position that all microbes belong to a single kingdom called *Protista* ("first life"). The thinking here is that a great many microorganisms are neither plant nor animal—hence, the special kingdom. The so-called *lower protists,* the most primitive organisms, include the blue-green algae, bacteria, and rickettsiae; and the so-called *higher protists* include the protozoa, fungi, and algae (exclusive of the blue-green algae).

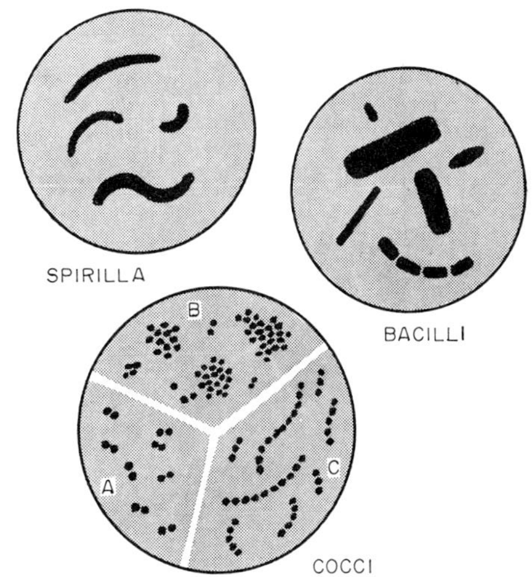

Fig. 6-2. Bacterial forms. **A,** Diplococci; **B,** staphylococci; **C,** streptococci. (From Brooks, S. M.: Basic facts of medical microbiology, ed. 2, Philadelphia, 1962, W. B. Saunders Co.)

BACTERIA

Bacteria compose the class *Schizomycetes* of the phylum *Protophyta* (according to Bergey).* The *orders* of this class of medical concern are presented below.

Eubacteriales. The members of this order, sometimes referred to as "true bacteria," cause the bulk of all infectious diseases. These organisms are single-celled forms of three basic morphologic types—rodlike, spiral, and spherical (Fig. 6-2). The rodlike forms are called *bacilli* (sing., *bacillus*) and the rigid, spiral forms are called *spirilla* (sing., *spirillum*). The spherical forms, called *cocci* (sing., *coccus*), are further characterized by the groupings they assume in the wake of cell division—that is, *diplococci* (cocci in pairs), *streptococci* (cocci in chains), *staphylococci* (cocci in grapelike bunches), *sarcina* (cocci in cuboidal packets of eight cells), and *gaffkyae* (cocci in cuboidal packets of four cells).

*Most texts in biology relegate bacteria to the special phylum *Schizomycophyta*.

The families of order Eubacteriales of chief medical concern are the following.

Enterobacteriaceae. This family is made up of a number of gram-negative (p. 143), saprophytic, and parasitic (p. 128) bacilli that inhabit the intestinal tract of man and animals. These organisms ferment certain carbohydrates, and an important feature within the family is the ability—or inability—to ferment lactose. The principal pathogens of the family are *Escherichia coli* (causes urinary tract infections), *Aerobacter aerogenes* (urinary tract infections), *Klebsiella pneumoniae* (respiratory infections), *Proteus vulgaris* (urinary tract and wound infections), *Salmonella typhosa* (typhoid fever), *Salmonella paratyphi* (paratyphoid fever), *Salmonella typhimurium* ("food poisoning"), and *Shigella* spp.* (bacillary dysentery).

Brucellaceae. This family is made up of small, nonmotile (p. 138), gram-negative bacilli that cause a number of diseases in man. The chief pathogens are *Pasteurella pestis* (causes plague), *Pasturella tularensis* (tularemia), *Brucella* spp. (undulant fever), *Haemophilus influenzae* (respiratory infections, meningitis), *Haemophilus ducreyi* (soft chancre), and *Bordetella pertussis* (whooping cough).

Micrococcaceae. This family is made up of gram-positive (p. 143), nonsporeforming (p. 137), nonmotile cocci that commonly inhabit the skin and mucous membranes. The species *Staphylococcus aureus* is one of the most troublesome and dangerous organisms known. Among other infections, it causes boils, abscesses, pyelonephritis, osteomyelitis, pneumonia, food poisoning, and septicemia ("blood poisoning").

Neisseriaceae. This family is made up of gram-negative, nonsporeforming, nonmotile cocci that have a tendency to arrange themselves in pairs. The chief pathogens for man are *Neisseria gonorrhoeae* (gonorrhea) and *Neisseria meningitidis* (epidemic meningitis).

Lactobacillaceae. This family is made up of microaerophilic and anaerobic bacteria (p. 139) that characteristically ferment sugars with the production of acid and gas. They occur in milk and dairy products and in the mouth and intestinal tract of man. The chief pathogens of the family are *Diplococcus pneumoniae* (a common cause of pneumonia) and *Streptococcus pyogenes* (the cause of septic sore throat and scarlet fever).

Corynebacteriaceae. This family is made up of parasitic and pathogenic bacteria that occur in dairy products and in the soil. The chief pathogen, *Corynebacterium diphtheriae,* is the cause of diphtheria.

Bacillaceae. This family is made up of gram-positive, sporeforming bacilli that are widely distributed in soil and decomposing organic matter. The chief genera are *Bacillus* (aerobes) and *Clostridium* (anaerobes), and the chief pathogens are *Bacillus anthracis* (causes anthrax), *Clostridium tetani* (tetanus), *Clostridium botulinum* (botulism), and *Clostridium perfringens* (gangrene).

Bacteroidaceae. This family is composed of gram-negative bacilli that require enriched media for growth. The chief patho-

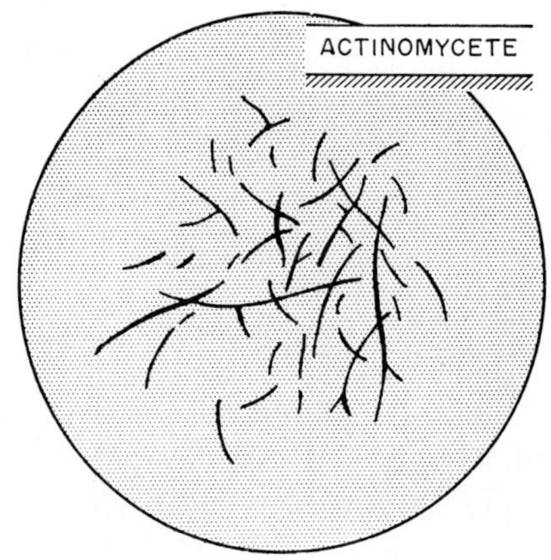

Fig. 6-3. Actinomycete. (From Brooks, S. M.: Basic facts of medical microbiology, ed. 2, Philadelphia, 1962, W. B. Saunders Co.)

*The abbreviation spp. indicates that two or more species are involved.

gens are *Bacteroides* spp. (wound infections), *Fusobacterium fusiforme* (associated with trench mouth), and *Streptobacillus moniliformis* (rat-bite fever).

Actinomycetales. This order is made up of moldlike bacteria with elongated cells, frequently filamentous, which have a tendency to branch (Fig. 6-3). There are three families. Family *Mycobacteriaceae* is constituted by *acid-fast* (p. 143), rodlike organisms that exhibit some branching. The chief species of the family are *Mycobacterium tuberculosis* (the cause of tuberculosis) and *Mycobacterium leprae* (the cause of leprosy). The family *Actinomycetaceae* is made up of organisms that grow in threadlike filaments. Pathogenic species belong to the genera *Nocardia* and *Actinomyces.* The family *Streptomycetaceae* is made up of organisms strikingly similar to true molds. This family is characterized by the fact that a dozen or more key *antibiotics* are produced by organisms of the genus *Streptomyces.*

Spirochaetales. The bacteria of this order (commonly called spirochetes) are slender, flexuous, spiral organisms that closely resemble protozoa (Fig. 6-4). For the most part, they are highly motile and differ from one another morphologically in length and number of spirals. The order is divided into two families—*Spirochaetaceae* and *Treponemataceae.* To the former belong the free-living spiral bacteria of water, and to the latter the slender spiral bacteria that are parasitic to man and animals. The chief pathogens are *Treponema pallidum* (the cause of syphilis) and *Treponema pertenue* (the cause of yaws).

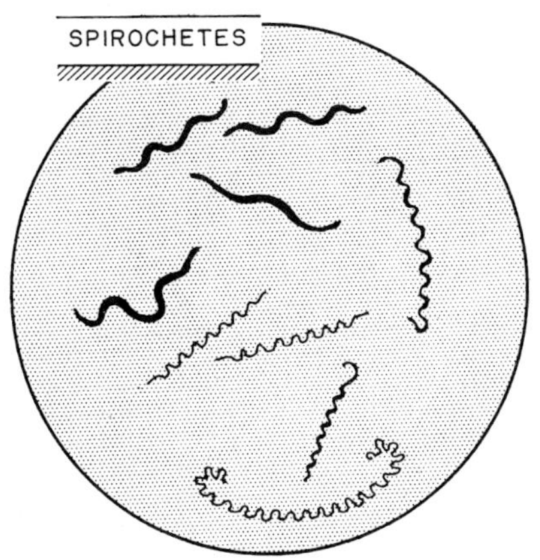

Fig. 6-4. Spirochetes. (From Brooks, S. M.: Basic facts of medical microbiology, ed. 2, Philadelphia, 1962, W. B. Saunders Co.)

Pseudomonadales. This bacterial order is made up of a number of species of bacilli and spirilla that are widely distributed throughout nature. Of medical importance are the families *Pseudomonadaceae* and *Spirillaceae.* The members of Pseudomonadaceae are short, nonsporing, bacilli that move by means of polar flagella. Most species are gram-negative. The chief pathogen, *Pseudomonas aeruginosa,* is a common invader of wounds, burns, urinary tract, and middle ear. The Spirillaceae family is made up of gram-negative spirilla with a polar flagellum. The chief pathogens are *Vibrio comma* (the cause of Asiatic cholera) and *Spirillum minus* (the cause of rat-bite fever).

Mycoplasmatales. This order is composed of delicate, nonmotile organisms without a cell wall. On solid media the cells are roundish, whereas in fluid media they occur as irregular filamentous forms. These bacteria are commonly referred to as *pleuropneumonia-like organisms* (PPLO for short) because the first species of the type to be discovered causes a disease in cattle known as bovine pleuropneumonia. The species *Mycoplasma pneumoniae* is a cause of pneumonia in man.

VIRUSES

Viruses may be regarded as infectious giant molecules that come alive only in the presence of *living cells.* Thus, they occupy the twilight zone between the living and the dead. No one pretends to know their relationship to free-living microbes, and it is merely for convenience that Bergey relegates them to the order *Virales* of the class *Microtatobiotes* (phylum *Protophyta*). Vi-

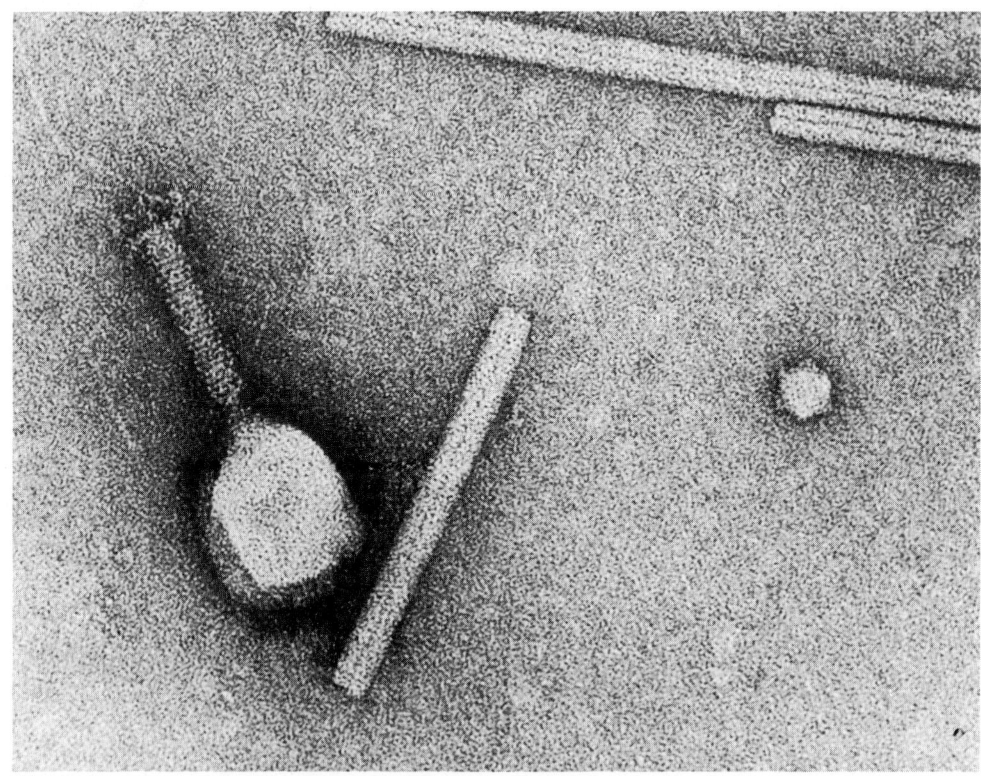

Fig. 6-5. This electron micrograph underscores exquisitely the differences in size and shape among the viruses. The flask-shaped virion is the T4 bacteriophage, the rod-shaped virions are the tobacco mosaic virus, and the spherical virion is the ϕX174 bacteriophage. ($\times$450,000.) (Courtesy F. A. Eiserling, Department of Bacteriology, University of California at Los Angeles.)

ruses range in size from about 10 to 350 millimicrons (mμ), and all under 200 mμ are beyond the reach of the *light* microscope. This explains the popular expression "ultramicroscopic." Viruses are particulate in nature and vary greatly in shape. Some are spherical, some are cuboidal, some are rod shaped, and there are those that remind one of a tadpole (Fig. 6-5).

The virion. A virus particle, or virion, is composed of a large coil of *either* deoxyribonucleic acid (DNA) or ribonucleic acid (RNA) tightly folded and packed within a protein coat called a *capsid.* In turn, the capsid is organized into subunits called *capsomeres.* Plant viruses contain RNA; animal viruses contain RNA or DNA; and most bacterial viruses contain DNA.

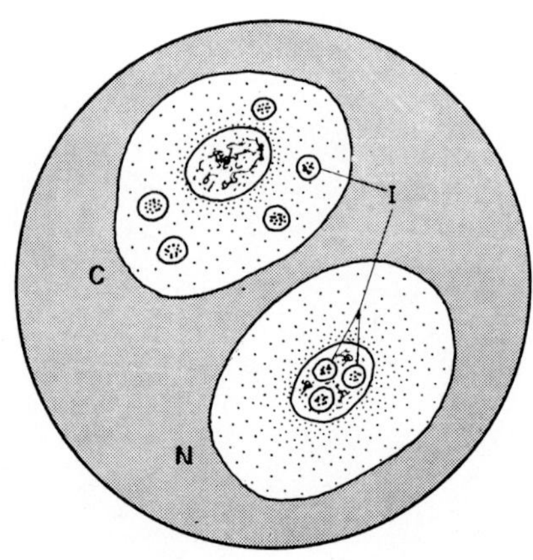

Fig. 6-6. Inclusion bodies in the cytoplasm, **C,** and nucleus, **N.** (From Brooks, S. M.: Basic facts of medical microbiology, ed. 2, Philadelphia, 1962, W. B. Saunders Co.)

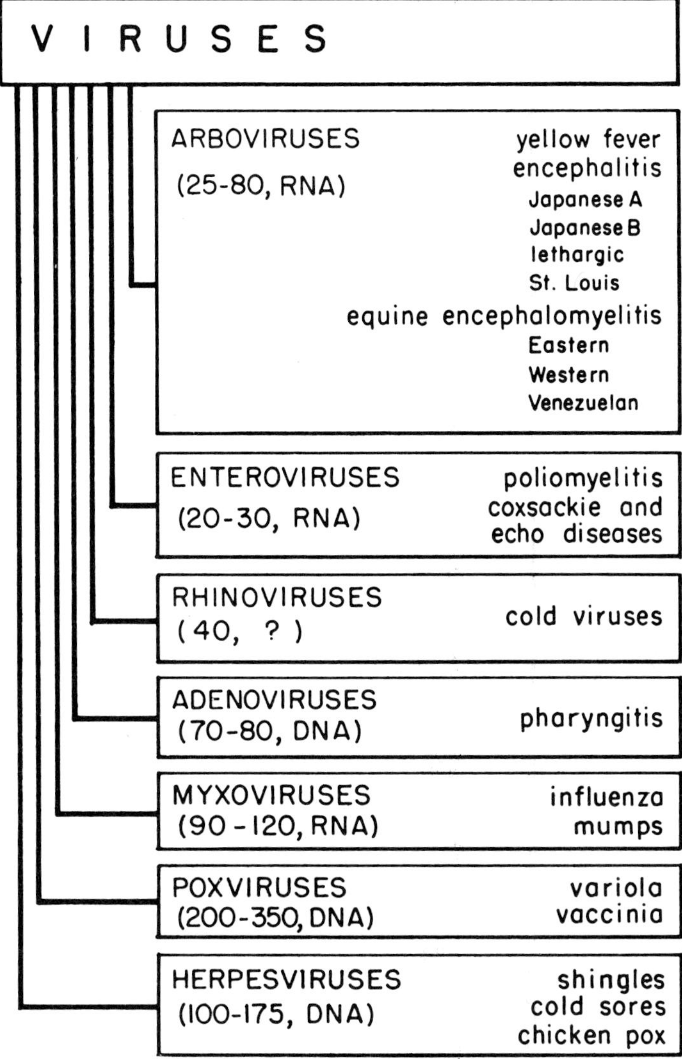

Fig. 6-7. Classification of viruses on the basis of particle size (in millimicrons), nucleic acid content (DNA or RNA), and diseases caused. (From Brooks, S. M.: A programmed introduction to microbiology, St. Louis, 1968, The C. V. Mosby Co.)

Bacteriophages and replication. Viruses that attack and bring about the destruction of bacterial cells are called bacteriophages (or simply "phages"). The action itself is often referred to as the *Twort-d'Herelle phenomenon* in honor of its discoverers. A great deal of what we know about viruses stems from phage studies, particularly in regard to the mechanism of replication within the host cell. In brief, a phage virion attacks the bacterial cell by injecting its nucleic acid through the cell membrane. Thereupon the viral nucleic acid takes over the cell's metabolic machinery and proceeds to turn out new virions at the expense of the host. In 10 minutes or so the cell ruptures (*lyses*), with the release of a hundred or so phage virions—virions all set to attack other bacterial cells in the same fashion. This is more or less the way viruses behave in the tissues of susceptible plants and animals.

Inclusion bodies. Cells that play host to viruses commonly show so-called inclusion bodies either in the cytoplasm or nucleus (Fig. 6-6). For the most part, inclusion bodies represent clusters or colonies of virions. Some inclusion bodies are so highly specific that they are of signal importance in the laboratory diagnosis of viral infections (for example, the *Guarnieri bodies* of smallpox and the *Negri bodies* of rabies).

Classification. Viruses that attack man and animals fall into seven major families: *poxviruses, herpesviruses, arboviruses, myxoviruses, adenoviruses, enteroviruses,* and *rhinoviruses* (Fig. 6-7). On a strictly clinical basis, human viruses are often grouped according to the area or part of the body chiefly involved in the disease, that is, *dermotropic* viruses (skin and mucous membranes), *pneumotropic* viruses (respiratory tract), *neurotropic* viruses (nervous system), *viscerotropic* viruses (some organ), and *pantropic* viruses (a variety of tissues and organs).

Cancer. Viruses cause certain malignant tumors (cancer) in animals. These include, among others, Rous sarcoma of chickens, myxomatosis of rabbits, leukemias of mice and chickens, and polyomas of rabbits, mice, and hamsters. In man the common wart (a *benign* tumor) is caused by a virus, but as yet no virus has been isolated from any type of human cancer. In the event such a virus is discovered it may be possible to develop a protective vaccine against the disease.

RICKETTSIAE

Rickettsiae are organisms that lie between bacteria and viruses in size and complexity. According to Bergey, they compose the order *Rickettsiales* of the class *Microtatobiotes* (phylum *Protophyta*). Rickettsiae are pleomorphic, gram-negative, bacilloid structures that can be cultured only in the presence of *living* tissue (Fig. 6-8). Like viruses, they are *intracellular* parasites, but otherwise rickettsiae more closely resemble bacteria. They attack both man and animals, with rodents and ticks serving as the chief reservoirs of infection. Mites, lice, and fleas serve as vectors, transmitting rickettsiae from animal to animal, from animal to man, and from man to man. The principal groups of rickettsiae of medical concern are presented in Fig. 6-9.

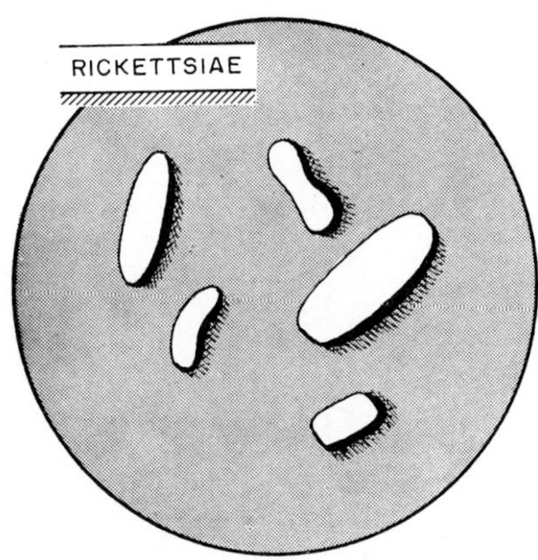

Fig. 6-8. Rickettsial forms as seen under the electron microscope. (From Brooks, S. M.: Basic facts of medical microbiology, ed. 2, Philadelphia, 1962, W. B. Saunders Co.)

FUNGI

The term *fungi* in common usage refers to any and all growths that to the unaided eye look like a *mold.* This includes the *true* molds (filamentous organisms with extensive branching), certain actinomycetes, and certain yeasts (Fig. 6-10). A true mold is a fuzzy growth composed of interlacing filaments (*hyphae*) that reproduce by means of spores. (A tuft of hyphae is called a *mycelium.*) Actinomycetes, as stated earlier, are moldlike bacteria that are often branched and sometimes form mycelia. Although so-called *true* yeasts usually do not form filaments, a number of pathogenic species are filamentous under certain conditions. The bulk of the pathogenic fungi belong to the class *Fungi Imperfecti* of the phylum Eumycophyta.

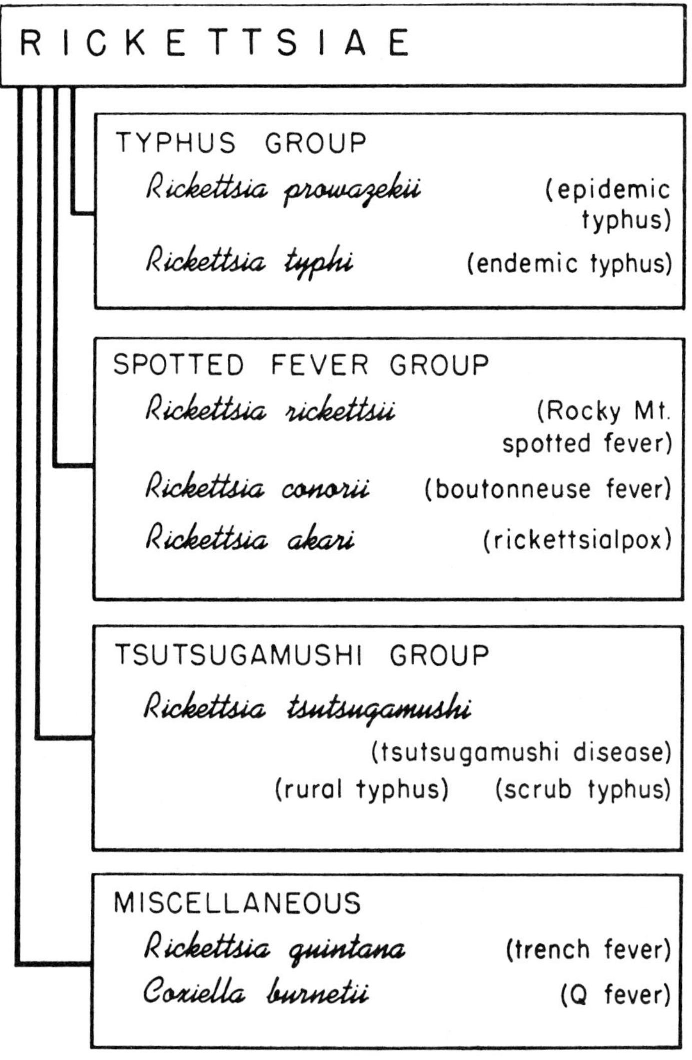

Fig. 6-9. Clinical classification of rickettsiae. (From Brooks, S. M.: A programmed introduction to microbiology, St. Louis, 1968, The C. V. Mosby Co.)

Yeasts. Though it has been and often still is common practice to define a yeast as a unicellular organism that reproduces by *budding,* in actual practice the definition is rather uncertain for a number of reasons. For example, some yeasts reproduce by fission, some (perhaps all) under certain conditions produce mycelia, and not uncommonly many molds, under the appropriate conditions, assume a yeastlike form. Thus, it seems more realistic to consider a yeast, or a true yeast, as an organism that *usually* exists in a single-celled or yeastlike form. In the same vein the expression *yeastlike mold* may be used to refer to a mold that, under certain conditions, becomes yeastlike. As used here, the true yeasts include the nonpathogenic organisms belonging to the genus *Saccharomyces* of the class *Ascomycetes* (phylum Eumycophyta).

The yeast cell, which is from 20 to 100

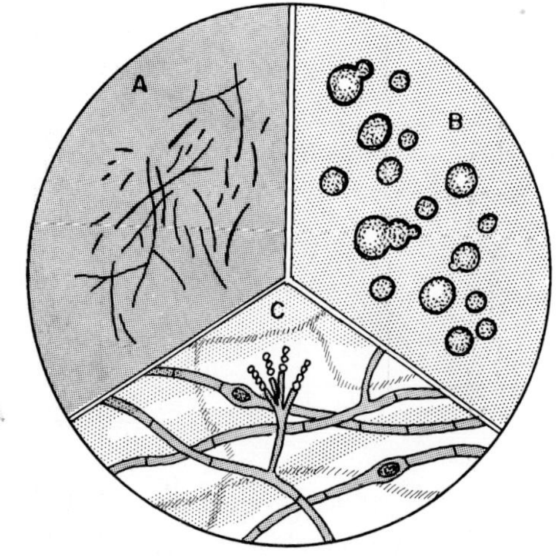

Fig. 6-10. Fungal types. **A,** Actinomycete; **B,** yeast; **C,** mold. (From Brooks, S. M.: Basic facts of medical microbiology, ed. 2, Philadelphia, 1962, W. B. Saunders Co.)

times larger than the bacterial cell and contains vacuoles and granules in the cytoplasm, reproduces by budding and by the formation of ascospores. The most common and useful of all yeasts is bakers' or brewers' yeast *(Saccharomyces cerevisiae),* an organism characterized by large, plump, oval, or round cells. Another species is *Saccharomyces ellipsoideus,* the common wine yeast that occurs on the skin of the grape. Both species release enzymes ("zymase") that catalyze the formation of ethyl alcohol (C_2H_5OH) from glucose ($C_6H_{12}O_6$) in the process of fermentation (p. 104).

PROTOZOA

Protozoa are *unicellular* animal organisms that vary considerably in structure and function (Fig. 6-11). They are much

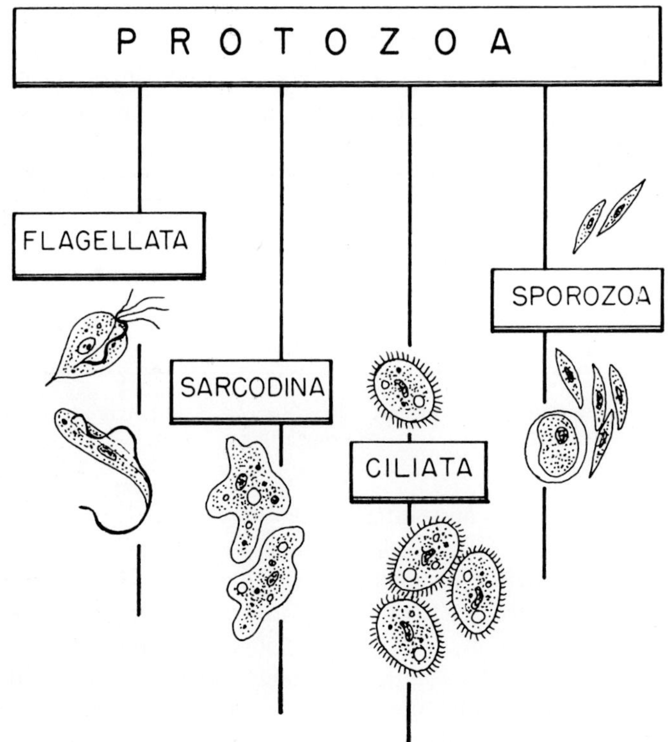

Fig. 6-11. Protozoa fall into five classes on the basis of their mode of locomotion. Class Suctoria (cilia only in early stages) is not shown. (From Brooks, S. M.: A programmed introduction to microbiology, St. Louis, 1968, The C. V. Mosby Co.)

larger than bacteria and possess well-defined nuclei. The chief groups of the phylum are *Sarcodina* (which move by means of pseudopodia), *Flagellata* (which move by means of flagella), *Ciliophora* (which move by means of cilia), and *Sporozoa* (which have no means of locomotion). Although most are harmless and beneficial, a number of species cause serious infection in both man and animals.

PARASITIC WORMS AND ECTOPARASITES

Although most parasitic worms and ectoparasites are not microbial in the usual sense of the word, they nonetheless cannot be studied in detail without the aid of the microscope. What is more, their infective stages for the most part are indeed microscopic. Parasitic worms belong to the phyla *Nematoda* (roundworms) and *Platyhelminthes* (flatworms). Nonsegmented flatworms (*flukes*) belong to the class *Trematoda* and segmented flatworms (tapeworms) belong to the subclass *Cestoda*. The term *ectoparasites* is used here to describe certain pathogens that live upon the surface of the body, namely, lice, fleas, and mites. These organisms belong to the classes *Insecta* (having three pairs of legs) and *Arachnida* (having four pairs of legs) of the phylum *Arthropoda*.

BACTERIAL MORPHOLOGY AND PHYSIOLOGY

The bacterial cell. The bacterial cell, ranging in size from 0.5 to 15μ in its greatest dimension, is basically like other cells except for the fact that it does not usually possess a well-defined nucleus. In most instances the nuclear material appears to be dispersed throughout the cell in the form of "nuclear bodies."

Capsule. The gelatinous outer wall that surrounds the bacterial cell is called the capsule (Fig. 6-12). Although it is difficult to demonstrate this structure in many species, most workers now believe that it surrounds all bacterial cells. It is generally held that the capsule serves as a protection against adverse environmental factors and thereby enhances the virulence of the cell. The capsule is also of some diagnostic significance, for its presence or absence serves as a mark of identification.

Spores. Certain bacilli have the ability to form round to oval resistant structures of "condensed protoplasm" called spores (Fig. 6-13). Within the cell they are called endospores; when released to the outside (as a result of disintegration of the cell wall), they are called free spores. In this connec-

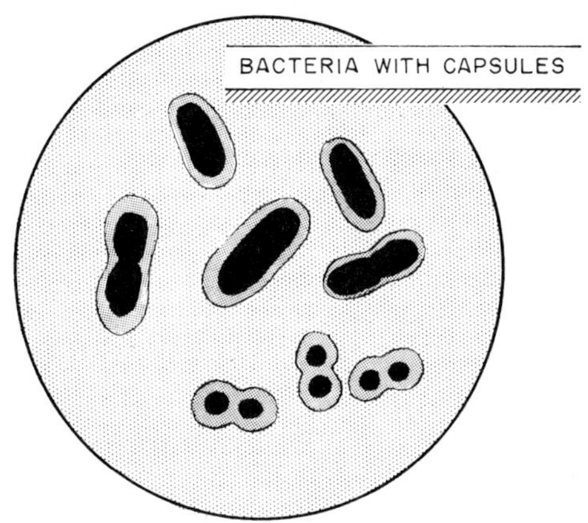

Fig. 6-12. Capsules. (From Brooks, S. M.: Basic facts of medical microbiology, ed. 2, Philadelphia, 1962, W. B. Saunders Co.)

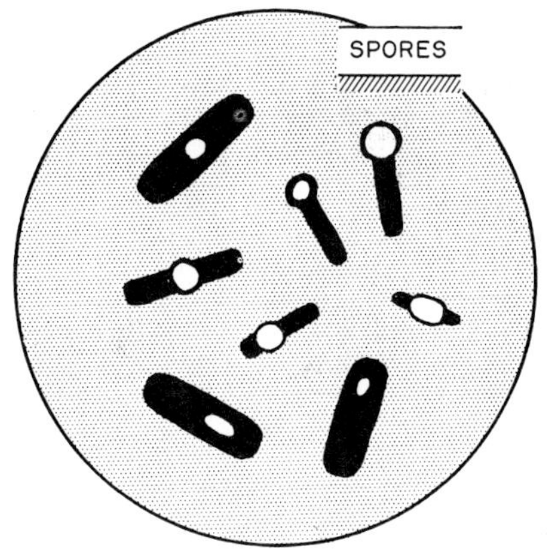

Fig. 6-13. Spores. (From Brooks, S. M.: Basic facts of medical microbiology, ed. 2, Philadelphia, 1962, W. B. Saunders Co.)

tion it is of interest to note that when a sporeforming species is observed microscopically, one generally sees endospores, free spores, and some bacilli with no spores at all. Not only the mere presence of spores but also their shape and position are of interest and diagnostic value; that is, a species that forms a large oval spore at the end of the cell always forms such a spore (Fig. 6-13).

Since spores are formed (one to a cell) in response to such adverse factors as high temperatures, desiccation, and the like, we can well appreciate that sporeforming pathogens are more difficult to destroy than nonsporeformers. This means that methods of sterilization must be aimed at the spores as well as at the vegetative cell. Unless a spore is destroyed, it will germinate back into the bacterial cell.

Flagella. Flagella, hairlike structures believed to be cytoplasmic extensions, are responsible for bacterial motility. Although rarely seen among the cocci, most bacilli and spirilla are equipped with these microscopic propellers. The manner in which flagella are distributed about the surface of the bacterial cell (Fig. 6-14) is of importance in identification.

Variation. The old saying that "the only thing constant is variation" certainly applies in full measure to bacteria. Indeed, we can expect morphologic or physiologic changes in any species. Microbial variation would be largely of theoretical interest if it were not for the fact that the change produced often is one of increased virulence or drug resistance. Most staphylococci, for example, which were initially highly sensitive to penicillin and certain other antibiotics, have acquired an alarming resistance. Further, some bacteria are able to pass on their resistance to other bacteria via a so-called resistance or R factor.

In the laboratory we encounter *pleomorphism,* or variation in shape. Thus, a species that possesses a coccal shape may, upon aging, display shapes ranging from spherical to bacillary. This explains why the age of a bacterial culture should always be known prior to microscopic examination.

Reproduction and growth. True bacteria reproduce by simple division, or *binary fission* (Fig. 6-15). When a few organisms are inoculated into some suitable culture medium such as meat broth, they proceed to divide (after an initial lag phase) about every 20 minutes. After a time, however, there ensues the resting phase in which the organisms are dying as fast as they divide, and finally the death phase sets in (Fig. 6-16). From the first stage to the last usually represents a period of about 24 hours.

Growth requirements. One should not be especially surprised to learn that bacteria

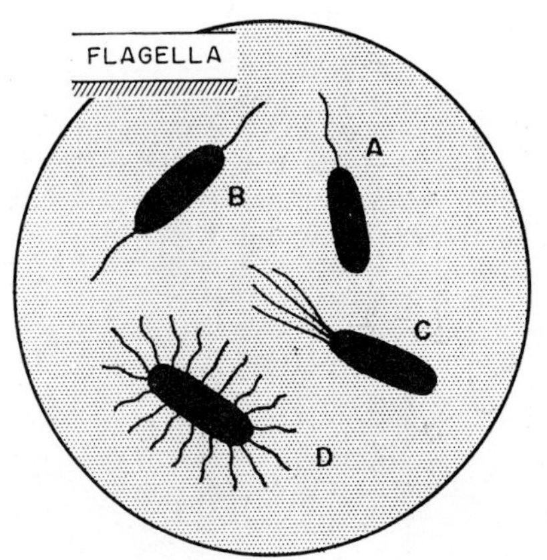

Fig. 6-14. Flagella. **A,** Monotrichate; **B,** amphitrichate; **C,** lophotrichate; **D,** peritrichate. (From Brooks, S. M.: Basic facts of medical microbiology, ed. 2, Philadelphia, 1962, W. B. Saunders Co.)

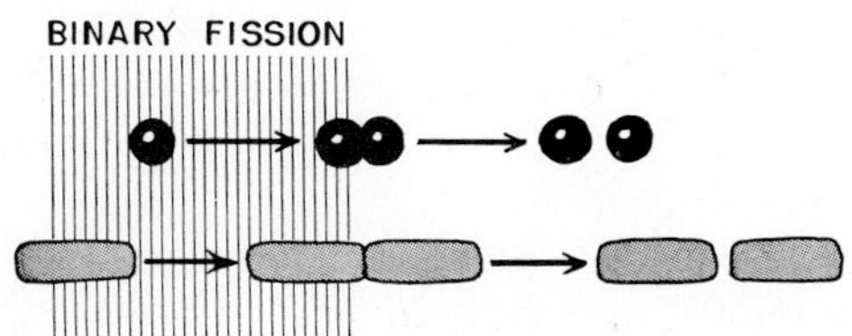

Fig. 6-15. Binary fission. (From Brooks, S. M.: Basic facts of medical microbiology, ed. 2, Philadelphia, 1962, W. B. Saunders Co.)

have a variety of growth requirements that must be met if they are to be cultured successfully in the laboratory. Although some, like people, are easy to please, others are quite fussy. The various factors relating to growth are discussed in some detail herewith.

Food. Relative to nutrition, there are two kinds of bacteria: those that can utilize carbon dioxide and simple inorganic compounds (*autotrophic* bacteria) and those that require organic matter (*heterotrophic* bacteria). Of medical importance is the fact that the former are nonpathogenic, whereas many species of the latter kind are pathogenic.

Heterotrophic bacteria that live on dead or decaying organic matter are called *saprophytes;* those that live in the tissues of living organisms are called *parasites.* Facultative saprophytes are bacteria that usually are parasitic but may be saprophytic. In contrast, facultative parasites are bacteria that are usually saprophytic but may be parasitic. Some bacteria, however, are strictly saprophytic *(obligate saprophytes),* and some are strictly parasitic *(obligate parasites).*

Water. Protoplasm, whether it be in the bacterial cell or in the big toe, must have water to survive. Like other forms of life, however, bacteria differ widely in their water requirements. The spirochete of syphilis, for instance, can last only a few hours without moisture. Some sporeformers, on the other hand, may survive for years.

Oxygen. Some bacteria cannot live without oxygen (*obligate aerobes*), and some cannot live with it (*obligate anaerobes*). In between are the *facultative anaerobes;* that is, organisms that can adapt to either condition. Finally, there are the *microaerophiles,* or organisms that require a reduction in the amount of oxygen present in the atmosphere.

Obviously, the culturing of a given species demands knowledge of its oxygen requirements. Obligate anaerobes, for instance, must be cultured in the absence of oxygen, and a variety of physical and chemical techniques have been developed for this purpose. An ultrasimple procedure is as follows: A tube of sterile broth is heated to drive out any oxygen absorbed from the air and then inoculated after being quickly cooled. A small piece of fresh sterile liver is then added (to act as a reducing agent) and the broth covered with a layer of sterile petrolatum (or paraffin) to prevent absorption of atmospheric oxygen.

Temperature. For each species of bac-

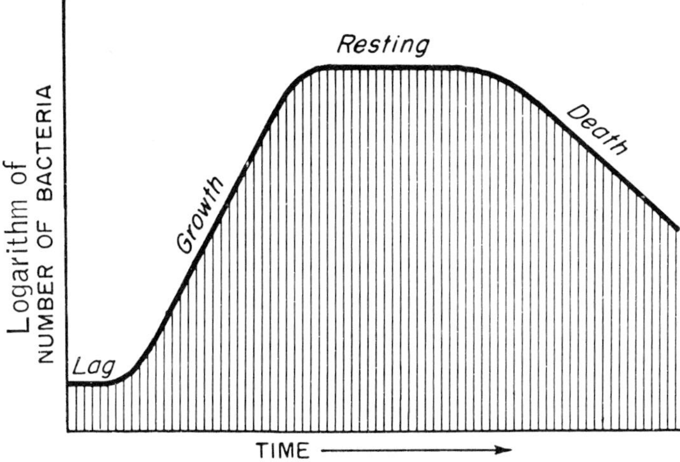

Fig. 6-16. Bacterial growth curve. (From Brooks, S. M.: Basic facts of medical microbiology, ed. 2, Philadelphia, 1962, W. B. Saunders Co.)

teria there are the so-called minimal temperature (the lowest temperature at which growth occurs) and the maximal temperature (the highest temperature at which growth can occur). Saprophytes have an optimal temperature range of 25° to 30° C., whereas the range for parasites is about 32° to 38° C. Certain autotrophic organisms, however, have optimal temperature ranges far below and above these figures. Bacteria with optimal temperature ranges of 4° to 10° C., 25° to 40° C., and 50° to 55° C. are called psychrophiles, mesophiles, and thermophiles, respectively.

pH. Microbes are quite sensitive to changes in pH, the majority doing best somewhere between pH 5 and 8. Generally speaking, the optimum for molds is pH 5, and for bacteria it is pH 7 to 7.5. Obviously, all media must be adjusted to the optimum pH of the organism that is to be cultured.

Osmotic pressure. Being semipermeable, the bacterial cell membrane is affected by changes in osmotic pressure. If exposed to solutions of a much higher pressure than its own (hypertonic solutions), the cell loses water and shrinks (plasmolysis) (Fig. 6-17). In hypotonic solutions the cell swells slightly but does not rupture because of the restraining *cell wall.*

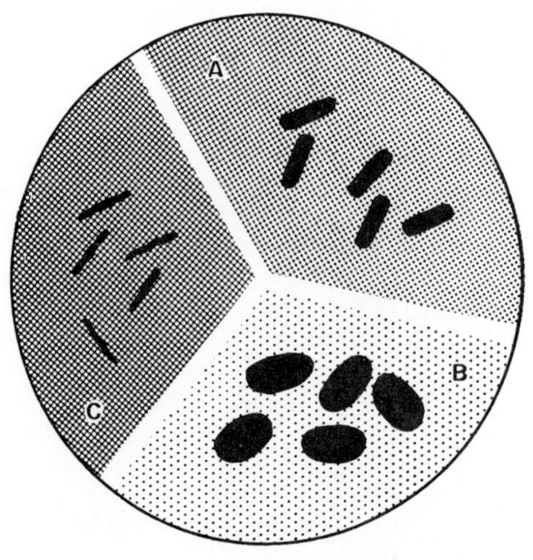

Fig. 6-17. The bacterial cell and osmosis. (Effects much exaggerated.) **A,** Isotonic solution; **B,** hypotonic solution, **C,** hypertonic solution. (From Brooks, S. M.: Basic facts of medical microbiology, ed. 2, Philadelphia, 1962, W. B. Saunders Co.)

Light. All microbes are either inhibited or killed by the ultraviolet rays of the sun. These rays and other short-wave electromagnetic radiations such as x rays and gamma rays are lethal to microbial protoplasm. The mode of injury might reside in the fact that certain enzyme systems are destroyed or altered. As one might expect, sporulating organisms are more resistant than the vegetative cells.

Microbial relationships. Like other biologic societies, microbes have their friends and their enemies. Some species live together in mutual satisfaction (*mutualism*) and some are unable to live together at all (*antibiosis*). Then there is the situation where one member is aided by the association, while the other is essentially unaffected (*commensalism*).

The phenomenon of antibiosis, of course, has given us one of our most powerful weapons against infection—the antibiotic. An antibiotic may be defined as a chemical agent produced by one microbe that inhibits or kills another microbe. We shall have more to say about these miracle drugs shortly.

THE LABORATORY

Microscopy. The microscope provides the magnification that enables us to see microorganisms. Such instruments are of two basic types—light (or optical) and electron. Light microscopy deals with five optical techniques—*bright field, dark field, phase contrast, ultraviolet,* and *fluorescence.* Electron microscopy, as its name suggests, uses a beam of electrons rather than light rays to effect magnification.

The bright-field microscope is the most commonly used instrument for routine work. The area, or microscopic field, to be observed is brightly illuminated and the objects appear dark against a light background. The general run of microscopes of this type can magnify up to about 1000 times. The bright-field microscope used in microbiology is commonly called the *compound* microscope (Fig. 6-18) because two or more lens systems are involved. Essentially, this instrument is a tube with a lens system called the *objective* at the bottom, and a lens system called the *eyepiece* (or ocular) at the top. A mirror directs a beam of light through the object on the stage, and the objective projects an enlarged image of the object up near the top of the microscope tube.* This image is viewed through the eyepiece, which acts much like a simple magnifying lens, the chief difference being that the eyepiece

*In some instruments the source of light is contained in the base (Fig. 6-18).

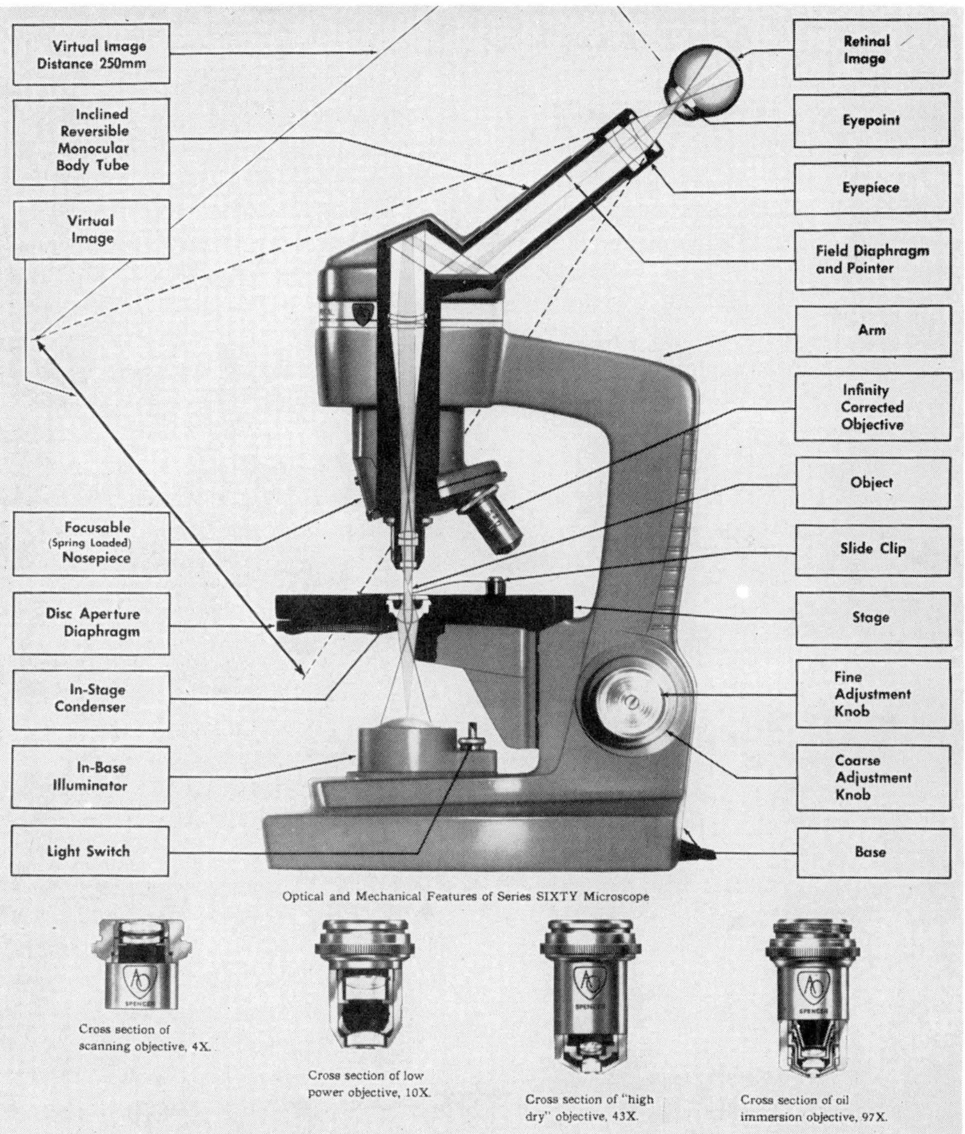

Fig. 6-18. Microscope. (Courtesy American Optical Co.)

magnifies an aerial image instead of the actual object. The final much-enlarged image formed by the eyepiece is referred to as the "apparent image," so called because the light rays do not actually come from the image. The final magnification obtained with the compound microscope is the product of the objective and eyepiece magnifications.

Most compound microscopes are equipped with three objectives: *low power* (10×), *high power* (43, 44, or 45×), and *oil immersion* (95 or 97×). The most commonly used eyepiece is 10×, although higher and lower magnifications are available. For most laboratory work the oil-immersion objective is used. This objective in combination with a 10× eyepiece magnifies an object almost 1000 times (for example, $97 \times 10 = 970$). Since the in focus working distance between the slide and the objective is very close, a wide cone of light is needed—hence, the use of oil immersion to keep the light rays from bending away from the objective (and thereby darken the microscopic field). The optical principle involved is the *refractive index;* that is, as light passes from one medium (for example, glass) into another of a higher or lower refractive index (for example, air) the rays are bent. Light rays are not bent when the two media have the *same* refractive index. (Immersion oil and glass have a refractive index of 1.52.)

Dark-field microscopy is used to examine microbes in the living state that cannot be seen by the bright-field microscope and to examine microbes that are so distorted by staining that their key characteristics are lost. Also, certain microbes cannot be stained by standard methods. This type of microscopy depends on the use of a substage condenser so constructed that the light rays do not pass directly through the object being examined (as is the case with the regular condenser) but strike it from the sides at almost a right angle to the objective. Thus, the microscopic field becomes a dark background against which microorganisms appear as bright silvery objects.

Ultraviolet microscopy permits a greater resolution and hence a greater magnification by virtue of the shorter wavelength of ultraviolet. The chief advantage of ultraviolet microscopy, however, lies in making visible various substances and structures not disclosed by visible light. Because ultraviolet light is invisible, special devices are used to render the images visible.

Fluorescence microscopy is a marriage of ultraviolet microscopy and fluorescent staining techniques. Certain dyes absorb ultraviolet energy and in so doing emit visible light of a characteristic color, a phenomenon called fluorescence. The technique is especially suited to the study of organisms that have an affinity for a specific fluorescent dye and to the "tagging" of antigen-antibody reactions in the serologic diagnosis of disease (p. 146).

Phase-contrast microscopy operates on the principle that light is bent or refracted in passing from one medium through another of a different optical density or refractive index. Whereas conventional microscopy does not make visible this effect, phase-contrast microscopy transforms refractive alterations into corresponding variations of brightness and thereby affords a more detailed examination of cellular structure.

The electron microscope employs electron waves instead of light waves and magnetic fields instead of lenses. Since electron waves are extremely short, the *resolving power* of the instrument is a hundred times or more than that of the light microscope. As a result, it is possible to magnify microbes several hundred thousand times.

To provide material suitable for microscopic examination, two techniques are used. One employs a suspension of organisms in a liquid ("hanging drop" and "wet-mount" preparations) and the other employs dried, fixed, and stained films or smears of the specimen. The suspension technique is used to demonstrate bacterial motility and to examine microbes distorted by drying and staining; stained smears are used in just about all other instances.

Staining. Since microbes are difficult to see and study unless stained, the bacteriologist has developed a great body of staining techniques. In general, these may be described as simple or special. A simple stain is one that is used merely to color the organism so that it can be more easily seen. On the other hand, a special stain is one used to elicit some special feature such as a spore or capsule. The stains commonly used for these procedures include methylene blue, crystal violet, carbolfuchsin, and safranine.

Simple stain. Simple staining is done by covering the fixed smear with the dye and then, after 30 seconds or so, carefully washing off the stain with water. When the technique is carried out properly, the bacteria are clearly seen as colored bodies against a clear microscopic field.

Gram stain. Perhaps the most useful stain employed in bacteriology is that devised by Gram. In this technique the fixed smear is first stained with crystal violet and is then washed in water. It is next covered with Gram's iodine and decolorized with 95 percent alcohol. Finally, the smear is counterstained with safranine and carefully washed with water. The air-dried slide is then examined microscopically.

When the staining technique is properly performed, gram-positive organisms are *blue* and gram-negative organisms *red.*

Though the precise mechanism of the gram stain is not understood, most studies point to the cell wall. Briefly, in the case of gram-negative bacteria the alcohol treatment is thought to dissolve away much of the lipid from the wall, thereby permitting escape of the crystal violet–iodine complex. In contrast, dehydration by alcohol of the cell of gram-positive bacteria reduces the size of the pores in the cell wall and makes decolorization much more difficult.

But whatever the details, the gram reaction is indicative of a profound difference between gram-positive and gram-negative bacteria, as shown by certain immunologic properties and variations in susceptibility to sulfonamides and antibiotics. For instance, with the exception of gram-negative cocci, the sulfonamides and penicillin are more effective in the treatment of infections caused by gram-positive organisms. On the other hand, streptomycin is much more effective against gram-negative bacteria.

Acid-fast stain. Acid-fast bacteria are those which retain their stain even though washed with acid-alcohol. This highly characteristic property is thought to be due to the presence of certain fatty substances in the cellular membrane. In the Ziehl-Neelsen procedure the prepared smear is first covered with carbolfuchsin and gently heated for about 5 minutes. Next, the slide is washed with water and then decolorized with acid-alcohol and allowed to dry. Finally, the smear is counterstained with methylene blue, washed in water, and air dried. When this procedure is properly carried out, acid-fast organisms are stained *red* and all others are stained *blue.*

Bacteriologic culture media. As indicated from what has gone before, a culture medium must meet the needs of the microbe under investigation. Because there are so many different media in use, about the best that we can do in a work of this type is to discuss the general principles and the more basic media.

Nutrient agar. Nutrient agar is a basic medium prepared from agar, peptone, meat extract, sodium chloride, and distilled water. The agar forms the gel; the peptone supplies digested protein; sodium chloride supplies the mineral matter; and the meat extract supplies an array of proteins, fats, and vitamins.

Blood agar. Blood agar is a solid medium

prepared by adding a little human or animal blood to nutrient agar. This preparation is excellent for culturing most bacteria and is perhaps the most commonly used medium in routine laboratory work.

Sabouraud's dextrose agar. Sabouraud's agar is a solid medium prepared from agar, dextrose, peptone, and water. Because of its low pH (about 5.5), molds may be easily cultured to the exclusion of bacteria.

Nutrient broth. Nutrient broth is a basic liquid culture medium. This preparation contains all the ingredients of nutrient agar except the agar.

Synthetic media. Synthetic media are preparations whose exact chemical composition is known. In distinction to the media just discussed, they are prepared from specific chemical compounds, namely, sugars, amino acids, salts, and vitamins. Through the use of this type of medium, the bacteriologist and the biochemist have learned a great deal about microbial physiology.

Selective media. Selective culture media, as the term indicates, are designed to stimulate the growth of some bacteria and to inhibit the growth of others. They are employed in those instances in which the laboratory worker is concerned with the growth and isolation of a particular species. For example, if the feces were being examined for the presence of *Shigella dysenteriae,* the pathogen of dysentery, a medium containing penicillin would facilitate the search. This antibiotic inhibits many species but does not interfere with the growth of shigellae.

Differential media. Differential media include a large number and variety of media upon which bacteria grow in some characteristic fashion. In litmus milk, for example, lactose-fermenting organisms cause the medium to turn pink.

Inoculation. Inoculation is seeding of a culture medium with an organism (or organisms), using a sterile platinum wire (straight or looped) or a sterile glass pipet. Since it is extremely easy to contaminate the medium with organisms from sources other than the one being investigated, considerable practice is necessary. The procedure, like all others in the laboratory, must be carried out with *aseptic technique.* By this we mean handling of laboratory materials in such a manner that contamination does not occur.

Fluid media are generally inoculated with a tiny amount of material, using a sterile platinum wire. If a cubic centimeter or so of some liquid is to be added, a sterile pipet is used. After the medium has been inoculated, it is incubated (usually for 24 hours) and is then examined grossly and microscopically. Some species of bacteria grow in such a characteristic fashion that the appearance of the broth is of diagnostic importance. *Bacillus subtilis,* for example, forms a heavy scum on the surface.

Solid media are inoculated by stabbing or streak plate. A stab inoculation is made by pushing a straight, sterile platinum wire (coated with the inoculum) vertically through a column of sterile medium contained in a bacteriologic tube. The manner of growth along such a stab is characteristic for many organisms.

For purposes of isolation, bacteria are best allowed to grow upon media contained in a Petri dish. In the streak plate method a loopful of inoculum is streaked across the surface of a sterile solid medium. Following incubation, colonies appear along the streak, each colony containing descendents of a single organism (that is, it is "pure").

Tissue cultures. Tissue (or cell) cultures are used for the propagation of viruses. Some of the more commonly used cell lines include chick embryo cells, monkey kidney cells, and human cancer cells. When a bottle or Petri dish is used, these cells (bathed in the appropriate culture fluid) attach to the bottom and grow as a thin sheet called a monolayer or lawn. In instances where the virus destroys the cells of the lawn (the "cytopathic effect"), colorless areas, or

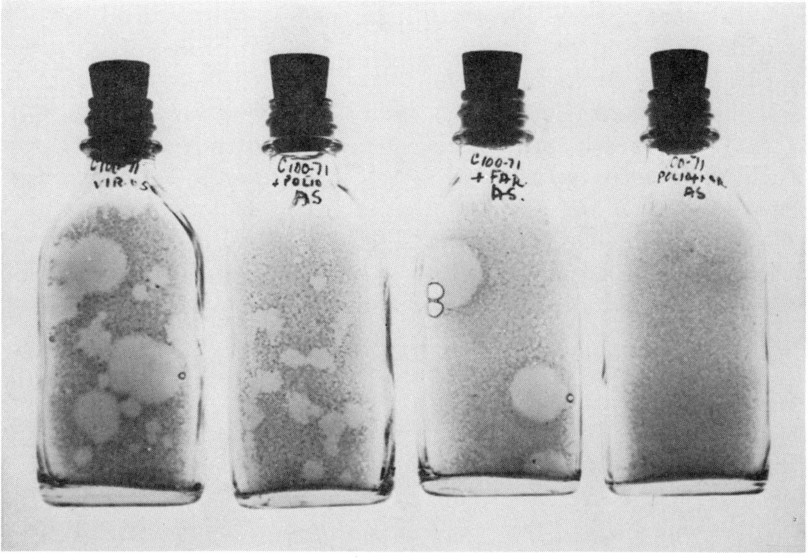

Fig. 6-19. Bottle cultures of monkey kidney cells (on which enteroviruses can grow) were used in detecting mixtures of viruses. The clear spaces (plaques) are areas in which the cells have been infected by virus and have degenerated. The bottle at the left contains two kinds of plaques: large ones characteristic of poliovirus and small, irregular ones typical of echovirus. In the second bottle, polio antiserum inhibited the growth of poliovirus, and only echovirus plaques appeared. In the third bottle, echovirus antiserum suppressed the growth of echovirus and permitted the isolation of poliovirus. In the bottle at the far right, antisera to both poliovirus and echovirus were present, and no plaques developed. (Courtesy M. Benyesh-Melnick and J. L. Melnick, Baylor University College of Medicine.)

plaques, form, each of which represents the progeny of a single virion. Tissue cultures are used in three ways: to determine the virus content of a specimen (on the basis of the number of plaques); to produce a virus in bulk amounts (for the preparation of vaccines); and to identify viruses. Identification is made on the basis of the type of plaque formed and/or cytopathic inhibition using type-specific immune serum (Fig. 6-19).

Biochemistry. Since most species of bacteria are morphologically indistinguishable, the microbiologist must usually employ biochemical and physiologic techniques in addition to the microscopic work. The more common biochemical tests depend upon the presence of such metabolic products as acids, gases, nitrites, indole, and acetylmethylcarbinol. When phenol red lactose broth (Fig. 6-20), for example, is inocu-

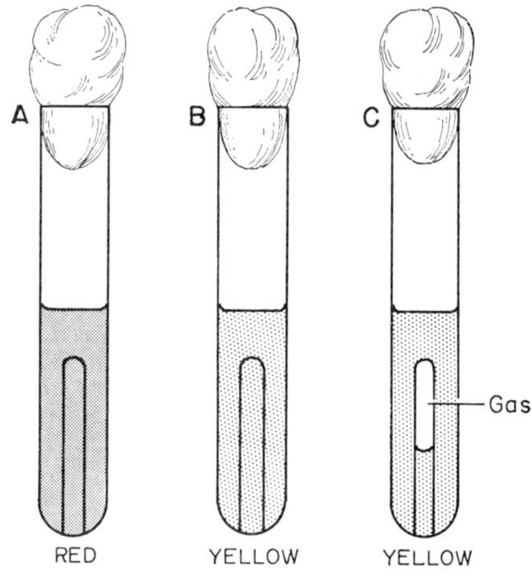

Fig. 6-20. Action of bacteria upon phenol red lactose broth. **A,** No acid or gas formed. **B,** Acid formed. **C,** Acid and gas formed. (See text.) (From Brooks, S. M.: Basic facts of medical microbiology, ed. 2, Philadelphia, 1962, W. B. Saunders Co.)

lated with an unknown species, there are three possible results: no color change, a yellow color change with no gas formation, and a yellow color change with gas formation. These results are based on the fact that some bacteria do not ferment lactose, whereas others do (some with acid and gas and some with acid only). Just this simple test alone is often of considerable help in narrowing down the field of investigation.

Serology. Serology refers to in vitro *antigen-antibody* reactions, and diagnostic serology refers especially to the various laboratory procedures used to demonstrate telltale antibodies in the patient's blood serum. The full meaning of all that serology has to offer will be noted shortly (p. 156).

ANTIMICROBIAL METHODS

We shall now discuss the principal points of interest relating to the inhibition and destruction of microorganisms. Generally, the various procedures in use may be conveniently characterized as physical or chemical. The former category includes such agents as heat, light, and radiation, and the latter includes antiseptics, germicides, antibiotics, and the like.

Hot-air oven. The hot-air oven used in the hospital and laboratory to sterilize glassware and certain metal objects is not unlike the cooking oven. In order to ensure complete sterilization, it is operated at a temperature of 170° to 180° C. for 1½ to 2 hours. Such a temperature destroys all vegetative cells and spores.

Boiling water. Although boiling water will easily kill organisms in the vegetative state, their spores may survive several hours of boiling. For this reason, the procedure is not suitable for sterilizing materials in the laboratory (such as culture tubes, Petri dishes, and culture media) that must be completely free of microbial cells and spores. Boiling may be used, however, to effect disinfection (that is, destruction of all pathogens) of such objects as hypodermic needles, syringes, certain instruments, and dishes. The accepted procedure calls for bringing the water to a boil before the materials are added and then continuing to boil for at least 15 minutes. Naturally, it is of prime importance that all objects be completely submerged.

Steam. Steam is used both "free" and under pressure to sterilize a wide variety of materials. The *autoclave* (Fig. 6-21), which employs steam under pressure, is nothing more than a large pressure cooker. The principle of operation is based upon the fact that as the pressure of the confined steam rises the temperature also rises. At a pressure of 15 pounds, the usual pressure used, the temperature is 121° C. When exposed to this temperature for 30 minutes, all objects are sterilized. Culture media, glassware, surgical dressings, sponges, parenteral solutions, and certain rubber articles are usually sterilized by autoclaving.

Free steam (100° C.) is used to sterilize articles and materials that are damaged by the high heat of the autoclave (for example, certain culture media). In this mode of sterilization, objects are placed in the Arnold sterilizer and exposed to steam for 30 minutes on each of 3 successive days. The process is based upon the fact that between exposures the unkilled spores germinate into heat-sensitive vegetative cells.

Pasteurization. Pasteurization is the disinfection of milk and other substances by heating at a moderate temperature for a definite time. In the *holding method,* milk is heated to 62° C. and held at this temperature for 30 minutes. In the *flash method,* milk is subjected to a temperature of 71° C. for 15 seconds. Immediately following heating, the milk is cooled and bottled. Although milk is still laden with microbes, the organisms are harmless and even contribute to the flavor.

Filtration. Filtration is a process whereby suspended particles are removed by some

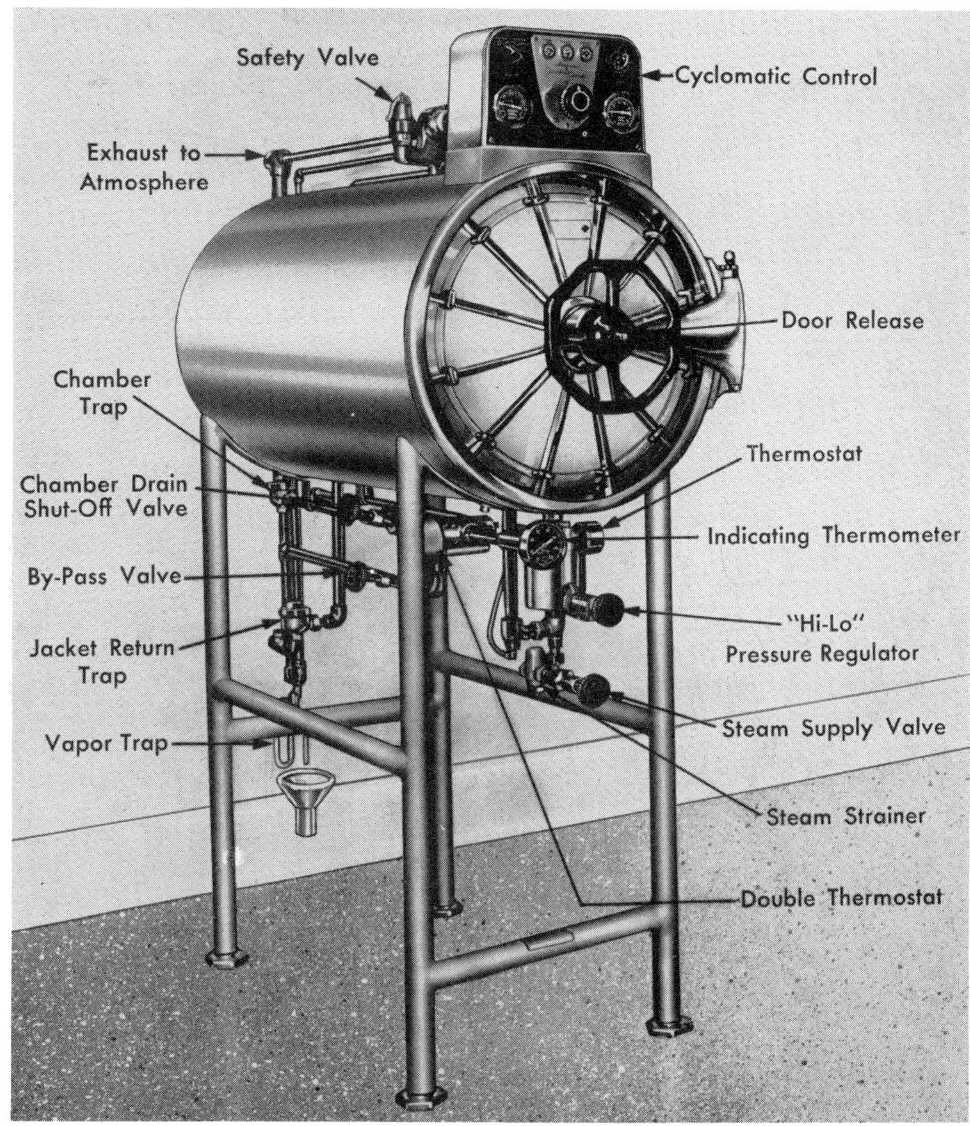

Fig. 6-21. Autoclave. (Courtesy American Sterilizer Co.)

material (the filter) that permits passage of the liquid but not the particles. Its effectiveness, of course, depends upon the size of the pores of the filter. For laboratory use, filters are available that remove certain bacteria but permit certain viruses and rickettsiae to run through. These so-called bacterial filters are highly useful for isolating filtrable viruses and bacterial toxins and for sterilizing certain preparations destroyed by heat. Among the more popular are the Berkefeld filter (Fig. 6-22), which is made of unglazed porcelain, and the Seitz filter, which is made of asbestos.

Radiation. In recent years certain forms of radiation have been turned against the microbe. Ultraviolet lamps, for example, are now widely used in hospitals and in industry for safe, quick, and reliable disinfection and sterilization. Other forms of radia-

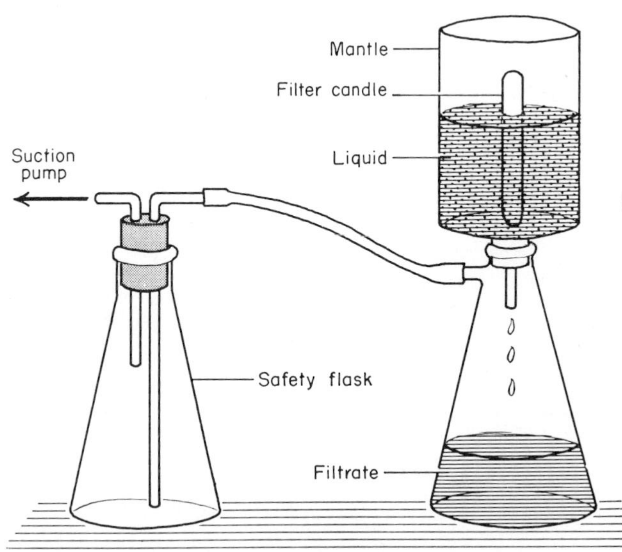

Fig. 6-22. Berkefeld filter. (From Brooks, S. M.: Basic facts of medical microbiology, ed. 2, Philadelphia, 1962, W. B. Saunders Co.)

tion under investigation for this purpose include high-speed electrons, x rays, and isotopes. In the not-too-distant future, radiation may supplant the more conventional antimicrobial methods.

The denaturing effect of energy rays is generally agreed to reside in their ability to ionize certain key cellular constituents. In this condition the normal metabolic processes are altered and with proper dosage the cell dies.

Ultrasonic waves. Sound waves with frequencies above the hearing limit of the human ear (20,000 cycles per second) can shatter microbes and effect sterilization. The article or material to be sterilized is merely exposed to a transmitter emanating ultrasonic waves. This unique mode of sterilization is already employed in certain industries and laboratories.

Desiccation. Desiccation, or drying, used since time immemorial to preserve perishables, is still one of our most important means of inhibiting microbial multiplication. However, by virtue of the fact that some dried spores retain their viability for years, the process by itself is not reliable for sterilization.

Refrigeration. Like desiccation, refrigeration cannot be relied upon as a mode of sterilization. Although a few species are destroyed by low temperatures, some pathogens may withstand temperatures as low as −70° C. The principal use of refrigeration, therefore, is to preserve perishables via microbial inhibition.

Chemical methods. A chemical agent inhibits or kills microbes either by the destruction of protoplasmic constituents or by selective action, that is, via mechanisms that interfere with a basic metabolic system. The latter mode of attack has proved the most successful for the simple reason that selective action is much less toxic to the host. Indeed, in some instances an anti-infective drug can be aimed at a molecular target unique to the microbe. The sulfonamides or "sulfa" drugs, for example, interfere with utilization of para-aminobenzoic acid (PABA), a nutrient vital to a number of bacterial species. The mechanism of action apparently is *competitive inhibition;* that is, by virtue of their very close molecular similarity, the bacterial cell accepts the drug as well as the PABA, thereby blocking the intake of the latter.

The chemical structures for PABA and sulfanilamide are as follows:

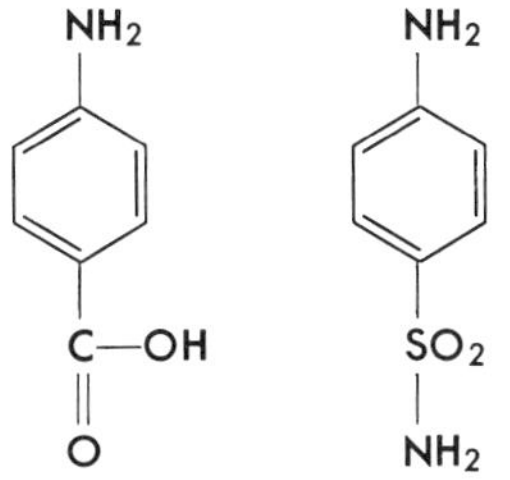

PABA: NH_2–C_6H_4–C(=O)–OH

Sulfanilamide: NH_2–C_6H_4–SO_2–NH_2

PABA Sulfanilamide

The idea of competitive inhibition is very much like putting the wrong key in the lock; although it fits, it prevents the entrance of the right key.

Local anti-infectives. By local anti-infectives we mean those chemical agents applied topically (locally) to arrest or destroy pathogenic organisms. These include such popular medicinals as antiseptics, disinfectants, germicides, and fungicides. Some of the more commonly used agents are presented in Table 6-1.

The ideal antiseptic, disinfectant, or germicide possesses certain obvious qualities. It should be effective in low concentration, it should not be irritating, and it should not lose its effectiveness in the presence of foreign material such as dead tissue and blood. The first quality—potency—is often expressed by the so-called *phenol coefficient.* This is a number that compares the action of a given anti-infective agent with that of phenol (carbolic acid) against the same test organism under the same conditions. Thus, a phenol coefficient of 4 means that the agent is four times more effective than phenol against a certain microbe under certain conditions. Since the coefficient does not take the other considerations (namely, irritation) into account, the expression obviously is of limited value.

Systemic anti-infectives. In contrast to the local anti-infectives, the systemic category includes medicinals that are safe enough to be administered orally or parenterally. The idea of fighting infection systemically with specific chemical agents was heralded by the monumental work of Paul Ehrlich, who in 1909 introduced arsphenamine (Salvarsan or 606) in the treatment of syphilis. Although this agent proved to be seriously toxic, it sparked the discovery of the sulfonamides (ca. 1933) and the antibiotics (ca. 1940).

Properly used, the term *antibiotic* refers

Table 6-1. Commonly used local anti-infectives

Agent	Strength of solution commonly used	Use
Ethyl alcohol	70%	Antiseptic-disinfectant
Chlorine	1:1,000,000	Disinfection of drinking water
DDT	10%	Ectoparasiticide
Furacin*	0.2%	Antiseptic-disinfectant
Gexane*	1%	Ectoparasiticide
Gentian violet	1%	Antiseptic-disinfectant
Hexachlorophene	3%	Antiseptic-disinfectant
Hydrogen peroxide	3%	Antiseptic-disinfectant
Mercurochrome*	2%	Antiseptic-disinfectant
Merthiolate*	1:1000	Antiseptic-disinfectant
Potassium permanganate	1:5000	Antiseptic-disinfectant
Silver nitrate	1%	Antiseptic-disinfectant
Sodium hypochlorite	0.5%	Antiseptic-disinfectant
Tincture of iodine	2%	Antiseptic-disinfectant
Undecylenic acid	1-10%	Fungicide
Zephiran*	1:1000 to 1:10,000	Antiseptic-disinfectant

*Trade name.

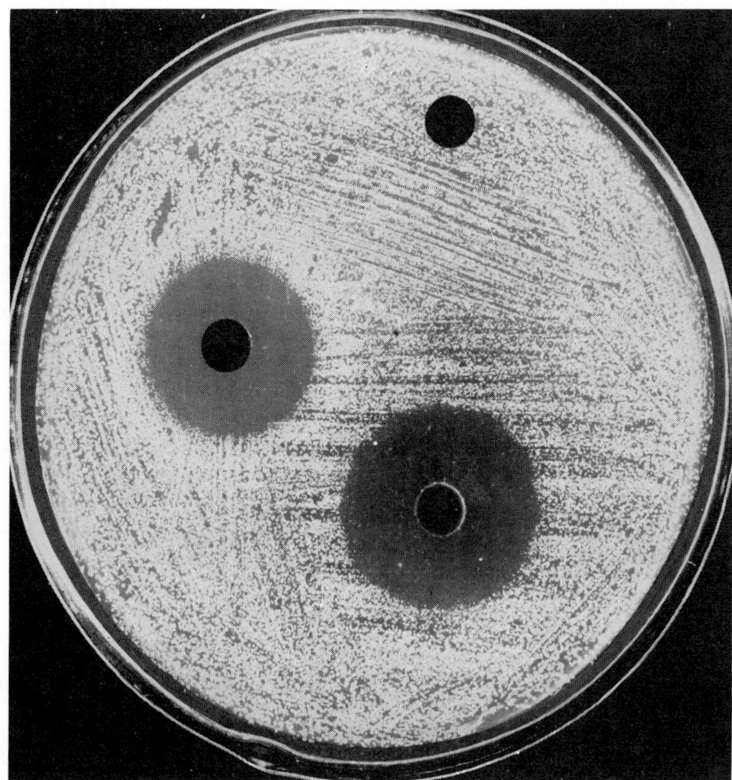

Fig. 6-23. Determination of sensitivity of bacteria to different antibiotics. A Petri dish of agar is heavily inoculated with the test organisms. Disks of filter paper impregnated with different antibiotics are dropped on freshly inoculated surface. The bacterial growth is white. Note that there is a zone of inhibition of bacterial growth around two of the disks, whereas there is no inhibition of growth around the third. The zone of inhibition indicates that growth of the organism would probably be limited in a patient receiving that antibiotic. (From Smith, A. L.: Principles of microbiology, ed. 6, St. Louis, 1969, The C. V. Mosby Co.)

to an anti-infective substance produced by one microorganisms that inhibits or kills another microorganism (Fig. 6-23). Commonly, however, the term is applied to any and all systemic anti-infectives (to the sulfonamides, for instance) that originate in the test tube. The penicillins (the basic molecule of which is derived from the mold *Penicillium chrysogenum*) continue to dominate the field. Nonetheless, their ineffectiveness against "resistant staph," gram-negative bacilli, rickettsiae, and protozoa has prompted the development of an ever-growing number of new antibiotics, the majority of which are derived from actinomycetes of the genus *Streptomyces.*

In addition to the sulfonamides and antibiotics, the organic chemist has synthesized other highly effective systemic agents. The sulfones against leprosy, isoniazid and para-aminosalicylic acid against tuberculosis, and chloroquine against malaria are only a few of a vast array of diversified chemicals. Many of these will be discussed elsewhere in those sections dealing with infection.

INFECTION

Infection, the central theme of medical microbiology, is essentially a tug of war between the pathogen and the host; in order to aid the latter at the calculated expense of the former, we must take stock of certain basic facts.

Etiology. By etiology we mean the sum of our knowledge regarding the cause of disease. Relative to infection, therefore, this might properly include the nature, source, mode of transmission, and avenue(s) by which the pathogen gains entrance into the body.

Koch's postulates. In order to stamp a given species as the cause of this or that infection with complete confidence, certain requirements (Koch's postulates) must be met. These may be stated as follows:

1. The organism must be present in every case of the infection.
2. The organism must be isolated and grown in pure culture.
3. In pure culture the organism must cause the disease when inoculated into susceptible animals.
4. The organism must then be recovered from the animal and must be shown to be the same as that inoculated.

With relatively few exceptions, the pathogens that cause disease in man meet these requirements. There is, for instance, some question regarding the etiology of Vincent's angina.

Source of pathogens. Man and animals serve as the permanent and primary reservoirs of infection. The human reservoir includes patients and carriers. Whereas the patient harbors a pathogen during the period of the infection, the carrier harbors a pathogen for months, years, or in some instances for life. Interestingly enough, a carrier may never have had the infection himself. Obviously, carriers are a serious threat to the health of the community for unless they can be identified and treated, such persons may easily infect thousands of others. Such was the case of Typhoid Mary, the cook who spread typhoid fever wherever she worked.

The animal world harbors a number of vicious pathogens. Rabies, tuberculosis, encephalitis, and brucellosis are only a few examples. Many of our public health laws and regulations are concerned with the control of this important problem. In general, they have been highly successful. Bovine tuberculosis, for instance, has been all but eliminated as a public health problem.

Transmission. The manner in which pathogens travel from the source to the host is obviously of paramount importance. Indeed, some of the great steps in the control of disease have been in this area. Generally, it may be said that transmission is effected either directly or indirectly. By the former we mean bodily contact and droplet infection (the spread of pathogens via talking, laughing, and coughing). By indirect transmission we mean the spread of infection via air, water, soil, food, contaminated objects (fomites), and vectors.

A vector is a carrier (usually an insect) that transmits a pathogen from one host to another. In the case of arthropod or insect vectors the infectious agent is carried in one of two ways—biologically or mechanically.

In biologic transmission the pathogen passes through part of its life cycle in the vector. In other words, such a vector not only transmits the infection but also is essential to the survival of the pathogen. This is especially significant, for it means that if we can eradicate the vector we can eradicate the disease. In a large measure, man has done this in the case of yellow fever and certain other mosquito-borne infections.

By contrast, a mechanical vector is not essential to the life cycle of the parasite. The common fly is a good example; for instance, it contaminates its feet by simply alighting on typhoid-laden feces. However, although fly control is helpful, it alone cannot eradicate typhoid fever.

Portals of entry and exit. The manner in which a pathogen gains entrance to and leaves the body is of considerable importance in prophylaxis. In the case of epidemic meningitis, for example, the nurse wears a mask when caring for the patient, since the chief portal of entry of the pathogen is the nasopharynx. By the same token, the sputum of a patient with pulmonary tuberculosis must be disinfected, for it is laden with tubercle bacilli.

Incubation period. The incubation period is the time between exposure to a given pathogen and the onset of the infection. This time varies considerably for different infections and even for the same infection. Fortunately, however, the incubation period is of sufficient constancy to be of real practical value in public health work.

Types of infection. Several adjectives are used to describe an infection. An infection is said to be *local* when it is confined to a given area (for example, a boil) and systemic when it involves the whole body (for example, "blood poisoning"). Often, however, the local manifestation is merely a prelude to *systemic* involvement and in this event the expression *focal infection* is frequently used.

If during the course of an infection by one pathogen the patient contracts another infection, the former is referred to as a primary infection and the latter as a secondary infection. In other words, the so-called secondary invaders, or opportunists, incite trouble as a consequence of lowered resistance occasioned by the primary infection. Pneumonia, for example, is not infrequently a sequel to a cold or a bad case of measles. Often the secondary invader is a member of the normal flora of the body, that is, those microbes habitually present in or upon the body.

Other terms used to describe an infection include *bacteremia, septicemia, pyemia,* and *toxemia.* Bacteremia refers merely to the presence of bacteria in the blood. Septicemia, in contrast, means that bacteria have not only entered the bloodstream but also are actively multiplying. By pyemia is meant the presence of pyogenic or pus-forming bacteria and toxemia refers to the presence of bacterial toxins, a condition that may prevail in such infections as diphtheria and tetanus.

Pathogenesis. Let us now consider the mechanisms by which disease-producing microbes attack and injure the body. Often we become so accustomed to saying that such and such an organism causes this or that infection that we forget about how it does this. The better-understood mechanisms will be described briefly.

Mechanical injury. The mere presence of microbes in the tissues is obviously of pathologic importance. Indeed, in some infections, this may be the principal feature. In tuberculosis, for example, the tubercle bacilli form such bulk as to "push away" the good tissue and interfere with normal function. As another example, we might cite intestinal worms that often cause dangerous obstruction.

Toxins. Toxins are highly dangerous and often lethal bacterial products. There are two kinds: *exotoxins* and *endotoxins.* Exotoxins, the most deadly biologic poisons known, are responsible for a number of diseases of man, including tetanus, diphtheria, gas gangrene, anthrax, plague, and "staph" and botulism food poisoning. It has been estimated that 7 ounces of the exotoxin produced by *Clostridium botulinum* could kill off the earth's entire human population. Endotoxins are usually much less deadly in nature, but nonetheless are capable of causing a violent response. Animals inoculated with lethal doses show dyspnea, profuse diarrhea, excessive weakness, and sometimes paralysis of the extremities. So far, endotoxins have been isolated only from *gram-negative* bacteria, most especially the virulent *enteric* bacilli responsible for typhoid fever, salmonellosis, and related infections.

Exotoxins are *heat-labile* proteins that are readily released from the bacterial cell, whereas endotoxins are *heat-stable* lipopolysaccharide-protein complexes much less readily released. Other key differences relate to *antigenicity* and *pyrogenicity.*

Exotoxins are highly antigenic and stimulate the output of neutralizing antibodies called *antitoxins;* endotoxins, in contrast, are *weakly* antigenic and poor stimulators of immunity. In regard to pyrogenicity, or ability to cause fever, endotoxins *are* highly pyrogenic and exotoxins *are not.* The mechanism of the temperature rise results from the interaction of endotoxin and white cells of the blood; that is, the endotoxin causes the white cells to release a *pyrogen* that acts upon the "thermostat" in the brain.

Fortunately, the formation of exotoxins by bacteria is relatively uncommon, confined mainly to *Clostridium botulinum, Clostridium tetani,* and *Corynebacterium diphtheriae.*

Other toxic substances. In addition to exotoxins and endotoxins, microbes form a variety of other substances that play a role in the disease process. Among others are included *hemolysins* (which destroy red cells), *leukocidins* (which destroy white cells), *coagulase* (which facilitates clotting), *hyaluronidase* (which dissolves intercellular cement), and *kinases.* The last agents bring about the dissolution of clots (or inhibit the clotting of plasma) by an activating mechanism. Streptokinase, for instance, a kinase produced by streptococci, converts plasminogen (of the plasma) into its active form, plasmin (or fibrinolysin), which thereupon dissolves the clot. Thus, it is not correct to say—as do many books—that streptococci release fibrinolysin. Another factor released by streptococci is streptodornase, which, together with streptokinase, decreases the viscosity of necrotic debris by the depolymerization of DNA. This action, however, does not appear to be related to virulence.

Diagnosis of infection. The diagnosis of infection is made from the signs and symptoms, immunologic tests, and laboratory findings. In some infections the signs and symptoms are so characteristic that a diagnosis may be made solely on this basis. A mother who has reared two or three children, for instance, can often "spot" a case of measles with no more difficulty than the young doctor.

As used here, immunologic tests refer to those procedures carried out on the patient employing either antigen or antibody. For example, in the Schultz-Charlton test, if an injection of scarlet fever antitoxin into an area of rash causes the latter to blanch, the individual is thus proved to have that particular infection.

And by laboratory findings we mean any and all procedures carried out in the laboratory for the purpose of aiding the physician in the diagnosis. Included are the microbiologic investigations of suitable specimens (blood, spinal fluid, feces, urine, and swabbings) and serology studies, that is, tests done on blood serum to disclose telltale antibodies.

Treatment. *Specific* treatment against an infection includes the use of anti-infective drugs, namely, the antibiotics and sulfonamides, and antisera. We must not, however, forget the patient; that is, things must be done to ameliorate the discomfort arising from the insult to the tissues. As a matter of fact, symptomatic treatment is all that can be given in many instances. All of us realize, for example, that the doctor can do little more for a cold than treat the symptoms and wait for the virus to leave the body.

Prophylaxis. The ultimate aim in medical microbiology is to discover ways and means of protecting the body against its microbial enemies. And this is a big order, for it entails immunization, isolation, identification of carriers, eradication of vectors, and good sanitation.

Drinking water. Perhaps the most important single item in public health is the procurement of *safe* drinking water, a problem that the United States itself is not solving fast enough. Indeed, the water situation for the world in general steadily worsens.

According to the United States Public Health Service, drinking water must be free of pathogenic organisms. Water containing one or two coliform organisms (p. 130) per 100 ml. in the piped supply that enters a distribution center is regarded as satisfactory, but counts above three and ten are regarded as suspicious and unsatisfactory, respectively.

The disinfection of water is generally carried out by the use of germicidal chemicals. Although bleaching powder (calcium hypochlorite) was at one time the most widely used agent for this purpose, it has been all but replaced in large-scale treatment by liquid chlorine, which is added to the water by an automatic feeding device. For ordinary clear surface water a concentration of available chlorine of 0.5 to 1 part per million gallons destroys ordinary intestinal bacteria and viruses. In the event of overchlorination the taste can generally be removed with such dechlorinators as sulfur dioxide and potassium permanganate.

In the field or where the public water supply becomes contaminated, disinfection becomes an individual problem. In such instances chemicals may be added (for example, hypochlorites or iodine compounds) or the water may be boiled. Boiling is not only the simplest method but also the only one to be relied upon completely when the water is exceptionally impure.

IMMUNITY

Up to this point we have directed our attention to the invader; now we shall discuss the defender. More to the point, we shall discuss what is known about immunity—the *resistance* of the body to infection (Fig. 6-24).

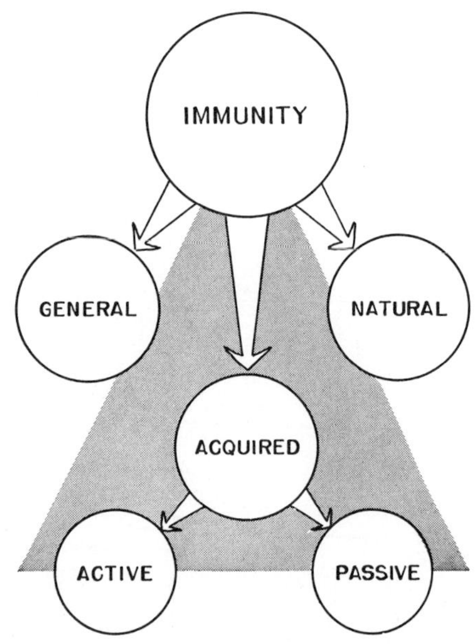

Fig. 6-24. Immunity. (From Brooks, S. M.: Basic facts of medical microbiology, ed. 2, Philadelphia, 1962, W. B. Saunders Co.)

General immunity. As used here, the term *general immunity* refers to those defenses possessed by all persons in *normal health.* These defenses include the cilia that cover the respiratory mucosa (Chapter 13), hydrochloric acid (Chapter 14), the blood (Chapter 12), the lymphatic system (Chapter 11), and certain "antibiotic" principles that appear in the tissues and body fluids, such as *lysozyme* (Chapter 13), *properdin* (present in the blood), and *interferon.* The latter agent, isolated just a few years ago, has considerable *antiviral* activity.

Natural immunity. Natural immunity as used here, is resistance to infection with which an individual is endowed by heredity. Of prime significance is the fact that this resistance may be at the species, racial, or individual level. As we know, some species are more resistant than others to a given pathogen. Man, for instance, is not affected by the distemper virus, a deadly enemy of the dog. There is also some difference relative to race. The Negro, for example, is considerably more resistant to malaria than the white person. At the individual level, common experience teaches us that some persons are more resistant than others to certain infections. Thus, a fair share of our defense against infection is traceable to our parents. Although the mechanism of natural immunity might well reside in the factors just cited in the discussion of general immunity, there is evidence to indicate that there is much more to it than this—hence, the expression *natural.*

Acquired immunity. In addition to our inborn ready-made resistance, nature has seen fit to delegate much immunologic responsibility to the process of living—to acquired immunity. By acquired *active* immunity, we mean the ability of the body to build up its resistance against the pathogen or its toxins. The accepted theory is that *antigens* (that is, toxins and certain chemical factors of the microbial protoplasm) stimulate the reticuloendothelial system (namely, the plasma cells of the spleen, liver, lymph nodes, and bone marrow) to produce *antibodies,* specific immune substances that appear in the *gamma globulin* fraction of the blood serum. And moreover, a specific antigen provokes a specific antibody. Of importance to the host, of course, is the fact the microbe, or its toxin, is destroyed or neutralized when it encounters the antibodies that it has provoked.

Actually, the microbial cell is considered a mosaic of antigens. For example, some antigens are characteristic of flagella, others of capsules, and still others of the cell proper. In most instances, however, it appears that only one microbial antigen is of immunologic significance. In tetanus, for example, the key antigen is clearly the exotoxin that provokes the output of the lifesaving antitoxin.

The body can acquire active immunity in one of two ways: by actually having an infection or artificially. As is well known, many diseases (for example, measles, poliomyelitis, and scarlet fever) usually attack only once; that is, certain pathogenic antigens provoke a lasting high concentration of antibodies. Ideally, of course, we would like to acquire immunity without experiencing an infection and, as we know, this has been accomplished in a number of severe maladies through the use of vaccines and toxoids. Indeed, artificial active immunization (first demonstrated by Jenner against smallpox) represents one of the great conquests of medical science.

Active vs. passive immunity. When the antibodies of one person are injected into another person, the result is acquired *passive* immunity. As we might suspect, active immunity lasts for a much longer time than passive immunity. In some instances the reticuloendothelial system, once stimulated, continues to produce antibodies throughout life. In contrast, injected antibodies start to disappear from the blood in a matter of days.

Passive immunity may be natural or artificial. It is artificial when the body is given a shot of antiserum and it is natural when antibodies from the mother's blood diffuse across the placenta into the circulation of the unborn child. Thus, for the first several weeks of life a newborn infant is protected by passive immunity acquired in utero. After this time, however, his body must shift for itself immunologically.

Vaccines. Vaccines are antigenic preparations made from killed or attenuated ("weakened") bacteria, rickettsiae, or viruses. They provoke *active* immunity and are highly useful in the prevention of disease. In order that the student will not wonder why some vaccines are attenuated while others are killed (the latter obviously are preferable), let it simply be said that certain organisms, when killed, lose either all or a good share of their *antigenicity.* The attenuated poliovirus, for example, has been shown to be a much better stimulator of antibodies than the killed virus.

The measures used in the preparation of killed vaccines include heat, ultraviolet light, and certain chemicals such as formalin and tricresol. Attenuated vaccines, on the other hand, are prepared from pathogens that have been grown and treated in a special way. For example, many pathogens lose their pathogenicity when continuously cultured and subcultured over a long period of time.

Toxoids. Toxoids are neutralized toxins. Like vaccines, they are employed to "vaccinate" the patient and to provoke *active* immunity. The principal toxoids in use today are those against tetanus and diphtheria.

Antisera. Therapeutically, antisera (or immune sera) are blood derivatives that contain antibodies against specific infections. Since these preparations provide immediate immunity, they are administered to susceptible persons who have been dangerously exposed to an infectious disease or to persons who are already ill.

The most important antisera include those against diphtheria, tetanus, gas gangrene, rabies, and botulism. These are prepared by vaccinating horses and then processing the blood removed from the animal after a high titer of antibody appears in the circulation. From human blood (of persons who have recovered from an infection) are also made antisera for use in those instances in which an individual is hypersensitive to horse serum. Human gamma globulin has proved of value in the treatment of measles, hepatitis, and poliomyelitis.

Interferon stimulation. Experimentally, synthetic RNA has proved of value in the prevention of certain viral infections. It works by entering the cell and there stimulating the output of interferon, a protein agent that inhibits the replication of virions. The implications of this mode of prophylaxis are great, and much research in this direction is being carried out in the hope of expanding our control over a wide variety of viral diseases.

ANTIGEN-ANTIBODY REACTIONS

The reaction between an antigen and its homologous antibody is of a chemical nature, and to demonstrate such reactions a variety of in vitro tests have been devised. These so-called serologic tests constitute one of the chief means of identifying organisms and of diagnosing disease (p. 153).

Types of antibodies. The central idea of a *serologic test* may be illustrated by the following example: When blood serum containing antibodies against the bacterium *Salmonella typhosa* (the cause of typhoid fever) is added to a suspension of that organism, clumping, or *agglutination*, of the bacterial cells occurs. Thus, if a suspension of *Salmonella typhosa* is agglutinated by a serum under study, it shows that antityphoid antibodies are present, and that the individual from whom the serum was taken has encountered *Salmonella typhosa* (and may indeed have typhoid fever). By the same token, if a bacterium under study is strongly agglutinated by *known* antityphoid serum, it pinpoints the organism as *Salmonella typhosa.*

By convention, antibodies are classified on a basis of the serologic tests used to demonstrate their presence. The principal kinds (of antibody) include *agglutinins* (agglutinate microbial cells such as in the above example), *precipitins* (produce a precipitate when added to a solution of the homologous antigen), *lysins* (cause dissolution of bacterial or other cells), *antitoxins* (neutralize toxins), *opsonins* (enhance phagocytosis), and *neutralizing antibodies* (deactivate viruses).

Although antigen-antibody reactions are characterized by specificity, there are a number of instances in which unrelated microbes react with the same antibody. This is because such microbes have antigens in common. A classic example concerns certain strains of the bacterium *Proteus vulgaris,* an organism that is agglutinated by antibodies provoked by several species of rickettsiae. Indeed, this is the basis of the *Weil-Felix* test used in the differential diagnosis of rickettsial diseases.

Haptens. Certain fatty or starchy substances of relatively low molecular weight act only *partially* as antigens; that is, they react with antibodies but are unable to stimulate antibodies. Such substances, called haptens, can be made complete antigens by combining them with the appropriate proteins. Thus, hapten A in combination with protein B provokes the production of an antibody that reacts with hapten A as well as the A-B complex. Typically, the antibody does not react with protein B alone, and for this reason, haptens are considered the "specificity" part of the antigen molecule.

Complement-fixation test. One of the most commonly used serologic procedures for the diagnosis of infectious diseases and the identification of microorganisms is the so-called complement-fixation test. This test is based on the fact that a protein substance in the blood called *complement* enters into the reaction between antigen and antibody. That is, antigen (A) plus antibody (B) plus complement (C) yields "A-B-C complex"—a chemical complex in which complement is said to be "fixed." Thus, when complement and *known antigen* are added to a specimen under investigation and the complement becomes fixed, this demonstrates the *presence* of the homologous antibody. To the contrary, if complement *does not* become fixed, it shows that the homologous antibody *is not* present. By the same token, complement and *known antibody* can be used to signal the presence —or absence—of the homologous antigen. The trick, of course, is to know when complement becomes fixed, and for this purpose, *sheep red cells* and *rabbit serum* containing anti-sheep *hemolysins* are used. In the presence of complement, hemolysins (commonly called *amboceptors*) cause red cells to *lyse*, thereby producing a red color as a result of the release of hemoglobin. And, as in all such antigen-antibody reactions, complement becomes *fixed*.

In practice (Fig. 6-25) the test is carried out in two steps. In step one, known antigen and unknown antibody—or vice versa—and a *measured* amount of complement are added to a tube and incubated. In step two, sheep red cells and rabbit antiserum are added to this mixture. Now, *if hemolysis occurs,* it shows that complement *was not* fixed in step one, meaning that the homologous antibody or antigen in question is *not present.* On the other hand, *if hemolysis does not* occur, it shows that the homologous antibody or antigen in question *is present.*

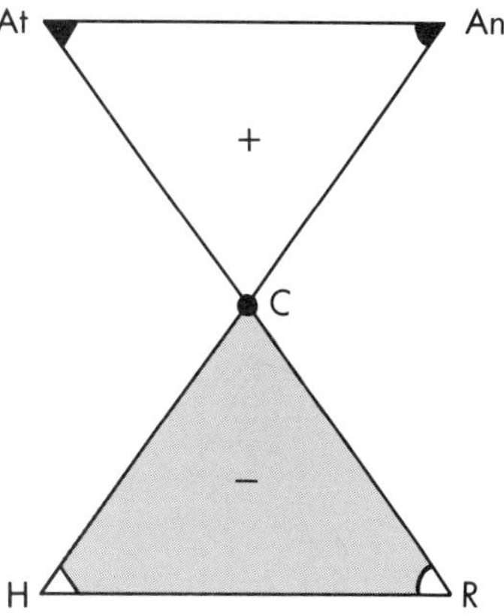

Fig. 6-25. Complement fixation at a glance. If patient's serum contains antibody, **At,** against the test antigen, **An,** complement, **C,** becomes *fixed* and hemolysin, **H,** is *unable* to lyse red cells (positive test, upper triangle). Conversely, if patient's serum *does not* contain antibody against the test antigen, complement is free to interact with **H** and **R** (red cells) to effect hemolysis (negative test, lower shaded triangle).

Hemagglutination inhibition test. This is one of the most commonly used serologic tests for the identification of viruses and viral antibodies. It is based on the fact that most viruses attach to the surface of red blood cells and in so doing cause the red cells to agglutinate. A virus that has been mixed with its specific antibody, however, cannot attach to red cells and cause agglutination. Thus, if a serum under study prevents a *known* agglutinating virus from producing agglutination, it proves that the individual has come in contact with this virus. By the same token, a virus that fails to agglutinate red cells after having been mixed with *known* antibody is thereby identified, provided, of course, said virus is known to produce agglutination in the absence of antibody.

Skin tests. A so-called "skin test" operates either on the principle of hypersensitivity or immunologic response. In the hypersensitivity test a dose of antigen (prepared from the pathogen in question) produces a reaction at the site of the injection in individuals who are infected by this particular pathogen. In the immunologic test a "skin dose" of some microbial toxin produces a reaction at the site of injection in individuals who are *not immune* to the disease in question. In immune individuals the homologous antitoxin neutralizes the toxin. Thus, the hypersensitivity test is useful in the *diagnosis* of infectious diseases, and the immunologic test is useful in determining *susceptibility* to infectious diseases.

Questions

1. To what phylum and classes do bacteria, viruses, and rickettsiae belong?
2. To what phyla do protozoa, fungi, and yeast belong?
3. According to many authorities, there are three kingdoms of living things. Explain.
4. Describe a typical bacterial cell.
5. Distinguish between spirilla and spirochetes.
6. Distinguish among diplococci, streptococci, and staphylococci.
7. Discuss the microbes belonging to the orders Eubacteriales and Actinomycetales.
8. Decribe a virus and the way in which it attacks living tissue.
9. What is a bacteriophage?
10. What is a yeast?
11. Discuss the chemical events in alcoholic fermentation.
12. Describe the different types of protozoa.
13. Describe the different types of parasitic worms.
14. Is a spore a "mode" of reproduction? Explain.
15. In the microscopic study of a bacterial culture, why is it important to know the age of the culture?
16. Compare mitosis and binary fission.
17. If a single bacterium is added to a sterile tube of broth, about how many organisms will be present 2 hours later?
18. All parasitic bacteria are heterotrophic. Explain.
19. Distinguish between an obligate aerobe and a facultative anaerobe.
20. Most pathogens are mesophiles. Explain.
21. Most bacteria do not grow in heavy syrups. Explain.
22. Distinguish between mutualism and commensalism.
23. What is an antibiotic?
24. What is the purpose of using oil with the 95× objective?
25. In the complement-fixation test, hemolysis signals a *negative* result. Explain.
26. Compare nutrient agar and nutrient broth.
27. Why must all laboratory media be sterilized before use?
28. Sabouraud's agar has a pH adjusted to 5.5. Why?
29. What are synthetic media?
30. Distinguish between selective and differential media.
31. Explain why gram-positive bacteria are blue and gram-negative bacteria are red.
32. Describe in detail the technique for doing a simple stain.
33. Describe the technique for doing an acid-fast stain according to the Ziehl-Neelsen method.
34. Discuss the use of the hot-air oven.
35. An object that has been boiled in water may not be sterile. Explain.
36. Discuss the use of the autoclave.
37. Discuss the use of radiation in sterilization and disinfection.
38. Pasteurized milk is not sterile. Explain.
39. What is meant by competitive inhibition?
40. Distinguish between local and systemic anti-infectives.
41. Distinguish among the following terms: antiseptic, disinfectant, germicide, and fungicide.
42. Discuss the limitations of the phenol coefficient.
43. Distinguish between a mechanical and a biologic vector.
44. What is a healthy carrier?
45. Discuss the significance of secondary invaders.
46. What is meant by the normal flora?
47. Distinguish between an exotoxin and an endotoxin.
48. A baby is born with acquired passive immunity. Explain.
49. Compare the composition and use of vaccines, antisera, and toxoids.
50. Discuss the relationship between an antigen and an antibody.
51. Define the following terms: dermatomycosis, mycosis, helminthiasis, trench mouth, spirochete, complement, cystitis, mastoiditis, ab-

scess, conjunctivitis, pneumonia, erysipelas, septicemia, carbuncle, aseptic technique, lumpy jaw, yaws, agglutinin, hapten, serology, pleomorphic, inclusion body, "phage," abiogenesis, lysozyme, interferon, opsonin, lysis, fluorescence, refractive index, resolving power, plaque, amboceptor, "cytopathic effect," antigenicity, virulence, plasma cell, and PPLO.

Chapter 7

The body as a whole

Before venturing into the fascinating details relating to human anatomy and physiology, one should first see the body as a whole. The present chapter is addressed to this idea.

GENERAL PLAN

Like other vertebrates, the human body is a bilaterally symmetrical structure with a backbone and an array of organs housed in two major cavities—the ventral and the dorsal.

Ventral cavity. The ventral or anterior cavity lies before the spinal column and contains the bulk of the viscera of the body. Quite conveniently, it is divided into the thoracic and the abdominal cavities, the latter separated from the former by the diaphragm.

Thoracic cavity. The thoracic cavity is subdivided by a serous membrane (the pleura) into the right and left pleural cavities, each encompassing a lung (Fig. 7-1). The other thoracic organs and structures—the heart, trachea, bronchi, esophagus, vessels, nerves, and thymus gland—lie between the pleural cavities in a third cavity called the *mediastinum.* Since the heart is encased in a membranous sac known as the pericardium, the anatomist also refers to the *pericardial* cavity.

Abdominal cavity. The abdominal or abdominopelvic cavity, which is bounded by the diaphragm above and the pelvis below, is lined with a membrane called the *peritoneum.* In this cavity are found the stomach, liver, gallbladder, pancreas, spleen, kidneys, intestines, bladder, rectum, and sex organs. However, since the kidneys lie behind the peritoneum (retroperitoneal), some anatomists do not include them among the abdominal viscera.

Pelvic cavity. The lower portion of the abdominal cavity is commonly referred to as the pelvic cavity—hence, the term *abdominopelvic.* Specifically, this cavity lies below an imaginary line drawn across the crests of the hipbone.

The pelvic inlet is said to divide the cavity further into the greater (or false) pelvic cavity above and the lesser (or true) pelvic cavity below. The former contains parts of the large intestine, and the latter contains the bladder, rectum, and certain reproductive organs. In general, the true pelvis lies below the peritoneum.

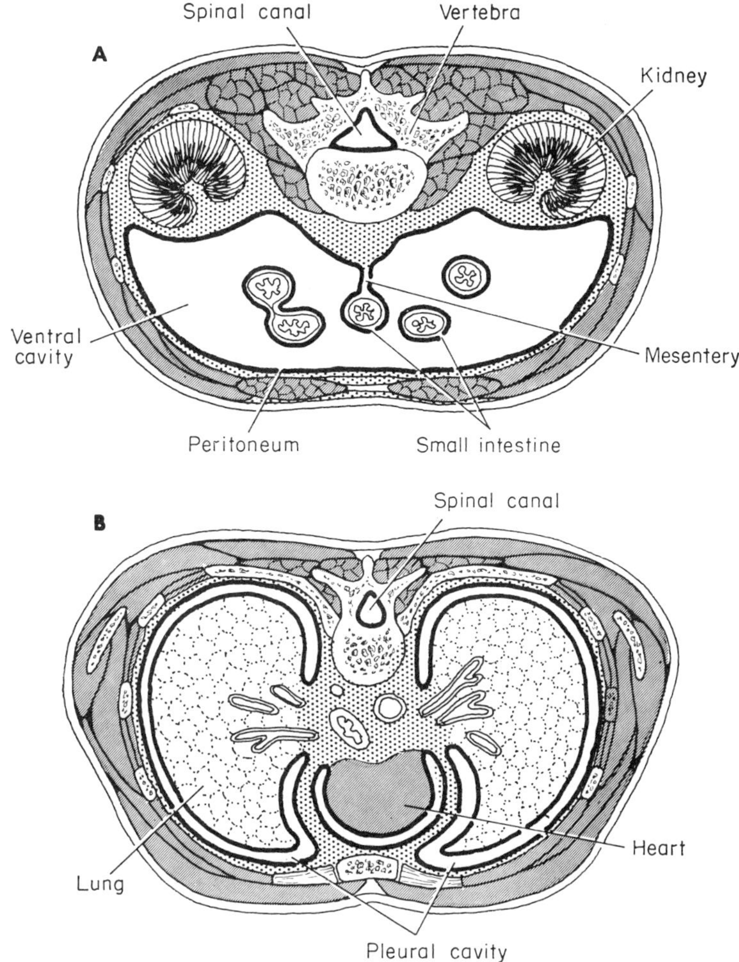

Fig. 7-1. The abdominal, **A,** and thoracic, **B,** cavities. (Adapted from Kimber D. C., Gray, C. E., Stackpole, M. A., and Leavell, C. E.: Anatomy and physiology, New York, 1961, The Macmillan Co. By permission.)

Dorsal cavity. The dorsal or posterior cavity is a continuous space enclosed by the bones of the cranium and vertebrae and lined by the meninges. It is divided into the cranial cavity, which houses the brain, and the spinal cavity, which houses the spinal cord.

THE CELL

The cell is the unit of living matter. About 100 trillion of these microscopic bits of life are formed and differentiated to make up an adult man. As in all higher forms of life, the cells of the human body are organized into *tissues,* the tissues into *organs,* and the organs into *systems.* In spite of this specialization, however, cells have the same basic structure and mode of survival. Thus, it will prove of basic value to review briefly the highlights of cytology.

Physical structure. All cells have certain constant or nearly constant features: *nucleus, cytoplasm,* and a variety of cytoplasmic *organelles* (Fig. 7-2). The typical cell has a single nucleus that contains hereditary bodies called *chromosomes* and one or more dense, round structures called *nucleoli.* The material that fills the remainder

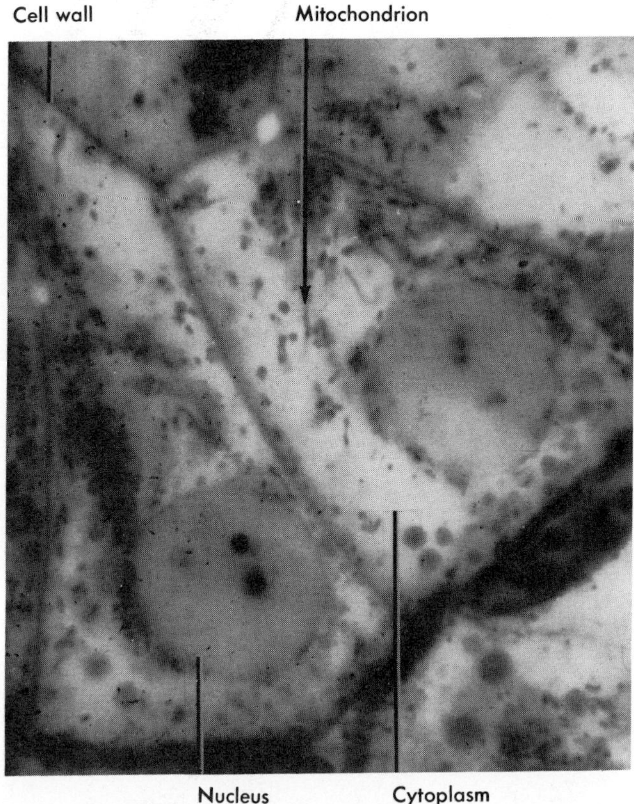

Fig. 7-2. Basic features of the cell. (Iron hematoxylin; ×1000.) (From Bevelander, G.: Essentials of histology, ed. 6, St. Louis, 1970, The C. V. Mosby Co.)

of the cell, the cytoplasm, contains within its hydrated matrix a system of vesicles known as the *endoplasmic reticulum,* studded (in most cells) with small granules called *ribosomes.* Also present are rodlike or spherical bodies called *mitochondria,* an array of lobed and laminated bodies called the *Golgi apparatus,* a *centrosome, vacuoles,* various "inclusions" (such as secretion granules and fat droplets), and *lysosomes.* The latter cytoplasmic organelles are membranous vesicles, or "sacs," containing a variety of enzymes that digest food particles and destroy bacteria and other foreign debris. In addition, the plant cell contains a *cell wall* and structures of variable size and shape called *plastids,* some of which engage in photosynthesis. Both the nucleus and the cytoplasm are enclosed by the nuclear and cell membranes, respectively.

Chemical structure. Whereas cytology in the recent past was predominantly morphologic, today it is becoming increasingly physical and chemical. According to F. O. Schmitt, there is a concept developing called the "morphology of molecular complexes."

The cytoplasm and the nucleoplasm (the substance of the nucleus) are collectively referred to as *protoplasm.* A chemical analysis of protoplasm reveals a galaxy of dissolved salts, carbohydrates, fats, and proteins. The latter compounds are the backbone of life. While carbohydrates and fats are used mainly for energy, the huge protein molecules not only serve as the "protoplasmic skeleton" but also, chiefly in the form of *enzymes,* control cellular metabolism, or the chemical reactions of life. But of all the astronomical number of substances, ribonucleic acid of the cytoplasm and the deoxyribonucleic acid of the nucleus are now known to play the most basic role.

As described earlier (p. 124), deoxyribonucleic acid (DNA) is the substance of the genes, the basic units of the chromosomes which, in conjunction with ribonucleic acid (RNA), direct the synthesis of new protein. The mechanism is briefly as follows: In the nucleus, DNA—in addition to replicating itself—also forms, when the occasion demands, RNA, which thereupon makes its way out into the ribosomes via the endoplasmic reticulum. Here the bases along the RNA chains (p. 124) "attract" certain amino acids (with the assistance of *transfer* RNA), which subsequently are clamped together by the appropriate enzymes. The newly formed protein now peels off, and the chain is set for another synthesis. Thus, a certain type of DNA produces a certain type of RNA which, in turn, produces a certain type of protein. Since protein is the "body and soul" of protoplasm, we can readily agree that DNA is life's molecular blueprint.

The cell and nuclear membranes are constructed of a meshwork of protein threads (stromatin) filled in with a matrix of cholesterol, phospholipids, and neutral fat. Those spaces, or pores, in the membrane that are not cemented over permit the diffusion of water, oxygen, carbon dioxide, and a few other substances. Any fat-soluble substance, on the other hand, whose molecules are too large to pass through the pores diffuses in and out of the cell by dissolving in the fat of the membrane wall. Most nutrients, however, probably enter the cell via active transport.

Metabolism. Cellular metabolism, as indicated, is the sum total of chemical activity in the cell. Essentially, this entails the release of energy to perform such physical functions as movement, secretion, nerve impulse transmission, and the synthesis of new protoplasm. The bulk of this energy release has now been shown to occur in the mitochondrion, the powerhouse of the cell. We shall take up the details of metabolism in Chapter 15.

Growth. Cells grow as a consequence of the synthesis of new protoplasm following the absorption of nutrients. However, when they attain a diameter somewhere between 10 and 20μ, they cease to grow, according to one view, because the surface (which is proportional to the square of the diameter) cannot keep pace with the cell volume (which is proportional to the cube of the diameter). In short, the need for nutrients outstrips the supply via the cell membrane. Nature solves the dilemma in a most simple way—via reproduction; that is, cells divide in order to survive.

Cellular reproduction. Cells of the *somatoplasm* (all body cells except germ cells) divide by a process called karyokinesis or, more commonly, *mitosis.* As shown in Fig. 7-3, the initial phases of the division process are characterized by the transformation of the chromatin network within the nucleus into a few or many threads, bars, or rods called *chromosomes.* The latter now divide lengthwise into equal parts, while the strands of the spindle are seen radiating toward them. As the strands shorten, the chromosome halves are drawn apart and collected together at the opposite poles of the cell to form two separate nuclei. Finally, the cytoplasm splits, and the chromosomes once again become organized into the chromatin network of two new nuclei. Thus, the daughter cells resemble each other by virtue of the fact that the chromosomes (with their genes of DNA)—the blueprints of heredity—have been equally divided between them.

Each species has a characteristic chromosome number that normally does not change during the complex mechanics of

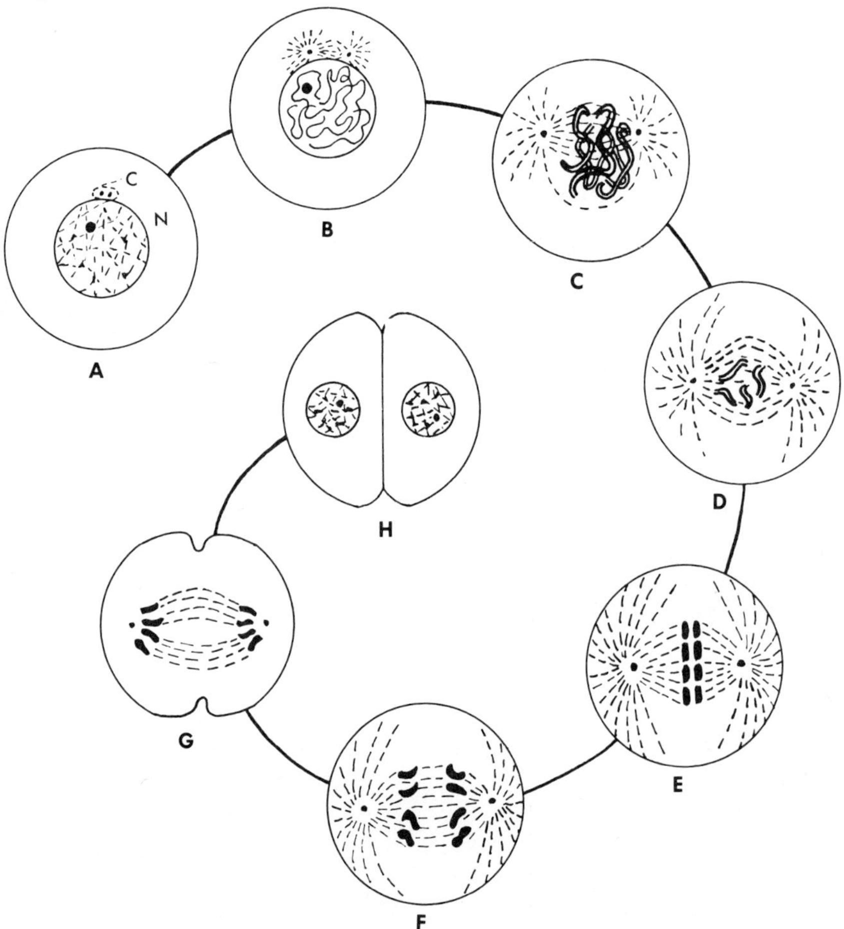

Fig. 7-3. Mitosis. **A,** Interphase, or "resting cell." **B** to **D,** Prophase. **E,** Metaphase. **F,** Anaphase. **G** and **H,** Telophase.

mitosis. In man there are *forty-six* chromosomes. The significance of this number has been recently underscored by the finding that certain developmental abnormalities and congenital malformations (a subject referred to as teratology), heretofore of unknown etiology, are due to an abnormal chromosome count. The cells of mongoloids (Down's syndrome), for example, contain forty-seven chromosomes.

Gametogenesis. In contrast to the somatoplasm, which functions for the individual, the germ plasm functions to preserve the species via sexual reproduction. This brings us to the subject of gametogenesis, that is, the formation of *gametes,* or sex cells, by the testis (*spermatogenesis*) and ovary (*oogenesis*). In this process the chromatin forms the same number of chromosomes as in mitosis, but instead of the chromosomes dividing lengthwise, they pair up and separate. Thus, instead of receiving forty-six chromosomes (the so-called *diploid number*), as in mitosis, each daughter cell receives twenty-three chromosomes (the *haploid number*). This manner of division is aptly called reduction division, or *meiosis.*

Just a little thought, of course, will disclose the reason for all this; that is, when the sperm with its twenty-three chromosomes fertilizes the ovum with its twenty-

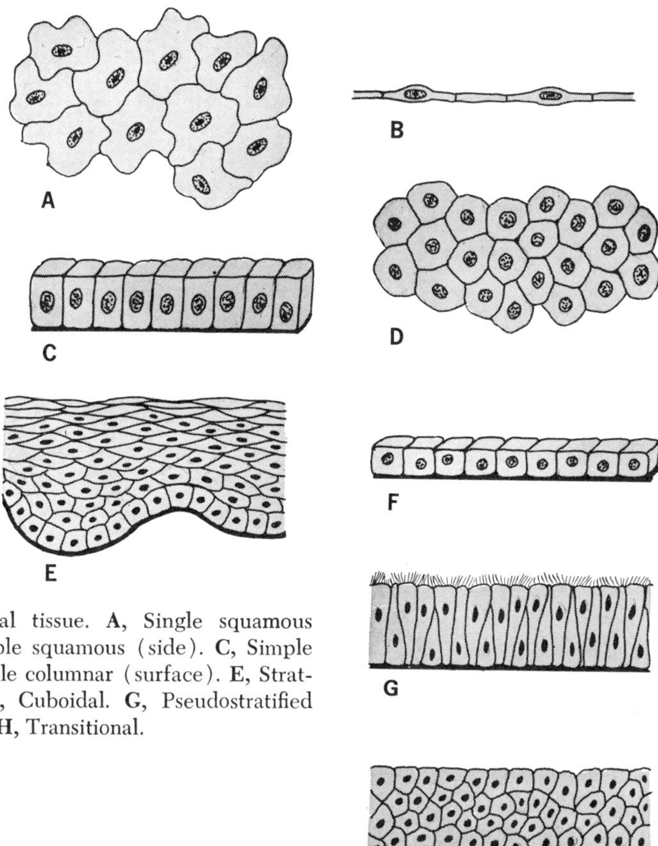

Fig. 7-4. Epithelial tissue. **A**, Single squamous (surface). **B**, Simple squamous (side). **C**, Simple columnar. **D**, Simple columnar (surface). **E**, Stratified squamous. **F**, Cuboidal. **G**, Pseudostratified ciliated columnar. **H**, Transitional.

three chromosomes, the proper diploid number of forty-six is maintained throughout future generations. In summary, then, the somatoplasm divides by mitosis, and the germ plasm divides by meiosis.

TISSUES

Histology, the microscopic study of tissues, is basic to an understanding of the body in health and disease. For this reason, the student should devote a fair amount of time to this particular area.

Considering the complexity of life, it is somewhat surprising to discover that the trillions of cells of the body are organized into four major kinds of tissue: epithelial, muscular, connective, and nerve. Although there are several variations of each, even the beginner can usually distinguish one kind from the other without too much difficulty. Tissues differ in relation to size, architecture, and arrangement of the cells, the type and quantity of intercellular substance, and location and function. The cardinal characteristics of the principal varieties are discussed here.

Epithelial tissue. Epithelial tissue, or epithelium, consists of cells joined tightly together by small amounts of intercellular cement (Fig. 7-4). The scarcity of intercellular space is highly characteristic. Since this tissue is devoid of a blood supply, it must derive its sustenance from the underlying tissue fluid.

Epithelial tissue is generally fashioned into a membrane covering external and internal surfaces, including vessels and other small cavities. In this manner it serves the functions of protection, secretion, excretion, absorption, and sensory reception. The chief types of epithelial tissue are discussed in the paragraphs that follow.

Simple squamous. Simple squamous epithelium consists of a single layer of platelike cells arranged in an attractive and highly characteristic mosaic. This type of tissue lines the alveoli, serous cavities, heart, vessels, crystalline lens of the eye, and labyrinth of the inner ear. The terms *endothelium* and *mesothelium* are applied to the simple squamous epithelium that lines the circulatory organs and serous cavities, respectively.

Stratified squamous. Stratified squamous epithelium consists of several layers of cells that, as a rule, range in shape from cylindrical in the deepest layer to simple squamous at the surface (Fig. 7-4). Stratified squamous epithelium forms the outer layer of skin and lines the nose, mouth, and anus.

The cells in the deeper layers are continually multiplying and migrating upward. In so doing they become flattened, dehydrated, and hard. As a consequence, the simple squamous cells at the top (the old cells) are continually being rubbed off to make room for a new surface. This remarkable sequence of events makes stratified squamous epithelium the most logical covering to protect body surfaces, particularly for those areas under constant environmental attack. Not only does this unique type of epithelium ward off outside forces, it also prevents the loss of body fluids. Furthermore, it contains certain microscopic structures (receptors) that serve to pick up environmental stimuli.

Transitional. Transitional epithelium is similar to stratified squamous epithelium in that the cells are arranged in layers, but it differs in that there are fewer layers and especially in that the surface cells are bloated, not flattened. Transitional epithelium lines most of the urinary tract.

Simple columnar. The simple columnar type of epithelial tissue is composed of a single layer of tall, upright, cylindrical, or prismatic cells fitted together in a very orderly fashion (Fig. 7-4). Also highly characteristic is the presence of so-called goblet cells, unicellular glands that secrete mucus. This signal fact accounts for the expression *mucous membranes* (p. 130).

In its truest form, simple columnar epithelium lines the gastrointestinal tract from the lower esophagus to the anal opening. Throughout this extensive area it serves to secrete digestive juices and absorb fluids and digested food.

Simple ciliated columnar. Simple ciliated columnar epithelium differs from the simple columnar type in possessing at its free or exposed surface protoplasmic projections called cilia (Fig. 7-4). These whiplike microscopic processes serve the unique function of impelling secretions and microscopic particles along the surface. This is accomplished not by the cilia lashing madly back and forth *en masse* but rather by a calculated succession of movements in one direction. Because of this and also because of their astronomical number, the cilia generate a current of fantastic power. Simple ciliated columnar epithelium lines the nose, the uterine tubes, and the upper part of the uterus.

Pseudostratified columnar. Pseudostratified columnar epithelium is really simple ciliated columnar epithelium modified by pressures occasioned by its location. The cells are squeezed in such a fashion that the displaced nuclei present a picture of stratification—hence, the expression *pseudostratified* (Fig. 7-4). Pseudostratified columnar epithelium lines the respiratory passageways.

Muscle tissue. Muscle tissue is characterized by its ability to contract. There are three types of muscle—skeletal, smooth, and cardiac.

Skeletal muscle. Skeletal muscle is composed of fibers marked by transverse bands (Fig. 7-5). For this reason, it is not infrequently referred to as striated or striped

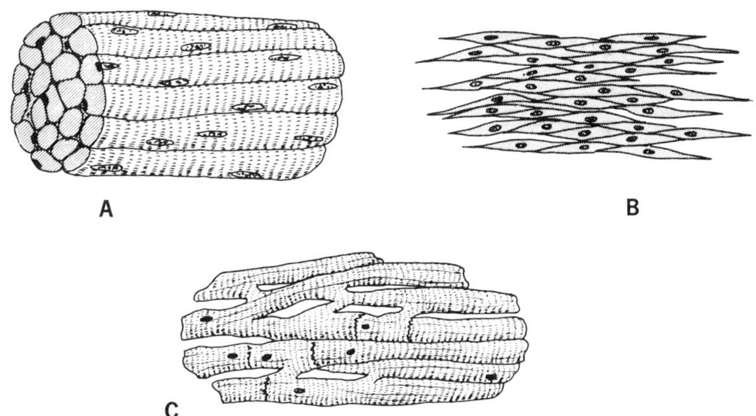

Fig. 7-5. Types of muscle. **A**, Striated. **B**, Smooth. **C**, Cardiac.

muscle. Also, since this is the type of muscle that is attached to the bones and under the control of the will, it is often called voluntary muscle.

By virtue of the fact that skeletal muscle constitutes two thirds of the weight of the body, we can readily appreciate the importance of this particular tissue to the anatomist and physiologist. The histologic and gross anatomic details will be presented in some detail in Chapter 10, which deals with the muscular system.

Smooth muscle. Whereas skeletal muscle is remarkably uniform in appearance and functional characteristics, smooth muscle is extremely variable. In general, however, smooth muscle is composed of elongated cigar-shaped cells without striations (Fig. 7-5)—hence, the expression *smooth.* Since it is the muscle of the viscera and is largely under involuntary control, we often use the terms *visceral* and *involuntary* to describe this particular tissue. In contrast to the powerful and energetic movements of skeletal muscle, smooth muscle generally contracts in a less forceful manner. The waves of motion throughout the intestine (peristalsis) are typical of its action.

Cardiac muscle. Cardiac muscle is the muscle of the heart. Although similar to skeletal muscle in having cross striations, it differs from the latter tissue in that its fibrous cells branch one into the other, producing a *syncytium,* or multinucleate mass of protoplasm (Fig. 7-5). In contrast to skeletal and smooth muscle, cardiac muscle is characterized by its rhythm and, above all, by its automatism.

Connective tissue. Connective tissue (Fig. 7-6) is the most variable and widespread of all the tissues. It houses the internal organs, sheathes the muscles, wraps the joints, and composes the blood and skeleton. Connective tissue, therefore, may be said to support, protect, and/or nourish the body.

Connective tissue is constituted by three basic histologic elements—cells, fibers, and intercellular substance (also called ground substance or *matrix*). Because these three elements are the basis for distinguishing one connective tissue from another, we shall say a word or two about each before proceeding to specific types.

The chief connective tissue cells include the fibroblasts, macrophages, mast cells, plasma cells, and blood cells. Although fibroblasts do not appear in the blood, they are the most common cellular element in the other varieties of connective tissue. Fibroblasts are flat, star-shaped cells (Fig. 7-6) that play the unique role of manufacturing fibers. Macrophages are large, ameboid cells that wander throughout the tissues, devouring foreign particles via *phago-*

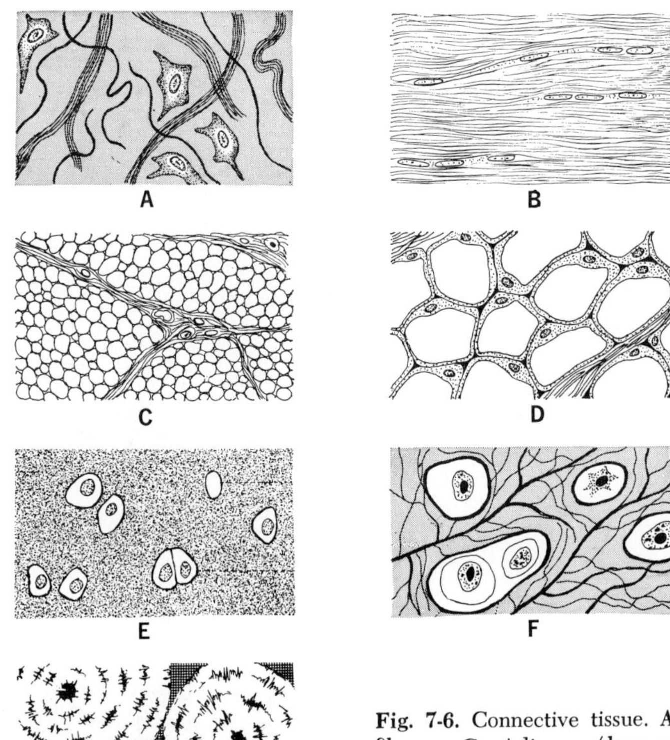

Fig. 7-6. Connective tissue. **A,** Areolar. **B,** White fibrous. **C,** Adipose (low power). **D,** Adipose (high power). **E,** Hyaline cartilage. **F,** Elastic cartilage. **G,** Bone.

cytosis. Mast cells are mononuclear, irregularly shaped structures with a granular cytoplasm. These cells store an anticoagulant substance called heparin (Chapter 12). Plasma cells, usually found in lymphoid and related tissues, are similar to mast cells; they are now generally recognized as the chief producers of antibodies. Cells of the blood, which are of several types, are discussed in detail in Chapter 12.

The fibers present in connective tissue are of three types—*white, elastic,* and *reticular.* White or collagenous fibers are fine and glistening microscopic strands that occur in interlacing bundles (Fig. 7-6). Elastic fibers, on the other hand, are yellow and coarser and occur as separate strands that branch and join with one another. Reticular fibers are immature strands that compose the netlike supporting framework in lymphoid and myeloid tissues.

The intercellular substance in connective tissue is highly characteristic and determines whether a particular type of tissue is fluid, jellylike, plastic, or hard. In contrast to epithelial and muscle tissue, the amount of intercellular substance in connective tissue exceeds the cellular elements. Indeed, we shall do well to consider connective tissue as one in which cells and fibers are distributed in a matrix of "water, jelly, or rock."

Areolar tissue. To the unaided eye, areolar connective tissue looks like tissue paper—delicate, thin, and easily torn. Histologically, it represents connective tissue in its truest form, that is, cells and white and elastic fibers scattered throughout a soft matrix. Areolar tissue forms the basis of subcutaneous tissue and runs between the organs. Thus, it serves principally to support and cement.

Adipose tissue. Human adipose tissue contains fat and looks like the fat on meat. Histologically, it may be described as a fine meshwork of areolar tissue with fat cells (cells with fat globules) distributed throughout the interspaces (Fig. 7-6). Present under the skin and about the viscera, adipose tissue serves to support, protect, insulate, and store energy. For the latter reason, this tissue is of vital interest to the calorie counter.

Fibrous tissue. Fibrous connective tissue is of three kinds—white, elastic, and fibroelastic. In white fibrous tissue, white fibers dominate the intercellular space. There are few connective tissue cells and little matrix. This beautiful pearl-white tissue is flexible but also amazingly strong. It composes organ capsules, deep fascia, aponeuroses, ligaments, tendons, muscle sheaths, periosteum, and the dura mater.

Elastic tissue, often called yellow fibrous tissue because of its color, is characterized by pronounced elasticity. This tissue composes certain ligaments of the vertebral column (ligamenta flava).

Fibroelastic connective tissue contains both white and elastic fibers. The large arteries such as the aorta are abundantly supplied with this particular variety.

Cartilage. Cartilage is an opaque, bluish white tissue with the consistency of a hard rubber ball; in short, it is gristle. Microscopically, cartilage is found to be composed of cells secluded in widely separated tiny spaces called lacunae. The matrix is a dense, translucent, homogeneous substance with or without fibrous elements. Cartilage is covered by a dense membrane, called the perichondrium, that serves to nourish and repair the tissue.

HYALINE CARTILAGE. Hyaline cartilage is a glasslike cartilage with a translucent pale blue matrix. It is found at the ends of bones (articular cartilage) and in the larynx; it composes the rings of the trachea and bronchi; and it forms the anterior nasal septum.

ELASTIC CARTILAGE. Elastic cartilage, or yellow fibrocartilage, is essentially hyaline cartilage with elastic fibers throughout the matrix. It is present in the external ear, eustachian cartilage, epiglottis, and certain arytenoid cartilages of the larynx.

FIBROUS CARTILAGE. Fibrous cartilage, or white fibrocartilage, is hyaline cartilage with interlacing bundles of white fibers running through the matrix. It is found between the vertebrae and composes the symphysis pubis.

Bone. With the exception of the bones of of the face and skull, most bone may be dramatically described as hyaline cartilage "turned to stone"; that is, the semisolid matrix of the latter tissue has given way to a hard, dense deposit of calcium salts. However, in contrast to the inaccessible cells in cartilage, bone lacunae intercommunicate through microscopic channels, called canaliculi, arranged concentrically about larger channels known as haversian canals. Each canal, with its concentric lacunae and lamellae (rings of matrix), constitutes a so-called *haversian system.* By this system the blood supply to bone is distributed to its matrix-locked cells via the canals and canaliculi.

Bone is either *compact* or *cancellous* (spongy). In compact bone the lamellae of the osseous matrix are put down layer upon layer, whereas in cancellous bone the lamellae form a delicate latticework pattern with a spongy appearance. The gross anatomy of bone will be discussed in detail in Chapter 9, in which the skeletal system is considered.

Reticuloendothelial tissue. Reticuloendothelial tissue, identified by the presence of reticular fibers, composes the so-called reticuloendothelial system, that is, the spleen, lymph nodes, bone marrow, and liver. The system is concerned with blood formation, storage of fatty materials, phagocytosis, and elaboration of antibodies.

Blood. Blood is a type of connective tissue characterized by a fluid matrix. Its histology and function will be discussed in detail later in the book (Chapter 12).

Nerve tissue. Just one look at nerve tissue is enough to indicate its function—the *conduction* of impulses. Nerve tissue composes the brain, spinal cord, and nerves. Although nerve cells, or neurons, vary considerably in architecture, they are all characterized by an octopus-like arrangement of cytoplasmic projections (processes) called *dendrites* and *axons.* In the brain and spinal cord there are supporting cells in addition to neurons. These cells, characterized by their small oval nuclei, constitute the so-called neuroglia. Macroscopically, nerve tissue is either white or gray in color and soft and friable to the touch.

MEMBRANES

Membranes are sheets of tissue that cover or line various parts of the body. They are composed of a layer of epithelium on a layer of connective tissue. The chief membranes of the body include the mucous, serous, and synovial membranes. The skin itself may be considered a membrane, and the term *membrane* is also used to describe various sheets of connective tissue that separate or connect certain structures, for example, the interosseous and thyrohyoid membranes.

Mucous membranes. Mucous membranes line cavities or passageways leading to the exterior, the most extensive including those lining the digestive tract, the genitourinary tract, and the respiratory passageways. That which lines the digestive tract has a stratified squamous epithelium from the mouth two thirds of the way down the esophagus and a simple columnar epithelium all the rest of the way. The mucosa of the respiratory tract is distinguished by its pseudostratified ciliated columnar epithelium. In the genitourinary mucosa we find both simple ciliated columnar and transitional epithelium.

We should not forget that the term *mucous membrane*, or *mucosa,* is derived from the word *mucus,* which means the lubricating and protective slime secreted by the goblet cells in the epithelium. Mucus is essential to life.

Serous membranes. In contrast to mucous membranes, serous membranes line closed cavities. The principal membranes of this type include the pleura, which lines the thoracic cavity, the peritoneum, which lines the abdominal cavity, and the pericardium, which surrounds the heart. The epithelium of serous membranes is of the simple squamous type and bears the name *mesothelium.*

A serous membrane not only lines a particular cavity but also wraps about the organ contained therein. This brings to the fore two terms of considerable anatomic significance—*visceral* and *parietal.* The visceral layer refers to the serous membrane about the organ, while the parietal layers refers to the layer that lines the cavity. Obviously, in the close quarters of our internal world this means that the visceral and parietal layers are in direct apposition, one rubbing against the other as the organs "move about." For example, when we breathe, the visceral pleura about the lung glides along the parietal pleura of the chest wall (p. 160). To reduce friction as a result of this continual movement, nature has placed a small amount of watery fluid (serous fluid) between the two layers. Thus, the body obeys a principle of engineering, namely, that where there are moving parts there must be lubrication.

Synovial membranes. Synovial membranes line tendon sheaths, bursae, and joint cavities. The epithelium is of the same type (mesothelium) that surfaces serous membranes. These membranes secrete a fluid called synovia or synovial fluid (similar in composition to serous fluid), which serves to lubricate the joints, tendons, and bursae.

GLANDS

A gland may be defined as an organ that produces a specific secretion. There are two major types: those that secrete via ducts (*exocrine* glands) and those that secrete directly into the blood (ductless or *endocrine* glands). Since endocrine glands secrete a variety of potent body regulators (hormones), they are discussed in detail in a special chapter (Chapter 22). Exocrines will be dealt with as the occasion arises.

Histologically, glandular tissue is modified epithelium. As a matter of fact, the simplest gland is the goblet cell (Fig. 7-7). Multicellular exocrine glands are classified according to the design of the ducts into which the cells pour their secretion (Fig. 7-7). The basic types include the tubular, saccular (also alveolar or acinous), and racemose or mixed (conbined tubular and saccular structures). These, in turn, are classified as simple or compound, depending upon the complexity of design. The more representative structures are shown in Fig. 7-7.

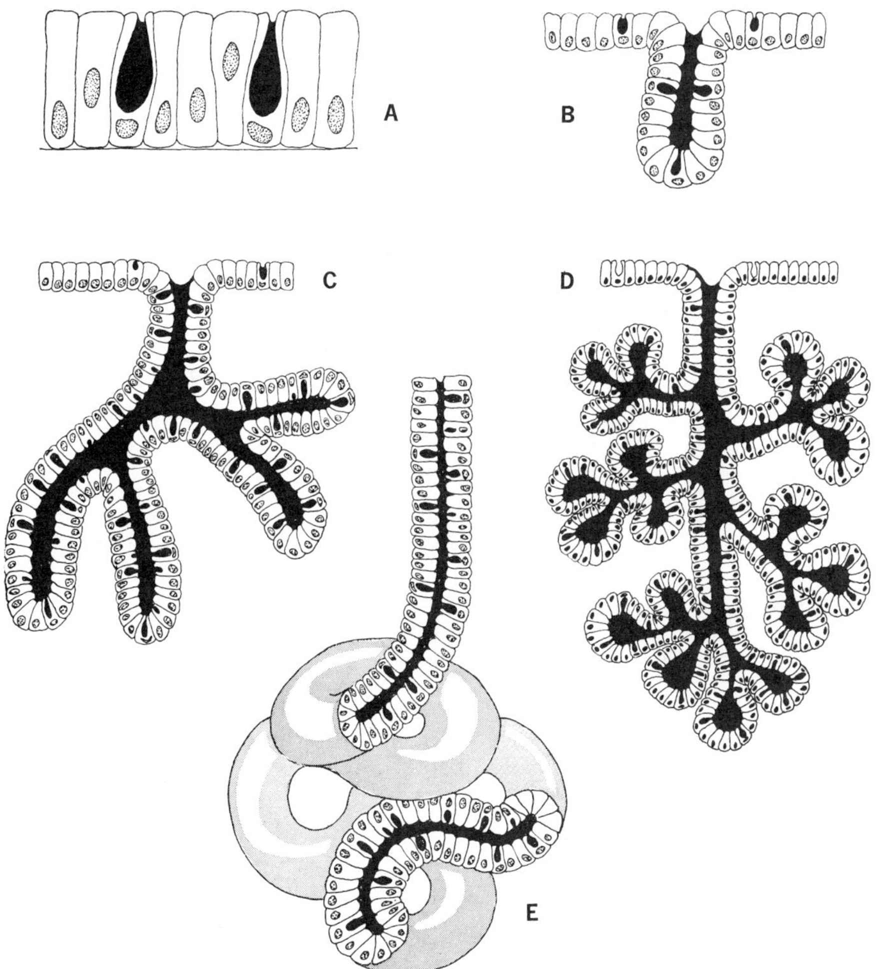

Fig. 7-7. Types of glands. **A,** Goblet. **B,** Simple tubular. **C,** Branched tubular. **D,** Compound tubuloalveolar. **E,** Coiled tubular.

BODY WATER

When we consider that water composes about two thirds of the weight of the human body, it is little wonder that physiology texts devote a chapter or two to the subject of water and fluids. Only in rather late years, however, have the physiologist and physician realized that water is not merely a cell-locked constituent of living tissue but one involved in the body as a dynamic whole. In short, water is "alive" and moving, and directly or indirectly is associated with health and disease.

For our present purpose, Fig. 7-8 will serve us well, for it shows how the water of the body is distributed. Even at this early stage in our study, however, we must appreciate that just because the percentage of water in a given compartment is so and so does not mean that water is static. Indeed, it merely indicates, for instance, that the water leaving the cells is equal to the amount entering the cells, and vice versa. So it is throughout the body. Later on, particularly in Chapter 18, we shall look into the rather elaborate forces concerned with this so-called *water balance.*

THE SYSTEMS

As indicated previously, we shall study the structure and function of the human body on the basis of systems. However, before setting out on this exciting journey, we shall first take a general look at the various systems and the way they operate in concert to produce the body as a whole.

Skeletal system. The skeleton not only forms the ageless framework of the body but also permits an almost endless variety of contortions, as the acrobat and the ballet dancer well know. The human skeleton is composed of 206 separate bones that articulate with one another at so-called joints. The location and design of the joint decide the type and extent of movement.

Contrary to first impressions, bone is very

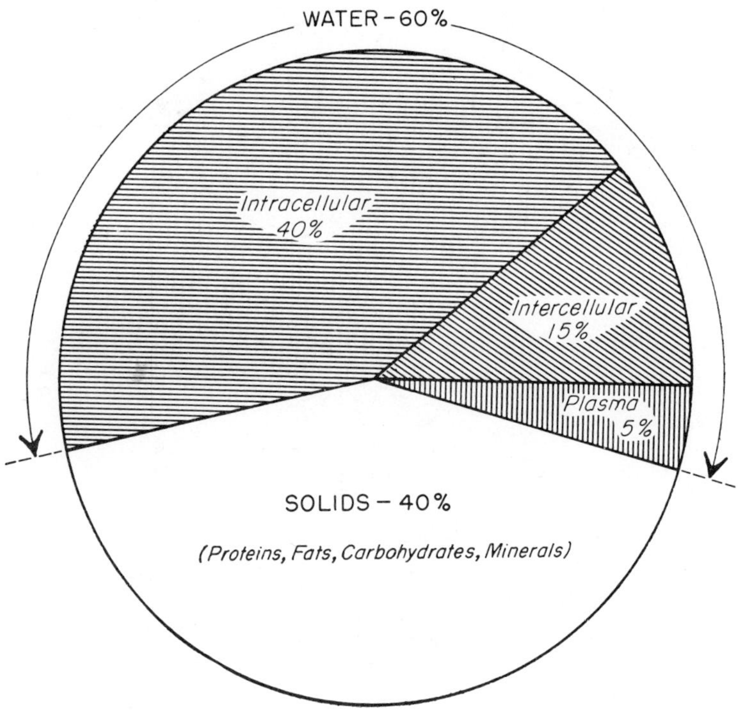

Fig. 7-8. Body water. (From Brooks, S. M.: Basic facts of body water and ions, ed. 2, New York, 1968, Springer Publishing Co., Inc.)

much alive and active and, in addition to its framework role, is the seat of hemopoiesis (blood formation) and calcium metabolism.

Muscular system. The muscular system here refers to the skeletal muscle of the body (p. 212), which is organized into more than 400 *muscles* of varying sizes and shapes. For example, the stapedius, a muscle of the inner ear, is only a fraction of an inch in length, whereas the sartorius muscle runs almost 2 feet down the thigh. Again, the sheetlike muscles of the abdomen are a far cry from the round, cigar-shaped muscles of the upper arm.

Muscles are attached to bones by white fibrous connective tissue called tendons, and when a muscle contracts in response to impulses from the central nervous system, tension is exerted upon the tendon and movement is thereby effected. Although the precise physicochemical mechanism by which muscle contracts is still a mystery, we do know that nerve impulses make the fibers shorten for a brief instant. This causes the entire muscle to shorten and contract.

Circulatory system. The circulatory system is composed of the blood, heart, and vessels. The right side of the heart pumps blood to the lungs (to pick up oxygen), and the left side pumps oxygenated blood to all parts of the body. We apply the term *pulmonary circulation* to the flow of blood between the heart and lungs and the term *systemic circulation* to the flow between the heart and the body as a whole.

A special division of the systemic circulation that brings blood from the intestines and spleen through the liver is called the portal circulatory system. In this manner the complex chemical machinery of the liver "works over" the nutrients that have been absorbed by the villi. Also, certain noxious agents are detoxified before they have an opportunity to insult the body at large.

Blood flows from the heart via the arteries and returns via the veins. "Between" these major vessels microscopic channels called capillaries permit diffusion of oxygen and nutrients from the blood into the tissues and diffusion of wastes from the tissues into the blood.

In addition to oxygen, nutrients, and wastes, the blood transports an endless variety of such substances as hormones, antibodies, and enzymes. Also, certain white cells destroy microbes and other foreign agents via phagocytosis. Not to be forgotten, too, is the fact that the blood plays a vital role in regulating body temperature.

Lymphatic system. An accessory system known as the lymphatic system transports lymph (a watery fluid derived from and similar to intercellular fluid) throughout the body. As the intercellular or interstitial fluid accumulates in the tissues, it forces its way into the lymphatic capillaries and thence into valved channels called lymphatic vessels. Finally, two major vessels lead the lymph to veins in the neck. Thus, the intercellular fluid, "squeezed" out from the blood, is returned to the blood via the lymphatic system.

A relatively recent development is the realization that blood protein escapes through the capillaries into the interstitial fluid. Thus, if this fluid were not returned to the circulation, via the lymph, blood protein would drop to dangerous levels in a day or two.

Unlike the circulation of blood, the lymphatic system does not require a pump. Instead, the movement of the body in general and the contraction of the muscles in particular are of sufficient force to "milk along" the lymph.

Located along the lymphatic vessels through which the lymph must pass on its journey to the blood are lymph nodes. Here, all large particles (old debris of dead tissue, giant molecules, and the like) are filtered out and bacteria are destroyed by the phagocytic cells. Moreover, it is principally here that the plasma cells manufacture antibodies. Thus, the lymphatic system turns out to be one of the chief defenses of the body.

Respiratory system. In a narrow sense the respiratory system refers to the exchange of gases (namely, oxygen, carbon dioxide, and water vapor) in the lung between the air and blood. In a broad and more realistic sense, however, respiration includes not only the exchange in the lungs but also the exchange of gases between the blood and tissues and the *transport* of gases (by the blood) between the lungs and the tissues. Anatomically, the fundamental portions of the system include the lungs, air passageways (nose, pharynx, larynx, trachea, and bronchi), and the respiratory muscles, namely, the intercostal muscles and the diaphragm.

Digestive system. Man's desire for food is adequately underscored by the fact that the digestive organs constitute the bulk of the abdominal viscera. The digestive apparatus includes the gastrointestinal tract (mouth, stomach, and intestines), salivary glands, liver, and pancreas. Physiologically, the system has a simple enough purpose, that is, the physical and chemical extraction of nutrients from the diet and the absorption thereof into the blood through the intestinal mucosa.

Digestion proper, or the breakdown of food, is brought about by digestive juices and enzymes secreted into the gut by the intestinal wall, salivary glands, pancreas, and liver. These agents split food into molecules small enough to edge their way into the intestinal villi. Such absorbable nutrients include water, minerals, vitamins, amino acids (from protein), glucose (from carbohydrates), and glycerol and fatty acids (from fat). Once in the blood these substances are transported throughout the body and ultimately enter the complex machinery of the cell where they are burned for energy or forged into the materials of life.

Metabolism. In its broadest and most accurate sense, metabolism simply means the sum total of life's chemical reactions. Put another way, but meaning exactly the same thing, metabolism is what the body does with what we feed it. In this context, one can hardly avoid the temptation to wonder philosophically how, on the one hand, an Einstein converts strawberry shortcake into a brain belonging to the ages and, on the other, a moron converts the same shortcake into a brain not far removed from that of an ape. This is not to say that one person's chemistry necessarily differs *drastically* from another's but, rather, that it *does* differ.

Metabolism includes *anabolism* (synthesis) and *catabolism* (degradation). The basic anabolic process is *assimilation* (the formation of new tissue), and the basic catabolic processes are *digestion* and *respiration*.

Urinary system. As the blood courses the organs and tissues, it collects the refuse of metabolism. Such unwanted and noxious substances as urea, uric acid, creatinine, phenols, sulfates, and phosphates must be taken out of the blood, and it is the job of the kidney to do it. The kidneys, situated as they are in the circulatory path, seem to "know" what to take out and what to leave in. In the process of this life-and-death picking and choosing, they yield urine, a concentrated aqueous solution of the waste products just mentioned. As urine emerges, drop by drop, from the microscopic collecting tubules of the kidneys, it works its way down the ureters to the bladder, where it waits to be discharged.

Sometimes substances appear in the urine that do not belong there. The presence, for instance, of sugar, blood, albumin, or pus is a strong indication that all is not well, either along the genitourinary tract or in some other area of the body. Thus, urine serves as a valuable aid in the diagnosis of disease.

Nervous system. The nervous system is composed of the brain, the spinal cord, and the peripheral nerves. It has two functions: (1) to permit the body to react to and act upon its environment and (2) to regulate its *milieu interne,* or internal environment. In responding to our environment we must be informed, first of all, about our environment via sight, hearing, smell, taste, touch, pressure, pain, vibration, position of the body, and tension in the muscles. The nerves that carry such stimuli and the parts of the brain that analyze them constitute the *sensory* portion of the nervous system. Being continually appraised of what is going on, the *motor* portions of the brain effect the response by transmitting impulses over the motor nerves supplying the skeletal muscles. So it is that we run when we see a snake!

Autonomic nervous system. The autonomic system refers to those peripheral nerves that supply smooth muscle, glands, and heart. Since it operates without conscious effort, the system is aptly named. In a typical situation an organ or gland receives two physiologically antagonistic autonomic fibers; that is, impulses over one will, in the case of muscle, cause contraction, whereas impulses over the other will cause relaxation. In the case of a gland, one type of fiber will stimulate secretion and the other will inhibit secretion. It is for this reason that the physiologist places the autonomic system into divisions—the *sympathetic* and *parasympathetic.* The former acts, as Cannon said, to prepare the body for "fight or flight." For example, stimulation of the sympathetic fibers going to the heart causes the heart to increase in rate and strength of contraction; the parasympathetic fibers slow the heart.

Endocrine system. Scattered throughout the body are islands of glandular tissue (ductless or endocrine glands) that release potent chemical agents, or *hormones,* directly into the blood. In concert with the autonomic nervous system, hormones regulate the metabolic profile and physiologic processes of the body. The importance of the system becomes immediately apparent when we realize that infinitesimal changes in the output of these tiny glands can mean the difference between health and disease—and sometimes between life and death.

Reproductive system. Whereas the other systems of the body are concerned exclusively with running the body, the reproductive system functions for posterity.

The ovum and sperm cell released by the ovary and testis, respectively, contain twenty-three chromosomes each, and in the act of fertilization the two gametes fuse into a forty-six-chromosome cell called a zygote. The zygote divides again and again and the morula stage attaches itself to the rich uterine lining where it proceeds to undergo rapid development and growth in the succulent tissue. By the embryo stage a full-fledged exchange of nutrients and wastes has been established via the umbilical cord and the placenta. Nine months following fertilization, the fetus is "ripe" and the mother's body is primed for birth. Powerful contractions of the uterine musculature now expel the new individual—and new student!

HOMEOSTASIS

In a very real sense the cells throughout the body are aquatic, being surrounded as they are by an aqueous medium called intercellular or interstitial fluid—a fluid having a very definite concentration of mineral matter, wastes, nutrients, and the like. Further—and as one would suspect—when the concentration of the constituents in this medium significantly depart from this "very definite concentration," the cells are in for trouble, and the body as a whole is headed away from normal toward disease. But central to our discussion here is that the myriad physiologic functions of the body are, in the long run, directly or indirectly concerned with maintaining the status quo of this internal environment, or *melieu interne*—a concept that the great physiologist Cannon expressed as *homeostasis.* For instance, the blood delivers nutrients to the interstitial fluid (which thereupon enter the cell) and removes (from the interstitial fluid) wastes, which in turn are removed by the kidneys. And so on with the other activities of the body.

Questions

1. In a single brief paragraph describe the human body.
2. Discuss the importance of histology in the diagnosis of disease.
3. Distinguish between a tissue and a membrane.
4. Distinguish between *mucus* and *mucous.*
5. Distinguish between secretion and excretion.
6. If a man weighs 150 pounds, how many quarts of water does his body contain? How much of this is held in the cells?
7. Discuss the statement "All life is aquatic."
8. Distinguish between a mucous and a serous membrane.
9. With a *single* word describe the function of the four basic tissues.
10. In one sentence describe the function of the skeletal, muscular, circulatory, respiratory, digestive, urinary, and nervous systems.
11. Define mediastinum, peritoneum, retroperitoneal, pelvis, pleura, mesothelium, goblet cells, cilia, anterior, gross anatomy, gene, mitochondria, viscera, adipose tissue, elastic fibers, perichondrium, synovial fluid, exocrines, dorsal, inferior, superficial, histology, cytoplasm, and mitosis.

Chapter 8

The skin

The skin or, more formally, the *integument,* is an organ of beauty and an anatomic and physiologic wonder. Among other things, it protects us against infection and injury; it prevents the loss of life-giving water; it expels noxious agents from the body; it cools us in the summer and warms us in the winter; and, via a galaxy of nervous receptors, it puts us in touch with the outside world. All this, mind you, plus its uncanny ability to bathe, oil, and give itself a new coat when the old one wears off.

LAYERS

The skin is composed of two distinct layers—the epidermis above and the dermis below (Fig. 8-1). The dermis is attached to the subcutaneous tissue and the latter, in turn, is attached to the superficial muscles and bones of the body.

Epidermis. The epidermis (sometimes called cuticle) is stratified squamous epithelium which, in the areas where it is thickest (palms of the hands and soles of the feet), is made up of four strata: from outward inward, the stratum corneum, the stratum lucidum, the stratum granulosum, and the stratum germinativum (Fig. 8-1).

The stratum germinativum consists of several layers of cells that are always in a state of rapid multiplication. As new cells are formed, they push upward and in so doing shove the strata above them forward. And in this upward march the cells become progressively squeezed, dehydrated, and scalelike. This accounts for the fact that the cells in the outermost layer—the stratum corneum—are dead and are constantly being shed to make room for those below. These dead cells are distinguished by the presence of a water-repellent protein called keratin, the principal protective chemical of the epidermis.

The epidermis receives no blood and, hence, must rely upon the underlying nutrient fluids. It does, however, possess fine nerve fibers between the cells of the inner layers.

Pigment. Color is skin deep and depends upon varying amounts of a pigment called *melanin,* formed by special cells in the stratum germinativum called melanocytes. The skin of the Negro and the darker areas on the white man (for example, about the nipple) contain large amounts of this pigment. Too, it must not be forgotten that the color of the skin is often influenced by the blood supply. The reason we blush,

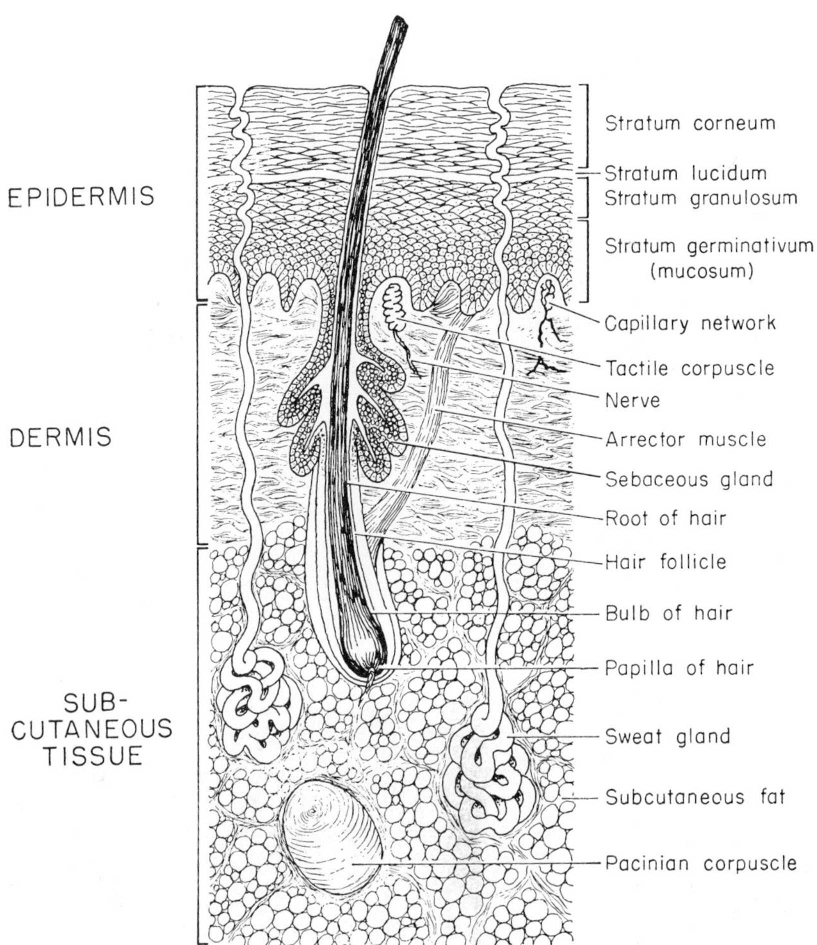

Fig. 8-1. The skin.

for instance, is that the cutaneous vessels dilate, thereby pooling more blood beneath the epidermis.

Dermis. Beneath the epidermis lies the dermis, or corium, composed of connective tissue well laced with elastic fibers, blood and lymph vessels, nerves, and accessory glandular structures. Characteristically, the dermis thrusts itself upward into peglike structures called papillae (Fig. 8-1), which serve to lock together the two layers of skin. Of no little concern to the criminologist is the fact that the papillae produce the ripples, or fingerprints, in the epidermis at the ends of the fingers and thumbs. Fingerprints are perhaps a person's most individualistic feature—they differ even between identical twins!—and they almost never change. On the other hand, as we grow older, the dermal elastic fibers progressively decrease and the skin starts to wrinkle.

Subcutaneous tissue. Subcutaneous tissue, or *superficial fascia,* anchors the skin to the muscles and bones beneath. It is composed of areolar connective tissue interlaced with fat, vessels, nerves, receptors, and glands. This tissue nourishes, supports, and cushions the skin, and its fat serves as food reserve.

Fat, the chief chemical constituent, is deposited and distributed according to the person's sex, and together with muscle and bone development, accounts for the difference in body shape between the sexes. Unhappily, the situation gets out of hand when we overeat, resulting in the piling up of fat beneath the skin. Conversely, when we diet, excess fat is burned and the skin is allowed to resume its normal texture and contour; thus, we "get our shape back."

Deep fascia. Beneath the superficial fascia lies the deep fascia, a thin layer of dense connective tissue without fat that covers the muscles and passes inward to form intermuscular septa. In certain areas the deep fascia thickens to produce ligaments, tendons, and aponeuroses.

ACCESSORY ORGANS

The accessory organs of the skin include nails, hair, microscopic glands, and receptors.

Nails. The nails are the horney distal appendages of the fingers and toes. They are made up of the epidermal cells developed from the stratum lucidum lying under the lunula, the white crescent-shaped structure situated at the proximal end of the nail.

Hair. Except for the palms of the hands and the soles of the feet, hair adorns the entire body. Although over the eye, in the nose, and in the ears hair serves an obvious function in screening out insects, dust, and other airborne debris, it has little physiologic value elsewhere. It is reasonable to assume, however, that primitive man was equipped with a "birthday coat" of sufficient quality to cope with colder climates.

Histologically, a shaft of hair grows upward as a consequence of extensive cellular multiplication at the papilla, a structure located at the base of the root (Fig. 8-1). The root (the portion of the hair that is embedded in the skin) and its coat of connective tissue constitute the hair follicle. As long as the epithelial cells near the papilla remain alive, a hair will continue to grow and regenerate, irrespective of the barber's efforts.

As we know, the "hair stands on end" and goose pimples appear in response to fright or cold. This somewhat primitive response is caused by contraction of the tiny muscles (arrectores pilorum) attached to the hair follicle. Also around the follicle are sebaceous glands that secrete an oil to "wet" the hair (Fig. 8-1). The color of hair is due to the presence of varying amounts of melanin within the shaft. Gray or white hair is a result of loss of pigment.

Sebaceous glands. For each hair there are at least two glands that secrete about the shaft an oily substance called *sebum.* (Modified sebaceous glands lying within the tarsus of each eyelid are referred to as meibomian glands.) Sebum oils the hair and also renders the skin soft and pliable.

Sudoriferous glands. Sudoriferous or *sweat* glands (Fig. 8-1) are distributed over the entire body, especially on the palms, soles, forehead, and axillary regions. These glands play an important role in regulating body heat and, in conjunction with the kidney, in ridding the blood of wastes. Sweat contains about 99 percent water, dissolved salts (chiefly NaCl), traces of urea, and miscellaneous other wastes. In abnormal conditions, however, bile pigments, albumin, sugar and even blood may appear. When the body becomes overheated, the sudoriferous glands step up the production of sweat, thereby enhancing evaporation and cooling of the skin. In the tropics as much as 10 to 15 liters of water may be lost daily through perspiration.

The sweat glands are governed by the autonomic nerves which, in turn, are under the direction of a presumed "sweat center" in the brain. As the temperature of the blood rises in response to the external temperature or to muscular activity, the center is triggered to send impulses to the glands, causing the production of sweat.

Insensible perspiration. Contrary to one's

first impression, the body loses water from the skin not only when we "sweat" but also every second of the day. Water that escapes as unnoticed vapor is called insensible perspiration. The cutaneous water output on a typical day averages about 0.5 liter. Obviously, this loss must be paid back by water intake.

Ceruminous glands. These are modified sweat glands located in the canal of the external ear. Instead of sweat, they elaborate cerumen, a waxlike secretion that aids the hairs in trapping dust, insects, and the like.

Receptors. As indicated, the skin places the body in sensitive "touch" with the outside world. This is accomplished through so-called external receptors, sensory nerve terminals that respond to pain, heat, cold, touch, and pressure (Fig. 8-2). Although these microscopic receivers are distributed over the entire body, they are more concentrated in some areas than in others. The back, for instance, has few receptors as compared with the fingertips.

Pain receptors. Pain receptors, or nociceptors, are naked nerve filaments found throughout the skin and in several other areas. They are the most numerous of all the five kinds of receptors. In contrast to the nociceptors in the viscera, those in the skin are sensitive to any type of stimulus, provided that it is strong enough to elicit a response. Generally speaking, visceral nociceptors respond only to pressure, contraction, and chemical agents.

Meissner's corpuscles. Encapsulated receptors called Meissner's corpuscles are lo-

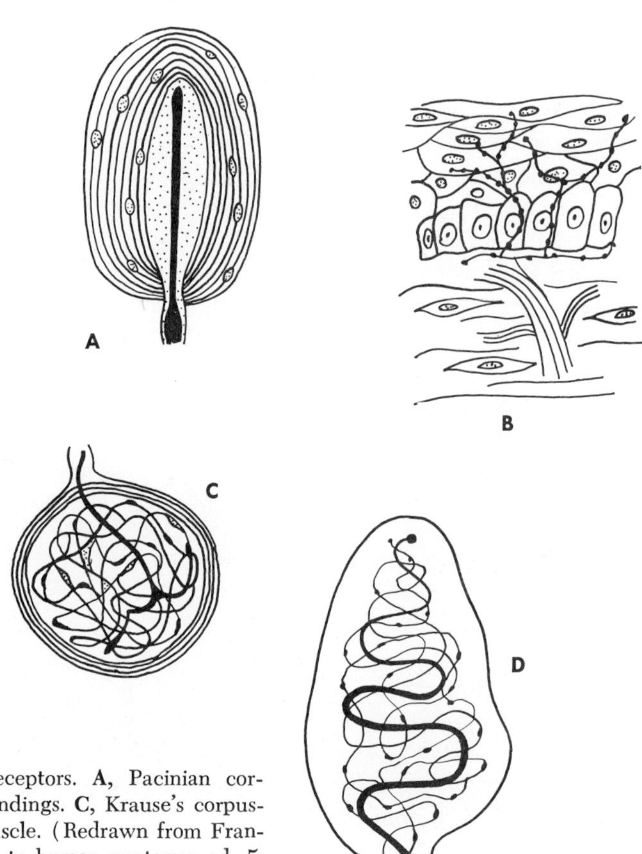

Fig. 8-2. Cutaneous receptors. **A,** Pacinian corpuscle. **B,** Free nerve endings. **C,** Krause's corpuscle. **D,** Meissner's corpuscle. (Redrawn from Francis, C. C: Introduction to human anatomy, ed. 5, St. Louis, 1968, The C. V. Mosby Co.)

cated in the dermal papillae of the fingers and toes, over the lips, in the mammary glands, and in the external genitals. They are "tuned" to the sense of touch.

Krause's corpuscles. Krause's corpuscles, also called the end bulbs of Krause, are cold receptors consisting of a spheroid capsule enclosing a granular mass and a terminal neurofibril. Krause's corpuscles are located in the mucous membranes of the mouth, nose, eyes, and genitals.

Ruffini's corpuscles. The receptors known as Ruffini's corpuscles are branching nerve endings in the skin that are sensitive to warmth. They are enclosed within a connective tissue sheath.

Pacini's corpuscles. Pacini's or pacinian corpuscles, the largest of the end organs, are pressure receptors found in the deeper parts of the skin covering the hands and feet. They also occur throughout the subcutaneous tissue, in the muscles, mesentery, and mesocolon. Pacinian corpuscles are ovoid in shape, and each contains a granular central bulb enclosing a single terminal neurofibril.

DISEASES AND DISORDERS OF THE SKIN

When we consider that the skin covers such an intricate and sensitive mechanism as the human body, it is little wonder that most of us cannot go through life without an occasional flare-up of this expansive organ. Such flare-ups may be caused by a microbial, physical, or chemical attack from without or by some microbial or metabolic attack from within. In the latter connection it is important to appreciate that a skin disease of internal cause may be due not only to forces within the skin itself but also, as is sometimes the case, to extracutaneous mechanisms.

Infection. Although the intact skin provides the body with an inimitable barrier against life's sea of microbial enemies, an injury, however minor, affords a portal of entry. The consequence may be a pimple or, in extreme cases, death. As stated, an infectious disease involving the skin does not have to attack from without. For instance, smallpox and measles, diseases that have cutaneous manifestations, are caused by inhaled or ingested viruses.

Staphylococcus. Sometimes pathogens pass through the intact epidermis via the hair follicle. The most common and nowadays potentially dangerous microbes of this character are the staphylococci, particularly *Staphylococcus aureus* (Fig. 8-3). An increasing number of strains of this species are becoming resistant to penicillin and other antibiotic agents. Staphylococci are common causes of pimples, sties, furuncles (boils), carbuncles, abscesses, and paronychia. Characteristically, these infections are marked by considerable pus formation, a hallmark of the staphylococci. At present there is no satisfactory vaccine against staphylococcal infections, but the chemist continues to plod away in the search for new and better antibiotics.

Streptococcus. Another invader of significance is *Streptococcus pyogenes* (Fig. 8-4), commonly referred to as "beta hemolytic strep" or "streptococcus hemolyticus." Among other infections, this pathogen causes cellulitis, erysipelas, septic sore throat, and scarlet fever. The latter dis-

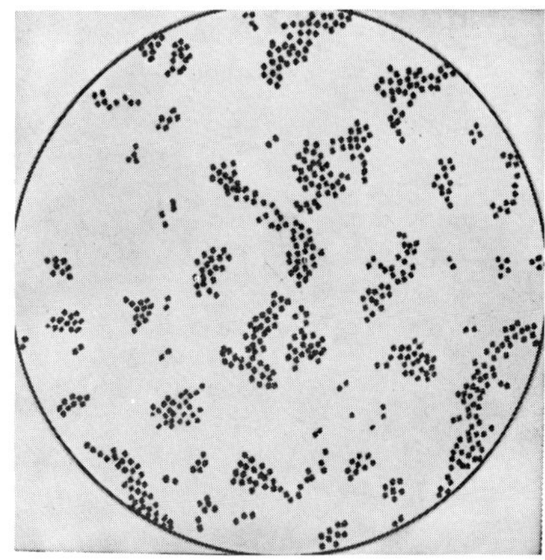

Fig. 8-3. *Staphylococcus aureus.* (From Smith, A. L.: Principles of microbiology, ed. 6, St. Louis, 1969, The C. V. Mosby Co.)

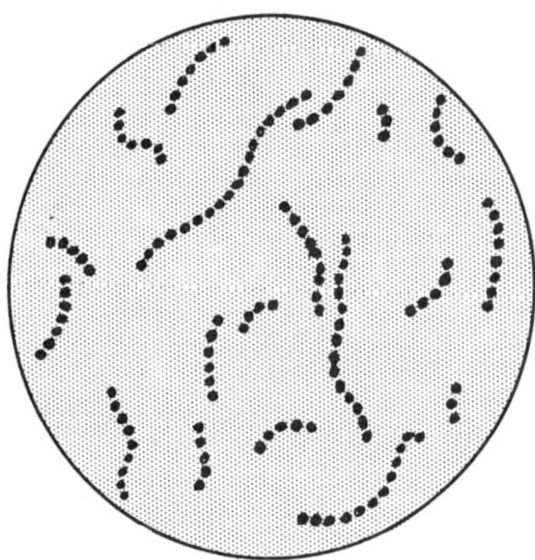

Fig. 8-4. *Streptococcus pyogenes.*

ease, characterized by a red rash and fever, is caused by the exotoxin. Since several conditions mimic scarlet fever, the Schultz-Charlton test is often used to establish a definitive diagnosis. In this test a "skin dose" of scarlet fever *antitoxin* is injected intradermally into an area of the rash, and if blanching occurs (as a result of neutralization of the toxin by the antitoxin), the diagnosis is positive.

Scarlet fever is successfully treated with penicillin. Patients should be isolated, and exposed susceptible persons should be given the drug for 3 to 5 days. Mass active immunization against the disease is not recommended, principally because scarlet fever has lost much of its former virulence.

An attack of scarlet fever engenders active immunity against the toxin, and immune persons react negatively to the *Dick test,* which is performed by injecting a very small amount of scarlet fever toxin intradermally into the forearm. In *susceptible* persons a "reaction" (red area) occurs within 24 hours at the site of the injection.

Pseudomonas aeruginosa. This bacterium is a motile, gram-negative, nonsporeforming bacillus often present in the intestinal tract, in sewage, and in polluted water. Though it does not incite a specific infection, the organism proves a troublesome secondary invader and commonly is responsible for abscesses, otitis media (middle ear infection), and infected wounds and burns. (Its involvement in urinary tract infections is discussed in Chapter 17.) Characteristically, *Pseudomonas aeruginosa* releases a *bluish green pigment* that tinges the pus of the infection. In regard to treatment, the antibiotics of choice are polymyxin B and colistin.

Other bacterial pathogens. Other bacterial pathogens of note associated with the skin include *Bacillus anthracis* (anthrax), *Pasteurella pestis* (plague), *Pasteurella tularensis* (tularemia or rabbit fever), *Actinobacillus mallei* (glanders), *Spirillum minus* (rate-bite fever), *Treponema pertenue* (yaws or frambesia), and *Mycobacterium leprae* (leprosy).

Smallpox. With a mortality rate between 10 and 30 percent, smallpox, or *variola,* is one of the most vicious viral infections. The malady is characterized by a disfiguring vesicular eruption that becomes pustular and finally crusty, leaving the well-known pockmarks. The virus is spread from man to man by direct contact, and it is spread indirectly via nasopharyngeal secretions and fomites. Smallpox is diagnosed on the basis of clinical appearance and the finding of inclusion bodies *(Guarnieri's bodies)* in the epithelial cells.

Since the infection always runs its course, it is highly significant that we possess a valuable vaccine for active immunization. The vaccine, a preparation containing so-called *vaccinia* virus* (Fig. 8-5), is usually applied to the outer aspect of the upper arm. In persons who have never been vaccinated or who have never had smallpox, an ugly vesicle develops at the site of vaccination (Fig. 8-6). This is an actual attack of *vaccinia,* and the body responds by elaborating antibodies—antibodies that are effective not only against vaccinia but also against smallpox. Immune

*An attenuated virus related *antigenically* to the viruses of variola and cowpox. Its origin is not known.

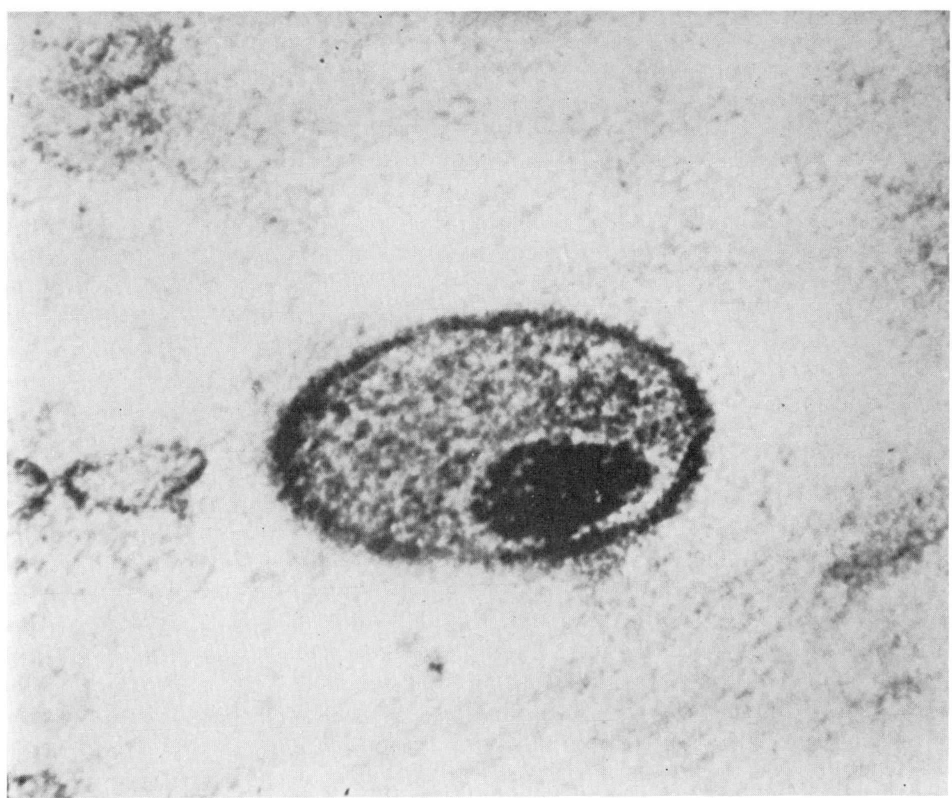

Fig. 8-5. Vaccinia virus. (×180,000.) (Courtesy Eli Lilly & Co.)

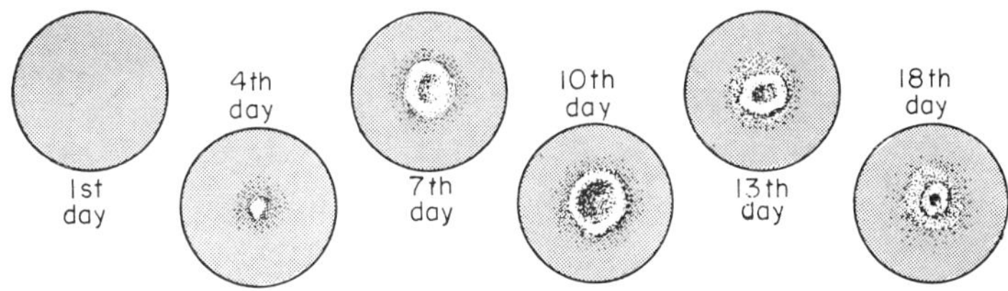

Fig. 8-6. Smallpox vaccination. (From Brooks, S. M.: Basic facts of medical microbiology, ed. 2, Philadelphia, 1962, W. B. Saunders Co.)

persons (that is, those previously vaccinated or those who have had the disease) develop only a red wheal. The absence of any reaction at the site of the vaccination almost always means an impotent vaccine.

Other prophylactic measures against smallpox include isolation of patients, concurrent and terminal disinfection, and quarantine. Treatment with methisazone, a new drug, may be of some value in prevention of the disease in exposed persons.

Measles. Measles, or *rubeola,* is a highly contagious viral disease characterized by skin rash, fever, and acute catarrhal inflammation of the eyes and respiratory passageways. The virus spreads easily through the air, particularly during the 3 or 4 days preceding eruption of the rash. Contagiousness ceases when the fever drops, and an attack usually provokes permanent immunity. Diagnosis is based upon clinical findings, especially the presence of small white areas inside the mouth called *Koplik's spots.*

Although measles is generally without serious consequence, one must be on guard against such secondary infections as pneumonia, mastoiditis, and otitis media. Should any of these complications occur, antibiotic therapy is indicated. Otherwise, the treatment is symptomatic. Active immunization against measles has been extensively investigated, and workable vaccines are now available. The attenuated or "live" vaccine is now generally considered the preparation of choice. According to recent reports, the disease in time may be completely eradicated.

Passive immunization with gamma globulin (Chapter 12) has been successfully used to treat persons with severe cases and to protect susceptible persons with low resistance.

German measles. German measles, or *rubella,* is a highly contagious but mild viral infection marked by a rash and swollen lymph nodes. Usually no treatment is necessary, and an attack almost always produces lasting immunity.

Because the virus causes congenital malformations (for example, cataract, microcephaly, deafness, and cardiac defects), *pregnant* women should avoid all contact with persons who have German measles. This is, indeed, the most important and serious aspect of the disease. A promising "live" vaccine is now about to go into general use.

Chickenpox. Chickenpox, or *varicella,* is a dermotropic viral infection characterized by fever and the appearance of vesicles after an incubation period of 1 to 3 weeks. The infection is generally mild, and an attack produces lasting immunity. There are no specific therapeutic or prophylactic measures.

Herpes zoster. Herpes zoster, commonly called *shingles,* is an acute, painful vesicular dermatitis. Since the virus follows the nerve trunks, the location and distribution of the lesions depend upon the particular nerves affected. An attack ordinarily confers lasting immunity. The treatment is symptomatic. At present nothing can be done to prevent herpes zoster.

Interestingly, both shingles and chickenpox are now known to be caused by the *same* virus. There is considerable difference of opinion among authorities as to the mechanism and explanation behind this rather strange situation, but the general feeling seems to be that the first invasion of the body by the so-called VZ (varicella-zoster) virus results in chickenpox, whereas shingles results from either the reinvasion or the activation of a latent virus. Support for this view stems from the fact that patients with shingles can produce no history of prior contact with an external source of the AZ virus and from the fact that certain stimuli and conditions are known to trigger a case of the infection—injury, drugs, leukemia, and hormones, for example.

Herpes simplex. Herpes simplex is an acute vesicular eruption of the skin and mucous membranes caused by a virus similar to the VZ virus (Fig. 8-7). Characteristically, the vesicles are soft and filled with a watery fluid. Although all areas are subject to attack, the most common site is the lips (the *cold sore*). Virulent strains of the virus have been known to turn neurotropic and attack the brain. There is no lasting immunity, and nothing specific can be done in the way of treatment.

Warts. Warts, or *verrucae,* are small benign skin tumors caused by a virus. Generally, they can be successfully removed by surgery or chemical treatment.

Rickettsial infections. Rickettsiae (p. 129) cause infections characterized by fever and a rash. The principal diseases include typhus fever (*endemic* and *epidemic*), rickettsialpox, and Rocky Mountain spotted fever (Fig. 8-8), the latter being the main

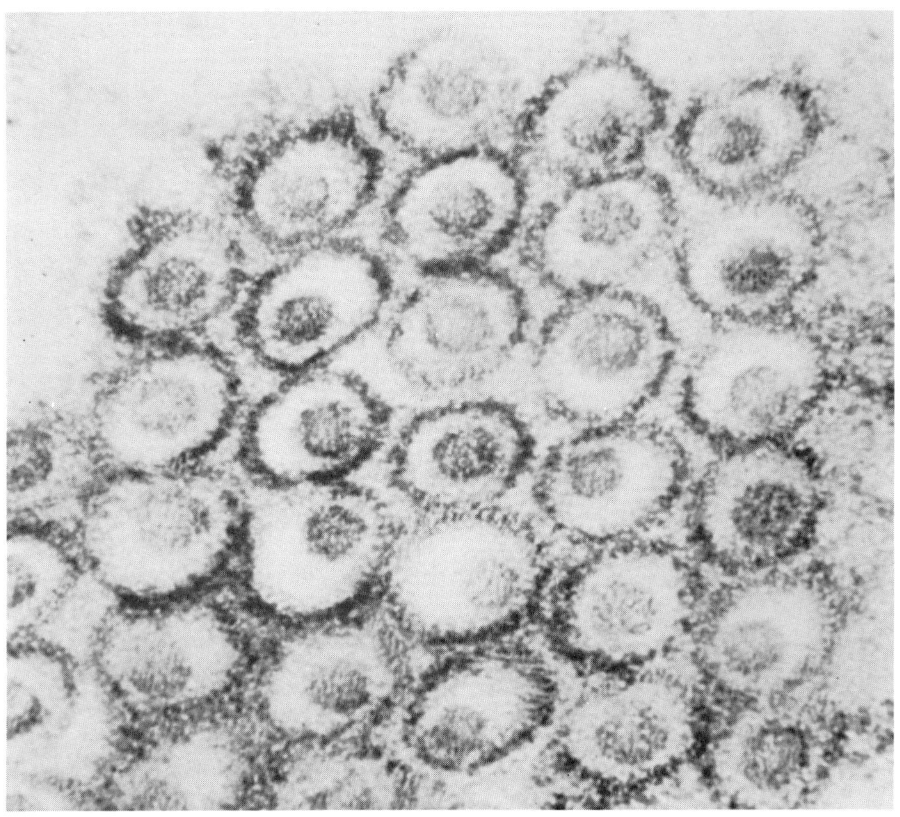

Fig. 8-7. Intranuclear crystal of the herpes simplex virus. (×90,000.) (Courtesy Eli Lilly & Co.)

rickettsial infection in this country. Diagnosis of these diseases is based on clinical findings, the demonstration of agglutinins in the blood via the Weil-Felix test, and complement-fixation tests. Therapeutically, the broad-spectrum antibiotics usually yield excellent results.

Fungal infections. An infection of the skin, hair, and nails caused by a pathogenic fungus (Fig. 8-9) is referred to as *dermatomycosis.* The typical skin lesion is characterized by the formation of ring-shaped, pigmented patches *(ringworm)* covered with vesicles or scales. Infected nails and hair, unless treated early, are ultimately destroyed. These changes are brought about by the mycelial filaments gradually creeping through the epidermal layers. The more

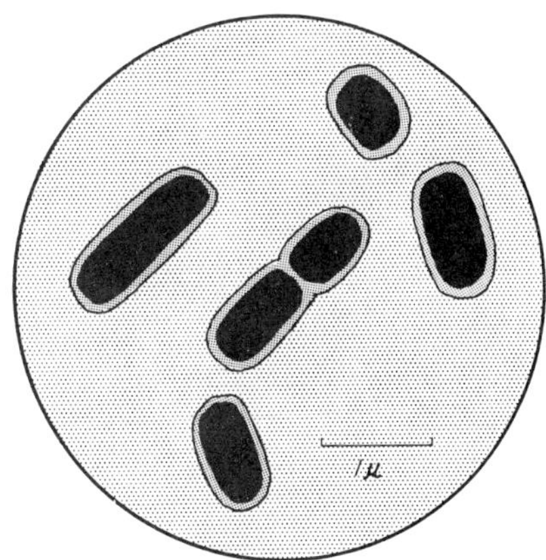

Fig. 8-8. *Rickettsia rickettsii,* the causative agent of Rocky Mountain spotted fever. (From Brooks, S. M.: Basic facts of medical microbiology, ed. 2, Philadelphia, 1962, W. B. Saunders Co.)

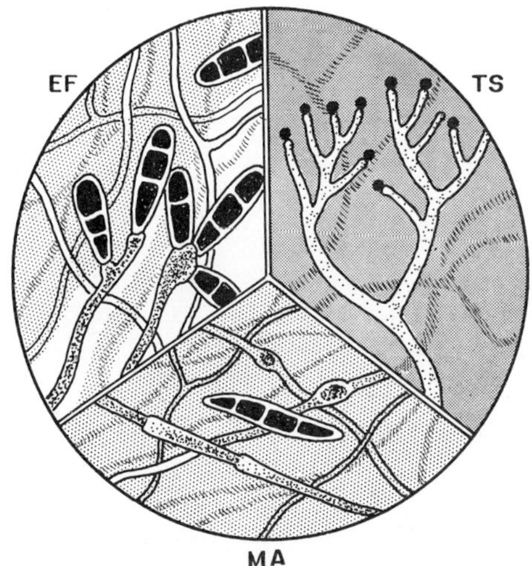

Fig. 8-9. Drawings from micrographs showing three species of dermatophytes (pathogenic fungi that attack the skin): *Epidermophyton floccosum,* **EF**; *Trichophyton shoenleini,* **TS**; *Microsporum audouini,* **MA.**

common dermatomycoses (named according to the affected area) include *tinea pedis* (athlete's foot), *tinea unguium* (fingernails or toenails), *tinea cruris* (groin), *tinea capitis* (scalp), *tinea corporis* (limbs or trunk), and *tinea barbae* (face and neck).

Until rather recently, the treatment of the dermatomycoses was not always satisfactory. The daily application of fungicidal powders, lotions, and ointments in many instances had to be continued for an extended period of time, often without a "sure cure." Now the antifungal antibiotic griseofulvin (Fulvicin; Grifulvin), available in tablet form, promises to drastically change the outlook in this medical area, complete cures having been effected in long-standing cases resistant to other modes of therapy.

Ectoparasites. Although not generally a threat to life, ectoparasites (p. 137) incite uncomfortable and troublesome infestations, often accompanied by secondary bacterial infections. Too, some species are vectors of viral and bacterial infections. The principal invaders include the itch mite (*Sarcoptes scabiei*), the chigger (*Trombicula irritans*), the head louse (*Pediculus humanus* var. *capitis*), the body louse (*Pediculus humanus* var. *corporis*), the crab louse (*Phthirus pubis*), and the human flea (*Pulex irritans*).

The itch mite and the chigger burrow into the skin, the flea and the body louse inhabit the surface of the skin, and the head louse and the crab louse infest the hair. Application of gamma benzene hexachloride (Gexane; Kwell) is the treatment of choice for scabies, and DDT preparations are used to destroy lice and fleas.

Noninfectious disorders. A great many skin conditions are caused by forces other than pathogenic microbes. For the most part, however, the etiology of these noninfectious dermatoses is poorly understood, and treatment necessarily falls short of the mark. Some of the more common and important conditions are briefly described here.

Allergy. When an antigen-antibody reaction takes place within the tissues themselves, the result is frequently an allergy. Locally, the cells may be injured or destroyed, and systemically, the body may suffer the ill effects of such breakdown products (released from the cells) as heparin, leukotaxine, and histamine, particularly the latter. An allergic reaction may be of any degree, ranging from a runny nose to a fatal anaphylactic shock.

As currently understood, an allergy results from weak immunity. That is, whereas microbial antigens stimulate such a high concentration of antibody that the antigens are destroyed or neutralized in the blood *before* they have a chance to penetrate the tissues, the antigens of allergy (called *allergens**) provoke so few antibodies (called *reagins*) that they escape such destruction in the bloodstream and enter the cells

*Almost any substance is a potential allergen. The most common, however, are certain foods (for example, milk, eggs, and strawberries), pollens, dander, and drugs.

where, as indicated, they cause trouble.

At present no one knows for certain why some persons are more susceptible to allergy than are others. One explanation, though, that seems to account for a good many facts is that some individuals, because of their peculiar genetic makeup, possess cells that are easily damaged by cellular allergen-reagin reactions. But this does not mean that all the tissues contain such cells, for an allergy is generally confined to localized areas such as the mucous membranes of the nose and eyes. Moreover, some allergic persons always develop a rash in exactly the same place, perhaps just the place where the cells are most susceptible to the reaction.

Until more is known about allergy, or hypersensitivity, the chief control of the condition will continue to center about the use of desensitization and antihistamines.

Allergic dermatitis, or allergic eczema, is the term applied to any inflammation of the skin caused by an allergy. The allergen may come from without or from within. In the former case the skin comes in contact with such substances as sensitizing chemicals or poison ivy, and in the latter, certain foods, dust, pollen, molds, and drugs are the culprits. Why certain persons are more sensitive than others is still a moot question.

The treatment of an allergic dematitis involves removal of the cause (elimination of strawberries or other food from the diet and avoidance of such allergenic agents as poison ivy), desensitization, and administration of antihistamines or corticosteroids.

Actinic dermatitis. Actinic dermatitis is an inflammatory condition of the skin caused by overexposure to ultraviolet radiation. Although this condition usually results from staying too long in the sun, one not infrequently encounters the hapless person who fell asleep under a sunlamp. Since sunburn, natural or artificial, can be extremely dangerous, one should always be on guard against it. This is especially true on cloudy summer days when large doses of ultraviolet rays, in contrast to visible light, filter through the atmosphere.

Psoriasis. Psoriasis, a dermatosis of many varieties, is marked by scaly red patches on the exterior surfaces. The cause is not known, and treatment is usually unsatisfactory.

Lupus erythematosus. Lupus erythematosus is a skin condition characterized by disklike patches with raised red edges and depressed centers. These are covered with scales that eventually fall off, leaving a white scar.

Disseminated lupus erythematosus is a more serious dermatosis with systemic repercussions. Indeed, it is often fatal, even when treated. The cause is unknown. At present the only treatment of significant value is periodic administration of corticosteroids (p. 414).

Pemphigus. Pemphigus, like disseminated lupus erythematosus, involves the general health of the patient and often proves fatal. The dermal features are characterized by successive crops of large blisters which, following absorption, leave deeply pigmented spots. These lesions often burn and itch. The cause is not known, and the only treatment of established value centers about the use of corticosteroids.

Scleroderma. In the frequently incurable dermatosis known as scleroderma, the skin becomes thick, hard, and rigid and is covered with pigmented patches. The cause is unknown. Once again, corticosteroids afford at present the principal avenue of hope.

Burns. A severe burn is a medical emergency of the first order, for destruction of the skin in this fashion causes shock, dehydration, electrolyte imbalance, renal damage, and unbelievable agony. Although burns covering less than 50 percent of the body are not generally considered fatal today, those involving larger areas afford a poor prognosis in many instances.

Obviously, treatment must be multidimensional. Analgesics to relieve pain, antibiotics to fight infection, and plasma and electrolyte solutions to replace lost fluid are all indicated. The correction of water and electrolyte imbalances may spell the difference between life and death, but the physician must exercise great care in giving just enough fluid to meet the need; too much will overload the circulation and lead to complications. One way to estimate the fluid requirement is by the following formula:

$$2 \times \text{Body weight (kg.)} \times \text{Percent of burn} + 2000 = \text{Cubic centimeters of fluid}$$

The percent of burn is obtained by the *rule of nines;* head, 9 percent (of body

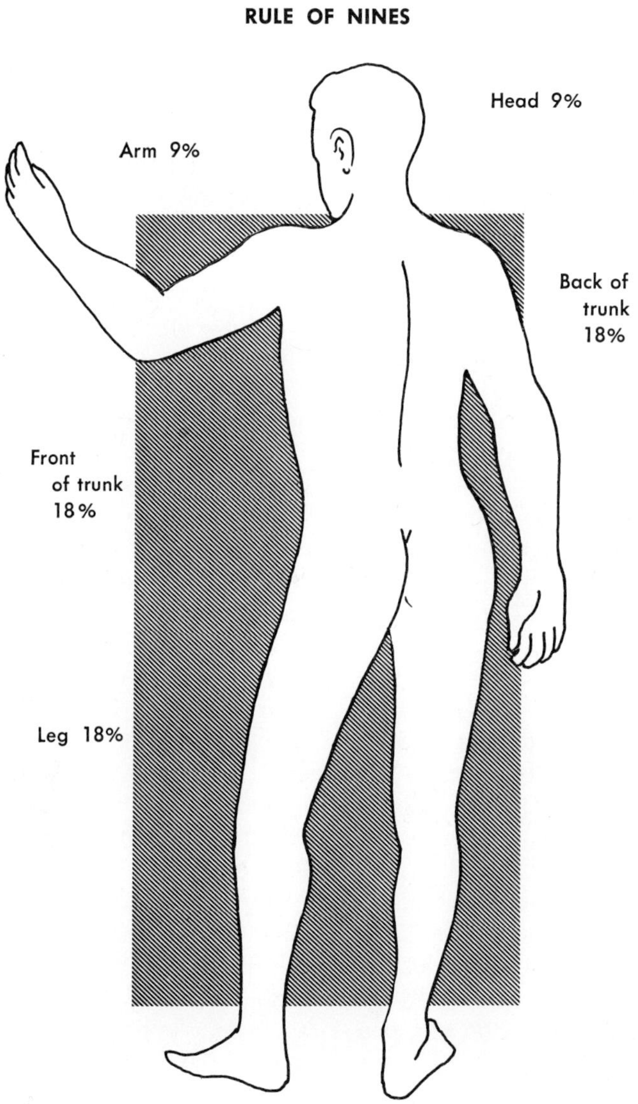

RULE OF NINES

Head 9%

Arm 9%

Back of trunk 18%

Front of trunk 18%

Leg 18%

Fig. 8-10. Surface areas of different parts of the body. (From Brooks, S. M.: The sea inside us, New York, 1968, Meredith Press.)

area); arm, 9 percent; leg, 18 percent; front of body, 18 percent; and back of body, 18 percent (Fig. 8-10).

The calculated volume represents the total volume of fluid (in the form of plasma, electrolyte solutions, and carbohydrate) to be given in the first 24 hours.

Questions

1. Describe in detail the structure of the epidermis.
2. Describe in detail the structure of the dermis.
3. Describe the composition of the subcutaneous tissue.
4. What makes some areas of the body darker than others?
5. Explain the fingerprint?
6. What is the principal change in skin as we grow older?
7. Describe the anatomy of the hair and its associated structures.
8. State the function of the sudoriferous glands.
9. Severe burns over a large area of the body may result in kidney damage. Explain.
10. What is cerumen?
11. Why are some areas of the body more sensitive than others?
12. What is the chief difference between the skin on the face and that on the sole of the foot?
13. Distinguish between skin and fascia.
14. Pimples, boils, and abscesses usually have a "common denominator." Explain.
15. A boil on the face is especially dangerous. Explain.
16. Explain the results of the Schultz-Charlton and Dick tests.
17. What is the morphologic difference between staphylococci and streptococci?
18. Discuss the prophylaxis of variọla.
19. Discuss the diagnosis, treatment, and prophylaxis of rubeola.
20. How does the physician distinguish between rubella and rubeola?
21. Discuss the diagnosis and treatment of the rickettsial infections.
22. What is ringworm?
23. What is an allergen?
24. Is it fair to say that most noninfectious diseases of the skin are of poorly understood etiology? Explain.
25. Discuss the injury and treatment of a severe burn.
26. Give the etiology, pathology (signs and symptoms), laboratory diagnosis, treatment, and prophylaxis for anthrax, plague, tularemia, glanders, and yaws.
27. Discuss in detail the mechanism of action of skin tests and desensitization in the management of allergies.
28. What is the association between shingles and chickenpox?

Chapter 9

The skeletal system

Without its skeleton the body would be a stationary bowl of jelly without the bowl. In short, the skeleton supports, protects, and permits positioning and movement of the body. Further, it produces the cellular elements of the blood and stores and releases calcium.

TYPES OF BONES

The 206 bones of the body are classified according to their shape into four categories: (1) long bones (for example, humerus and femur), (2) short bones (for example, carpals and tarsals), (3) flat bones (for example, parietal and sternum), and (4) irregular bones (for example, vertebrae and ethmoid).

BONE MARKINGS

Learning the name and position of a given bone is only the beginning. Bones have characteristic markings (determined by location and function), and it behooves the student of anatomy to know the major depressions, openings, and projections (or processes) of each. To this end, the following terms should be committed to memory:

condyle a rounded knob at the end of a bone.
crest generally, a ridge running along the surface of a bone.
foramen (pl., **foramina**) a hole.
fossa (pl., **fossae**) a depression or hollow.
head applied to the skeleton, a rounded process at the end of a bone by which it articulates with another bone.
meatus a passageway or tunnel into the interior.
sinus a cavity or space within a given structure.
spine, spinous process a slender, pointed projection of a bone. (The spinal column, or "spine," derives its name from the fact that the majority of the vertebrae possess prominent spinous processes.)
tubercle an expression commonly used in anatomy to describe a small nodule or eminence.
tuberosity a large, broad process of a bone.

BONE STRUCTURE

Bone is composed of about two-thirds inorganic matter and one-third organic matter. The former, present chiefly as mineral crystals of *hydroxyapatite,* occurs in the matrix along with a tough protein. The organic matter comprises principally the bone cells and blood vessels. The manner in which the cells lay down the matrix determines whether bone is *compact* or *cancellous.* Compact or hard bone looks and feels a good deal like ivory. Cancellous or *spongy* bone, on the other hand, is light and porous. Compact bone constitutes the shafts of long bones and the outsides of flat bones. The ends of long bones and the insides of most flat and irregular bones consist of spongy bone. (The spongy bone of the cranial bones is commonly called the *diploe.*)

The histologic features of bone were presented earlier (p. 169). For the gross architecture the student will do well to consider a typical long bone (Fig. 9-1). As stated previously, the shaft, or *diaphysis,* is composed of hard bone, and the ends, or *epiphyses,* consist of spongy bone. Since the epiphyses meet other bones at the joints, they are covered with hyaline or articular cartilage.

Except at its cartilaginous extremities, a long bone is covered with a tough membrane called the *periosteum.* If this membrane is carefully stripped from a fresh bone, tiny beads of blood appear on the surface. These beads represent the entrance of Volkmann's canals, microscopic channels that carry blood from the periosteum to the *haversian canals.* From the latter, tissue fluid makes its way to the bone cells in the lacunae via the canaliculi (p. 169). Thus, the periosteum and the *haversian system* serve to keep bone "alive."

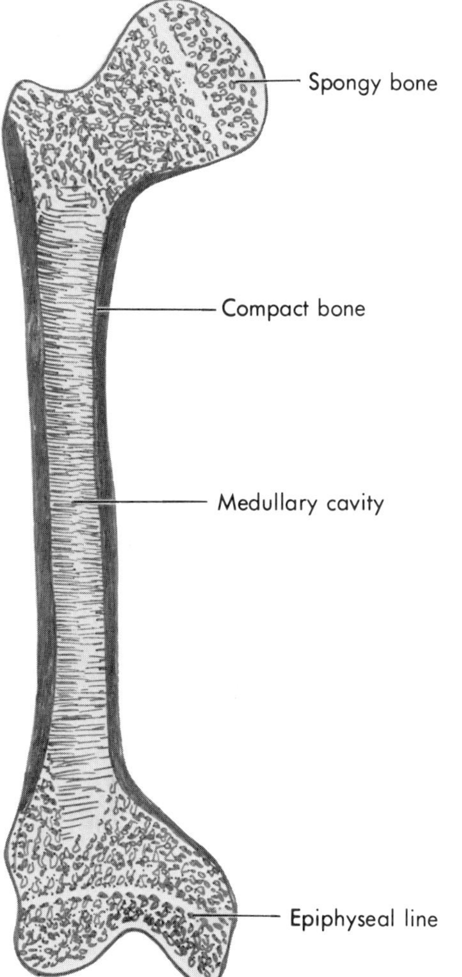

Fig. 9-1. Diagrammatic longitudinal view of a typical long bone.

Marrow. Running through the diaphysis is the central or *medullary* cavity (or canal), which is lined with a vascular tissue, the *endosteum,* and filled with a soft, fatty, yellowish substance called *yellow* marrow.

Red marrow. Red marrow is found at the ends of long bones and throughout the cancellous tissue of flat and irregular bones, particularly of the skull, vertebrae, ribs, sternum, and ilia. In contrast to the yellow variety, red marrow contains little fat and an abundance of so-called marrow cells—*erythroblasts, myeloblasts,* and *megakaryoblasts.* The erythroblasts, by undergoing a series of transformations, mature into erythrocytes, or red cells. In a like manner, the myeloblasts develop into the granular leukocytes (Chapter 12). The megakaryoblasts, or gaint cells, split up and become the blood platelets. Thus, red marrow, particularly that located in the vertebrae and sternum, is the principal tissue engaged in *hemopoiesis.*

OSSIFICATION

The growth from the miniature skeleton of the embryo to the full-sized skeleton of the adult takes about 25 years—a long, tedious, and complex process. Actually, the "bones" of the embryo are not real bones; they are skeletal structures composed of hyaline cartilage or fibrous membranes. As growth continues, the membranes become the flat bones (*intramembranous ossification*), and the cartilage becomes the long bones (*endochondral ossification*). The soft spots, or fontanelles, of the infant's head are fibrous membranes that have not yet undergone ossification.

The ossification of a long bone starts in the diaphysis and both epiphyses and progresses in all directions. The term *epiphyseal cartilage* is applied to the cartilage between the diaphysis and the epiphyses. As long as this cartilage remains (and its presence can be established via x-ray examination), a bone continues to grow in length. When the cartilage finally disappears, the remaining external line of juncture between the epiphyses and the diaphysis is referred to as the *epiphyseal line* (Fig. 9-1).

Osteoblasts and osteoclasts. Histologically and chemically, ossification means the deposition of a bony matrix, a process accomplished through the uncanny activities of the *osteoblasts,* the bone cells located in the lacunae and beneath the periosteum. First, these cells secrete a protein substance that forms a tough but not as yet bony matrix. Second, in this proteinaceous base they bring about the deposition of calcium salts, producing the marblelike apatite referred to earlier. This latter step is carried out largely through the agency of the osteoblastic enzyme alkaline phosphatase. By splitting the phosphate radical ($PO_4^{\equiv}$) away from organic phosphates, the enzyme effects the synthesis of Ca^{++}, $CO_3^{=}$, and $PO_4^{\equiv}$ into apatite.

Bone is continually being torn down as well as being built up, for if bone did not have some way of dissolving itself on the inside, the skeleton would become solid rock, squeezing out the marrow and life itself. But there is another reason for the dissolution of bone, and that is to supply calcium (Ca^{++}) to the extracellular fluids when the concentration of that ion drops below the normal value (10 mg.%).

The dissolution of bone is effected by multinucleated giant bone cells called *osteoclasts.* These cells, located in almost all the cavities of bone, secrete an enzyme that digests the protein matrix, thereby releasing Ca^{++} and $PO_4^{\equiv}$ into the blood.

Effect of stress. Obviously, osteoblastic and osteoclastic activity must remain in balance if the body is to maintain a healthy skeleton, and it is of interest to note that stress causes the osteoblasts to become more active. This helps to explain why the femur—a bone subjected to great pressure and bending—is so thick and strong.

Paradoxically, but fortunately, crooked leg bones tend to straighten out over the years; for example, pressure along the inner curvature and stretching along the outer curvature stimulate the osteoblasts and osteoclasts, respectively. As a result, the inner curvature becomes filled with bone, whereas the outer curvature loses bone.

Another powerful stimulant of osteoblastic activity is a break in bone. The injured osteoblasts in the vicinity of the break become very active and multiply in all directions, making protein and alkaline phosphatase available for ossification. This accounts for the rapid repair of a broken bone, particularly in the youngster.

Regulating factors. As indicated, the formation, growth, and repair of bone involve several factors, especially calcium, phosphorus, hormones and vitamins.

Vitamin D. At least 99 percent of the calcium of the body (estimated to be about 3½ pounds in an adult) is deposited in the skeleton. The major physiologic forces directing this deposition are vitamin D and alkaline phosphatase. Vitamin D accelerates the absorption of calcium and phosphate from the gastrointestinal tract. Though of much less importance than vitamin D, vitamin A also plays a role in mineralization of the skeleton (Chapter 16).

Parathyroid hormone. The parathyroid hormone, or *parathormone,* released by the parathyroid glands (Chapter 22), helps to regulate the concentration of ionic calcium in the extracellular fluids by increasing both the number and size of the osteoclasts, thereby stimulating the release of Ca^{++}. The parathyroids are triggered to secrete the hormone when the concentration falls below normal values. A severe deficiency of calcium or vitamin D, for instance, will stimulate the glands and bring about the release of Ca^{++} and $PO_4\equiv$ from the bony matrix. Since a drop in the ionic concentration of calcium causes embarrassment to the tissues, particularly to the heart and muscles (Chapter 10), the hormone plays a vital physiologic role.

ARTICULATIONS

The place of junction between two or more bones is called a joint, or articulation. The articulating surfaces may be separated by a thin membrane, by strong pads of connective tissue, or in the freely moving joints, by fluid. Joints are perhaps best classified according to the degree and variety of movement.

Synarthroses. In the synarthrotic type of joint there is close contact between the two adjacent bones; there is no joint cavity and there is no movement.

Sutures. Sutures are the synarthrotic articulations of the skull (p. 196) characterized by the presence of a thin layer of fibrous tissue uniting the margins of the contiguous bone.

Synchondroses. A synchondrosis is a synarthrosis in which the union of two bones is effected by hyaline cartilage. Synchondroses are found in growing bones between the diaphysis and the epiphysis. With the cessation of growth, this type of joint disappears.

Amphiarthroses. In the amphiarthrotic type of articulation there is limited movement. The union is effected by fibrocartilage and the joint is enveloped by ligaments. There may be a joint cavity. Amphiarthroses include the joints between the bodies of the vertebrate, the joints between the sacrum and ilium, and the joint between the two pubic bones.

Diarthroses. Diarthrotic joints permit variable degrees of movement. At a typical diarthrosis, the articulating surfaces are covered with hyaline cartilage, and the entire joint is invested by a ligament. Characteristically, there is a joint cavity lined by a synovial membrane and filled with synovial fluid (Fig. 9-2). As a matter of fact, we often refer to a diarthrosis as a synovial joint.

Diarthroses are subdivided according to degree of movement. The major types will be described briefly.

Gliding joints. In the gliding type of articulation one bone moves or glides across another. The joints between the carpals and tarsals are examples.

Pivot joints. The pivot joint is characterized by movement in the long axis of a bone. The best example is the articulation between the radius and the ulna.

Biaxial joints. A diarthrosis that permits movement in two planes at right angles to each other is called a biaxial joint. The wrist and the saddle joint at the base of the thumb are good examples.

Hinge joints. The articulation at the elbows and knees are typical diarthrotic hinge joints.

Ball-and-socket joints. The ball-and-socket type of diarthrosis permits full free-

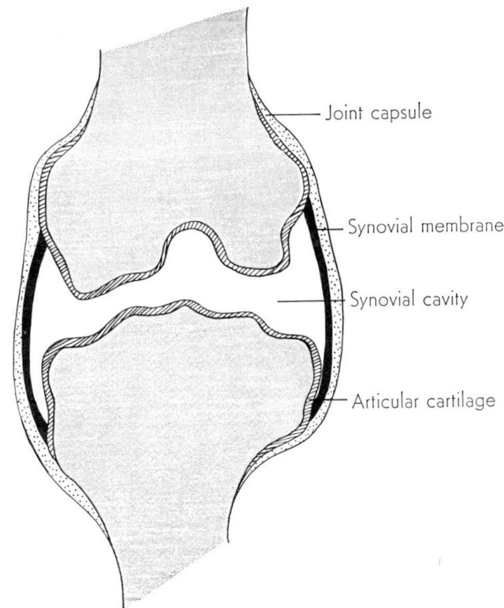

Fig. 9-2. Diagram of a typical diarthrosis.

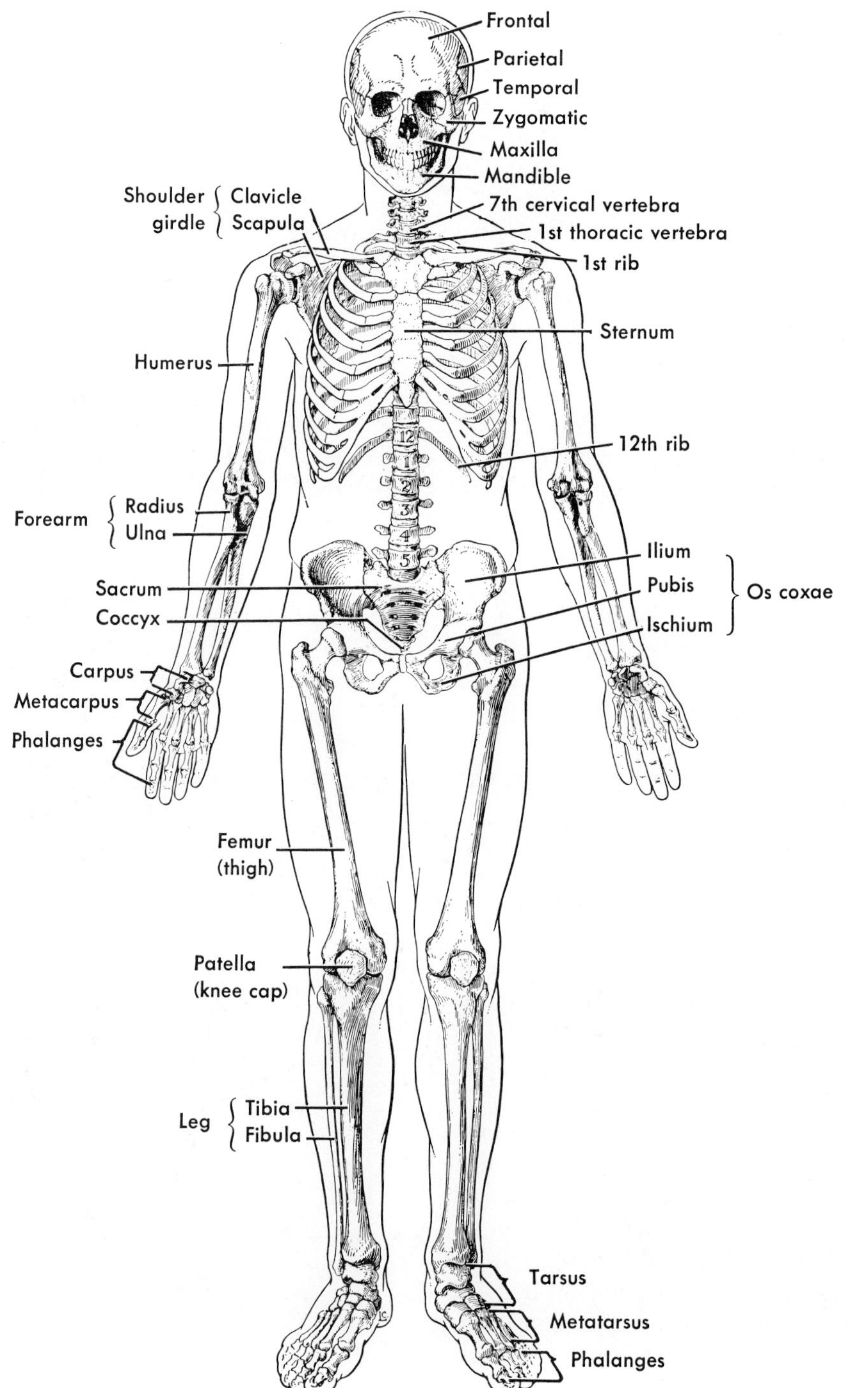

Fig. 9-3. Anterior view of the human skeleton. (After King and Showers; from Dorland's Illustrated Medical Dictionary, ed. 24, Philadelphia, 1965, W. B. Saunders Co.)

dom of movement. The hip and shoulder joints are the best examples.

Diarthrotic movement. The various possible movements at the diarthroses are given special names:

flexion decreasing the angle of a joint.
extension increasing the angle of a joint.
abduction drawing a part away from the midsagittal plane.
adduction drawing a part toward the midsagittal plane.
circumduction circular movement of a limb at a ball-and-socket joint.
rotation movement at a pivot joint.
gliding movement at a gliding joint.

AXIAL SKELETON

There are two main divisions of the skeleton (Fig. 9-3): (1) the *axial,* including the bones of the head, neck, and trunk, and (2) the *appendicular,* including the bones of the extremities. The salient features of the axial skeleton will be discussed first.

Skull. The skull consists of twenty-two irregularly shaped bones, excluding the ossicles of the ear (Table 9-1). The two divisions of the skull are the cranium and the face.

Cranium. The cranium houses the brain. Its roof (Fig. 9-4) is formed by the *frontal, parietal,* and *occipital* bones and its sides by the *temporal* bone and the great wings of the *sphenoid* (Fig. 9-5). These same bones, plus the tiny cribriform plate of the ethmoid bone, also form the floor (Fig. 9-6).

The outstanding surface features of the cranium are the foramen magnum, sutures, auditory meatus, and mastoid, styloid, and zygomatic processes. Inside the skull, looking down at the floor, the chief points of interest include a number of small foramina for nerves and blood vessels, the *sella turcica* (saddle-shaped depression in the sphenoid bone), and the crista galli (a tiny process of the ethmoid). The large opening in the occipital floor—the *foramen*

Table 9-1. Bones*

Bone	Single	Paired
Skull		
Cranium		
Frontal	1	
Parietal		2
Occipital	1	
Temporal		2
Sphenoid	1	
Ethmoid	1	
Face		
Nasal		2
Lacrimal		2
Maxilla		2
Inferior nasal concha		2
Zygoma		2
Palatine		2
Vomer	1	
Mandible	1	
Vertebrae		
Cervical	7	
Thoracic	12	
Lumbar	5	
Sacrum (5 fused)	1	
Coccyx (4 fused)	1	
Thorax		
Ribs		24
Sternum	1	
Upper extremity		
Clavicle		2
Scapula		2
Humerus		2
Radius		2
Ulna		2
Carpus		16
Metacarpus		10
Phalanges of hand		28
Lower extremity		
Hip (3 fused)		2
Femur		2
Patella		2
Tibia		2
Fibula		2
Tarsus		14
Metatarsus		10
Phalanges of foot		28
Miscellaneous		
Ossicles of the ear (3 in each)		6
Hyoid	1	
Total		206

*Adapted from Francis, C. C.: Introduction to human anatomy, ed. 5, St. Louis, 1968, The C. V. Mosby Co.

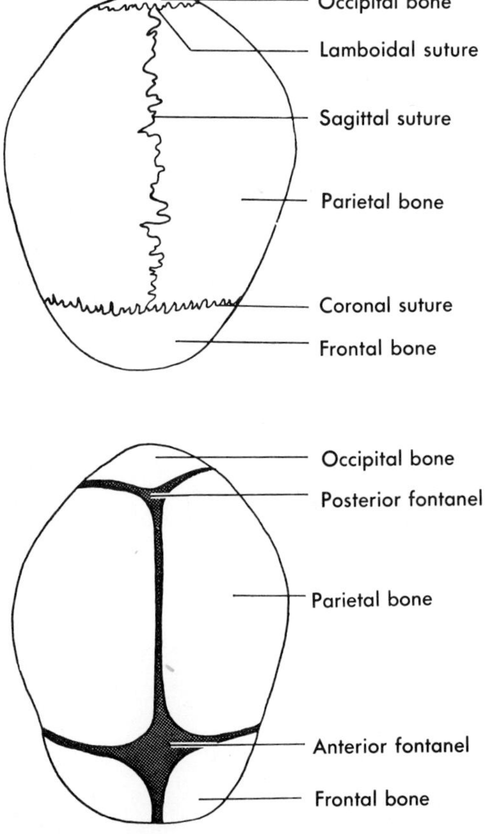

Fig. 9-4. Skull, top view. Upper drawing, adult skull. Lower drawing, fetal skull.

magnum—permits the spinal cord to join the brain.

Face. Although the face is said to be made up of fourteen bones, the frontal and ethmoid bones of the cranium are really needed to fill out the complete framework.

Like the batlike sphenoid of the cranium, the maxillae serve as the keystones of the face. All bones except the mandible articulate with these two bones. They join together at the midline, forming part of the *orbits,* part of the *hard palate,* and part of the floor and sidewalls of the nose. In contrast to the two bones of the upper jaw (the *maxillae*), the lower jaw consists of a single bone—the *mandible.* This is the largest, strongest, and most powerful bone of the face. The sockets (*alveoli*) of the maxillae and mandible, which hold the teeth, constitute the so-called *alveolar processes* of these bones.

The cheek is formed by the centrally located zygomatic (*malar*) bone, which articulates with the maxilla of the face and with the temporal, frontal, and sphenoid bones of the cranium.

The bony roof of the mouth, or *hard palate,* is formed anteriorly by the pro-

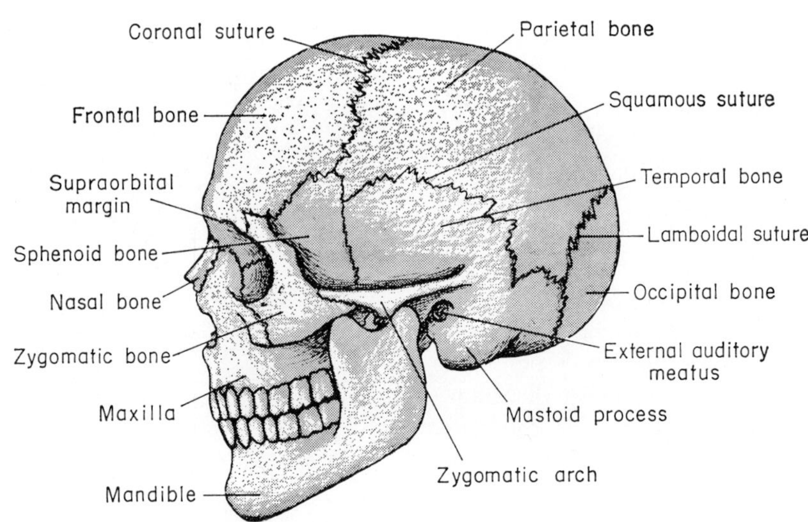

Fig. 9-5. Skull, side view. (Styloid process not shown.)

cesses of the *maxillae* and posteriorly by the two *palatine* bones. These bones are fused together so tightly that the hard palate sometimes looks like a single structure.

The remaining bones of the face—the *nasal, lacrimal, inferior conchae,* and *vomer* —help to form the nose. The key nasal bone, however, is the *ethmoid,* a cranial bone. This delicate and highly irregular bone forms the upper septum, the sidewalls, and part of the roof of the nose. The vomer, which arises perpendicularly along the midline of the hard palate, meets the *perpendicular plate* of the ethmoid posteriorly to form the *bony nasal septum* (Fig. 9-7). The anterior portion of the septum is composed of cartilage.

Into each nasal cavity (formed by the septum) project three scroll-shaped structures called *conchae,* or *turbinates.* The *inferior* conchae are separate bones; the *middle* and *superior* conchae are processes of the ethmoid. The conchae divide each nasal cavity into passageways, or *meati* (Chapter 13).

Sinuses. The air cavities within the bones of the skull include the *paranasal* and *mastoid* sinuses. The paranasal sinuses, which include those of the *frontal, sphenoid, ethmoid,* and *maxillary* bones, communicate with the nose; the mastoid sinuses (the

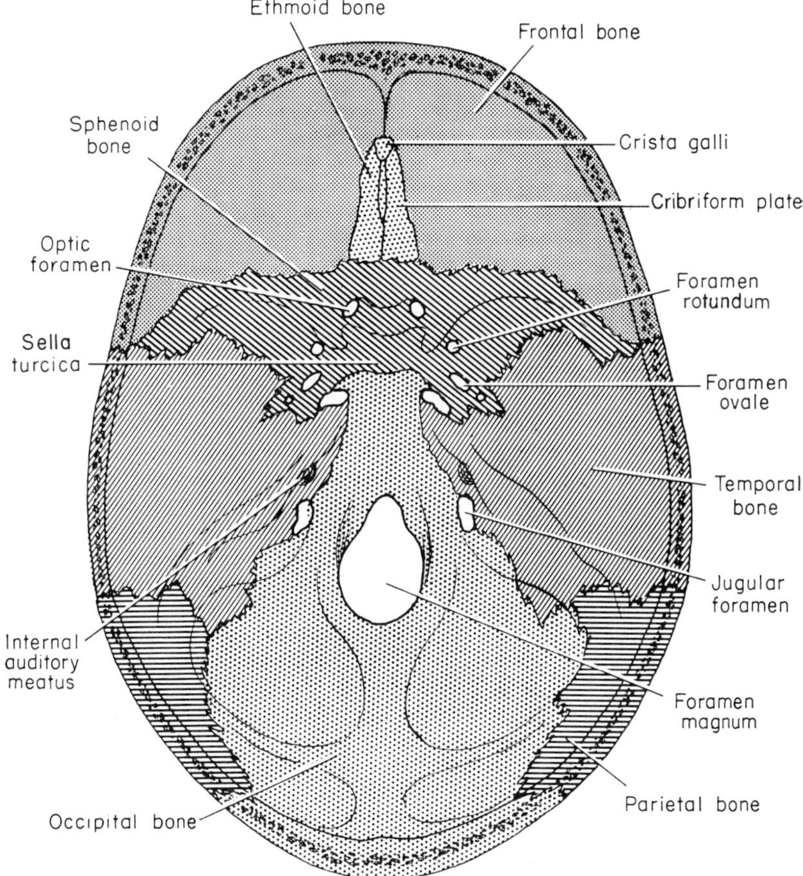

Fig. 9-6. Floor of the skull as seen from above. (Modified from Francis, C. C: Introduction to human anatomy, ed. 5, St. Louis, 1968, The C. V. Mosby Co.)

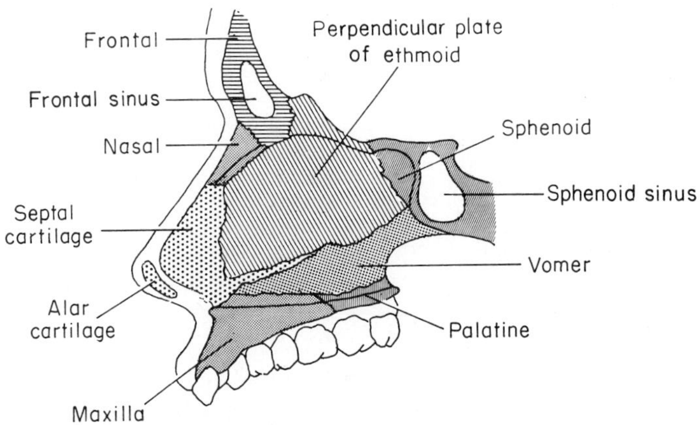

Fig. 9-7. Nasal septum and hard palate. (Modified from Francis, C. C: Introduction to human anatomy, ed. 5, St. Louis, 1968, The C. V. Mosby Co.)

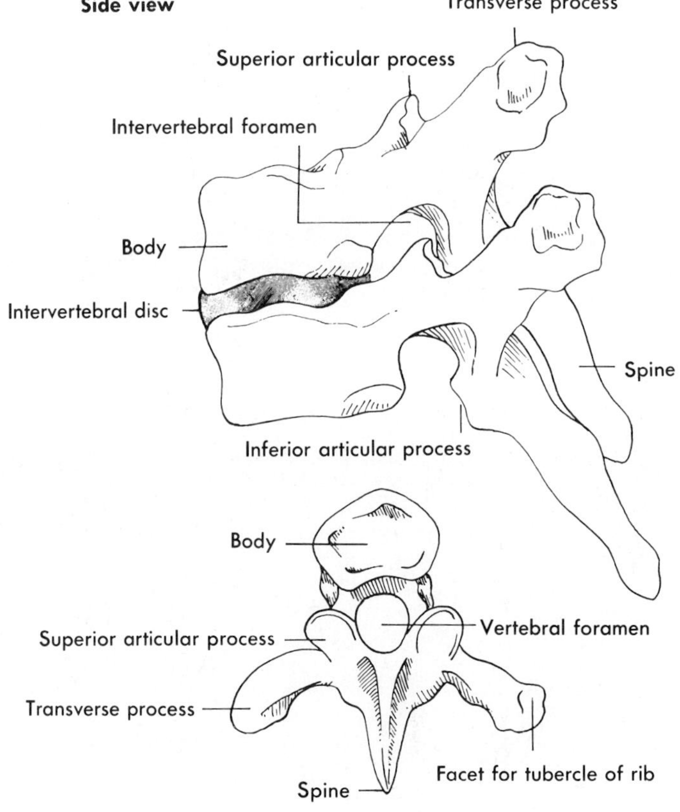

Fig. 9-8. Anatomy and articulation of the thoracic vertebrae.

tiny cavities within the mastoid process of the temporal bone) communicate with the middle ear. The maxillary sinus, the largest of the skull, is sometimes referred to as the *antrum of Highmore.*

Ear bones. Located within the middle ear cavity (in the petrous portion of the temporal bone) are three very tiny bones, or ossicles—the hammer (*malleus*), the anvil (*incus*), and the stirrup (*stapes*). These bones, so named because of their respective shapes, participate in the transmission of sound (Chapter 21). We should note that the six ossicles are not counted among the bones composing the skull.

Hyoid. The hyoid is a slender horseshoe-shaped bone situated at the upper border of the larynx, and by pressing in with the index finger just above the Adam's apple, one can easily feel it. Suspended from the styloid processes of the temporal bones, the hyoid has the unique distinction of being the only bone in the body that does not articulate with another bone. Attached to the hyoid are the extrinsic muscles of the tongue and a few muscles at the floor of the mouth.

Vertebrae. The vertebrae are the highly irregular bones that form the so-called spinal column. They are separated from each other by discs of fibrocartilage and are closely bound together by ligaments. Each vertebra is "equipped" with an opening (*vertebral foramen*), and together they form the so-called *vertebral* or *spinal canal* through which the brain thrusts the spinal cord. The nerves that issue from the cord pass through the *intervertebral* foramina,

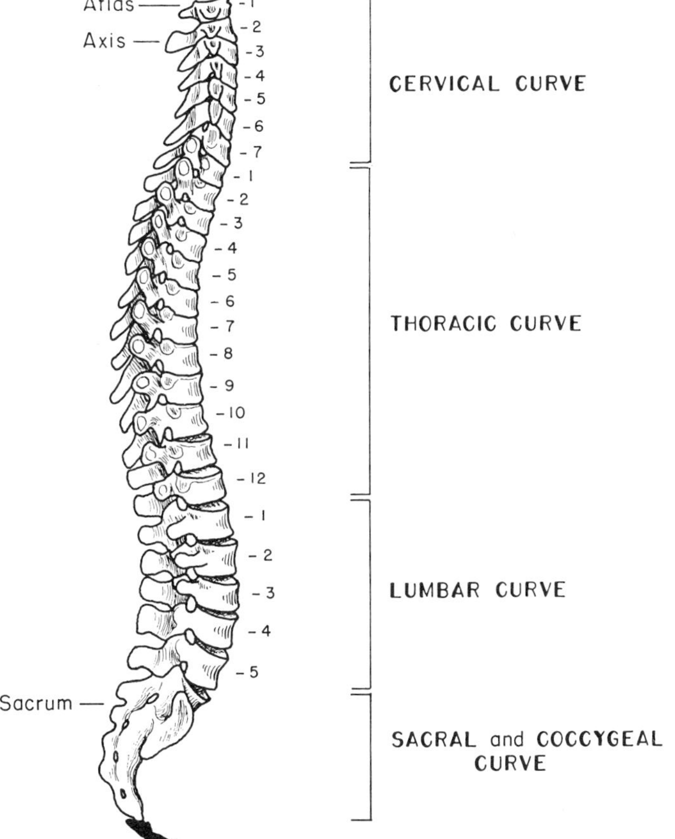

Fig. 9-9. Vertebral column.

openings formed by the vertebral notches (Fig. 9-8).

The vertebrae differ in size and shape but generally have similar features. A typical vertebra possesses a body (a solid cylinder of spongy bone), articular processes, a spine, and, as just mentioned, a foramen.

While in the embryo there are *thirty three* or *thirty-four* vertebrae, in the adult, the terminal vertebrae have fused, reducing the number to *twenty-six.* They are named according to their location in the column: cervical, thoracic, lumbar, sacral, and coccygeal (Fig. 9-9).

Cervical vertebrae. These are the seven movable vertebrae of the neck and are characterized by small bodies and stubby, spinous processes. The first cervical vertebra, aptly called the *atlas,* supports the head via two cup-shaped articular depressions that articulate with the two occipital condyles. The second vertebra (called the *epistropheus* or *axis*) sends up a projection, the odontoid process, around which the atlas rotates, permitting the head to move from side to side.

Thoracic vertebrae. There are twelve thoracic vertebrae. Compared to those of the neck, the thoracic vertebrae are larger and stronger and possess a well-developed, downward-pointing spinous process; and the *transverse* processes of all except the eleventh and twelfth vertebrae are equipped with facets for articulation with the tubercles of the ribs.

Lumbar vertebrae. The five lumbar vertebrae, which pass through the loin, are larger and heavier than the thoracic vertebrae. Their spinous processes are characteristically short, thick, and blunt.

Sacrum. In the adult the sacrum is a single bone formed by the fusion of five sacral vertebrae. The first vertebra is the largest, and each succeeding vertebra becomes progressively smaller in size. The smooth and concave anterior surface helps form the hollow of the pelvis. In contrast, the posterior surface is rough and uneven to permit attachment to the muscles of the back. The sacrum articulates with the ilia at the *sacroiliac joints.*

Coccyx. The coccyx, or "tail," a small triangular bone at the end of the vertebral column below the sacrum, is formed by the fusion of *four* (sometimes five) coccygeal vertebrae.

Ribs. The twelve pairs of ribs (Fig. 9-3), together with the sternum in the front and the thoracic vertebrae in the back, form the skeletal framework of the thorax. A typical rib is a long, slender, curved bone with its head joined to a vertebra and its other end joined to the sternum by a band of cartilage.

The first seven ribs are joined to the sternum by separate *costal cartilages,* whereas the cartilages of the ninth and tenth ribs are fused with the cartilage of the eighth rib. Accordingly, the first seven pairs are often referred to as "true" ribs, and the remaining five as "false" ribs. The costal cartilages of the eleventh and twelfth ribs do not meet the sternum at all and, for this reason, are commonly called "floating" ribs. The tips of these ribs may be felt by working the fingers along the lower border of the thoracic cage.

Sternum. The sternum, or *breastbone,* is a dagger-shaped bone forming the chest wall at the midline in front. The upper handlike portion of this bone is called the *manubrium,* the middle portion, or "body," is called the *gladiolus,* and the tip (not ossified in early life) is called the *xiphoid process.* At the manubrium the sternum articulates with the first rib and the clavicle (*collarbone*).

APPENDICULAR SKELETON

The appendicular division of the skeletal system includes the bones of the upper and lower extremities.

Upper extremity. The parts of the upper extremity include the shoulder, upper arm, elbow, forearm, wrist, and hand.

Scapula. Commonly called the shoulder

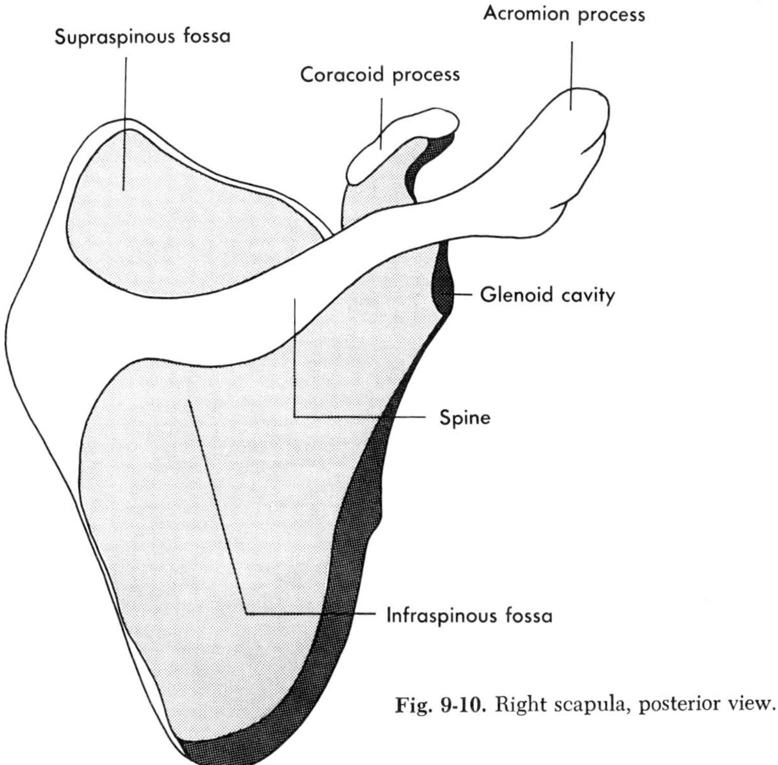

Fig. 9-10. Right scapula, posterior view.

blade, the scapula is largely a flat, thin, triangular bone possessing a well-developed spine and two prominent processes—the *coracoid* and the *acromion* (Fig. 9-10). The latter forms the tip of the shoulder and articulates in front with the lateral end of the clavicle. Below the coracoid process is an oval shallow fossa called the *glenoid cavity,* which accommodates the head of the humerus.

Clavicle. The clavicle, or collarbone, forms the bony root of the neck in front. A long, curved, slender bone, the clavicle swings from its articulation with the *acromion process* to the manubrium at the midline.

Humerus. The humerus is the bone of the upper arm (Fig. 9-3). One of the best examples of a long bone, the humerus has a well-rounded head at one end and epicondyles at the other. The head articulates with the *glenoid cavity* of the scapula, and the capitulum and trochlea (rounded surfaces below the epicondyles) articulate with the radius and the ulna, respectively.

Between the epicondyles are the *coronoid* fossa in front and the *olecranon* fossa behind. The former accommodates the coronoid process of the ulna during flexion, and the latter accommodates the olecranon process of the ulna during extension.

Ulna. The longer of the two bones composing the lower arm, the ulna (Fig. 9-3) lies on the side of the little finger. This may be easily proved by running the fingers from the tip of the elbow to the small projection at the side of the wrist.

The ulna is characterized principally by the coronoid and olecranon processes, the latter constituting the elbow. Between these two processes is the so-called semilunar notch that receives the trochlea of the humerus.

Radius. The radius runs parallel to the

ulna on the outer or thumb side of the lower arm. At the proximal end its head articulates with the ulna and the capitulum of the humerus. At the distal end the radius articulates with the wrist and the head of the ulna.

Carpal bones. The wrist, or *carpus,* is composed of eight bones, arranged in two rows (Fig. 9-3). The proximal row includes the navicular, lunate, triquetrum, and pisiform bones; the distal row includes the greater multangular, lesser multangular, capitate, and hamate bones. The prominence at the front of the wrist on the side of the little finger is produced by the pisiform bone.

Hand bones. The bones of the hand include the *five metacarpals* of the palm and the *fourteen phalanges* of the fingers (Fig. 9-3). With the exception of the thumb (which contains two), there are *three* phalanges in each finger. The metacarpals, beginning with the thumb, are numbered I through V. The phalanges are named the first or proximal phalanx, the second phalanx, and the third phalanx.

Lower extremity. The lower extremity includes the hip, thigh, knee, leg, ankle, and foot. The term *leg* is commonly used to designate that part between the knee and the ankle.

Os innominatum. The os innominatum is commonly called the *hipbone* or *innominate bone.* Actually, this large, powerful, and highly irregular bone is made up of three other bones—the *ilium,* the *ischium,* and the *pubis* (Fig. 9-11). These bones are so completely fused in the adult, however,

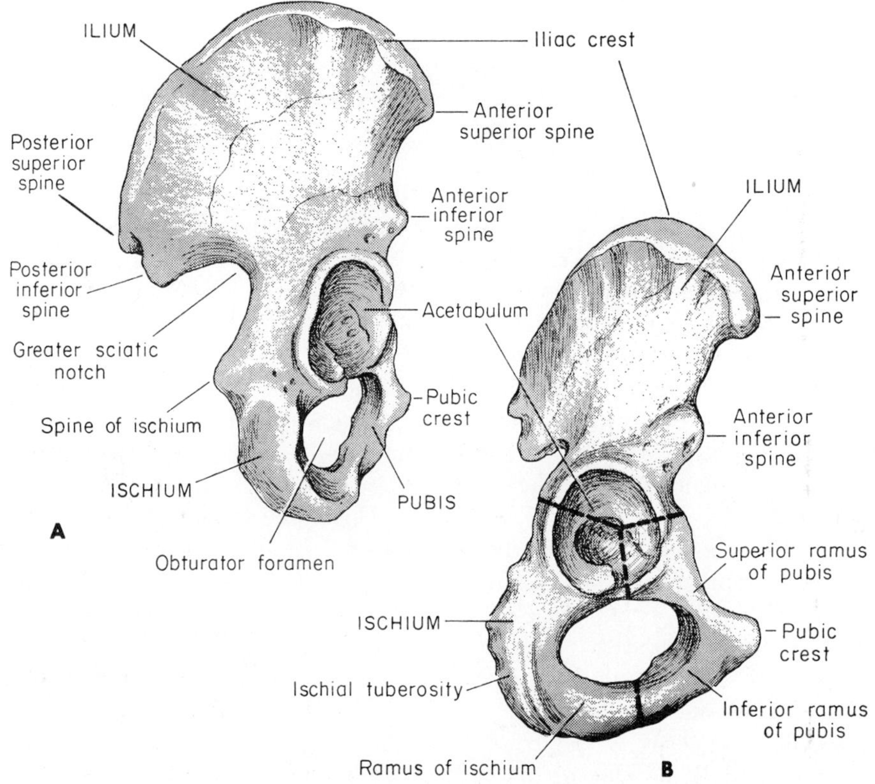

Fig. 9-11. Hipbone. **A,** Lateral view of right hipbone. **B,** Lateral view looking directly into acetabulum. Broken lines indicate where the three bones have joined together, usually obliterated by the age of 16 years. (Modified from Francis, C. C: Introduction to human anatomy, ed. 5, St. Louis, 1968, The C. V. Mosby Co.)

that it takes a while to detect the lines of juncture.

The principal features include the iliac crest, the acetabulum, the obturator foramen, and the greater sciatic notch. The iliac crest borders the ilium at the top and terminates in front and behind as the *anterior* and *posterior superior spines*, respectively. Below these are two other projections of the ilium—the *anterior inferior* spine and the *posterior inferior* spine. The *acetabulum*, a deep socket that receives the head of the femur, is formed by the fusion of the ilium, ischium, and pubis. The obturator foramen, "the largest hole in the skeleton," is bounded by the ischium and the pubis.

Strong ligaments unite the two hipbones with the sacrum at the *sacroiliac* joints to form the pelvis (Fig. 9-3). Anteriorly, the pubic bones articulate with each other at the *symphysis pubis* to form the pubic arch. The female and male pelves differ in two major respects: in the female the pubic arch is broader and the pelvic cavity is wider and more capacious.

Femur. The femur, or *thighbone,* is the largest, heaviest, and most powerful bone in the body. At its upper end it is equipped with a smooth spherical head that fits neatly into the acetabulum (Fig. 9-11). At the base of its neck are two prominent processes—the *greater trochanter,* a massive projection lateral to the shaft, and the *lesser trochanter,* a smaller projection on the inner side. The shaft itself is round and, with the exception of the *linea aspera,* smooth. The latter, a ridge that runs down along the back of the shaft, serves to attach muscles to the femur.

At the distal end the femur forms the lateral and medial condyles, which articulate with the patella and the tibia. Between these processes is the *intercondylar fossa.*

Patella. The patella, or *kneecap,* is a shell-shaped bone embedded in the tendon at the front of the knee (Fig. 9-3). (Because it resembles a grain of sesame, it is often said to be *sesamoid.*) When the leg is flexed, the patella is forced forward; when the leg is extended, the patella sinks back into the intercondylar fossa.

Tibia. The tibia, or *shinbone,* is the larger of the two leg bones. Its proximal end is thickened and forms two smooth articular surfaces—the lateral and medial condyles —which support the lateral and medial condyles of the femur. At the distal end on the inner side is the *medial malleolus,* the prominence on the *inner* side of the ankle.

Fibula. The fibula is a long slender bone that runs lateral and parallel to the tibia (Fig. 9-3). Proximally, it articulates with the tibia; distally, it terminates as the *lateral malleolus,* the *outer* prominence of the ankle.

Foot bones. The bones of the foot include seven tarsals, five metatarsals, and fourteen phalanges. The metatarsals are numbered I through V, beginning with the big toe. With the exception of the big toe (which has two), there are three phalanges in each toe and, like the phalanges in the hand, they are named the first (proximal) phalanx, the second phalanx, and the third phalanx.

DISEASES OF BONE

Some of the principal diseases of bone and the skeletal system are briefly described in the paragraphs that follow.

Arthritis. Arthritis is an inflammation of a joint. Since there are so many varieties of the condition and so many ambiguous and confusing clinical terms, we are in need of a better system of classification. Until the causes are known, however, any classification is tentative. For the present the categories presented here will have to do.

Rheumatoid arthritis. Rheumatoid arthritis is a chronic systemic involvement characterized by painful inflammatory changes in the joints. Deformity and generally invalidism occur as the disease progresses. Histologically, the main lesions are lymphocytic infiltration and excess connective tissue in and about the joints. The incidence of the malady in women is just about double that in men.

Rheumatoid arthritis is one of the major causes of disability in this country. Although its cause remains unknown, recent developments point to some highly interesting and perhaps significant biochemical findings. Treatment centers about rest, physiotherapy, and drugs (for example, aspirin and steroids).

Infectional arthritis. Infectional arthritis is an acute secondary infection of the joint marked by pronounced redness, heat, swelling, and pain. The usual etiologic factors are staphylococci, gonococci (Chapter 23), and tubercle bacilli (Chapter 13). Treatment consists of giving the appropriate anti-infective agent, both systemically and directly into the joint.

Other forms. Other important forms of arthritis result from rheumatic fever, injury, degenerative changes, gout, and tumors. Treatment in each instance naturally depends upon correction of the underlying cause. Although much remains to be learned about rheumatic fever, abundant experience has shown that it can be prevented by prompt administration of penicillin in all streptococcal infections.

Osteitis deformans. Osteitis deformans, or *Paget's disease,* is a chronic inflammation of bone with marked deformity. Muscle pain, bone pain, and hearing impairment are also commonly experienced. Initially, there is decalcification and softening of the skeleton that results in bending and bowing of the weight-bearing bones. To make matters worse, in the late stages of this strange disease there is unbridled recalcification, resulting in a thickened, enlarged, and twisted skeleton. The cause of osteitis deformans is unknown, and its treatment is nonspecific.

Osteitis fibrosa cystica. Osteitis fibrosa cystica, also known as *von Recklinghausen's disease* of bone, is a grotesque bone disorder resulting from hyperparathyroidism (p. 413). The excess parathyroid hormone "washes out" the calcium from the skeleton into the blood, leaving a flimsy framework that bends, bows, and breaks under the weight of the body. Also, stones may appear in the kidneys as a result of *hypercalcemia.* In the early days of medicine, before the cause of this disease was discovered, the patient eventually grew into an unrecognizable twisted mass of flesh and bone. Today, removal of the hyperplastic or tumorous parathyroid(s) offers an excellent prognosis.

Osteomalacia. Osteomalacia is a disease of adulthood in which the skeleton becomes soft because of inadequate calcification. As a result, the bones become flexible, brittle, and deformed. There is also considerable rheumatic pain and malaise. The etiologic factor is a calcium-phosphorus (vitamin D) deficiency.

Rickets. Rickets is a disease of childhood caused by a deficiency of vitamin D (Chapter 16). Insufficient deposition of calcium salts in the bones causes malformation and deformities, particularly bowing and bending of the leg bones. Another characteristic and important feature of rickets is *tetany* (Chapter 22).

Tumors. Some of the most incapacitating and deadly neoplasms are those of bone. The primary growths may be benign or malignant; the secondary ones are metastatic and always malignant. The more destructive are osteogenic sarcoma and multiple myeloma. Both are insidiously progressive and always fatal, death in the majority of patients occurring within about 3 years following diagnosis. Treatment includes administration of pain relievers, radiation, and antineoplastic drugs.

Infections. The most important infections of bone are osteomyelitis and tuberculosis. Osteomyelitis, which is marked by fever plus tenderness and pain over the affected bone, usually arises from invasion by staphylococci, streptococci, pneumococci, or typhoid bacilli, especially the first *(Staphylococcus aureus).* These organisms gain access to bone either by way of the blood as a result of an acute focal infection or directly following compound fracture or other trauma. Before the advent of chemotherapy, osteomyelitis frequently proved fatal. Today, early treatment with the appropriate drug affords a favorable prognosis.

Tuberculosis of the bones and joints occurs as a secondary infection; that is, the pathogen *(Mycobacterium tuberculosis)* makes its way to these sites from a focus of infection elsewhere in the body (Chapter 13). The course of the disease is chronic and destructive. Therapy includes a thorough search for the primary infection, appropriate surgical procedures, and administration of antitubercular drugs (namely, streptomycin, isoniazid, and PAS).

Questions

1. Describe the histologic characteristics of bone.
2. Describe the gross anatomy of a typical long bone.
3. Explain the importance of calcium and phosphorus in the diet.
4. Discuss the composition and function of bone marrow.
5. What is the function of alkaline phosphatase in ossification?
6. Discuss the reabsorption of bone.
7. Explain the mechanism by which crooked bones tend to straighten out with age.
8. Discuss the mending of a broken bone.
9. What are the roles of vitamin D and the parathyroid hormone in bone metabolism?
10. Describe the various types of diarthrotic joints and cite three examples of each.
11. Describe the skeletal features of the face.
12. Describe the ethmoid bone in detail and explain the role that it plays in the anatomy of the face and cranium.
13. Distinguish between a foramen and a meatus.
14. Describe the structure of the hard palate.
15. Describe the nasal septum.
16. Describe the backbone of the embryo.
17. Discuss the relationship of the spinal cord and spinal nerves to the vertebral column.
18. Describe the skeletal features of the thorax.
19. Describe the structure of the pelvis and its principal features.
20. Compare the bones of the hands and feet relative to their structure and number.
21. Discuss the term *arthritis.*
22. Discuss the etiology of von Recklinghausen's disease.
23. Distinguish between osteomalacia and rickets.
24. Discuss the major tumors of bone.
25. Discuss the major infections of bone.

Chapter 10

The muscular system

In this chapter we shall discuss the highlights of the structure and function of the skeletal muscles of the body. Attached as they are to the skeleton and controlled by nervous impulses from the brain, skeletal muscles permit us to talk, breathe, make funny faces, run, dance, wave good-by, type, turn somersaults, and perform any other physical activity dictated by the will. This explains why these muscles are commonly described as voluntary.

MUSCLE FIBER

The multinucleated muscle fiber is considered to be the anatomic unit of skeletal muscle. A single muscle is made up of thousands of these basic units. Each fiber has a diameter between 5 and 150μ and a length anywhere from a few millimeters to 4 inches or so.

The details of a single muscle fiber are shown in Fig. 10-1. In this idealized illustration it will be seen that each fiber is composed of smaller units called *myofibrils* and that these, in turn, are composed of two types of *myofilaments.* The delicate cell membrane that encloses the fiber is called the *sarcolemma.* The *sarcoplasm* separates the myofibrils.

Sarcomere. The light and dark bands along the muscle fiber are constituted of thin myofilaments and thick myofilaments, respectively. A so-called sarcomere is the muscle unit delimited by the so-called Z lines that cut across the center of the light bands. (The dark bands are called *anisotropic* or A bands, and the light ones are known as *isotropic* or I bands.) Great progress in muscle physiology has resulted from the discovery of the two proteins *actin* and *myosin.* Whereas actin molecules are present in the isotropic bands and extend part of the way into the anisotropic bands, myosin is found only in the anisotropic bands. The role these proteins play in muscle contraction will be discussed shortly.

MYONEURAL JUNCTION

When a nerve arrives at a muscle, its fibers part company and terminate among the muscle fibers at sites called myoneural junctions (Fig. 10-2). Generally, each muscle fiber is supplied with at least one myoneural junction and not infrequently with several. When a nerve impulse reaches a myoneural junction, *acetylcholine* is formed and contraction ensues.

But once acetylcholine has sparked the impulse along the muscle fiber, it ceases

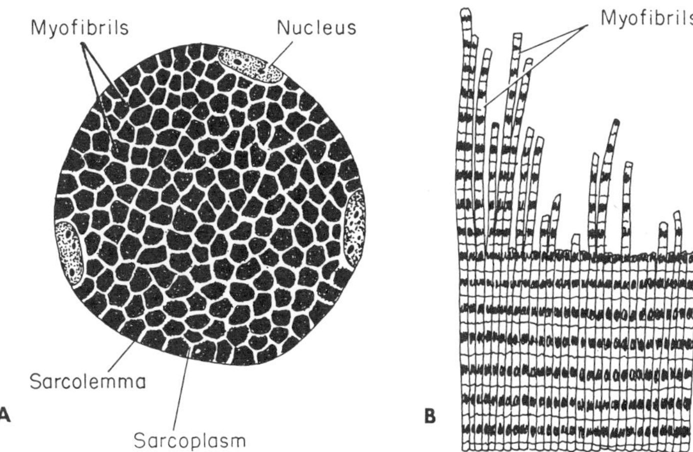

Fig. 10-1. Muscle fiber in cross section, **A**, and longitudinal section, **B.** (Modified from Maximow, A. A., and Bloom, W.: A Textbook of histology, ed. 7, Philadelphia, 1957, W. B. Saunders Co.)

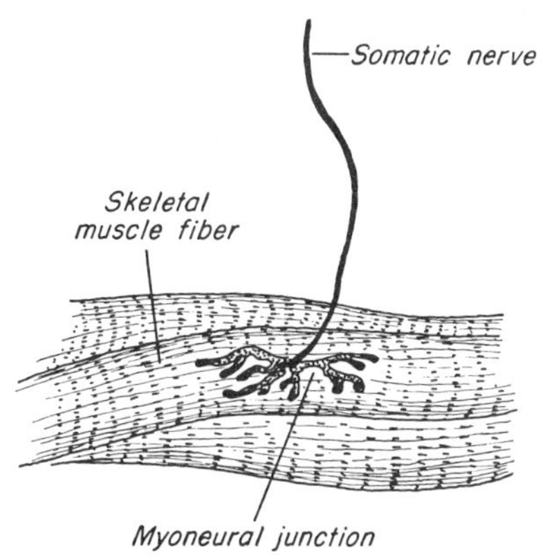

Fig. 10-2. Diagram of the myoneural junction. (From Brooks, S. M.: Basic facts of pharmacology, ed. 2, Philadelphia, 1963, W. B. Saunders Co.)

to be useful. As a matter of fact, if it is not soon "erased," the fiber will not have an opportunity to repolarize, or recharge, itself, and thus be ready to fire when triggered the next time. To this end, the body employs the enzyme *cholinesterase,* which is present throughout the body, especially at the myoneural junction. In a flash, cholinesterase splits acetylcholine into acetic acid and choline, metabolites that in due course are resynthesized into acetylcholine.

Motor unit. Each of the several thousand nerve fibers entering a muscle branches a number of times before coming to rest at the myoneural junctions. On the average a single fiber will cause contraction of 150 or so muscle fibers. Since the muscle fibers innervated by a *single* nerve fiber contract in unison, they constitute a so-called *motor unit.* Muscles that perform delicate movements have only about one tenth the number of fibers per unit as those engaged in gross movements.

CHEMISTRY OF CONTRACTION

Once acetylcholine initiates the impulse, or *action potential,* along the sarcolemma, calcium ions (in the sarcoplasm) enter the myofibrils. The calcium ions thereupon trigger an enzyme action that brings about the hydrolysis of *adenosine triphosphate* (Chapter 15), breaking it down into adenosine diphosphate with the release of energy. And as now understood, it is this energy that powers the shortening—or contraction—of the myofibrils. All of this takes place within a few thousandths of a second!

The source of energy needed for resynthesis—and replenishment—of adenosine triphosphate (ATP) from adenosine diphosphate (ADP) apparently is provided by the breakdown, or dephosphorylation, of *creatine phosphate* (phosphocreatine). This substance, too, must be replenished, and the view for many years has been that the energy for this synthesis derives from the breakdown of muscle *glycogen,* granules of which are distributed throughout the sarcoplasm. Specifically, glycogen, via the *anaerobic* process of *glycolysis* (p. 309), is degradated to lactic acid, one fifth of which is *aerobically* oxidized in the *Krebs cycle* (p. 311) for the purpose of providing energy to resynthesize the other four-fifths back into glycogen. Thus, the ultimate source of energy for contraction depends upon oxygen. The latter is "stored" in muscle as *oxymyohemoglobin;* that is, oxymyohemoglobin breaks down into myohemoglobin and oxygen. Myohemoglobin has a much greater affinity for oxygen than does the hemoglobin of the blood and thus serves to provide oxygen to muscle even when the oxygen content of blood is low.

Fatigue and oxygen debt. There is a limit to what muscle can do, and during extreme exertion there are both fatigue and an "oxygen debt," both effects relating to the accumulation of lactic acid. In other words, the oxygen intake falls short of the oxygen requirement of the muscles, with the result that the body goes into debt. Thus, the runner continues to breathe heavily *after* the race to pay this oxygen debt or, metabolically speaking, to oxidize lactic acid and thereby replenish glycogen, creatine phosphate, and ATP, in that order.

HEAT OF CONTRACTION

From the standpoint of physics, muscle is not efficient in converting energy into work. The normal person has an efficiency of only about 20 percent, and even athletes cannot top 35 percent. This is according to nature's will, however, for the energy not utilized in contraction appears as *heat.* Indeed, it is chiefly the heat liberated in muscle that keeps the body warm.

ALL-OR-NONE LAW

The all-or-none law applies to both nerve fibers and muscle fibers. This law states that when a *fiber* is stimulated it responds *maximally or not at all;* that is, over and above a certain critical value, the response does not depend upon the strength of the stimulus.

MUSCLE TWITCH

A classic way to study muscle contraction is to produce a so-called muscle twitch, that is, a single contraction elicited by a single instantaneous stimulus. The required materials include a freshly excised muscle (for example, the frog gastrocnemius), a kymograph, and a stimulating electrode.

If the muscle is stimulated with the kymograph at rest (Fig. 10-3), the result will be a straight vertical line. If the muscle is stimulated with the drum turning, however, we note that a curve is produced (Fig. 10-4). Note especially the delay between application of the stimulus and onset of the response. This period, which is only a fraction of a millisecond, represents the events leading up to the interaction between actin and myosin, or the actual contraction.

Isotonic vs. isometric contraction. The setup shown in Fig. 10-3 produces an *isotonic* twitch, so called because the weight, or force, applied to the muscle remains the same throughout contraction. In contrast, an *isometric* (same length) twitch is produced by stimulating a muscle suspended between two rigid points. The difference between the two types of contraction is rather significant, for whereas in the isotonic contraction the muscle changes shape and shortens, in the isometric contraction the muscle does not change shape or shorten but only creates force. Characteristically, too, the isometric twitch is much faster in action.

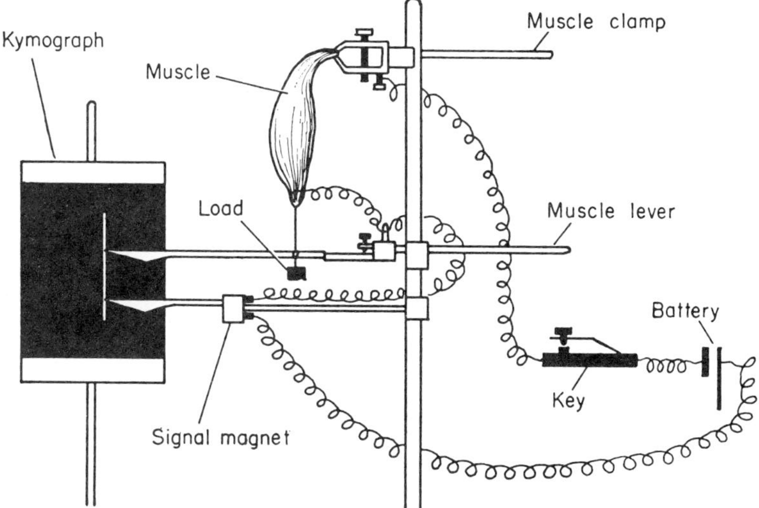

Fig. 10-3. Laboratory apparatus used to study muscle contraction. (Modified from Tuttle, W. W., and Schottelius, B. A.: Textbook of physiology, ed. 15, St. Louis, 1965, The C. V. Mosby Co.)

In the body, muscle contraction is both isotonic and isometric. Lifting the arm, for example, is largely an isotonic act; standing is an isometric act.

STRETCHING

Stretching has considerable bearing on the force of contraction. If the length to which a muscle is stretched is less than normal, the force of contraction is decreased. On the other hand, the force is decreased if a muscle is stretched too much. Thus, for each muscle there exists a stretch value that permits the most forceful contraction.

MOTOR SUMMATION

Once again let us turn to the laboratory setup shown in Fig. 10-3 to demonstrate the physiologic principle known as motor summation. With the drum turning very slowly, a series of stimuli of increasing intensity are applied to the muscle every 10 seconds or so, producing a pattern like the one shown in Fig. 10-5. This shows quite vividly that the force of contraction, up to a point, depends upon the strength of the stimulus. Since the all-or-none principle still holds true (that is, a muscle fiber contracts maximally or not at all), the only way that we can account for this effect is to assume that the number of motor units called into play depends upon

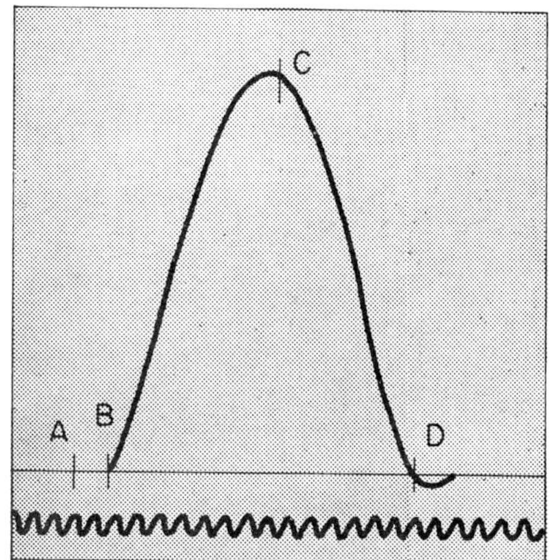

Fig. 10-4. Kymographic record of the muscle twitch. **A-B,** Latent period; **B-C,** contraction; **C-D,** relaxation. Time (1/100 second) indicated by lower tracing. (After Sterling and Howell; adapted from Best, C. H., and Taylor, N. B.: The human body, ed. 3, New York, 1956, Holt, Rinehart & Winston, Inc. By permission.)

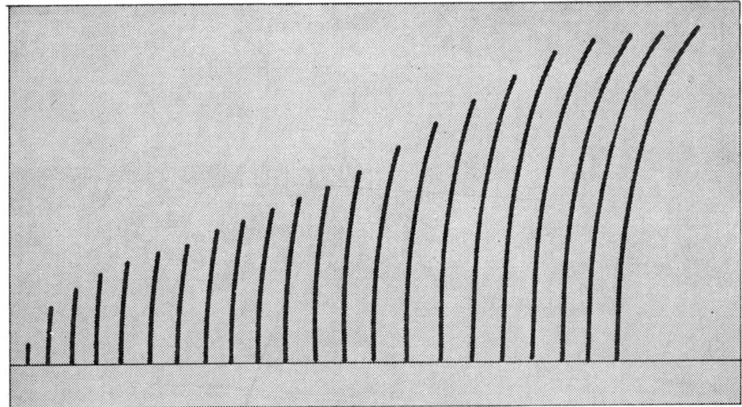

Fig. 10-5. Motor summation. Record of a series of contractions caused by stimuli of increasing strengths. (Adapted from Best, C. H., and Taylor, N. B.: The human body, ed. 3, New York, 1956, Holt, Rinehart & Winston, Inc. By permission.)

the strength of the stimulus. Motor summation, therefore, may be defined as the adding or summing up of the motor units of a muscle in response to a stimulus. In other words, all gradations of contraction between the weakest and the strongest are attained by varying the number of motor units contracting simultaneously.

TETANIZATION

The kymographic tracings that we have dealt with up to this point were obtained either by a single shock or by series of single shocks with an appreciable rest period in between. The result is drastically different if we stimulate a muscle at such a rate that it is not permitted to relax between shocks. Now we have so-called *wave summation;* as the rate of stimulation increases, the "waves" blend into a smooth, continuous contraction (Fig. 10-6). This response, called tetanization, can be predicted from the duration of a single contraction. For example, if it takes a certain muscle $\frac{1}{60}$ second to contract, a stimulating current delivering a volley of sixty or more shocks per second will produce tetanization.

Under normal conditions the muscles of the body perform their duties via a combination of summation and tetanization; that is, the different motor units are fired one at a time but rapidly enough to produce the smooth tetanic type of response rather than the jerky twitch.

TONUS

A freshly killed animal is as limp as a piece of string because its muscles have lost their tone. By tonus, or muscle tone, we mean the slight degree of tension under which the spinal cord maintains the muscles of the body; that is, most of the time the cord is sending out a few impulses over the motor nerves. This prevents the muscles from becoming flabby and prepares them for optimum performance when they are called upon to contract. The muscles relax during sleep because the cord "goes to sleep."

Excitement, fear, and other emotions enhance muscle tone because the nervous system steps up its impulse transmission. Perhaps the reason that we are "jumpy" under such circumstances stems from the sensitivity of hypertonic muscle.

THE MUSCLES

There are 327 paired and 12 unpaired skeletal muscles; they vary greatly in size and shape (Figs. 10-7 and 10-8). For example, whereas the gluteus maximus forms

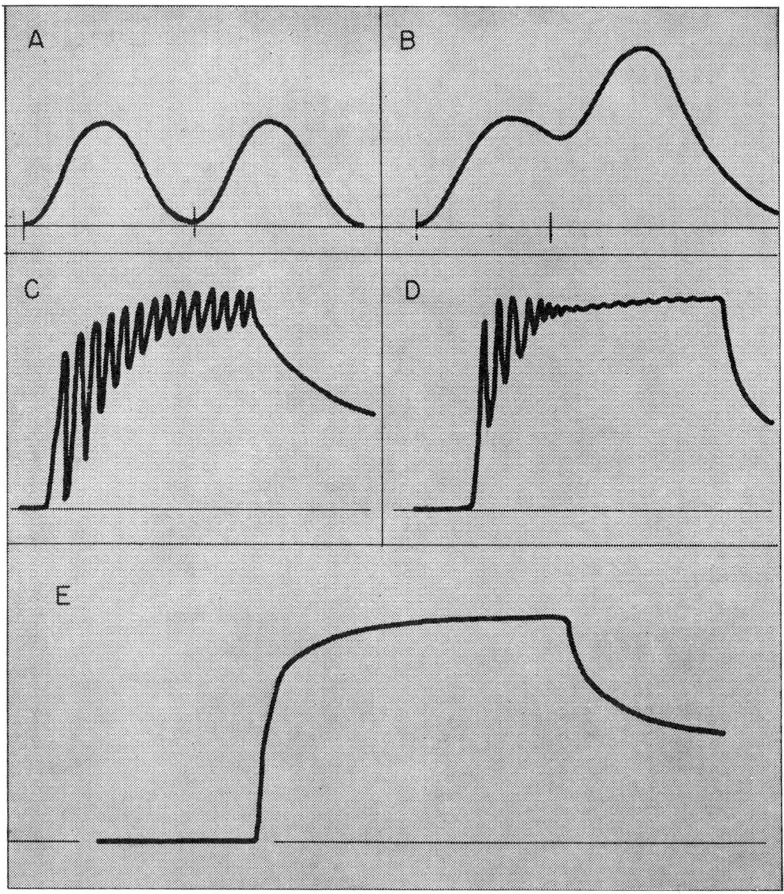

Fig. 10-6. Wave summation and tetanization. **A,** Second stimulus applied after relaxation of muscle. **B,** Second stimulus applied after a shorter interval than that represented in **A. C** to **E,** Still shorter intervals. Note complete tetanus in **E.** (Adapted from Best, C. H., and Taylor, N. B.: The human body, ed. 3, New York, 1956, Holt, Rinehart & Winston, Inc. By permission.)

the bulk of the buttocks, the stapedius muscle of the middle ear is composed of only a few tiny strands. Regardless of these gross differences, however, the muscles are all histologically the same, that is, parallel fibers organized into microscopic bundles, or *fasciculi.*

Typically, a muscle consists of a main portion called the body and two extremities, the origin and insertion, which are attached by the *epimysium* to bone, cartilage, or fascia. When the epimysium terminates as a strong white cord, we call the attachment a *tendon.* On the other hand, if the attachment takes the form of a white or ribbonlike expansion, it is called an *aponeurosis.*

Origin vs. insertion. When a muscle contracts, one of the bones to which it is attached moves and the other remains stationary. By convention, the end of the muscle attached to the stationary bone is called the origin, and the "movable" end is called the insertion. In not a few circumstances, however, the origin and the insertion are interchangeable, depending upon the movement being effected.

Agonist vs. antagonist. An agonist is a

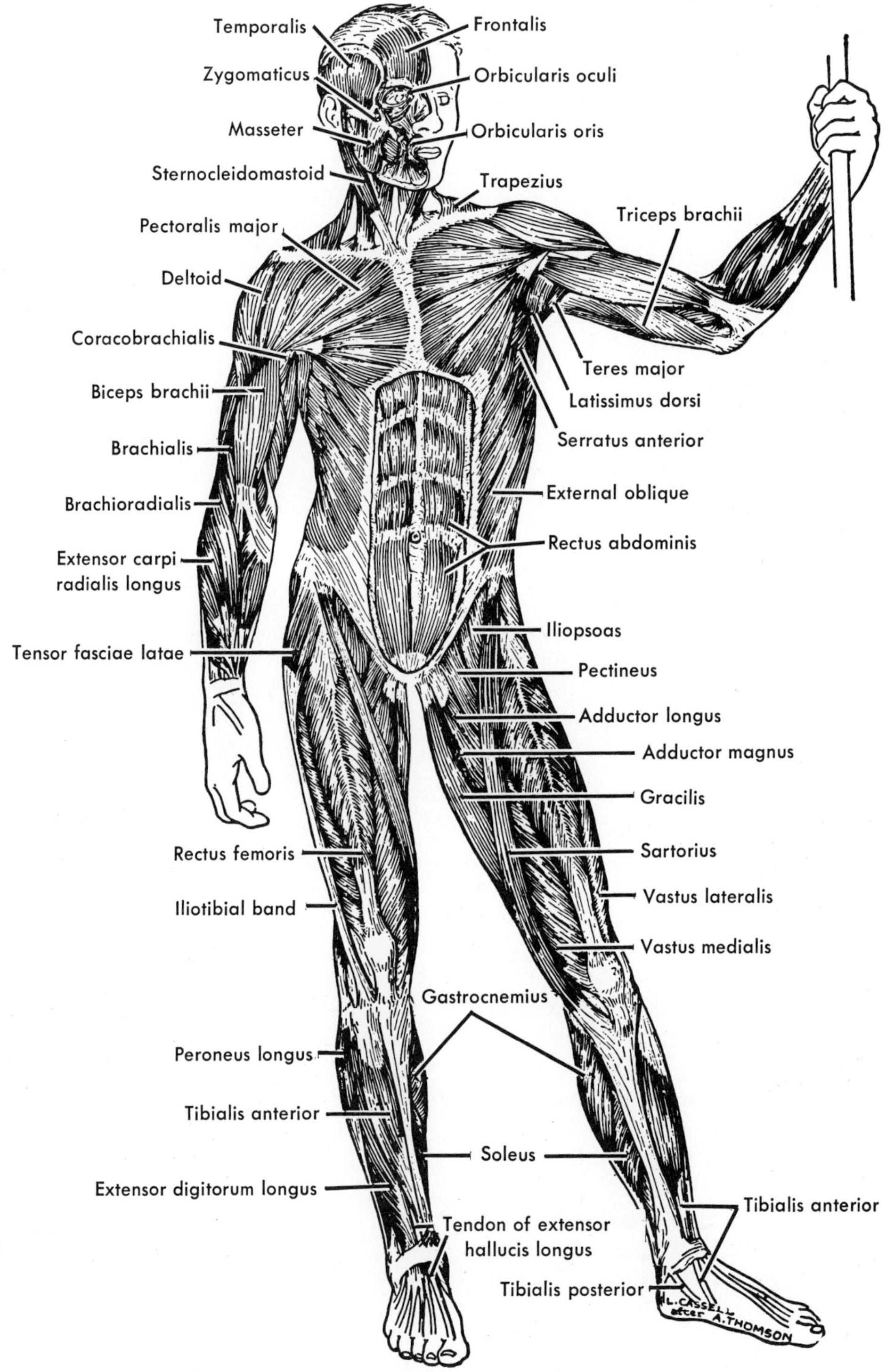

Fig. 10-7. Anterior view of muscles of the body. (From Millard, N. D., King, B. G., and Showers, M. J.: Human anatomy and physiology, Philadelphia, 1956, W. B. Saunders Co.)

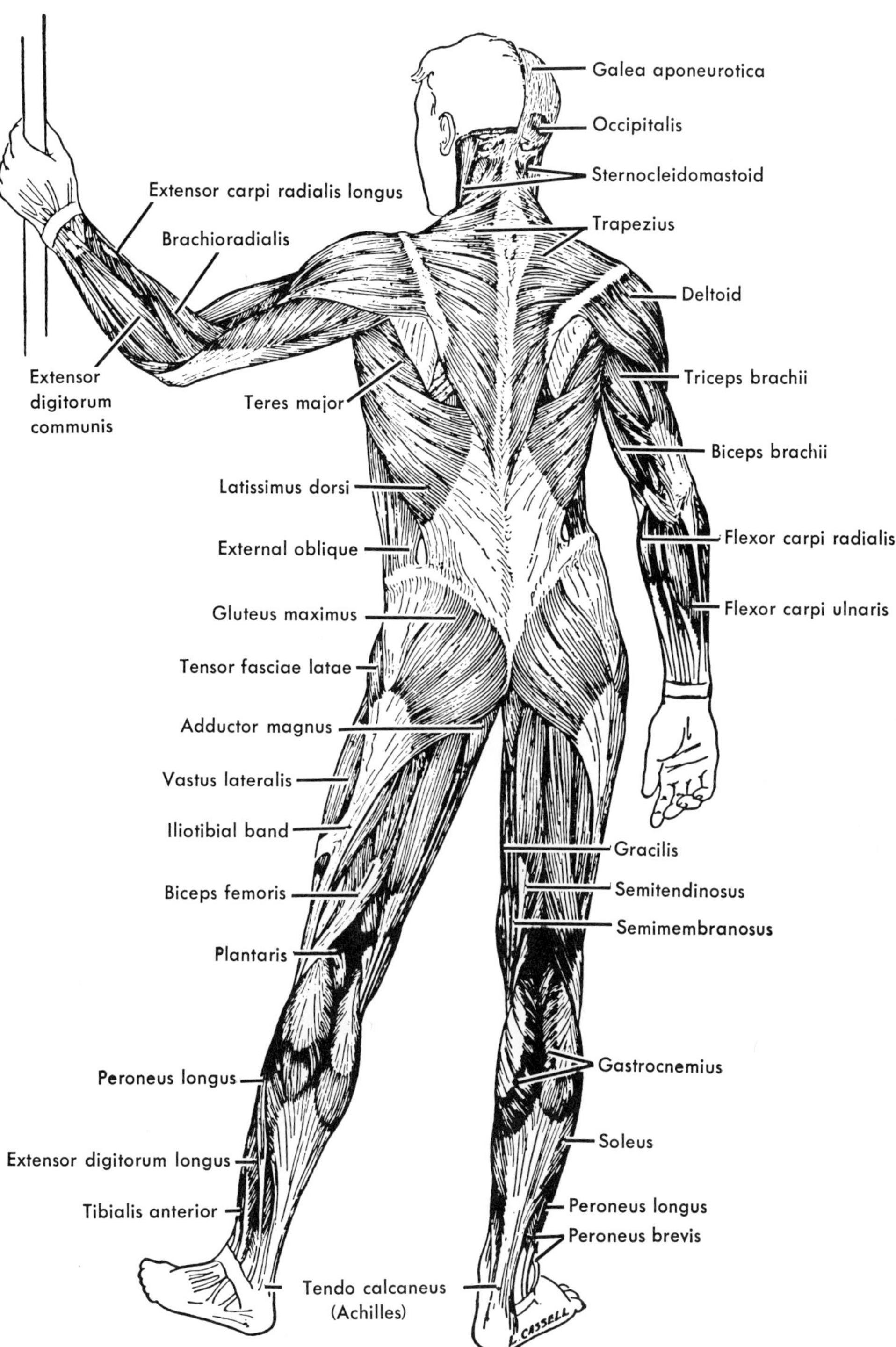

Fig. 10-8. Posterior view of muscles of the body. (From Millard, N. D., King, B. G., and Showers, M. J.: Human anatomy and physiology, Philadelphia, 1956, W. B. Saunders Co.)

prime mover, or a muscle whose contraction actually produces the movement. Conversely, an antagonist is a muscle that relaxes while its agonist contracts. "Antagonistic" muscles not only have an opposite action but also by necessity an opposite location; for example, if a flexor lies anterior to a given bone, the extensor lies posterior to the bone.

Synergists. Rarely is a single muscle responsible for a given movement. For the sake of smoothness, muscles are so arranged that the agonist is aided by neighboring muscles called synergists. In extending the leg, for example, four large muscles are called into play.

Classification. Skeletal muscles are perhaps best grouped according to their principal action:

flexors muscles that decrease the angle of a joint.
extensors muscles that increase the angle of a joint.
abductors muscles that move a part away from the midsagittal plane.
adductors muscles that move a part toward the midsagittal plane.
supinators muscles that turn the palm upward.
pronators muscles that turn the palm downward.
levators muscles that raise a part or an area.
depressors muscles that lower a part.
rotators muscles that cause a part to pivot upon its axis.
tensors muscles that tense or make a part more rigid.
sphincters muscles that reduce the size of an opening.
dorsiflexors muscles that pull the foot backward.
plantar flexors muscles that pull the foot downward.

Flexors. Flexor muscles effect *flexion* or sagittal plane movement in which the angle of a joint is decreased (Fig. 10-9). The more important include the *sternocleidomastoideus, pectoralis major, biceps brachii, iliopsoas, rectus abdominis,* and the flexors of the wrist, fingers, leg, and foot (Table 10-1).

Extensors. Extensor muscles effect *extension* or sagittal plane movement in which the angle of a joint is increased (Fig. 10-9). Some of the chief extensors are the *latissimus dorsi, triceps brachii, gluteus maximus, quadriceps femoris, sacrospinalis,* and the extensors of the wrist and fingers (Table 10-1).

Abductors. Abductors are muscles that effect *abduction* or bring a part of the body away from the midline (Fig. 10-9). Mus-

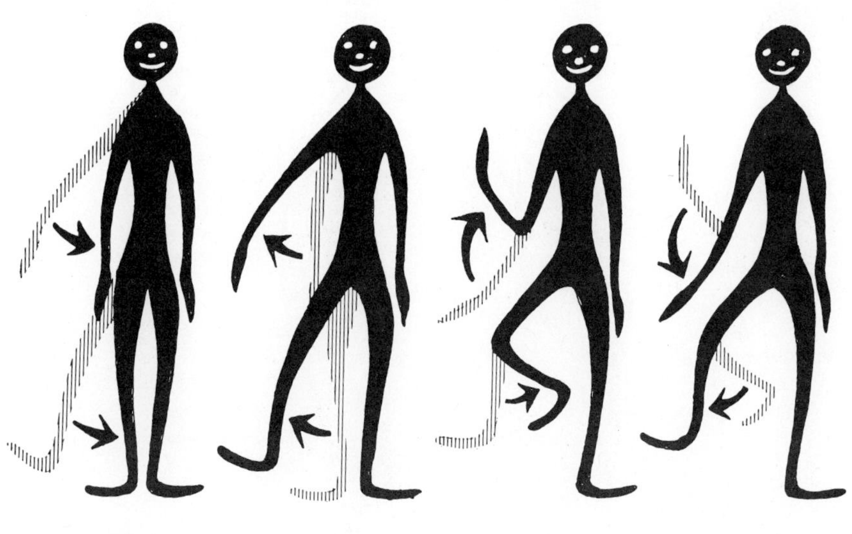

Fig. 10-9. Examples of "muscle action."

Table 10-1. Major muscles

Muscle	General origin	General insertion	Chief function
Adductors of thigh	Ilium and pubis	Femur and tibia	Adduct thigh
Adductor magnus			
Adductor longus			
Adductor brevis			
Anterior tibial group	Tibia and fibula	Foot	Dorsiflexes foot
Biceps brachii	Scapula	Radius	Flexes and supinates forearm
Buccinator	—	—	Aids in chewing
Deltoid	Clavicle and scapula	Humerus	Abducts arm
Epicranius	—	—	Wrinkles forehead
External oblique	Lower costal cartilages	Crest of ilium	Flexes trunk
Gastrocnemius	Condyles of femur	Heel bone	Plantar flexes foot
Gluteus maximus	Sacrum and ilium	Femur	Extends thigh
Hamstring group	Ischial tuberosity	Tibia and fibula	Flexes leg
Biceps femoris			
Semitendinosus			
Semimembranosus			
Iliopsoas	Ilium and lumbar vertebrae	Femur	Flexes thigh
Internal oblique	Iliac crest	Lower costal cartilages	Flexes trunk
Latissimus dorsi	Lower vertebrae and ilium	Humerus	Extends and adducts arm
Orbicularis oculi	—	—	Closes eyes
Orbicularis oris	—	—	Closes mouth
Pectoralis major	Clavicle and chest wall	Humerus	Flexes and adducts arm
Posterior tibial group	Tibia and fibula	Foot	Plantar flexes foot
Quadriceps femoris	Ilium and femur	Tibia	Extends leg
Rectus femoris			
Vastus intermedius			
Vastus lateralis			
Vastus medialis			
Quadratus lumborum	Ilium and lumbar vertebrae	Lumbar vertebrae	Flexes vertebrae
Rectus abdominis	Pubis	Sternum and costal cartilages	Flexes trunk
Risorius	—	—	Extends corners of mouth
Sacrospinalis	Vertebrae	Vertebrae and ribs	Extends trunk
Sartorius	Anterior superior iliac spine	Tibia	Turns thigh outward
Serratus anterior	Chest wall	Scapula	Draws shoulders forward
Sternocleidomastoideus	Clavicle and sternum	Occiput	Flexes head
Tensor fasciae latae	Ilium	Tibia	Abducts thigh
Transversus abdominis	Lower ribs	Linea alba	Compresses viscera
Trapezius	Upper vertebrae	Scapula and clavicle	Braces shoulders
Triceps brachii	Humerus and scapula	Ulna	Extends forearm

cles of this character include the *deltoid* and *tensor fasciae latae* (Table 10-1).

Adductors. Adductors are muscles that effect *adduction* or bring a part of the body toward the midline. The principal adductors include the *pectoralis major, latissimus dorsi,* and adductors of the thigh (Table 10-1).

Abdominal muscles. The sides of the abdominal wall are formed by three sheets of muscle—the *external oblique,* the *internal oblique,* and the *transversus abdominis.* The wall has great strength because the fibers of these muscles run in three different directions. The front, central wall of the abdomen is formed by the *rectus abdominis* and the aponeuroses of the muscles at the sides (Fig. 10-10).

The rectus abdominis arises from the pubis and passes upward as a strong column of muscle to be inserted into the xiphoid process and the fifth, sixth, and seventh costal cartilages. Cutting across the rectus abdominis transversely are three or four fibrous bands called *inscriptiones tendineae* which, together with the *linea alba,* produce the gridlike appearance of the skinned abdomen (Fig. 10-7). The linea alba (white line) results from the meeting of the aponeuroses of the external oblique muscles at the midline.

The posterior abdominal wall is formed by the bony vertebral column and the *quadratus lumborum,* a strong column of muscle that arises from the iliac crest and the lower lumbar vertebrae and inserts into the twelfth rib and the upper lumbar vertebrae.

Inguinal canal. The inguinal canal is a channel, 1 inch or so in length, that tunnels obliquely through the lower abdominal wall just above the *inguinal ligament.* In the male the spermatic cord passes through the inguinal canal on its way to the testis. In the female the canal serves to anchor the round ligament of the uterus.

The inguinal canal is the weakest site in the abdominal wall, which accounts for the common occurrence of inguinal *hernias.* In this type of hernia in the male the parietal peritoneum makes its way through the canal and finally into the scrotum. As this outpouching continues, a portion of the abdominal contents, such as the omentum or a loop of intestine, may follow and aggravate the condition.

Other weak areas in the wall occur about the umbilicus and along the linea alba above the umbilicus.

Muscles of scapula. The *trapezius* and the *serratus anterior* are the most important muscles that act upon the scapula. The trapezius (Fig. 10-8), a broad, triangular muscle that arises from the occipital bone and vertebrae (seventh cervical to twelfth thoracic) and inserts into the clavicle and the spine of the scapula, braces the shoulders and rotates the scapula. The serratus

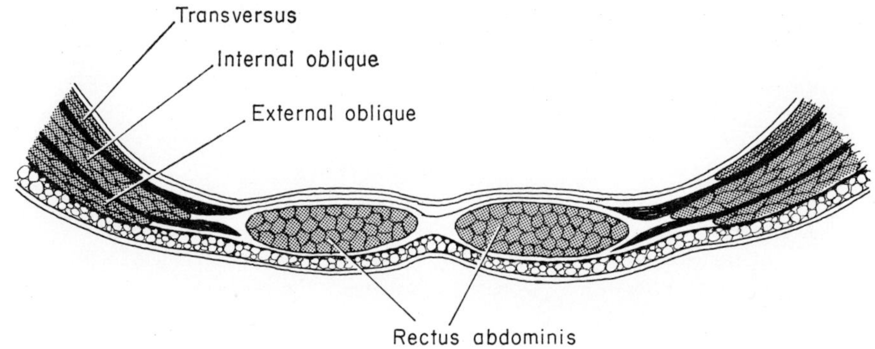

Fig. 10-10. Abdominal muscles in cross section. (Modified from Anthony, C. P.: Textbook of anatomy and physiology, ed. 7, St. Louis, 1967, The C. V. Mosby Co.)

anterior (Fig. 10-7) originates from the lateral chest wall (second to eighth ribs) and inserts into the vertebral margin of the scapula. This muscle serves to draw the scapula forward.

Muscles of head. Whereas most muscles of the body are concerned solely with the performance of work, those of the face are also concerned with expression, an effect singularly perculiar to human beings. Of special interest are the *orbicularis oculi, orbicularis oris, buccinator, masseter, risorius,* and *epicranius* muscles. The orbicularis oculi closes the eye, the orbicularis oris closes the mouth, the masseter and buccinator assist in chewing, the risorius draws the mouth, and the epicranius raises the eyebrows.

DISEASES OF MUSCLE AND RELATED DISORDERS

Muscular dystrophy. A variety of heredofamilial disorders falls into the category of muscular dystrophies and atrophies. Perhaps the most important is progressive muscular dystrophy, the cause of which remains unknown. As indicated by its name, the onset is gradual and insidious. In the early stages the child walks awkwardly and tends to fall easily. In time he is not able to get up unless helped. Examination shows wasting away of some muscles and enlargement of others. This enlargement is a result of pseudohypertrophy, however, for histologic examination reveals that the affected muscle has deposits of fat in between the muscle fibers. Other than massage and understanding care, there is no specific treatment for muscular dystrophy. The patient usually is confined to a wheelchair and dies at an early age.

Myasthenia gravis. Myasthenia gravis is marked by fatigue and exhaustion of the muscles. Characteristically, there is progressive paralysis without atrophy or sensory disturbance. Although any muscle may be affected, those of the head and neck are most commonly involved. This explains the expressionless face and drooping eyelids of the person who has this disorder.

For some reason, the nerve impulse fails at the myoneural junction. Some workers have suggested that this is due either to a lack of acetylcholine or to the presence of too much cholinesterase, particularly because parasympathomimetic drugs afford considerable relief (p. 379). As to the reason behind this defect, present evidence indicates some sort of "autoimmune disease" involving the *thymus gland* (p. 242). About one third of the patients with myasthenia gravis have either an abnormal persistence of the gland (which normally disappears during childhood) or else a *thymoma* (thymic tumor). Also, about one half of the patients with thymoma display the signs and symptoms of myasthenia gravis. In such cases thymectomy (removal of the gland) may afford some relief.

Bursitis. Bursae are fluid-filled cavities within the tissues that develop when there is repeated movement and friction. This explains why they are generally situated near the joint cavities. As a result of trauma or infection, they become inflamed and bursitis ensues. Not only is bursitis fairly common, but it is also extremely painful and not infrequently refractory to conservative treatment. Some of the more common sites of the disorder include the elbow, shoulder, and knee (housemaid's knee). In addition to drugs for relieving pain and fighting infection, the physician may prescribe massage, diathermy, or x-ray therapy. In cases in which there is no specific infection the corticosteroids often give considerable relief.

Tetany. This disorder of neuromuscular tissue is marked by muscle twitchings, cramps, and convulsions. Any situation that produces a drop in blood calcium (*hypocalcemia*) can cause tetany. The usual etiologic factors include alkalosis (Chapter 18), vitamin D deficiency (Chapter 16), and hypoparathyroidism (Chapter 22). To terminate an attack, the physician injects intravenously a 10 percent solution of calcium gluconate or similar preparation. To prevent further episodes, however, the underlying cause must be dealt with.

Tetanus. Tetanus, or *lockjaw,* a most vicious infection, is caused by the *exotoxin* released by *Clostridium tetani,* a slender, motile, gram-positive, anaerobic bacillus with terminal spores. The latter structures, being considerably wider than the body of the bacillus, make the organism appear as microscopic tennis rackets (Fig. 10-11). The exotoxin appears to act like strychnine, facilitating the transmission of nerve impulses across all synapses (that is, junctions between the neurons). As a result, there is generalized *hypertonus* with intermittent convulsions. Stiffness of the jaw, the most common symptom, is of utmost diagnostic significance. Death may be due to respiratory failure. As in many conditions, the heart continues to beat for several minutes after breathing has stopped.

As should be well known, the omnipresent *Clostridium tetani* is introduced into the tissues via contaminated wounds, particularly wounds of the puncture type (for example, those sustained in stepping on a nail, stab wounds, gunshot wounds, bites, and the like). The deeper the wound, the greater is the likelihood of tetanus because *Clostridium tetani,* being an anaerobe, thrives in the absence of air. Soon after the bacilli have established a foothold in the underlying tissues, they start to multiply and turn out the deadly exotoxin. Since it takes fantastically little of the toxin to destroy life, time is of the essence. Statistics show that when treatment is delayed 1 day after the onset of symptoms the mortality rate is about 50 percent. On the other hand, if the victim survives, he usually is free of all ill effects in a month or so.

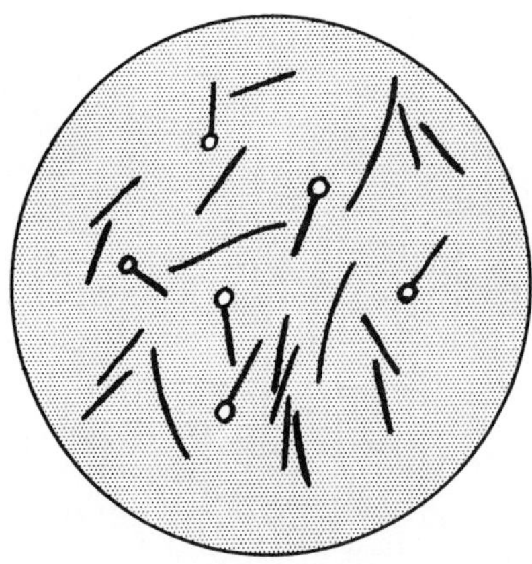

Fig. 10-11. *Clostridium tetani.* Note terminal spores. (From Brooks, S. M.: Basic facts of medical microbiology, ed. 2, Philadelphia, 1962, W. B. Saunders Co.)

World War II demonstrated that tetanus *toxoid* affords 100 percent protection, which means that no one need die at the hands of this disease. The recommended procedure is to give a primary injection, followed by booster shots 1 year later and every 3 to 5 years thereafter. Because one third to one half of tetanus cases occur with no history of injury, such precaution is highly desirable.

Tetanus prophylaxis in injured patients centers upon whether such patients have been previously immunized. The recommended procedure is as follows:

Patients previously immunized

1. Adequate cleansing and debridement of wound.
2. Toxoid booster.
3. Antitoxin*—may be needed rarely (along with toxoid) for very extensive wounds, for persons seen more than 48 hours after injury, and for patients whose last toxoid booster had been given more than 20 years previously.
4. Antibiotics—given if danger of clostridial infection is very great or if indicated for other bacterial infection.

Patients not previously immunized

1. Adequate cleansing and debridement of wound.

*Since tetanus antitoxin derived from *horse* serum is not without danger, particularly in allergic patients, the availability of *human* antitoxin (for example, Hyper-Tet) is of considerable significance.

2. Antitoxin—may be omitted for trivial wounds; indicated for all tetanus-prone wounds.
3. Antibiotics—given if clostridial infection is likely or if indicated for other bacterial infection.
4. Toxoid—first dose gives no protection for wound being treated but provides opportunity to start active immunization.

Gas gangrene. Gas gangrene is caused by *Clostridium perfringens* and several other species of the genus. Like the organism that causes tetanus, this bacillus is a gram-positive sporulating anaerobe that thrives when introduced into the tissues. This explains its common occurrence in dirty lacerated wounds. As indicated by the name, there is death of cells *en masse* (*gangrene*) as well as considerable amounts of gas in the affected area. Both effects result from the elaboration of toxins and enzymes by the bacilli. Treatment includes thorough cleansing of wounds and administration of gas gangrene antitoxin and penicillin. These measures were dramatically effective in treatment and prevention of the infection during World War II and the Korean War.

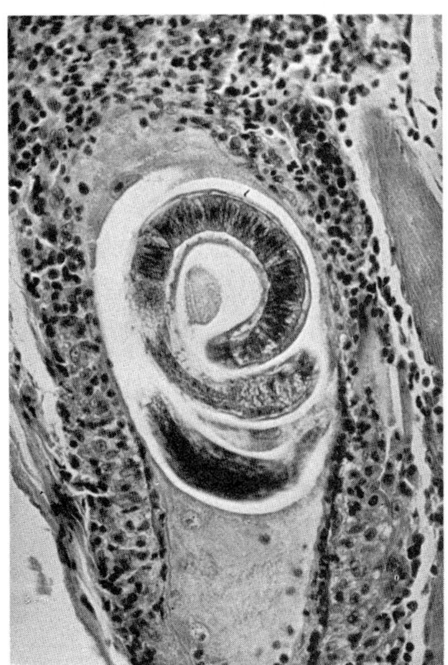

Fig. 10-12. Microscopic section of muscle showing embedded *Trichinella spiralis.* (From Ivey, M.: Helminths. In Frankel, S., Reitman, S., and Sonnenwirth, A.: Gradwohl's clinical laboratory methods and diagnosis, ed. 7, St. Louis, 1970, The C. V. Mosby Co.)

Trichinosis. Trichinosis is an infestation caused by the nematode *Trichinella spiralis,* one of the smallest of the parasitic worms. Its life cycle is briefly as follows: The encysted larvae in infested meat are released in the intestine during the course of digestion. From here they make their way into the lymphatic vessels and ultimately penetrate and encyst in the muscles (Fig. 10-12). Man acquires the infestation by eating infested poorly cooked pork, and the pig acquires it by eating infested rats and raw garbage containing infested pork wastes.

The early manifestations of infestation include fever, nausea, abdominal pain, and diarrhea. Later on, when the larvae take up residence in the muscles, the patient experiences stiffness, pain, and swelling. Insomnia is also a characteristic feature. Other than the drug *thiabendazole,* for which tests are promising, treatment remains symptomatic. Fortunately, the prognosis is good in most cases.

Trichinosis is an excellent example of a malady that can be extinguished completely by prophylactic means. This includes thorough cooking of all fresh pork and sterilization of all garbage fed to pigs.

Questions

1. Discuss the role of acetylcholine and cholinesterase at the myoneural junction.
2. Outline the major chemical events relating to muscle contraction.
3. Why do we shiver in an extremely cold environment?
4. The force of contraction up to a point varies with the strength of the stimulus. Is this laboratory fact in conflict with the all-or-none law?
5. Describe the isotonic muscle twitch.
6. Discuss the value of stretching in the contraction of muscle.
7. Distinguish between motor summation and wave summation.

8. Name the chief agonist and the chief antagonist in flexing of the arm.
9. Describe the basic anatomy of a skeletal muscle.
10. Cite two good examples of movements in which the origin becomes the insertion and vice versa.
11. Distinguish between plantar flexion and dorsiflexion.
12. What is meant by muscle tone?
13. What evidence can you cite to support the theory that myasthenia gravis is caused by a lack of acetylcholine or too much cholinesterase.
14. Discuss the etiology, treatment, and prophylaxis of tetanus.
15. Describe the life cycle of *Trichinella spiralis.*
16. Discuss the cause and treatment of tetany.
17. Which muscles are passed through in a McBurney incision?
18. Is there any physiologic basis for the so-called warm-up in athletics?
19. Explain the effect of exercise upon muscle.
20. Distinguish between a ligament and a tendon.
21. Human tetanus antitoxin contains no heterologous protein. Explain.
22. Biopsy is used in the diagnosis of trichinosis. Explain.
23. Distinguish between clonic and tonic convulsions.
24. What is the purpose of using both penicillin and antitoxin in the treatment of an actual case of tetanus?
25. How is tetanus toxoid made?
26. In severe cases of gas gangrene the hyperbaric chamber may be lifesaving. Explain.

Chapter 11

The cardiovascular and lymphatic systems

Modern medicine was born in 1628, for in that year the English physician William Harvey published his findings that the heart pumps the blood about the body through a well-channeled and well-organized system of vessels. Although since that time a tremendous body of facts and figures has been amassed concerning the workings of the cardiovascular system, there are still many outstanding questions in dire need of solution. Indeed, diseases of the heart and blood vessels are the leading causes of death.

THE HEART

The heart (Figs. 11-1 and 11-2) is a sac-enclosed, muscular pump located in the lower mediastinum directly behind the sternum. It is about the size of the individual's fist and somewhat pear shaped, with the apex directed to the left between the fifth and sixth intercostal spaces (about 3 inches from the sternum).

Pericardium. The sac that surrounds the heart, known as the pericardium, consists of an external layer of dense fibrous tissue and an inner serous layer (the visceral pericardium) that surrounds the heart directly and is reflected over the inner surface of the fibrous coat forming the parietal pericardium. The base of the pericardium is attached to the diaphragm, and the cavity between the visceral and parietal layers is filled with a thin serous liquid measuring between 5 and 20 ml.

Chambers. The heart is a mass of specialized muscle (myocardium) organized into four chambers—two atria and two ventricles. These chambers are lined on the inside and outside by the endocardium and the epicardium, respectively. (The epicardium is just another term for the visceral pericardium.)

Atria. The atria (sing., *atrium*), the two upper chambers, are much smaller than the ventricles and have relatively thin walls. Characteristically, on the outer side of each atrium there is an ear-shaped or auricular appendage—hence, the use of the word *auricle* for atrium. In the wall between the two atria is a small oval depression, the *fossa ovalis,* which marks the site of an opening, the *foramen ovale,* in the fetal heart (Chapter 23).

The right atrium receives the *venae cavae* (the great veins that return blood from all parts of the body) and the coronary sinus (the heart vein that returns

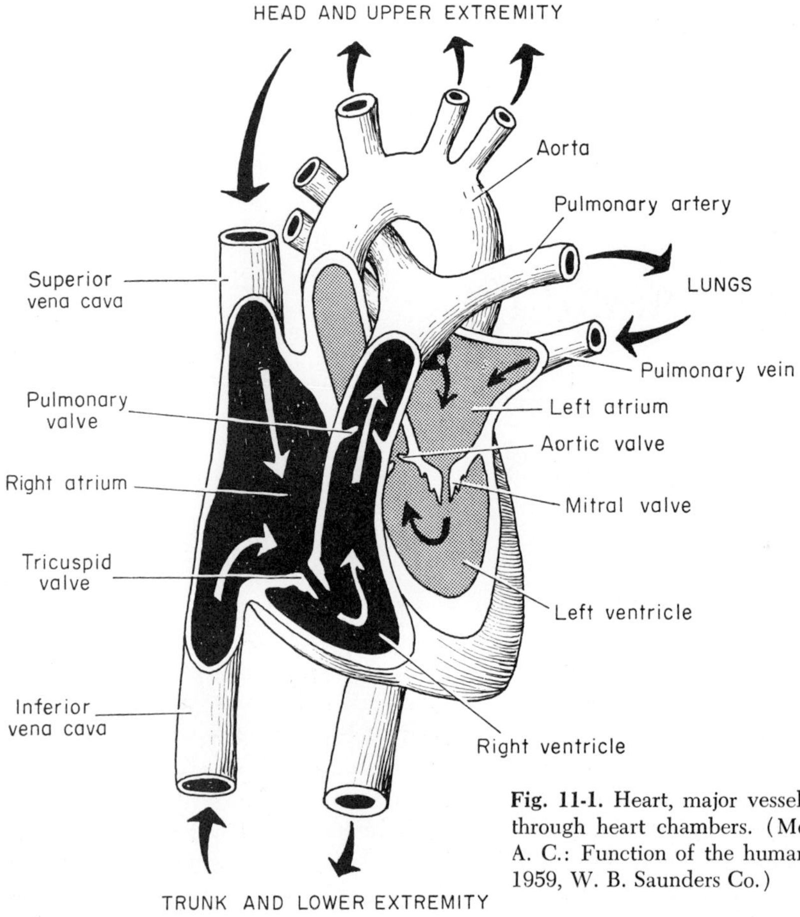

HEAD AND UPPER EXTREMITY
Aorta
Pulmonary artery
LUNGS
Superior vena cava
Pulmonary vein
Left atrium
Pulmonary valve
Aortic valve
Right atrium
Mitral valve
Tricuspid valve
Left ventricle
Inferior vena cava
Right ventricle
TRUNK AND LOWER EXTREMITY

Fig. 11-1. Heart, major vessels, and path of blood through heart chambers. (Modified from Guyton, A. C.: Function of the human body, Philadelphia, 1959, W. B. Saunders Co.)

Common carotid artery
Internal jugular vein
Subclavian artery and vein
Subclavian artery and vein
Superior vena cava
Aortic arch
R. auricle
L. auricle
R. ventricle
L. ventricle
Inferior vena cava
Abdominal aorta

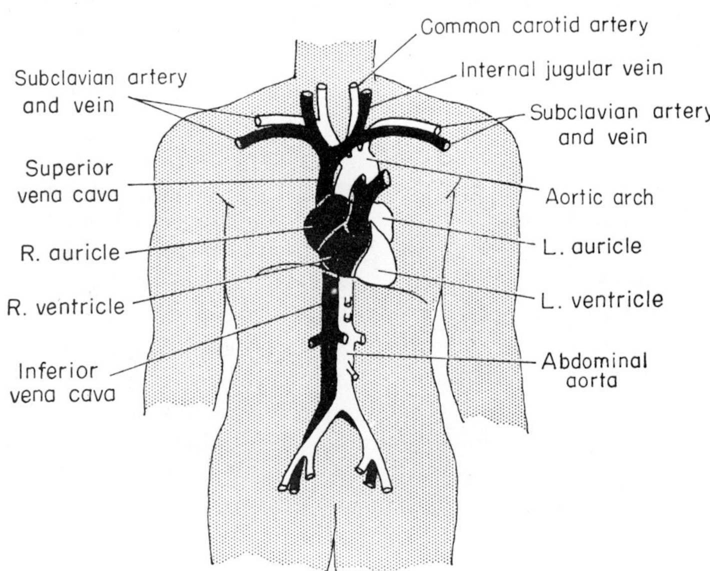

Fig. 11-2. Heart and associated vessels.

blood from the heart muscle itself). Below, the right atrium leads into the right ventricle through an opening guarded by the right *atrioventricular valve.* Because this valve has three cusps, it is commonly referred to as the *tricuspid valve.*

The left atrium receives the four pulmonary veins from the lungs. Below, it leads into the left ventricle past the left atrioventricular valve, also called the *bicuspid* (two cusps) or *mitral valve.*

Ventricles. The inside wall of the right ventricle is arranged into interlacing bundles of muscle called *trabeculae carneae* and finger-shaped projections called the *papillary muscles.* Strong white cords, the *chordae tendineae,* run from the apices of the papillary muscles to the edges of the tricuspid valve, serving to prevent the latter from being swept up into the atrium during contraction. Blood leaves the right ventricle via the pulmonary artery, and to prevent the blood from flowing back into this chamber once it has been pumped out, the opening is guarded by the *semilunar valve* (Fig. 11-1). When the blood bumps back against this valve during ventricular relaxation, its three flaps fill out and close the opening.

The left ventricle is the largest chamber and forms the apex of the heart. Its thick, powerful wall must develop great pressure to force out the blood, via the aorta, to all parts of the body. Like the right chamber, its internal architecture is characterized by trabeculae carneae, papillary muscles, and chordae tendineae. Also, the aortic opening is equipped with a semilunar valve similar to the one in the pulmonary artery.

Purkinje system. In watching the heart beat, one gets the impression that it is contracting *en masse,* and this is as it should be, for unless the muscle fibers contract almost simultaneously the heart loses its compression and pumping power. However, cardiac fibers would not contract as they do if it were not for the Purkinje system. This system, composed of modified cardiac fibers (Purkinje's fibers), transmits the cardiac impulses to all areas of the ventricles four times as fast as the regular muscle. As shown in Fig. 11-3, these fibers begin at the tiny *atrioventricular node* (AV node) in the right atrial wall, continue for a short way as the *bundle of His,* divide at the top of the ventricular septum into the right and left branches, and finally break up into separate fine strands that pass into the muscle proper.

Cardiac cycle. The heart is characterized by automatic and rhythmic beating, which can be simply and dramatically demonstrated by hooking up a piece of frog or turtle heart muscle to a kymograph. Also, excised muscle from the human atrium and ventricle beats about sixty and

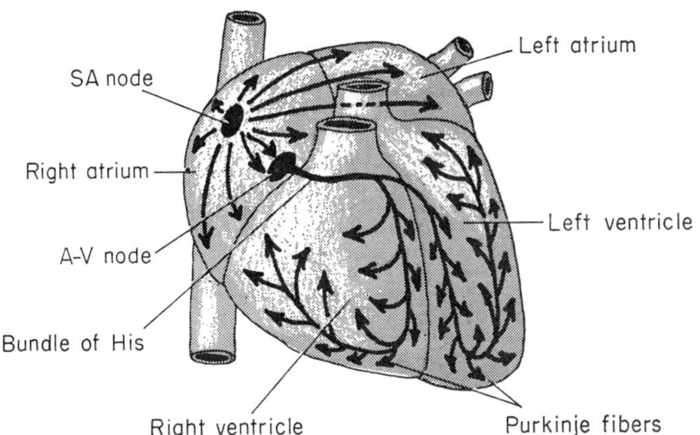

Fig. 11-3. Purkinje system. (See text.)

twenty-five times per minute, respectively. Therefore, how do we account for the fact that the heart "as a whole" is said to beat seventy-two times per minute? The answer lies in the *sino-auricular node* (SA node), located in the right posterior atrial wall just below the opening of the superior vena cava. This bit of nervous tissue, aptly called the *pacemaker,* beats and emits electrical impulses at the rate of about seventy-two times per minute. These impulses instantly flash over the atria and ventricles, stimulating these chambers to beat at the same pace. Thus, even though the atria and ventricles do have their own inherent rhythms, under normal conditions they "keep tune" to the pacemaker.

The cardiac cycle (which lasts about 0.8 second) starts with the initiation of an electrical impulse at the SA node and ends following ventricular relaxation. The impulse spreads first over the atria and then over the ventricles via the Purkinje system. This takes only about 0.2 second! In the wake of this excitation the atria and the ventricles contract, in that order.

Electrocardiograph. As the electrical impulses pass through the cardiac muscle, very weak currents are transmitted to the surface of the body. Since these currents are a reflection of the electrical happenings in the heart, they have proved of tremendous value to the researcher and the physician. To pick up, amplify, and record these currents, "recording leads" from the electrocardiograph are connected to the body via smooth metal plates moistened with a conductive paste. The sites of the body to which a given set of leads are attached yield characteristic electrical wave patterns, and so it is essential to specify the lead number: lead I, right arm–left arm; lead II, right arm–left leg; lead III, left arm–left leg; and precordial (or chest) leads, V_1, V_2, and so forth. Since heart disease is generally accompanied by abnormal

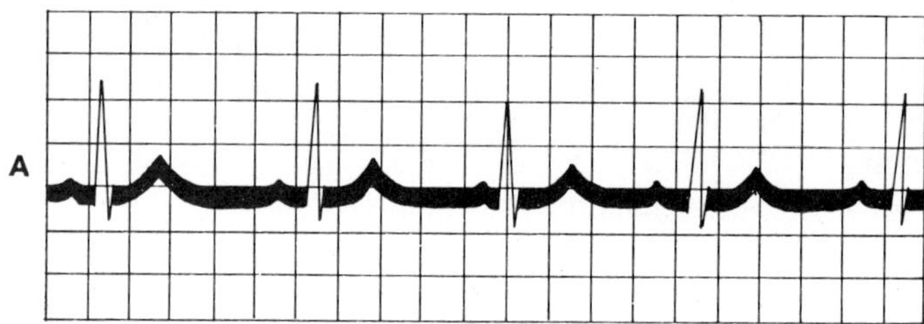

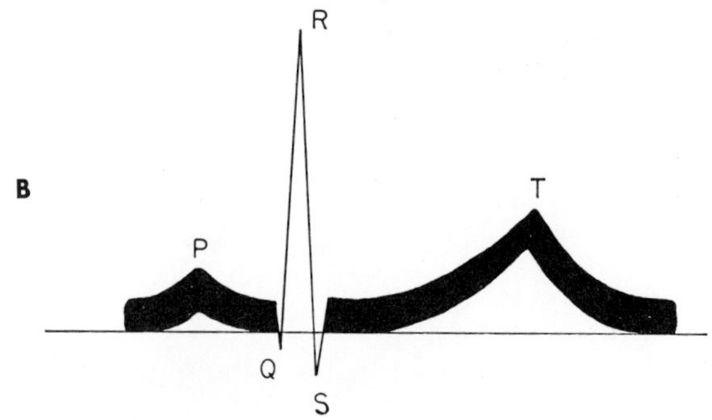

Fig. 11-4. Normal electrocardiogram. **A,** Record showing four complete cardiac cycles (lead I). **B,** Electrical waves of a single cardiac cycle. (See text.) (Adapted from Best, C. H., and Taylor, N. B.: The human body, ed. 3, New York, 1956, Holt, Rinehart & Winston, Inc. By permission.)

electrical events, the *electrocardiogram* (ECG) is of singular diagnostic importance.

A normal electrocardiogram for lead I is shown in Fig. 11-4. The *P wave* corresponds to the impulse passing through the atria, the *QRS complex* corresponds to the impulse passing through the ventricles, and the *T wave* corresponds to ventricular electrical recovery, or the return of displaced ions into the ventricular muscle fibers following the refractory period. The latter is the time during which the muscle is inexcitable.

Heart sounds. During the cardiac cycle the stethoscope discloses two sounds that resemble the syllables "lub" and "dub." The first sound (lub) is caused by the sudden closing of the atrioventricular valves when the ventricles contract; that is, the sudden closing creates vibrations in the blood and heart walls that are transmitted to the surface of the chest.

The second sound (dub) is caused by the blood bumping back against the semilunar valves at the end of systole just as the diastolic relaxation begins. Once again, this sets up vibrations in the blood and walls of the heart.

Now that we have discussed the cardiac cycle in relation to muscle contraction, electrical impulses, and audible sounds, the events shown in Fig. 11-5 can be fully appreciated.

Systole and diastole. Systole and diastole are very important expressions used in talking about the heart. Unless qualified otherwise (for example, *atrial* systole), systole means contraction of the *ventricles.* Likewise, diastole means relaxation of the ventricles. The systolic and diastolic periods can be noted by either the stethoscope or the electrocardiogram. *Mechanical* systole starts with the first sound and ends with the second, whereas *electrical* systole starts with the beginning of the QRS complex and ends with the T wave (Fig. 11-4). Conversely, electrical diastole starts with the end of the T wave and lasts until the outset of the QRS complex, and mechanical diastole starts with the second heart sound and lasts until the first heart sound.

Starling's law. Perhaps the most basic fact relating to the action of the heart is Starling's law, which states *that the volume of blood pumped by the heart is normally determined by the volume of blood returned to the heart.* Put another way, up to a point cardiac muscle contracts with greater force the more it is stretched. The diseased heart, however, frequently does not follow the "law of the heart." Indeed, in congestive heart failure the heart fails to pump effectively even normal volumes of blood.

Nervous control. Though the heart can continue to beat without nervous control, optimum performance depends upon regulatory impulses from the autonomic nervous system.

Parasympathetic nerves. The parasympathetic nerves (Chapter 19) make their way to the heart as the *vagus nerve.* Stimulation of the vagus decreases the rate of impulse formation at the SA node, decreases the rate of impulse conduction over the muscle fibers, and decreases the flow of blood through the coronary arteries. In short, parasympathetic stimulation *slows* the heart.

Sympathetic nerves. The sympathetic nerves supplying the heart act in opposition to the parasympathetic nerves; that is, they cause the heart to beat *faster* and *harder.* Sympathetic impulses are called forth in stressful situations when the body demands a more rapid flow of blood.

The pump in action. Blood returns to the heart via the *venae cavae,* which enter the right atrium. The atrium now contracts and sends the blood through the *tricuspid valve* into the relaxed right ventricle. Ventricular systole follows, and the blood is forced out through the *semilunar valve* into the *pulmonary artery* leading to the

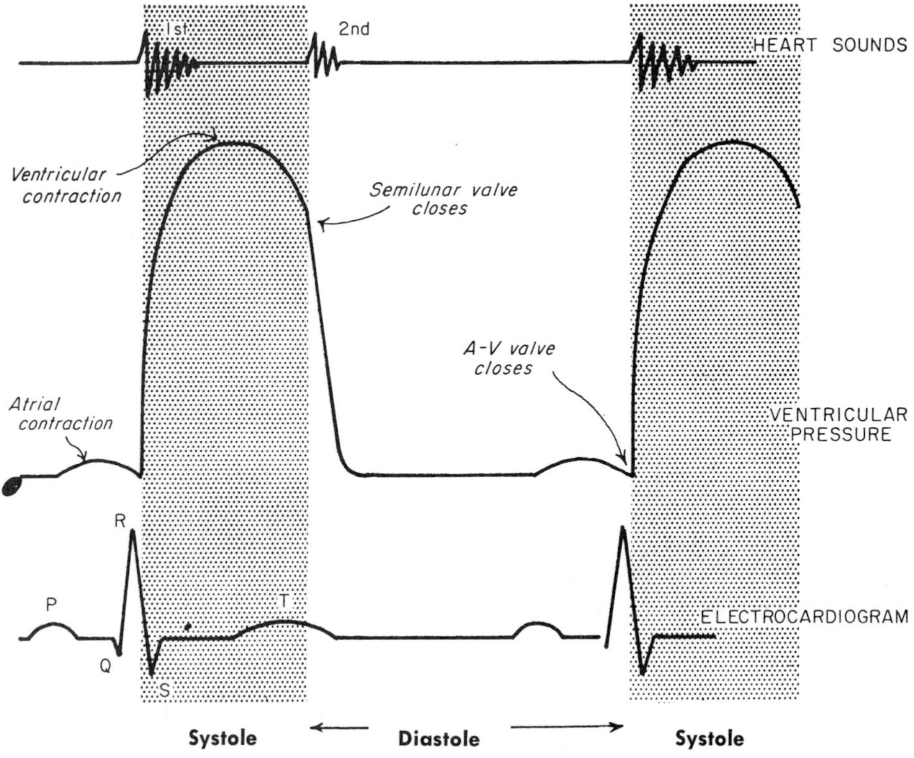

Fig. 11-5. Summary of events of the cardiac cycle as described in the text. (Modified from Guyton, A. C.: Function of the human body, Philadelphia, 1959, W. B. Saunders Co.)

lungs. Here the blood is purified and returned to the left atrium via the *pulmonary veins.* Atrial systole now forces the blood through the *bicuspid valve* into the left ventricle, whence it is ejected under great pressure to the systemic circulation via the *aorta.* These events are presented diagrammatically in Fig. 11-5.

BLOOD VESSELS

The vessels through which the blood flows include the arteries, arterioles, capillaries, venules, and veins, in that order.

Arteries. An artery is a vessel that carries blood *away* from the heart. Its thick, tough wall is composed of three coats—the *tunica intima,* the *tunica media,* and the *tunica externa* (Fig. 11-6). The tunica intima, the smooth inner lining of endothelium, is unique in that it runs uninterrupted throughout the vascular system; that is, it forms the lining of all the vessels. The tunica media, or middle coat, contains variable amounts of elastic tissue and smooth muscle. The aorta, for example, contains a great deal of elastic tissue and almost no muscle. The tunica externa, or outer coat, is composed of connective tissue. Interestingly, the larger arteries have within their walls smaller vessels, known as *vasa vasorum,* to nourish the thick tunics.

Generally, the arteries and their accompanying veins run along the flexor side of the extremities so as to be well protected against injury and stretching during movement. Also, in most cases the artery is more deeply placed than the vein.

The role of the arteries in circulation is by no means a passive one. Their elastic tissue permits them to give a little during systole, and their smooth muscle (under the direction of nervous impulses) per-

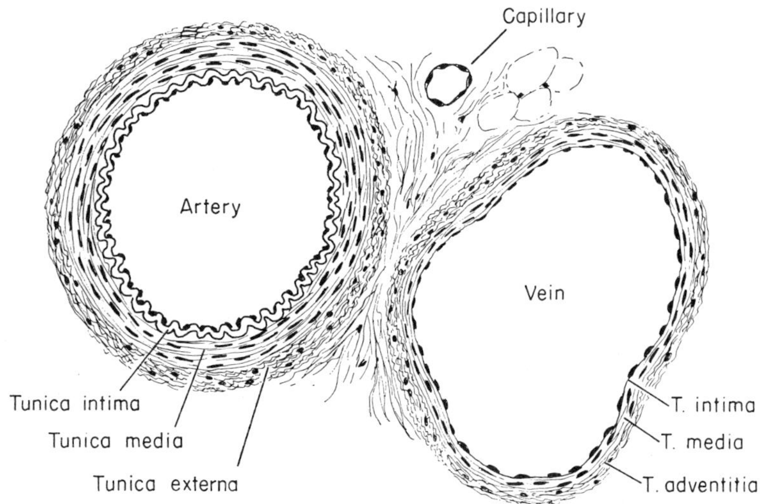

Fig. 11-6. An artery, a vein, and a capillary in cross section. (The terms *tunica externa* and *tunica adventitia* are used interchangeably.)

mits them to constrict or dilate. Indeed, nerve fibers form extensive plexuses about the arteries. As we shall soon see, these features have a life-and-death bearing on blood pressure.

Veins. A vein is a vessel that carries blood *toward* the heart. Like an artery, it has the three tunics (Fig. 11-6), but the vein wall is not as thick, as strong, or as elastic as that of an artery. Also, unlike arteries, veins collapse when empty, and many of the larger veins are equipped with *valves.* The latter structures are semilunar folds of the intima, with their free ends pointed toward the heart so as to prevent backflow. Valve-equipped veins are particularly common in the lower extremities.

Arterioles. As indicated by the suffix, arterioles are the smallest arteries. Because of the relatively large amount of smooth muscle in their walls, they are capable of being constricted or dilated well beyond the limits of the other vessels. This feature plus their great number account for the fact that, next to the heart, they play the most vital role in the control of blood pressure. By the laws of physics the arterioles *increase* the pressure when they are *constricted* and *lower* it when they are *dilated.*

Venules. As the name indicates, venules are the smallest veins. They deliver the blood from the capillaries to the veins proper.

Capillaries. Capillaries are the endothelial, one-cell thick microscopic blood channels (Fig. 11-7) omnipresent throughout the body. They are all that remain of the arterioles after the outer two coats have been removed; that is, the capillaries are essentially an interlacing network of "tunica intimas."

In a sense the capillaries are the "heart" of the circulatory system, for it is *through their walls* that the materials of life pass *into the tissues* and the cellular wastes pass into the blood. Also, the capillaries are a keystone in the maintenance of fluid balance. According to the *law of the capillaries,* the volume of fluid leaving the capillaries (through the walls) is balanced by the fluid returning through the walls. In this fashion the volume of blood and the volume of intercellular fluid are kept at a constant value. The details of this vital balancing process are discussed in Chapter 18 (inorganic metabolism).

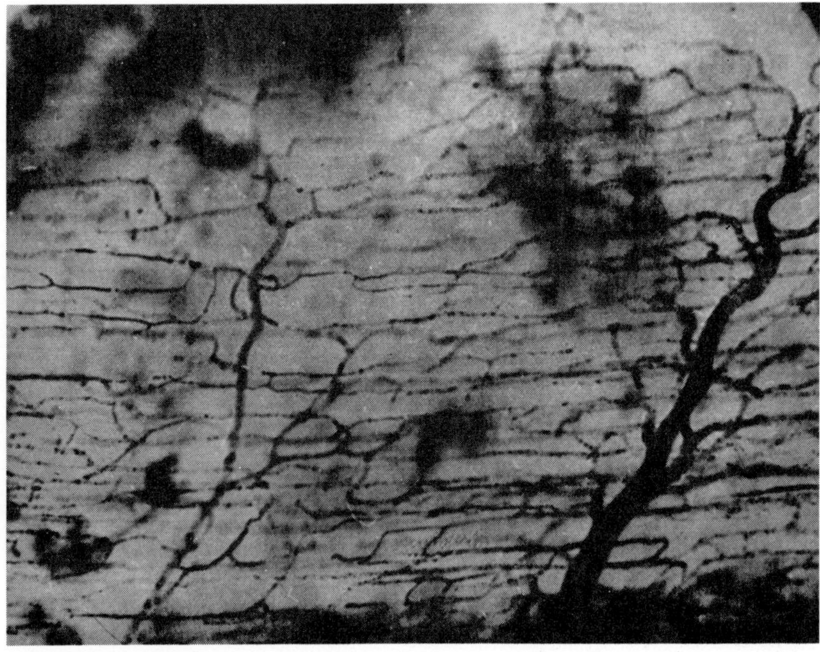

Fig. 11-7. Capillary bed of striated muscle. (×200.) (Courtesy Dr. Benjamin W. Zweifach, New York University School of Medicine.)

BLOOD PRESSURE

The blood pressure reaches its highest point during systole and its lowest point during diastole. Thus, instead of flowing along under constant pressure, arterial blood in a sense "jerks along" in sympathy with the heart.

In normal young adults the systolic pressure measures approximately 120 mm. Hg (120 millimeters of mercury), and the diastolic pressure about 80 mm. Hg. (By convention, this is expressed as 120/80.)

Measuring blood pressure. The classic and still the most commonly used device for measuring blood pressure in the laboratory is the *mercury manometer*. As shown in Fig. 11-8, a rubber tube leads an anticoagulant solution from the left arm of the instrument to a glass cannula inserted into the animal's carotid artery. Thus, the pressure of the blood is transmitted directly to the mercury. By convention, the blood pressure is taken to be the level of the mercury in the right column above that in the left, expressed in millimeters. For example, if the difference in the two levels is 100 mm., the pressure is said to be 100 mm. Hg.

For the purpose of "putting the pressure on paper," a recording arm is floated on the mercury and adjusted to write on the kymograph. As the level of the mercury bobs up and down in concert with the beating of the heart, the kymograph records not only the pressure but also affords a vivid picture of the heart in action.

In the doctor's office a special type of manometer called the *sphygmomanometer* records blood pressure indirectly (Fig. 11-9). An inflatable cuff, connected to the manometer by a rubber tube, is placed about the upper arm and pumped up by means of a rubber bulb to cut off the blood supply to the lower arm. (At all times the pressure within the cuff is registered on the manometer.) A stethoscope is then

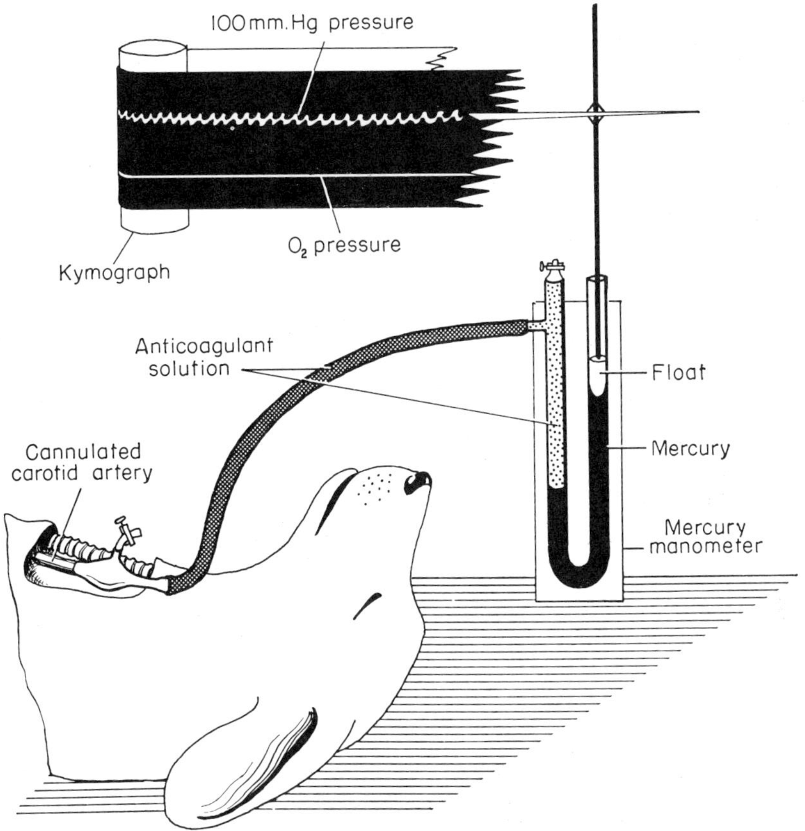

Fig. 11-8. Laboratory setup for taking blood pressure of anesthetized dog. (Modified from Guyton, A. C.: Function of the human body, Philadelphia, 1959, W. B. Saunders Co.)

placed on the flexor surface just below the cuff, and the latter is *slowly* deflated. At the instant the operator hears the first thumping sounds, he notes the reading on the manometer. This is taken as the highest or *systolic* pressure. (The sound is caused by the spurts of blood overcoming the pressure in the cuff.) The pressure in the cuff is now further reduced, and the pressure is noted on the manometer at which the sounds suddenly become dull and muffled. This is taken as the lowest or *diastolic* pressure. The reason the sounds disappear, of course, is that the blood, no longer obstructed by the cuff, flows along smoothly.

Pulse pressure. The pulse pressure is the difference between the systolic and diastolic pressures. Thus, a blood pressure of 120 over 80 (120/80) produces a pulse pressure of 40 mm. Hg. The chief factors affecting the pulse pressure are the cardiac stroke volume and arterial elasticity.

Cardiac stroke volume. The cardiac stroke volume is the volume of blood ejected by the heart at each beat. It averages about 70 ml. and ranges anywhere from 10 to 160 ml. Obviously, the greater the stroke volume, the greater will be the systolic pressure and, in turn, the greater the pulse pressure.

The relationship of stroke volume to heart rate is singularly interesting; to wit, the greater the stroke volume, the slower the heart has to beat to maintain adequate circulation. The heart rate of the well-trained athlete, for example, is often below the normal rate. In contrast, the weak

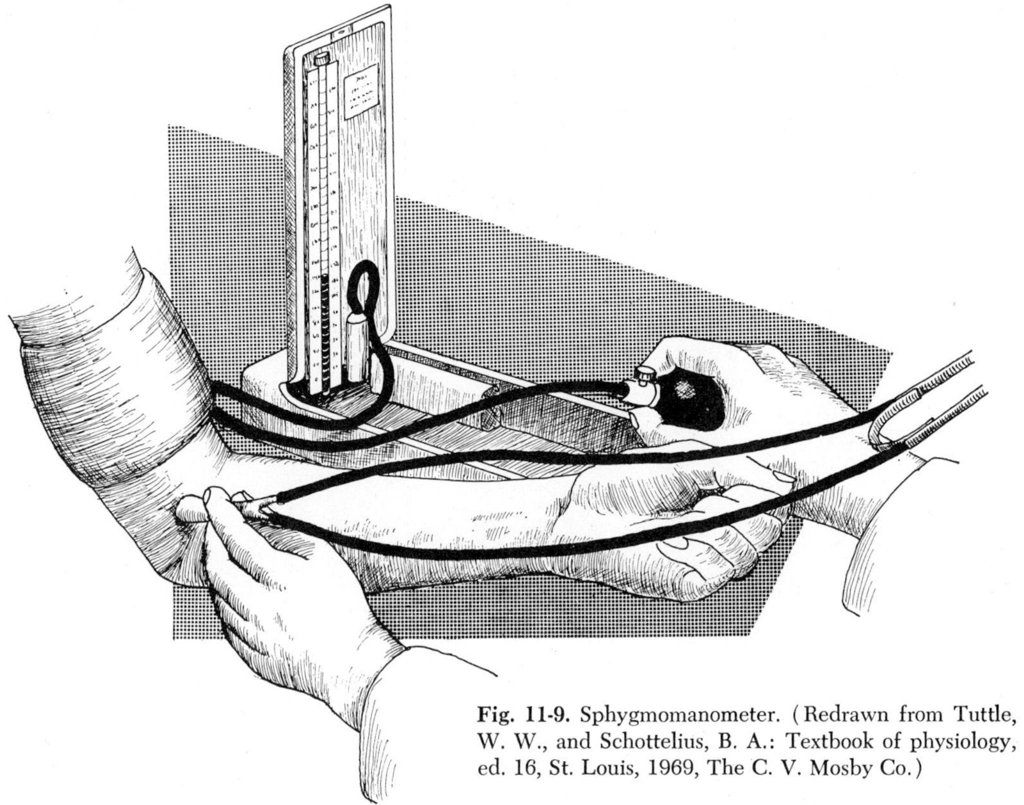

Fig. 11-9. Sphygmomanometer. (Redrawn from Tuttle, W. W., and Schottelius, B. A.: Textbook of physiology, ed. 16, St. Louis, 1969, The C. V. Mosby Co.)

heart must increase its rate to compensate for an inadequate output.

Arterial elasticity. The more elastic the arteries, the more easily the arterial system can accommodate the stroke volume; that is, by giving a little, the systolic and pulse pressures are lessened. Advancing age brings about a rise in the pulse pressure because of the gradual decrease of elastic tissue in the arterial wall. In arteriosclerosis, or hardening of the arteries, the pulse pressure may go as high as 100 mm. Hg.

Pulse wave. When a stone is thrown into the middle of a quiet pond, a wave travels out in all directions, losing its vigor the farther it goes. Also, when this wave hits the shore, it will be reflected backward and its contour will be changed.

This situation is very much like the transmission of a pulse wave; that is, with each beat a "wave of blood" spreads out through the arteries and, upon reaching the smaller arteries, is reflected backward. What happens to both the pulse pressure and the pulse wave from the aorta to the venae cavae is shown in a most vivid fashion in Fig. 11-10.

As the blood travels away from the heart, there is not only a dampening of the pulse pressure and pulse wave but also a fall in arterial pressure, dropping almost to zero (Fig. 11-10) in the great veins. This is easy to understand if we recall that the *total* cross section of the vessels increases tremendously in passing from the aorta to the capillaries. That is, since the *overall* resistance to the flow of blood progressively decreases, the pressure decreases.

Mean pressure. As we have seen, the arterial blood pressure throughout the cardiac cycle is not even, jumping from a low of 80 mm. Hg to a high of 120 mm. Hg. Physiologically, the so-called mean

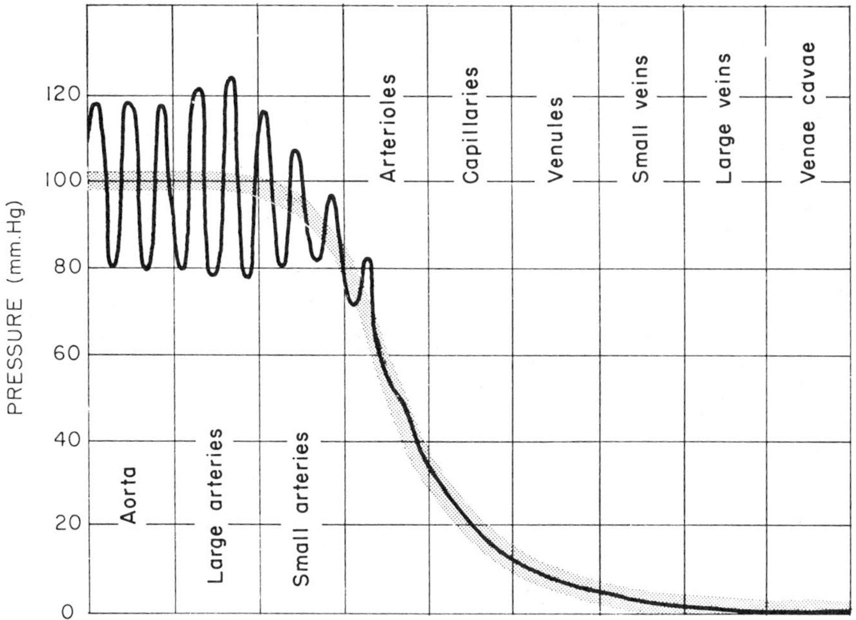

Fig. 11-10. Blood pressure curve showing the pressure gradients in different divisions of the circulatory system.

pressure is more significant than either the systolic or or diastolic pressure because this is the pressure that determines the average rate at which blood flows through the body. The mean pressure, found by averaging the pressures at all stages of the cardiac cycle, is about 100 mm. Hg in the resting condition. Generally, this figure can be arrived at by averaging the systolic and diastolic pressures.

Factors affecting arterial blood pressure. The mean arterial blood pressure depends upon the *cardiac output, total peripheral resistance, blood volume,* and *arterial elasticity* (p. 230). Cardiac output, or the rate at which blood is pumped, depends essentially upon the *heart rate* and the *stroke volume* (p. 229), the latter in turn depending upon the forcefulness of the contraction of the heart and the inrush of blood to be pumped. Peripheral resistance, or resistance to blood flow in the vessels, depends principally upon the *caliber* of the arterioles, the *number* of open capillaries, and blood viscosity. As stated previously, vasoconstriction increases blood pressure and vasodilatation decreases blood pressure. The number of open capillaries—the more open, the lower the pressure—depends upon such factors as temperature, metabolites, and blood flow through the arterioles supplying the capillary bed.

Capillary regulation. When for some reason the blood volume becomes too great, the concomitant rise in capillary pressure forces more fluid through the capillary walls (into the tissues), thereby *lowering* the blood volume and blood pressure. Conversely, loss of blood from the circulation lowers the blood pressure and *decreases* capillary filtration. As a result, the *relatively greater osmotic pressure* of the *blood will draw water from the tissues into the circulation.* (The mechanism of fluid movement across the capillary wall is presented in detail in Chapter 18.) Thus, the shift of fluid across the capillary wall plays an important role in regulating the blood volume and thereby the *blood pressure.*

Kidney regulation. Like the capillaries,

the kidneys regulate arterial pressure by acting upon the blood volume. After an excessive intake of fluid the kidneys step up the production of urine. On the other hand, they stop putting out urine following hemorrhage so that ingested fluid will remain in circulation.

The mechanisms involved in this renal control are the blood pressure itself and two hormones—the *antidiuretic hormone* and *aldosterone* (Chapter 22). In brief, an *increase* in blood pressure, resulting from an *increase* in blood volume, enhances glomerular filtration, the first step in the production of urine. Obviously, a drop in pressure has the opposite effect. The antidiuretic hormone and aldosterone decrease the output of urine by acting upon the renal tubules (Chapter 22). Both hormones are released when there is a drop in blood volume.

Nervous regulation. A variety of nervous reflexes regulate *heart rate* and degree of *arteriolar constriction* and thereby the arterial pressure. These reflexes operate through the *vasomotor center* in the medulla oblongata. This center has four areas which, upon stimulation, cause *vasoconstriction, vasodilatation, cardio-acceleration* (increased heart rate), and *cardio-inhibition* (decreased heart rate). The majority of impulses from these areas are transmitted down the spinal cord and over the sympathetic nervous system to the heart and blood vessels. To a lesser degree, impulses are carried by the parasympathetic system.

The vasomotor center is stimulated directly and most powerfully by medullary *ischemia* (deficiency of blood) and by an *increase* in the blood concentration of *carbon dioxide;* that is, the vasoconstriction and cardio-acceleration areas are caused to step up the transmission of impulses to the blood vessels and heart, respectively. The result, of course, is an *increase* in ar-

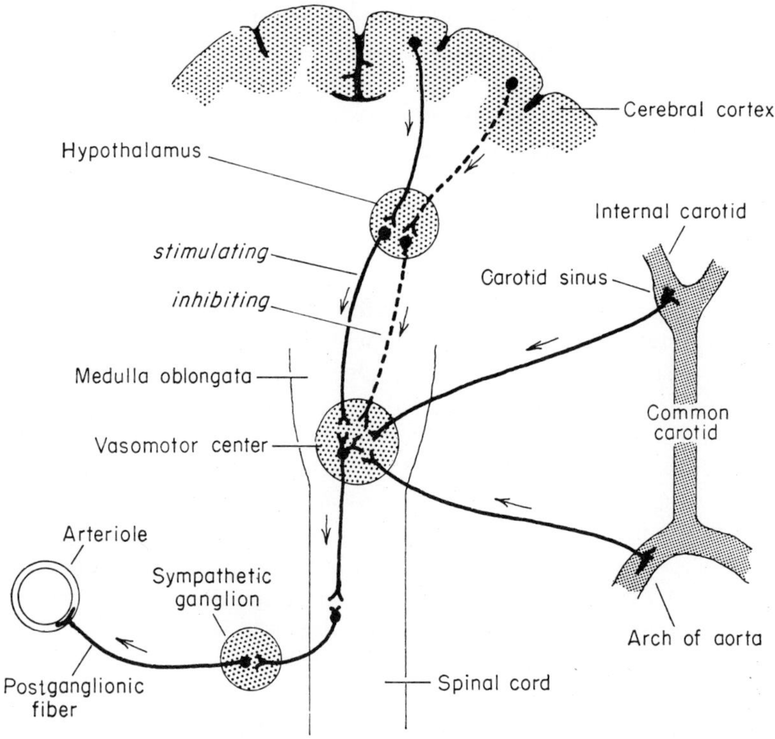

Fig. 11-11. Nervous regulation of blood pressure via the vasomotor center. (See text.)

terial pressure. In this fashion the body rids its tissues of accumulated waste products (of which carbon dioxide is only one) and remedies an embarrassed circulation, particularly to the brain.

Indirectly, the vasomotor center is affected by specialized sensory nerve endings, called *pressoreceptors* or *baroreceptors*, located in the walls of the *aortic arch* and *carotid sinuses* (Fig. 11-11). When the arterial pressure starts to rise, the pressoreceptors are stimulated and step up their transmission of impulses which, upon arriving at the center, trigger the vasodilatation and cardio-inhibition areas and thereby *lower* arterial pressure. Conversely, when the arterial pressure *drops* below normal, the pressoreceptors send fewer impulses to these areas and the pressure *rises* as a result of impulses released by the cardio-acceleration and vasoconstriction areas. These feedback moderating reflexes are commonly referred to as *Marey's law*.

Another possibility not to be ignored is the influence of the higher brain centers, as indicated in Fig. 11-11. In other words, emotion, rage, and "nervousness" elevate blood pressure by stimulating the cardio-acceleration and vasoconstriction areas via the hypothalamus.

Venous blood pressure. The venous pressure is the blood pressure in the veins, and in the standing position it varies from about −10 mm. Hg in the head to +90 mm. Hg in the feet. When a person is moving about, however, muscle contraction "milks along" the blood so that the hydrostatic pressures in the legs and feet are greatly reduced. This action, of course, depends upon the proper functioning of the valves, for if the valves are faulty, the blood slips back, thereby elevating the hydrostatic pressure and producing varicose veins.

Venous pressure throughout the body is determined mainly by the pressure in the right atrium. Since this pressure is just about zero, venous blood always flows toward the heart. Obviously, if the atrial pressure should rise significantly above zero, the venous return would be interfered with and the circulation would be embarrassed. As a matter of fact, increased atrial and venous pressures are the cardinal features of heart failure (p. 243).

As venous pressure within the right atrium increases, certain pressoreceptors in the great veins and atrial wall are stimulated and impulses are relayed to the cardio-acceleration center, thereby *increasing* the heart rate. The opposite occurs when venous pressure decreases. This response to changes in venous pressure is called the *Bainbridge reflex*.

BLOOD FLOW

The purpose of circulation is to effect a flow of blood through the tissues. At rest the normal heart pumps about 5000 ml. (over 5 quarts) of blood a minute. However, during exercise the flow can reach the phenomenal value of 35,000 ml. (36 quarts!) a minute? It is of interest to note that the flow of blood from the heart is equal to the *stroke volume times the heart rate*. For example, if we take the normal volume and rate to be 70 ml. and 72, respectively, the heart pumps 5040 ml. per minute.

Of the 5000 ml. of blood leaving the heart per minute, approximately 25 percent (1250 ml.) flows through the muscles, 25 percent through the kidneys, 15 percent (750 ml.) through the abdominal region, 10 percent (500 ml.) through the liver, 8 percent (400 ml.) through the brain, 4 percent (200 ml.) through the coronary vessels, and 13 percent (650 ml.) through the remaining areas.

The flow of blood through any given vessel of the body can be expressed according to Poiseuille's law:

$$\text{Blood flow} = \frac{\text{Pressure} \times (\text{Diameter})^4}{\text{Length} \times \text{Viscosity}}$$

In succinct language this formula states that blood flow is *directly* proportional to the blood pressure, *directly* proportional to the fourth power of the vessel's caliber, *inversely* proportional to the vessel's length, and *inversely* proportional to blood viscosity. All these factors, of course, can be easily demonstrated in the physics laboratory.

Vessel diameter. Of the physical factors shown in the formula, diameter, or caliber, is by far the most important, for in a flash the autonomic system can produce vasoconstriction or vasodilatation.

Exercise. During exercise the muscles demand extra oxygen and nourishment, and in an attempt to meet this demand, new capillaries open and the arterioles throughout the muscles dilate to enhance the blood flow. However, since vasodilatation reduces blood pressure, it is obvious that the vessels in other areas of the body (the skin, kidneys, liver, and gastrointestinal tract) must be constricted. In essence, then, the body is *shunting* blood from its *reservoirs* to where it is most needed.

Temperature control. The shifting of blood to and from the skin plays a vital role in temperature control. When the body temperature rises, the vasomotor center dilates the arterioles of the skin and thus shunts more warm blood to the surface. This steps up heat loss and restores the temperature to normal. On the other hand, when the temperature starts to drop, the arterioles are constricted and more blood is shunted from the skin to the interior. In this manner heat is conserved and temperature is maintained.

Hemorrhage. When large amounts of blood are lost, the blood pressure falls to dangerously low levels. In this instance the body defends itself by constricting the vessels in the less vital areas so as to assure an adequate flow of blood through the brain and heart muscle.

Reactive hyperemia. Reactive hyperemia is a classic example of the ability of the body to perform a difficult job in a simple way. Our present concern involves the task of increasing the blood flow to a given area without disrupting the whole circulation. As the metabolism in a given tissue increases, the need for more blood (to bring nutrients and remove wastes) is met simply and effectively by local vasodilatation, or reactive hyperemia. Conversely, in a low state of metabolism, the vessels constrict and thereby reduce the blood flow. In this way the tissues of the body are supplied with no more or no less than they need. This ingenious mechanism is thus the epitome of not only simplicity but also efficiency.

The exact mechanism responsible for reactive hyperemia is not known. It could be that vessels dilate because the muscles in their walls relax due to lack of nutrients, or it could be that they dilate in response to such waste products as lactic acid or carbon dioxide.

THE CIRCULATION

Let us now turn our attention to the general circulation (Fig. 11-12) and the major arteries (Fig. 11-13) and veins (Fig. 11-14).

Coronary circulation. It always comes as a surprise to some to learn that the blood does not pass directly from the chambers into the heart wall. Like other organs, the heart has its own blood supply system.

Immediately above the aortic valve two small arteries—the *left* and *right coronaries* (Fig. 11-15)—take leave of the great vessel and run along the surface of the heart, branching as they go and finally penetrating the myocardium. From the venules within the muscle the blood is directed into the coronary veins and thence into the right atrium via the *coronary sinus.*

The flow through the coronary arteries depends upon cardiac activity and sympathetic control. As in other tissues, increased activity will speed up the flow via reactive hyperemia. Also, the movement of the beating heart massages the vessels, thereby moving along the blood inside. Sympathetic stimulation improves coronary flow directly by vasodilatation and indirectly by increasing the heart rate.

It is of singular interest to learn that the coronary blood flow is greater during diastole than during systole. This is in stark contrast to the circulation in other areas of the body. The reason, of course, is that during systole the vessels are squeezed and occluded. An adequate coronary flow, therefore, is more dependent upon diastolic pressure than upon systolic pressure.

Pulmonary circulation. The pulmonary circulation refers to the flow of blood between the heart and the lungs (Fig. 11-12) for the purpose of absorbing oxygen and releasing carbon dioxide. The blood leaves the right ventricle via the *pulmonary artery* (guarded by a semilunar valve) and returns to the left atrium via the four *pulmonary veins.* In the lungs the capillaries surround

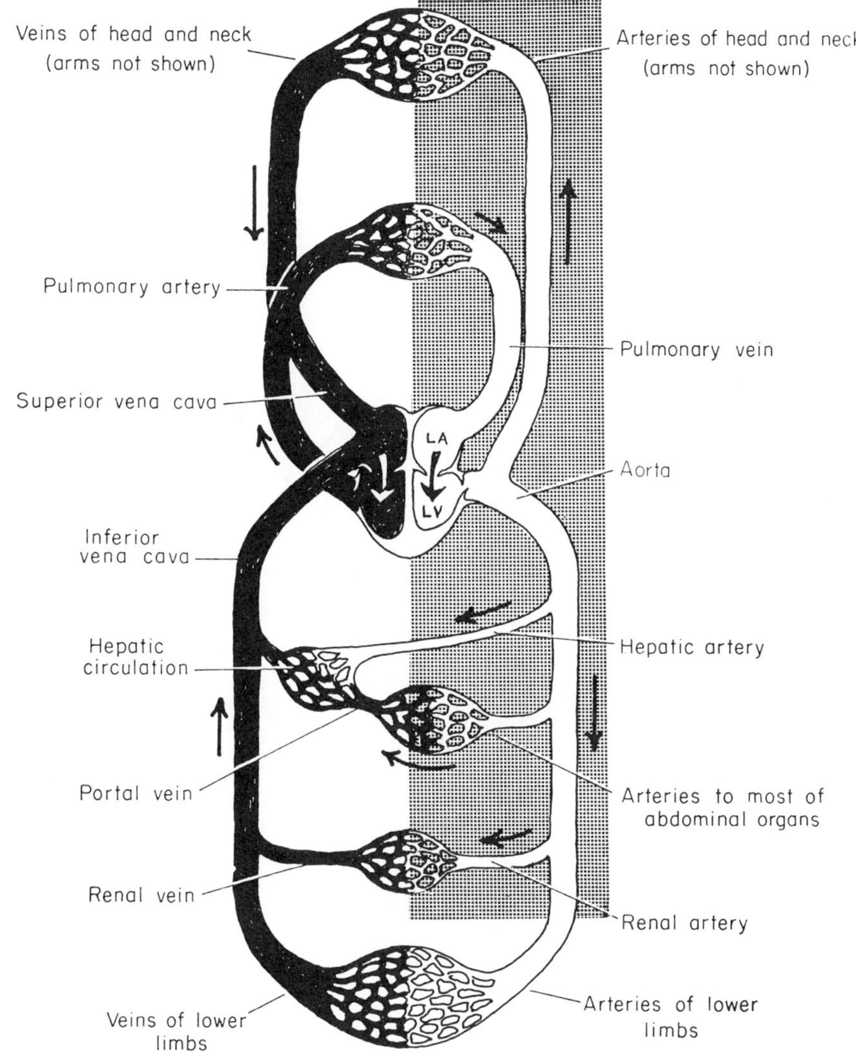

Fig. 11-12. General circulation.

the alveoli so as to make possible the exchange of gases. These respiratory features are discussed in Chapter 13.

The resistance to the flow of blood in the pulmonary circuit is so low that the arterial pressure in this area averages from about 13 to 87 mm. Hg less than the mean systemic arterial pressure! As a matter of fact, the vessels of the lung dilate so easily that the pulmonary pressure does not rise greatly even during exercise when the heart is pumping out several quarts of blood a minute. In general, the pulmonary flow follows the systemic flow; that is, the greater the flow through the systemic vessels, the greater is the flow through the pulmonary vessels, and vice versa.

Cerebral circulation. Relatively speaking, the brain receives a rich blood supply. Blood is pumped to the undersurface through the two *internal carotid* arteries and the two *vertebral* arteries. The former

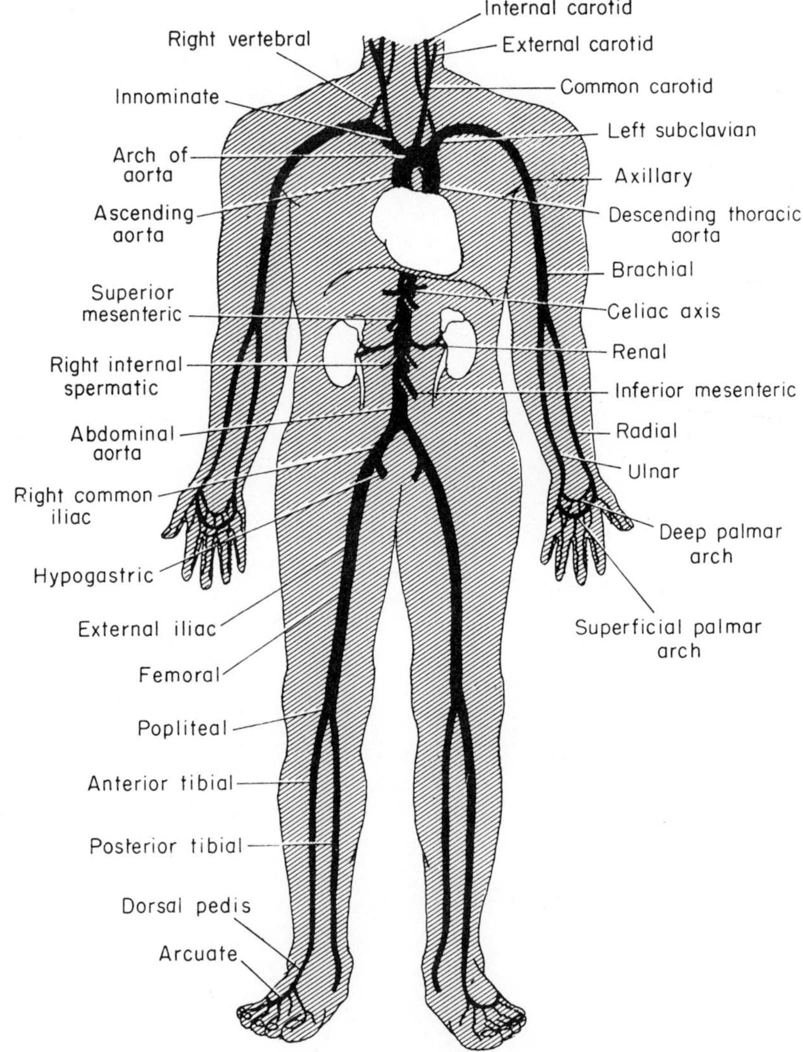

Fig. 11-13. Major arteries of the body. Note that there is only *one* innominate artery. (Modified from Anthony, C. P.: Textbook of anatomy and physiology, ed. 6, St. Louis, 1963, The C. V. Mosby Co.)

join the *circle of Willis* and the latter join the *basilar* artery, from which branches arise and spread over the surface of the brain (Fig. 11-16).

The veins of the brain are highly characteristic. In contrast to the usual architecture, they are actually *sinuses* that have been channeled in the fibrous lining, or dura mater, of the skull. Also, in contrast to the veins in most other regions of the body, the cerebral sinuses do not collapse. The sinuses drain into the jugular veins.

The flow of blood through the brain depends upon reactive hyperemia and sympathetic control. However, although activity or inactivity can bring about a change in blood flow in a localized area, it is of singular interest to note that the overall cerebral flow changes very little indeed. This is certainly fortunate, for nervous tissue can easily become excited by a sharp

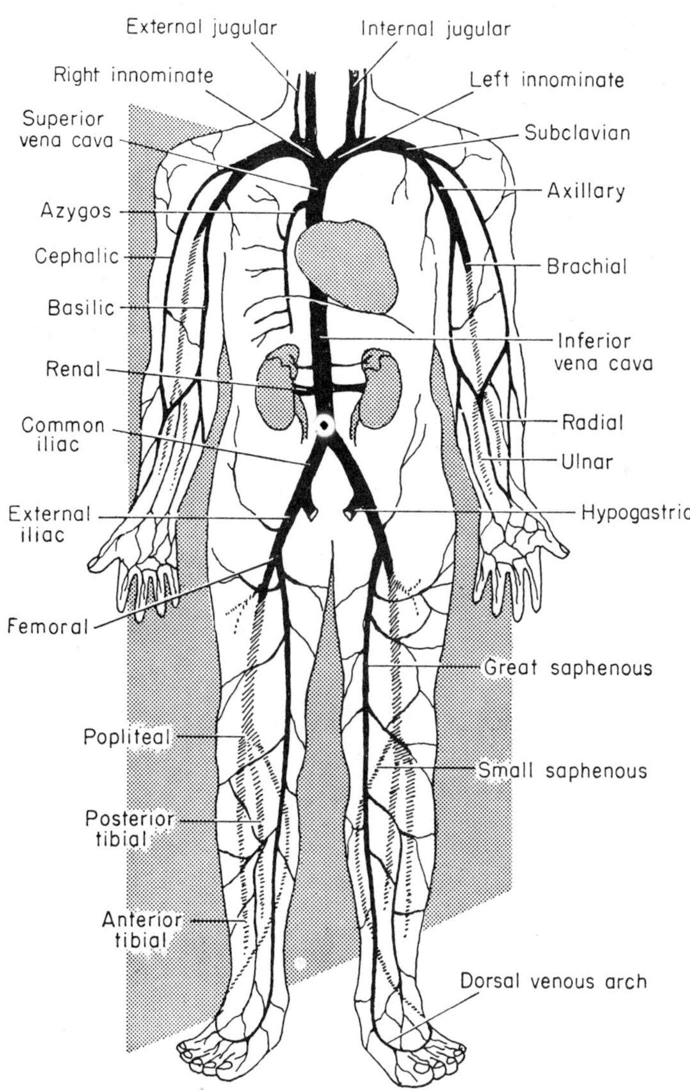

Fig. 11-14. Major veins of the body.

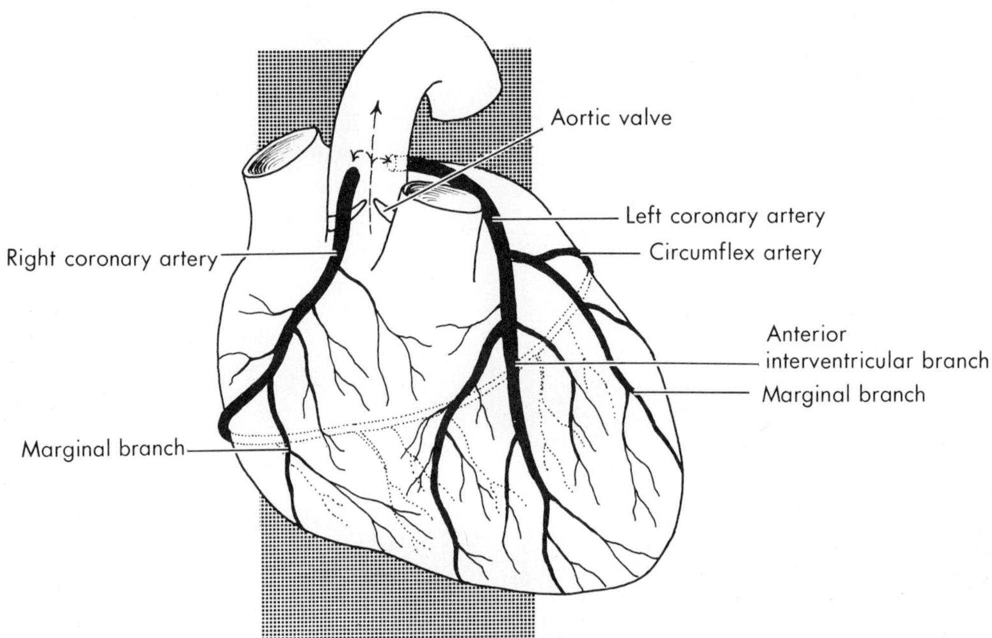

Fig. 11-15. Coronary circulation.

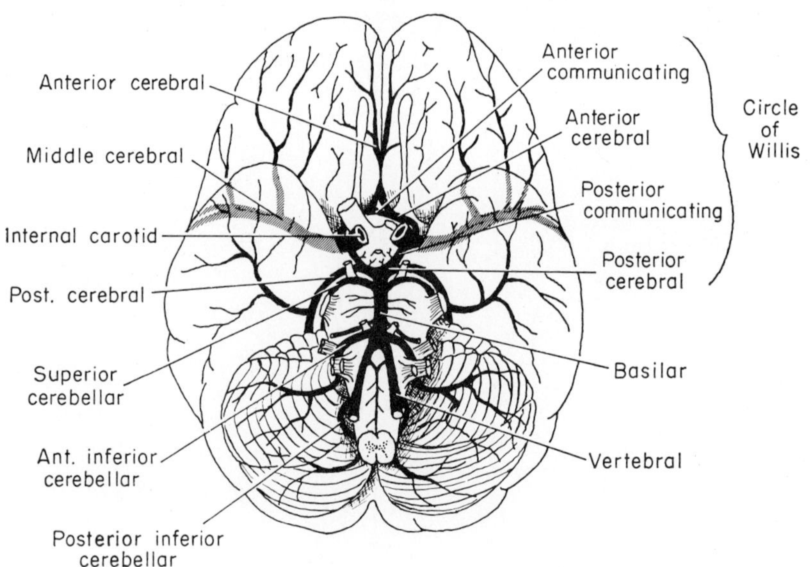

Fig. 11-16. Cerebral circulation. (Modified from Francis, C. C., and Farrell, G. L.: Integrated anatomy and physiology, ed. 3, St. Louis, 1957, The C. V. Mosby Co.)

rise and depressed by a sharp drop in blood pressure.

Portal circulation. The major anatomic features of the portal system are shown in Fig. 11-17. As can be seen, the system is composed of veins leading blood from the spleen and intestines through the liver and eventually into the *inferior vena cava.*

Intestinal blood is heavily laden with microbes from the gastrointestinal tract, and if it were to pass directly into the general circulation, infection would be the rule and not the exception. To remove these microbes (and other abdominal debris), the minute blood sinuses of the liver are equipped with Kupffer's cells, miraculous scavengers that devour everything in sight via phagocytosis. In addition to this defense mechanism, the liver also detoxifies an endless variety of ingested poisons and toxins. Once again, insult to the general circulation is prevented.

The liver is placed in the path of intestinal blood for another reason, too, and that is to remove and store absorbed nutrients, particularly glucose and amino acids. In this unique fashion the liver prevents fluctuations in the blood concentrations of these nutrients between meals.

Muscular circulation. Blood flow through the muscles is proportional to the amount of work being performed. That is, as contraction increases, the metabolites increase, which, in turn, causes vasodilatation (and an increased flow) via reactive hyperemia. Also, muscle contraction releases more carbon dioxide to the circulation, which increases the arterial pressure by acting on the vasomotor center. During exercise the latter mechanism is especially important in bringing blood to the muscles.

Cutaneous circulation. The flow of blood through the skin serves not only to supply nourishment but also to regulate body temperature and blood pressure.

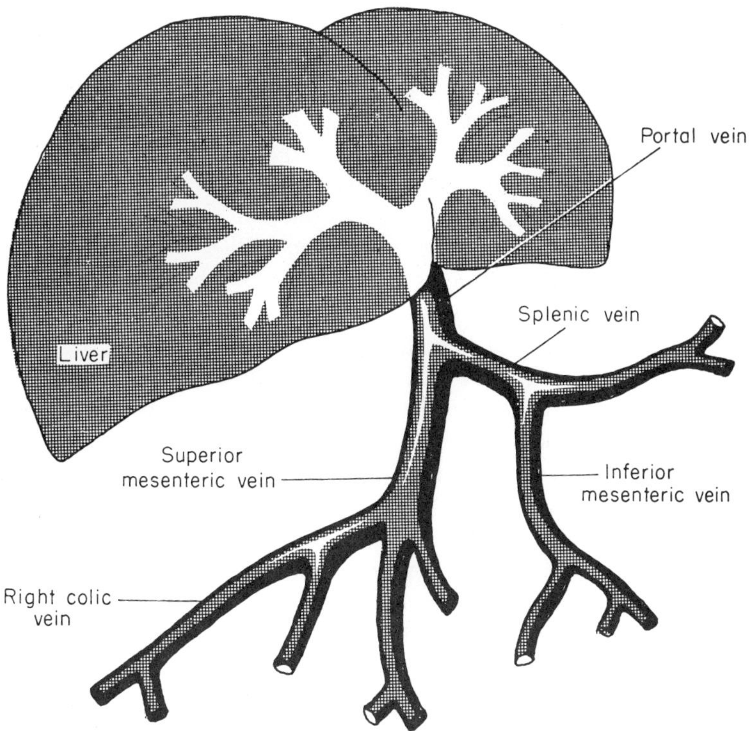

Fig. 11-17. Portal circulation.

LYMPHATIC SYSTEM

The lymphatic system includes the lymph, lymphatic vessels, and lymph nodes—the "system proper"—and an assortment of structures and glands characterized by the presence of lymphocytic cells—namely, the *spleen, tonsils, thymus,* and *lymphatic nodules (Peyer's patches)* of the intestine.

The lymphatics originate among the cells as microscopic capillaries that come together to form the progressively larger lymphatic vessels, much as twigs on a tree coalesce into branches. Finally, these vessels join together to form two main channels—the *thoracic duct* and the *right lymphatic ducts.* The thoracic duct is about 16 inches in length and originates in the lumbar region as a dilated structure called the *cisterna chyli.* It runs up the trunk and finally empties its lymph into the bloodstream at the juncture of the *left* internal jugular and subclavian veins. The right lymphatic ducts (sometimes there is just one) join the venous system at the juncture of the *right* internal jugular and subclavian veins. Except for the right arm, right upper chest, and right side of the head, which are drained by the right lymphatic ducts, all lymph flows into the thoracic duct.

Located along the lymphatic vessels, particularly in the inguinal, abdominal, cervical, and axillary regions, are small organs called *lymph nodes* (Fig. 11-18). These structures, composed mainly of lymphoid tissue compartmentalized by fibrous partitions, are situated in the path of the lymph as it flows from the afferent lymphatics into the efferent lymphatics (Fig. 11-18).

For all practical purposes, lymph is nothing more than intercellular or interstitial fluid that has left the tissue spaces and passed into the lymphatics. This fluid enters the lymphatic capillaries whenever the tissue pressure rises. Once within the vessels, lymph is massaged onward by the pressing of the muscles against the walls of the vessels. This action would be of no avail, however, if it were not for the presence of valves similar in structure and function to those found in the veins.

Obviously, lymph flows at a snail's pace. Whereas 5 to 6 quarts of blood pass through the heart per minute, only a fraction of an ounce of lymph passes through the lymphatics per minute. Also, the rate of flow varies greatly, depending upon the degree of physical activity.

Function. From the foregoing it can be seen that one function of the lymphatic system is the removal of excess tissue fluid. But this is by no means its only role, for as the fluid is removed, dead cells, bacteria, and other intercellular debris are swept away and filtered out in the lymph nodes. Here special cells digest the debris, converting it into harmless breakdown products.

Too, the lymph plays the vital role of returning to the blood the *protein* that is continuously seeping through the capillary walls into the intercellular fluid. If this were permitted to accumulate, the interstitial osmotic pressure would progressively rise and draw fluid from the circulation into the tissues, producing edema. Thus, the lymphatic system plays a key role in fluid balance. Further, certain cells within the nodes—called *plasma cells*—bolster the immunity of the body by producing *antibodies.* Finally, the nodes—along with the spleen—manufacture the *lymphocytes* of the blood (Chapter 12).

Spleen. The spleen is an ovoid organ located in the left hypochondrium directly below the diaphragm (Chapter 14). Histologically, it resembles a lymph node and is characterized by numerous venous sinuses. Indeed, it is the sinuses that allow the spleen to swell up with blood to a volume of 1000 ml. or shrink to a volume of 100 ml. In this way the spleen serves as one of the chief *blood reservoirs* of the body, removing blood from the circulation during times of quietude or plenty and releasing it in times of stress or deprivation.

The spleen also functions to cleanse the blood. Throughout the pulp and lining of the sinus walls are special phagocytic cells that devour bacteria and the debris remaining from the breakdown of fragile red cells. Another known function is the manufacture of *lymphocytes* (a type of white blood cell), a function it shares with other lymphoid tissue such as lymph nodes. Also, in the fetus the spleen, along with the liver

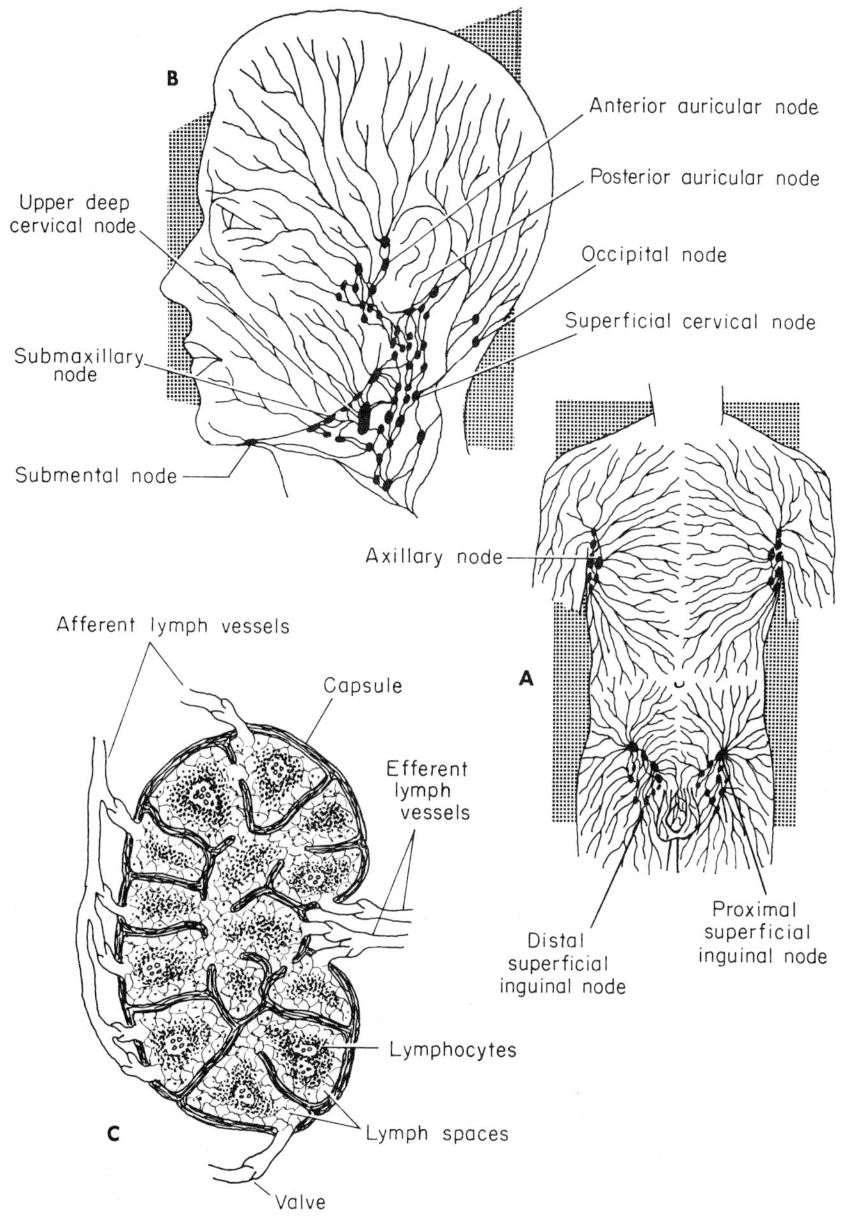

Fig. 11-18. Lymphatic system. **A,** General distribution of lymphatic vessels of the trunk. **B,** General distribution of lymphatic vessels of the head. **C,** Structure of a lymph node. (**A** and **B** after Sappey; modified from Francis, C. C: Introduction to human anatomy, ed. 5, St. Louis, 1968, The C. V. Mosby Co.)

and bone marrow, aids in the production of *red cells.*

Tonsils. The tonsils are aggregates of lymph nodules situated beneath the epithelium of the mouth and pharynx. Those of chief concern are the *palatine* tonsils (p. 266), *pharyngeal* tonsils (p. 265), and *lingual* tonsils. The tonsils produce monocytes, lymphocytes, and other scavenger cells that serve to protect the mouth, nose, and throat against bacterial attack.

Thymus. The thymus is a flat, pinkish gray, two-lobed gland lying high in the chest behind the sternum. Large in relation to the rest of the body in fetal life and in early childhood, by the age of puberty it has stopped growing and begins to atrophy. The thymus is the *source* of the small lymphocytes of the lymph nodes that are involved in *delayed hypersensitivity* and the *rejection* of skin grafts. This is underscored by the fact that infants born without the thymus develop no delayed hypersensitivity in response to various antigens and sometimes completely fail to reject a graft of skin from an unrelated donor. Interestingly, however, these infants *are not* deficient in antibodies, which indicates that the lymph node plasma cells *do not* originate in the thymus. Thus, there appears to be two separate immunologic systems—one dependent upon the thymus and the other independent of it. The plasma cells originate in the bone marrow and perhaps mature elsewhere before taking up residence in the lymph nodes.

CARDIOVASCULAR AND LYMPHATIC DISEASES

Diseases of the heart and vessels are the leading causes of death. Although a tremendous amount of money and effort has gone into cardiovascular research, many of the basic questions remain unanswered. As we learn more about the challenging complexities of the body, however, the answers will be found in due time. Indeed, in certain areas major breakthroughs appear to be coming in the foreseeable future.

Diseases of the heart. Heart disease may strike the valves, the endocardium, the pericardium, or the myocardium. Also, the patient may be born with an opening between the chambers. Any defect that is present at birth is referred to as congenital heart disease. Abnormalities of the heart inhibit its function as a pump and thereby endanger the body as a whole.

Congenital heart disease. In contrast to the high incidence of acquired heart disease, congenital diseases are relatively—and fortunately—uncommon. These conditions are caused by failure of normal development in utero. Since cyanosis in many instances is the first symptom to appear (because of poor oxygenation), we often hear the expression *blue baby.* Of singular interest is the fact that clubbing of the fingers frequently accompanies congenital heart disease.

Some of the more common congenital disorders of the heart are *pulmonary stenosis, atrial-septal defect,* and *patent interventricular septum.* The former condition, a *narrowing* of the opening between the pulmonary artery and the right ventricle, decreases the flow of blood through the lungs, on the one hand, and the return of blood to the heart, on the other. The "patent" defects embarrass the circulation by permitting the blood to flow directly between the atria and between the ventricles.

Other congenital defects include faulty valves, absence of valves, and a bizarre malformation called *tetralogy of Fallot.* The latter condition is characterized by four lesions—pulmonary stenosis, patent interventricular septum, enlargement of the right ventricle, and displacement of the aorta to the right.

Since it involves the heart indirectly, another congenital defect of interest is *patent ductus arteriosus* (Chapter 23). When the ductus arteriosus fails to close after birth, the heart has the added burden of pumping more blood than is needed

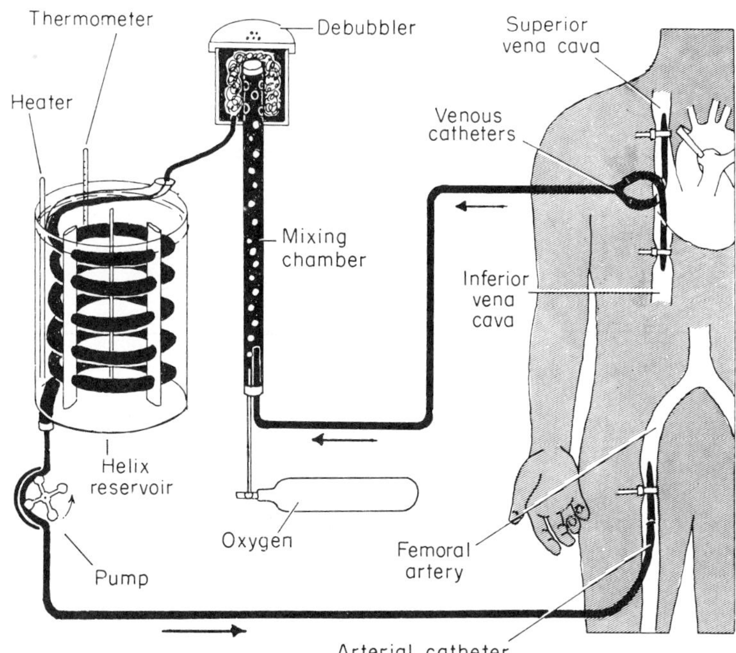

Fig. 11-19. Heart-lung machine. The blood flows from the two catheters inserted in the venae cavae to the bottom of the mixing chamber. Bubbles of oxygen rising through the chamber are removed in the debubbler. The blood then flows into the helix reservoir and is pumped back into the femoral artery of the patient.

through the lungs. This abnormal situation not only strains the heart but in later life also damages the lungs as a result of the high pressure in the pulmonary vessels.

In no other area of cardiovascular research have there been more fruitful or more dramatic results than in the surgical management of congenital heart disease. The surgeon can now ligate a patent ductus arteriosus, repair and replace bad valves, and patch openings between the chambers. Indeed, even the tetralogy of Fallot has yielded to the needle and scalpel. Such procedures demand an artificial heart and an artificial lung to keep the body alive during the operation. The essentials of the so-called *heart-lung machine* are shown in Fig. 11-19.

Rheumatic heart disease. The relationship between rheumatic heart disease (rheumatic fever) and streptococcal infections now appears to be etiologic. The essential lesion in this condition concerns the valves, generally the *mitral* and the *aortic*. Damage to these structures leads to either stenosis or regurgitation. In mitral or aortic stenosis the narrowed opening causes damming of blood in the lungs, with the result that the elevated pressure in the capillaries forces fluid into the alveoli. In the end the patient drowns in his own water. On the other hand, if the valves fail to close properly because of erosion, there is regurgitation, or the leaking backward of blood. The heart, in attempting to "correct itself" by beating harder and faster, becomes strained and weakened.

The prompt use of penicillin in *all* streptococcal infections is now recognized as the best defense against rheumatic heart disease. Treatment is continued until the last threatening organism has departed, and then some.

Congestive heart failure. The term *con-*

gestive heart failure is applied to the inability of the heart to pump at top efficiency. Although the condition can result from more blood returning to the heart than the heart can pump out (for example, overloading the circulation with intravenous fluids), the usual cause stems from heart damage; that is, either the valves are faulty (as in rheumatic heart disease) or the muscle is weakened by coronary disease or other injury.

The signs and symptoms of congestive heart failure are referable to poor circulation. A rapid, weak pulse, bluing of the skin, shortness of breath, fatigue, and edema are the classic features. Edema results from the increased venous pressures forcing fluid through the capillaries into the tissues and from poor filtration through the kidneys. Also, the presence of the adrenal hormone aldosterone (Chapter 18) stimulates the kidney to retain additional water and salt. Since salt "holds" water, this is a singularly aggravating feature.

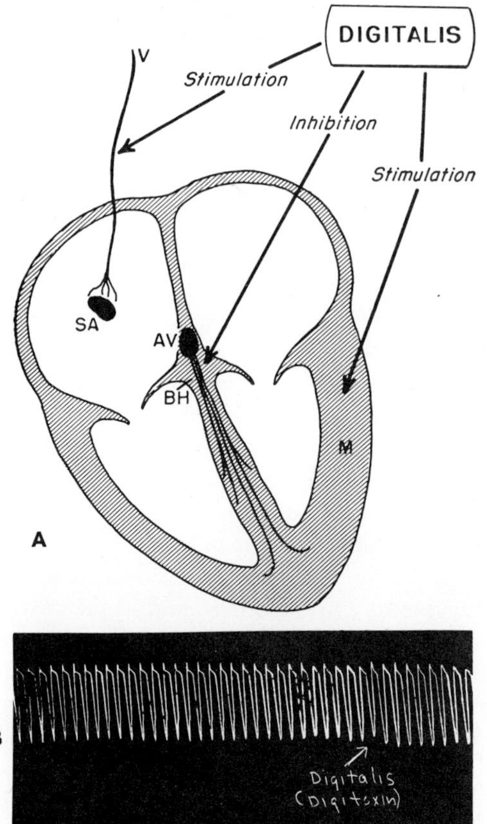

Fig. 11-20. Digitalis. **A,** Mechanism of action. **B,** Action upon the frog heart; note increase of strength of beat. **SA** and **AV,** Nodes; **BH,** bundle of His; **M,** myocardium. (From Brooks, S. M.: Basic facts of pharmacology, ed. 2, Philadelphia, 1963, W. B. Saunders Co.)

The treatment of congestive heart failure centers about the use of digitalis preparations to strengthen the myocardium (Fig. 11-20), diuretics to flush out the water and salt held in the tissues, and a salt-free diet.

Endocarditis. Endocarditis, a dangerous and often fatal heart disease marked by inflammation of the endocardium and valves, is usually caused by either streptococci or staphylococci. One of the more serious and common forms of the disease is *subacute bacterial endocarditis.* The etiologic microbe here is generally *Streptococcus viridans,* alone or in association with other microbes. Administration of penicillin and other antibiotics represents the treatment of choice.

Pericarditis. Pericarditis, inflammation of the pericardium (the sac about the heart), is characterized by fever, pain over the heart, rapid pulse, cough, and labored breathing. The condition usually follows in the wake of rheumatic fever, pneumococcal infection, and tuberculosis.

Coronary occlusion. Coronary occlusion means simply the blocking of a coronary artery. Not only is it the leading cause of death but also most of us develop the condition in old age. The area of the heart supplied by the blocked vessel dies from a lack of oxygen (*infarction*). Whether the victim survives an "attack" naturally depends upon the size of the vessel and the speed of occlusion. If death does not occur, the heart is weakened for several months and often for life.

Almost all cases of coronary occlusion result from *atherosclerosis,* one of the great medical challenges of our time. Apparently, atherosclerosis is caused by some defect in fat metabolism, for fatty deposits, containing chiefly cholesterol, form in the walls of the arteries. With age, fibrous tissue and calcium penetrate these deposits, causing them to harden—hence, the term *arteriosclerosis,* which literally means hardening of the arteries.

As the coronary arteries become atherosclerotic, danger is just around the corner. A fatty deposit may rip through the tunica intima and trigger a clot or thrombus (*coronary thrombosis*); a protruding fat deposit may break off; or a deposit may erode a vessel of the vasa vasorum, producing a tiny hemorrhage within the wall that pushes out the tunica intima. In any case a vessel becomes suddenly plugged, causing an *acute* coronary occlusion.

There is also the slowly developing variety of coronary occlusion in which nothing occurs except gradual narrowing of the vessel. This condition does not ordinarily precipitate an acute heart attack, but it does cause constricting and spasmodic pain in the chest (*angina pectoris*) following exertion, excitement, or emotion.

Coronary occlusion is treated by weeks or months of absolute rest to permit recovery of the damaged heart. Also, vasodilators to enhance the flow through the collateral circulation and anticoagulants (for example, *Coumadin*) to prevent enlargement of the clot are useful. In selected cases surgery may be lifesaving. The three main approaches are providing the heart muscle with an alternative supply of blood, repairing the diseased artery, and repairing the diseased heart.

In regard to prevention, there is now abundant evidence that obesity, smoking, and a high intake of cholesterol and *saturated* fats contribute significantly to coronary heart disease. *Unsaturated* fats and oil *work against* atherosclerosis, and it is the general feeling today that they should constitute the bulk of the fat in the diet.

Heart transplantation. In hopeless cases of heart disease, transplantation is now a recognized approach, albeit a tremendously difficult one on moral as well as medical grounds. The chief technical problem concerns "rejection" of the transplant by the forces of immunity, but to some degree this has been controlled through the use of drugs and antiserums to inhibit the host's plasma cells and lymphocytes. Obviously, the best answer is a mechanical heart and the day does not seem to be too far off when science will develop such a device.

Hypertension. Hypertension, or high blood pressure, is another ominous medical enigma. It occurs in about one out of every five persons, causing misery and not infrequently death. Hypertension kills by rupturing a vessel in a vital organ or by causing the heart or kidneys to fail.

About 90 percent of all cases of high blood pressure involve *essential* hypertension ("cause unknown"). However, possible causes have been postulated. Some researchers, for example, believe that essential hypertension is caused by a genetic defect in the areas where the sympathetic nerve fibers innervate the arterioles, causing excessive constriction. (As we know, arteriolar vasoconstriction is the most effective means of elevating blood pressure.) This attractive hypothesis is supported by the strong tendency for essential hypertension to be inherited and by certain recent laboratory developments. *Known* causes of hypertension include arteriosclerosis, certain brain abnormalities, kidney failure (Chapter 17), and an excessive output of adrenal hormones (Chapter 22).

The treatment of essential hypertension centers on the use of drugs to effect vasodilatation and rid the body of excess salt. In cases of known etiology, for example, a tumor of the adrenal gland, surgery may effect a cure.

Phlebitis. Phlebitis, or inflammation of the veins, is a potentially dangerous condition marked by infiltration of the vein walls and formation of a blood clot. The disease is accompanied by redness, edema, stiffness, pain, and sometimes infection in the affected area. Vasodilators, anticoagulants, and antibiotics are commonly prescribed for this condition to enhance the flow of blood in the affected part (usually the leg), to prevent enlargement of the clot, and to fight infection, respectively.

Phlebectasia. Phlebectasia, or *varicose* veins, is a common condition in which the veins are weak and dilated. Although such factors as continuous standing and congestive heart failure (factors that elevate the venous pressure) are usually associated with the disease, there may be an inherited weakness of the walls. Since varicose veins bleed easily, a slight injury to the affected areas may incite formation of a clot. Treatment is directed against the underlying cause; surgical intervention and, if the need arises, anticoagulant drugs are employed.

Thromboembolism. Thromboembolism, or embolism, is the blocking of a blood vessel with a thrombus that has broken loose from its site of formation. If the lung is affected, death is often instantaneous. Embolism is always a threat in such peripheral vascular diseases as phlebitis and phlebectasia. The treatment centers on the use of anticoagulants.

Shock. Shock is perhaps the most baffling medical emergency. Moreover, the ominous signs (hypotension, pallor, clammy skin, feeble and rapid pulse, decreased respiration, anxiety, and often unconsciousness) are frightening even to the seasoned physician. Morbidly interesting is the fact that shock is triggered not by one situation, but by many. A severe blow, a burn, a hemorrhage, a heart attack, an unpleasant experience, or even a bee sting may result in shock and death.

From the clinical picture just cited it is quite obvious that shock centers about the circulation. Moreover, most forms of shock can be explained, at least in part, on the basis of circulatory dynamics. In a severe hemorrhage or burn, for example, the reduced blood volume leads to reduced venous return and, in turn, to reduced cardiac output. Also, a severe heart attack causes a drastic cut in cardiac output because the pump is damaged.

In mild shock the body does a remarkable job of protecting itself by constricting the vessels and venous reservoirs. Thus, even though blood may be lost, the constricted vessels effect a normal venous return and cardiac output. If more than a quart of blood is lost, however, this mechanism cannot cope with the task, and cardiac output starts to fall.

The treatment of shock, to be successful, demands speed and proper choice of restorative measures. To correct volume deficiency, whole blood, plasma, or a plasma expander (for example, dextran) is used. If one of these is not available, electrolyte solutions or 5 percent glucose may be employed. Digitalis is indicated if the heart has been weakened. Also, such potent vasoconstrictors as *Levophed* and *Aramine* are commonly used to elevate a fallen blood pressure.

Lymphatic diseases. As the drainage system of the body for removal of bacteria and toxic materials, lymphatic tissue not infrequently becomes a seat of infection and inflammation.

Lymphadenitis. Lymphadenitis is inflammation of the lymph nodes. Generally, the condition accompanies local or systemic infection. Characteristically, the nodes of the involved area become swollen, painful, and tender. Treatment centers about the use of anti-infective drugs.

Lymphangitis. Lymphangitis, or inflammation of the lymphatic vessels, is usually accompanied by lymphadenitis. Considering the fact that the lymphatics lead into the nodes, this is quite understandable. As infection creeps along the vessels from the portal of entry, the underlying area becomes red, swollen, and painful. In addition, there may be chills and fever. Antibiotics and sulfonamides are commonly used against the microbial invader.

Tonsillitis. Tonsillitis is inflammation of the palatine tonsils. The acute form, usually caused by certain strains of nonhemolytic streptococci, can be a severe infection in which the tonsils become red, swollen, and painful and the crypts filled with noxious debris and pus. The throat is severely sore and swallowing is agonizingly painful. Systemically, the repercussions include muscular pains, malaise, fever, and chills. Bed rest, aspirin, and antibiotics are the generally prescribed therapeutic measures.

Although tonsillectomy was formerly the fashion of the day, this is no longer the case. Since the tonsils are a natural defense mechanism (perhaps much more so than has been realized), many authorities believe that they should be removed only in cases in which these organs are a chronic focus of infection.

Infectious mononucleosis. This acute infectious disease is characterized by fever, weakness, lymphadenitis, enlargement of the spleen, and a moderate leukocytosis due almost entirely to abnormal mononuclear cells (commonly referred to as *Downey's cells*). The cause is thought by some to be the so-called "EB virus," which also is associated with Burkitt's lymphoma (a cancerous condition peculiar to children of central Africa). Infectious mononucleosis is most common among young adults, especially students, and there is much evidence that it is passed along through "deep kissing." The treatment is purely symptomatic.

Hodgkin's disease. Hodgkin's disease is a progressive and fatal enlargement of the lymph nodes, spleen, and other lymphoid tissues. Typically, the involvement begins in the neck and spreads over the body. The treatment centers on the use of x rays and such chemotherapeutic agents as nitrogen mustard, chlorambucil, chlorphosphamide, and related compounds.

Filariasis. Filariasis is a tropical infestation caused by the so-called filarial worm (a nematode), two species of which are pathogenic to man—*Wuchereria bancrofti* and *Wuchereria malayi.* The adult worms, which are threadlike in shape and measure 1 to 3 inches in length, seek out the lymph vessels and nodes, particularly those of the pelvis and groin. The result is obstruction of the flow of lymph and (thereby) *elephantiasis* (tremendous swelling in the legs).

The life cycle of the filarial worm involves certain species of mosquitoes that inject the larval stage into the blood upon biting, the mosquito having itself been infected by another stage of the worm (microfilaria) present in the bloodstream of infected persons. The chief prophylactic measure in this helminthiasis, therefore, is mosquito control.

The diagnosis of filariasis is made by the finding of microfilariae in blood smears, and treatment consists chiefly in the administration of anti-infective agents, especially *Hetrazan.*

Questions

1. Describe the heart valves.
2. Compare the atria and the ventricles.
3. Distinguish between the papillary muscles and the trabeculae carneae.
4. Describe the Purkinje system.
5. Describe the electrical events in the cardiac cycle.
6. Describe and explain the heart sounds.
7. Discuss the law of the heart.
8. What is meant by systole and diastole?
9. Compare the effects of the sympathetic and parasympathetic nerves upon the heart.
10. Compare the structure of an artery and a vein.
11. What is meant by *vasa vasorum*?
12. Describe the role of the capillaries in fluid balance.
13. What is the meaning of a blood pressure of "140 over 100"?
14. What is meant by the pulse pressure?
15. What is the relationship of heart rate to stroke volume?
16. Assuming a blood volume of 5 liters and a heart rate of 70, what would be the average stroke volume?
17. What is the relationship of arterial elasticity to blood pressure.

18. Discuss the term *peripheral resistance.*
19. What is meant by the mean pressure?
20. What role do baroreceptors play in the regulation of blood pressure?
21. What is the relationship between atherosclerosis and acute myocardial infection?
22. Venous pressure throughout the body is determined mainly by the pressure in the right atrium. Explain.
23. Drugs that produce vasodilatation (for example, amyl nitrite) also increase the heart rate. Explain.
24. Mention four physiologic factors that cause vasodilatation.
25. What are the effects of viscosity and blood pressure upon blood flow?
26. Starting at the inferior vena cava, trace the blood to the aorta.
27. Describe the general features of the coronary circulation.
28. Describe the general features of the pulmonary circulation.
29. Describe the general features of the flow of blood to and from the brain.
30. Discuss the purpose of the portal circulation.
31. Describe the structure and function of the spleen.
32. Describe the general features of the circulation of blood in the muscles and skin.
33. Follow the flow of lymph from the lacteal vessels to the left subclavian vein.
34. What are the functions of the lymphatic system?
35. Name two congenital heart diseases and describe each.
36. Discuss the cause, manifestations, and treatment of congestive heart failure.
37. Discuss the relationship of atherosclerosis to coronary occlusion.
38. What is the purpose of using anticoagulants in coronary occlusion?
39. What is meant by renal hypertension?
40. What is a pheochromocytoma?
41. Write a short theme on the nature and causes of shock.
42. Why is phlebectasia potentially dangerous?
43. What is Hodgkin's disease?
44. Locate the palatine tonsils.
45. Discuss tonsillitis.
46. Naming all the major vessels, trace a red cell from the small intestine to the right foot.
47. Describe the histology of the myocardium.
48. Why is the left ventricle larger than the right?
49. What is the difference between the fossa ovalis and the foramen ovale?
50. Describe the basic features and operation of the electrocardiograph.

Chapter 12

The blood

Blood is the viscous red fluid of the body composed of cells suspended in plasma. This scarlet humor nourishes the tissues, carts away metabolites, fights infection, and plays a vital role in the adjustment of temperature, pH, and fluid balance. Thus, blood is the central element in homeostasis.

PLASMA

By centrifuging blood in a calibrated tube, we learn two basic facts: (1) that the plasma is a clear, almost colorless fluid and (2) that the cellular elements constitute about 45 percent of the total volume, a value referred to as the *hematocrit* (Fig. 12-1).

Chemically, plasma is a complex mixture of water (90 percent) and a galaxy of miscellaneous substances, including proteins, inorganic salts, lipids, glucose, waste products, vitamins, gases, enzymes, hormones, and antibodies. With the exception of proteins, whose molecules are largely confined to the circulation, the other constituents easily diffuse into the intercellular fluid. By the same token, intercellular constituents diffuse into the circulation. Thus, protein notwithstanding, plasma and intercellular fluid are practically identical. Indeed, they are classified together as the *extracellular fluid* (Chapter 18).

Plasma proteins. Since protein is the major force maintaining blood volume, it is the plasma's chief "solute"; that is, forced to remain within the capillaries, it prevents (by osmotic action) the escape of abnormal amounts of fluid into the tissues. The mechanics of this action are discussed in Chapter 18.

The plasma proteins fall into three types—albumins, globulins, and fibrinogen. Albumins, which make up the bulk of the 6 to 8 percent protein concentration in plasma, are responsible for practically all the osmotic force of the blood. The globulins are concerned with immunity, for practically all antibodies are *gamma* globulins. Fibrinogen participates in the vital process of clotting. Whereas albumin and fibrinogen are manufactured principally in the liver, globulins are formed by the *plasma cells* of the reticuloendothelial system.

Serum. When freshly drawn blood is placed in a tube and allowed to coagulate, a clot forms that gradually draws away from a clear liquid called the serum. Serum differs from plasma in only one significant

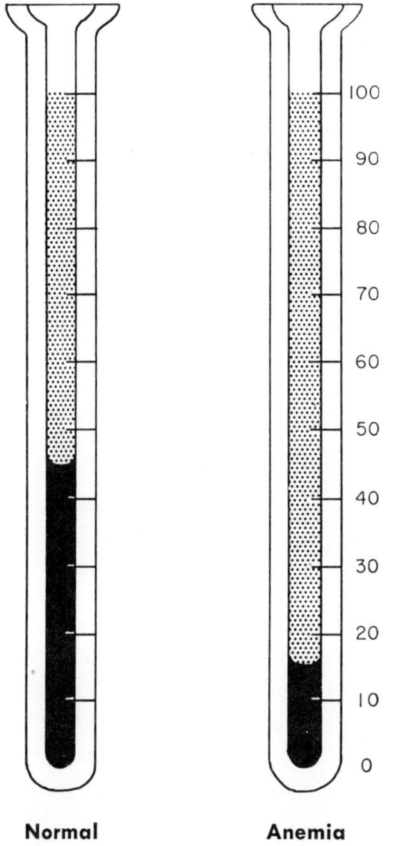

Fig. 12-1. Hematocrit of normal (45 percent) blood and anemic (15 percent) blood. (Modified from Guyton, A. C.: Function of the human body, Philadelphia, 1959, W. B. Saunders Co.)

respect; that is, it contains no fibrinogen. Thus, although the two expressions are often used as synonyms, there is this difference. If plasma is desired, therefore, blood must be treated with an anticoagulant (to prevent coagulation) and then centrifuged.

Edema. Whenever the concentration of plasma proteins falls below normal, the osmotic pressure of the blood falls and thereby permits passage of abnormal amounts of fluid into the tissues. The upshot is edema. A number of pathologic avenues lead to hypoproteinemia and edema. The more common causes are nephrosis, hepatitis, and malnutrition. In nephrosis, protein is lost in the urine; in hepatitis, the liver does not produce sufficient protein; in malnutrition, there is an absence of protein in the diet.

RED BLOOD CELLS

In each cubic millimeter of blood there are about five million red cells, or *erythrocytes,* in the male and four and one-half million in the female. Since the red cells outnumber the white cells by about 500 to 1, the hematocrit, for all practical purposes, is a reflection of the former cellular elements.

The red blood cell is characterized by the absence of a nucleus and the presence of an iron-bearing red protein called *hemoglobin.* Hemoglobin makes up approximately 33 percent of the cell and averages between 14 and 16 gm. per 100 ml. of whole blood. Other components of the red cell include the proteins and lipids, which make up the internal framework, as well as an assortment of minerals and enzymes.

The principal function of the red cell is to transport oxygen. Since this role is in the province of respiration, we shall reserve the details for Chapter 13.

Formation. The formation of blood cells is called *hemopoiesis.* In the fetus, red cells are manufactured by the liver, spleen, and bone marrow. By the time of birth the job is taken over exclusively by the marrow, and it is interesting to note in this connection that the flat and irregular bones produce more cells than do the long bones. Indeed, although there is a gradual decrease in blood cell production in all the bones with advancing age, the marrow of the long bones is engaged in this chore only during preadolescence.

There are several stages in the development of a red cell, beginning with the large *hemocytoblast* and ending with the erythrocyte, or mature red cell (Fig. 12-2). Once formed, they squeeze their way into the capillaries and enter the circulation at large. Sometimes, however, when the red cells are being produced at an accelerated

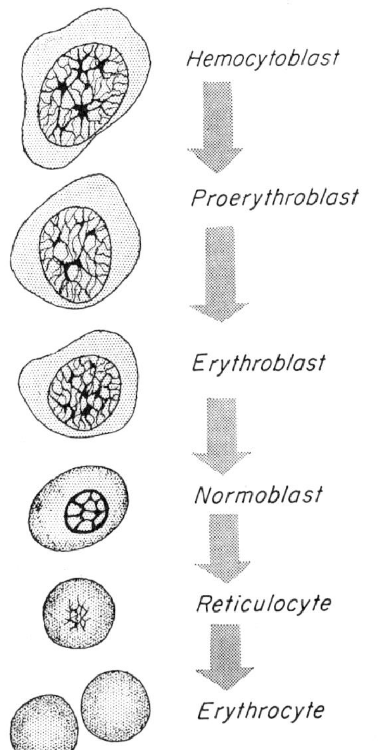

Fig. 12-2. Development of the red cell. (Modified from Guyton, A. C.: Function of the human body, Philadelphia, 1959, W. B. Saunders Co.)

rate, reticulocytes and sometimes even normoblasts enter the circulation before they have fully matured. As a matter of fact, the number of reticulocytes in the circulation is indicative of hemopoietic activity.

Special agents, particularly vitamin B_{12} and folic acid, are needed for the proper development of red cells. If either of these two vitamins is lacking, the erythroblasts fail to mature; instead, they grow into oversized cells called megalocytes. The presence of this particular type of cell in the blood indicates a so-called megaloblastic anemia.

Life of the red cell. It has now been established that a red cell has a life of about 120 days. At the end of this time it becomes fragile and finally breaks down, releasing hemoglobin to the circulation. The cellular fragments are engulfed and done away with by the reticuloendothelial cells that line the capillaries and liver sinuses.

Oxygen regulation. The production of red cells is controlled chiefly by the oxygen in the tissues. If the concentration drops, hemopoietic activity in the marrow becomes increased; if the concentration rises, hemopoietic activity becomes decreased. Thus, persons living at high altitudes or engaged in hardy exercise may have a red blood cell count as high as eight million or more. In contrast, the sedentary, sickly person may have a count as low as three million.

The mechanism of this regulation is as yet unknown. However, recent investigation indicates that diminished oxygen triggers the release of some hormone that stimulates the bone marrow.

Anemias. Anemia may be defined as a deficiency in red cells and/or hemoglobin. Quite understandably, the hematocrit will generally be below 45 percent (Fig. 12-3).

Anemia causes damage to the body in two ways. The most obvious insult will be a lack oxygen in the tissues due to the impaired ability of the blood to carry that gas. As a result, the cells, especially those of the nervous system, undergo degeneration. This explains such early symptoms as disinterest, fatigue, and loss of energy. The second way in which anemia damages the body has to do with viscosity. Decreased hematocrit values mean decreased viscosity, which in turn enhances the blood flow (p. 233). This results in excessive return of blood to the heart, causing overwork and, not infrequently, heart failure.

There are various anemias, depending upon the cause. Some are easily treated, and some lead to early death. The major types are discussed here.

Blood loss anemia. The sudden drop in blood volume that follows hemorrhage will normally be restored within 24 hours via ingested fluids and tissue fluid drawn into the circulation as a result of hemoconcentration. Since the lost red cells will not be replenished for several weeks, however, the hematocrit drops and anemia ensues.

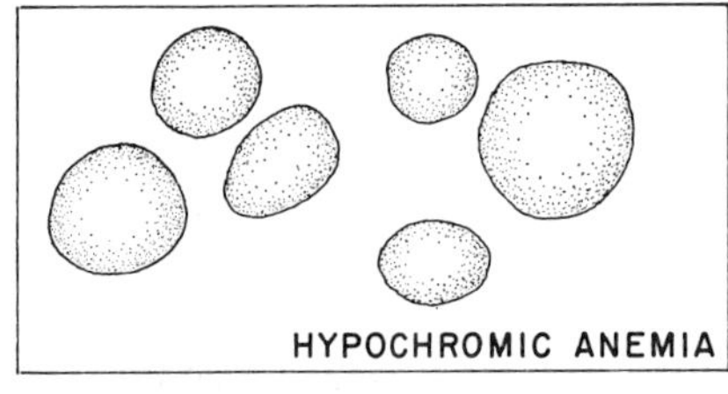

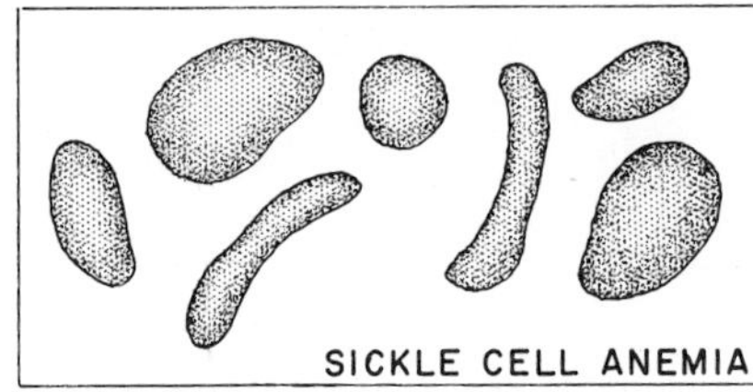

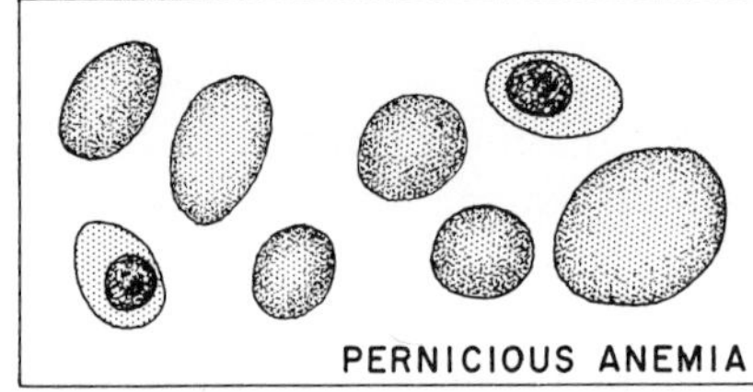

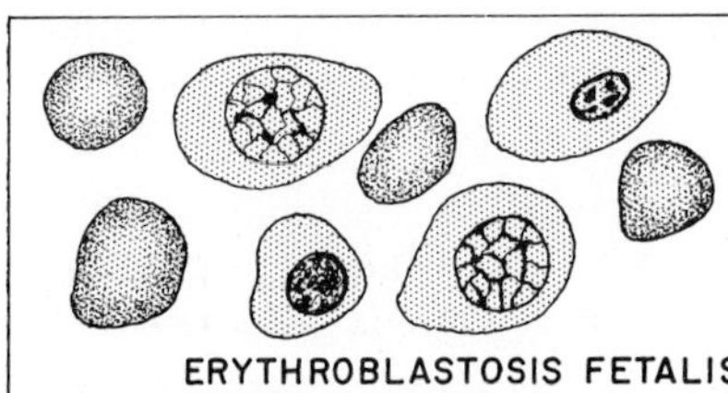

Fig. 12-3. Red cells as they appear in four types of anemia.

Chronic loss of blood will also produce anemia. Although the marrow may be able to maintain a nearly normal red blood count, the iron stores of the body become progressively decreased. Consequently, this type of anemia is marked by a mild drop in the number of red cells but a severe drop in hemoglobin.

Hemolytic anemias. By hemolytic anemia we mean excessive destruction of red cells. The most common forms include sickle cell anemia, erythroblastosis fetalis, and poisoning due to drugs and chemicals. Sickle cell anemia is a hereditary disease marked by distorted red cells (Fig. 12-3). Since the membranes of these cells are fragile, they are easily damaged and destroyed.

In erythroblastosis fetalis the pregnant mother builds up destructive antibodies against the red cells of the fetus. Consequently, the baby is born with a severe anemia. The reason for this incompatibility will be discussed shortly in connection with blood typing.

Iron-deficiency anemia. An insufficient intake of iron leads to a deficiency of hemoglobin and thus to anemia. Although the cell count is usually near normal, the concentration of hemoglobin in each cell is greatly reduced—hence, the expression hypochromic anemia (Fig. 12-3). This condition is rather common and is successfully treated with iron compounds such as ferrous sulfate.

Pernicious anemia. Pernicious anemia is a megaloblastic anemia that proves fatal if not treated. The highly characteristic blood picture is shown in Fig. 12-3.

The consensus now is that most cases of pernicious anemia result from a deficiency of a so-called *intrinsic factor* present in the mucosa of the stomach and duodenum. Since this factor serves to enhance the absorption of vitamin B_{12} (the *extrinsic factor*) into the circulation, a deficiency will severely curtail the manufacture of red cells in the marrow. The treatment of choice is parenteral administration of vitamin B_{12}. Some physicians, however, still employ liver extract, the active principle of which is vitamin B_{12}.

Another constituent of liver is folic acid, a member of the B complex, and for some time it was believed that this agent was the extrinsic factor. Clinical practice, however, has shown this not to be the case, because folic acid—in contrast to vitamin B_{12}—does not control the neurologic lesions of the disease. But folic acid is needed to treat the anemias of malnutrition, pregnancy, and infancy.

Aplastic anemia. In the event the bone marrow is destroyed, the manufacture of red cells stops completely, a fatal condition referred to as aplastic anemia. The usual

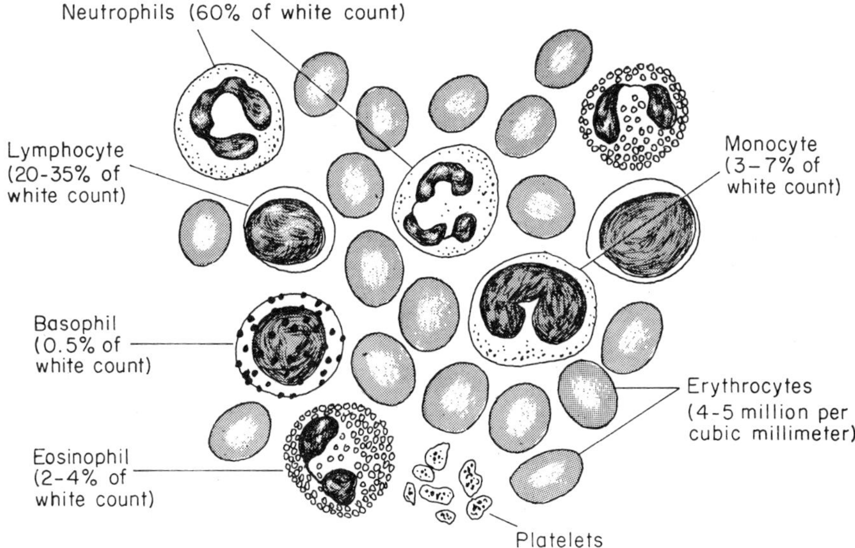

Fig. 12-4. Cellular elements of the blood. (Platelets average about 300,000 per cubic millimeter.)

causes are certain drugs, poisonous chemicals, and overexposure to such ionizing radiations as x rays and gamma rays.

Polycythemia. As stated previously, an increased red cell count, or polycythemia, is a normal response during strenuous exercise and at high altitudes. In polycythemia vera (or erythemia), however, the elevated count results from tumorous bone marrow. A tremendous number of red cells are poured into the circulation, and the hematocrit and viscosity are thereby dangerously increased (p. 249). The blood "flows like molasses," and there is a tendency to thrombosis. The treatment includes judicious use of blood letting and administration of radioactive phosphorus and anticoagulants.

WHITE BLOOD CELLS

White cells, or *leukocytes,* average in the neighborhood of 8000 per cubic millimeter of blood. These cells are called "white" simply because they are colorless.

Leukocytes are divided into *granulocytes** and *agranulocytes* (Fig. 12-4). The granulocytes, so called because of the granules in the cytoplasm, include the *neutrophils, eosinophils,* and *basophils.* The agranulocytes (which contain no granules) include the lymphocytes and monocytes.

Formation. With the exception of the lymphocytes, which are produced in lymphoid tissue (namely, the lymph nodes), leukocytes are formed in the bone marrow, along with the red cells, from the same basic stem cell—the hemocytoblast. Unlike the red cells, leukocytes can leave the circulation in great numbers by squeezing through the pores in the capillary wall, and in this manner they infiltrate the tissues and aid in fighting infection. It has been demonstrated in the laboratory that the average white cell remains in the blood for no longer than 3 or 4 days.

Neutrophils. Neutrophils are among the most spectacular cells in the human body. They move about like amebas and fight like soldiers. The involved, fantastic events that take place during inflammation, for instance, never cease to amaze even the most seasoned observer.

*Also called polymorphonuclear leukocytes because of their multilobed nucleus.

The inflammatory response runs essentially as follows: Damaged tissue releases a substance called leukotaxine that increases the permeability of the capillaries in the affected area. The neutrophils now line up along the inside wall (margination) and slowly but surely squeeze through the enlarged pores *(diapedesis)*. Once through, they head straight for the center of conflict, apparently in chemotaxic response to leukotaxine. Here they gobble up, or *phagocytize,* all foreign substances, including bacteria and tissue debris (Fig. 12-5). A single neutrophil may devour as many as fifty or more bacteria before falling victim to its belligerent meal. The aftermath, pus, is composed mainly of dead neutrophils that have fallen in defense of the body.

Neutrophilia. Aside from the local events already described, damaged tissues also release into the blood a leukocyte-promoting factor that stimulates the marrow to increase the output of leukocytes. This brings about an increase in the number of all the white cells *(leukocytosis),* but particularly of the neutrophils *(neutrophilia).* Pronounced neutrophilia, therefore, is an indication that all is not well. Because of the stepped-up production, many neutrophils leave the marrow in an immature form. The more commonly encountered early forms include the so-called *juvenile* and *stab* cells.

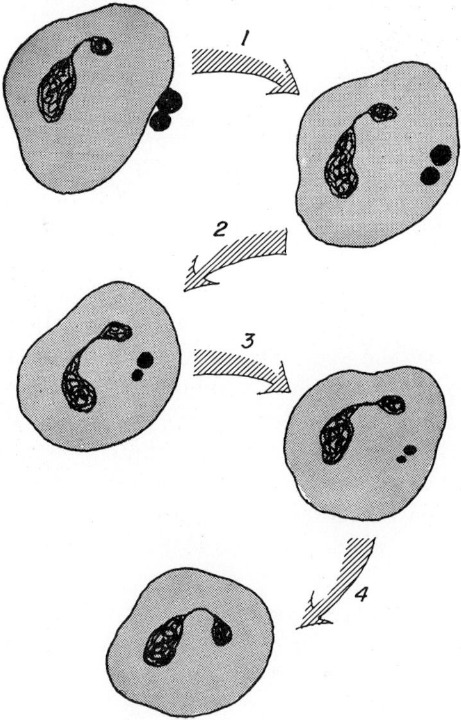

Fig. 12-5. Phagocytosis. Progressive engulfment and destruction of two staphylococci by a phagocytic leukocyte.

Eosinophils. Eosinophils are generally quite similar to neutrophils but may be distinguished from the latter by their larger granules, which take *acidic* dyes such as eosin—whence derives their name. Since these cells move about and scavenge to a much less extent than do neutrophils, one wonders what role they play in the defense of the body. It could be, of course, that they perform some vital activities unknown to the researcher. It is certainly quite significant, for instance, that eosinophils increase greatly *(eosinophilia)* in cases of hypersensitivity and parasitic infestation.

Basophils. The basophils are similar to neutrophils and eosinophils in most respects, except that their cytoplasmic granules take a *basic* dye. These cells possess relatively little movement and do not actively engage in phagocytosis.

Monocytes. Monocytes differ from granulocytes both morphologically and functionally. Indeed, in chronic infections the monocytes engaged in phagocytosis in a particular area often outnumber the neutrophils. Moreover, monocytes are able to mop up tissue debris that proves indigestible to the neutrophils. In short, the monocytes are an important part of the defense system of the body.

Lymphocytes. As stated previously, the lymphocytes are not formed in the marrow but in the lymph nodes and other lymphatic structures throughout the body. It is believed that certain lymphocytes (in the lymph nodes) differentiate into *plasma cells.* Further, it is held that the latter cell forms antibodies within its cytoplasm that are released upon the rupture of the cellular membrane. The fact that the lymphocytes in the blood have comparatively little cytoplasm lends considerable support to the theory.

Leukopenia. Leukopenia is the decrease in the number of white cells in the blood. The most serious form is agranulocytosis, or a lack of granulocytes. This condition results when the bone marrow is damaged by poisons, certain drugs, and radiation. Since the body is deprived of one of its major defenses against bacterial infection, the upshot is ulceration of the gastrointestinal and respiratory tracts. Unless anti-infective drugs are administered, the patient usually dies in a day or two.

Leukemia. Leukemia is a cancerous condition of the hemopoietic system characterized by a white cell count often as high as twenty-five times the normal value. Death is caused by interference with normal bodily functions.

Leukemias fall into at least three categories: myelocytic, caused by cancer of the bone marrow; lymphocytic, caused by cancer of the lymphoid tissue; and monocytic, characterized by a predominance of monocytes. The acute forms usually kill the patient in less than a year's time. The chronic varieties also lead to death, but often much more slowly. Although such antineoplastic drugs as aminopterin and the nitrogen mustards often prolong life, they do not offer cures. However, current research indicates that one day the chemist may devise drugs of greater value—perhaps even a cure.

THROMBOCYTES

Thrombocytes, or *platelets,* are minute, granular, disc-shaped structures in the blood that average around 300,000 per cubic millimeter. Not really cells, thrombocytes are believed to be fragments of giant cells in the red bone marrow called megakaryocytes. The role that thrombocytes play in clotting is included in the discussion that follows.

CLOTTING

Clotting *(coagulation)* prevents the escape of blood. The process looks simple, but research has disclosed that a galaxy of physicochemical gymnastics is involved. There is, indeed, a great deal that we do not know, but most authorities agree on the fundamental steps.

Basic mechanism. As shown in Fig. 12-6, the platelets at the site of the ruptured vessel disintegrate, thereby releasing, among other things, an enzyme called *thromboplastin.* The reason this occurs is of singular interest: Platelets and the endothelial cells lining the vessels both possess a negative charge; hence, platelets ordinarily are "pushed" away from the vessel walls. When a vessel is damaged, however, the endothelial cells lose this charge, thus permit-

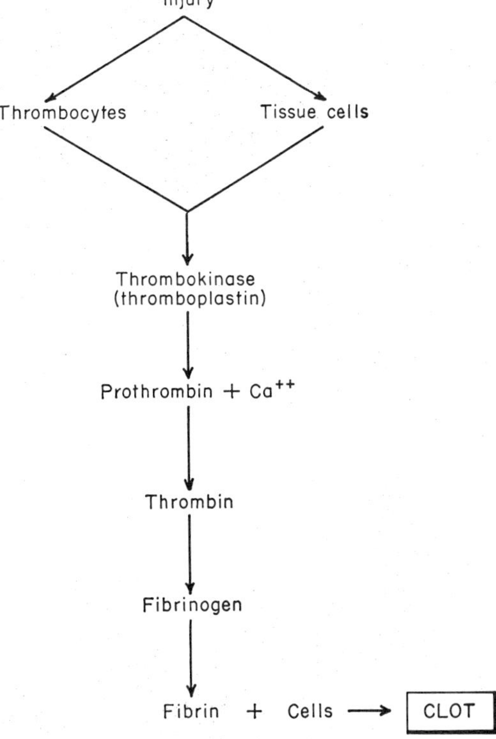

Fig. 12-6. Basic mechanism of clotting.

ting the platelets to stick to the walls. In so doing the platelet membrane ruptures and thromboplastin is released. A certain amount of thromboplastin is also released from regular tissue cells in the injured area. To speed up disintegration of the platelets, normal blood contains a so-called antihemophilic factor (factor VIII), the absence of which causes hemophilia (p. 257).

Thromboplastin, once released, starts to work rapidly on a plasma protein called *prothrombin,* converting the latter into the enzyme *thrombin.* In order for this reaction to take place, however, ionic calcium, factor V, and an array of other factors must be present. Also, it is important to know that prothrombin is synthesized in the liver with the aid of vitamin K.

Once formed, thrombin catalyzes the polymerization of the *soluble fibrinogen* molecules of the plasma into interlacing threads of an *insoluble* protein called *fibrin.* The later entraps the cellular elements, and a clot is born.

Heparin. As a safeguard against intravascular clotting, the blood contains a variety of *antithrombins* that inhibit the formation and/or action of thrombin. One such agent is heparin, which is present in most tissues throughout the body.

Fibrinolysin. In the event *antithrombins* do not hold their own and intravascular coagulation ensues, the blood calls forth a proteolytic enzyme called fibrinolysin (plasmin). In less than a day following clot formation, some mechanism triggers the release of this enzyme from a plasma precursor called *plasminogen.* Fibrinolysin dissolves the clot by digesting the fibrin threads.

Coagulation tests. A number of tests are employed to appraise the ability of the blood to coagulate. The more important are described here.

Bleeding time. By bleeding time is meant the time that it takes for a prick delivered to the finger or earlobe to stop bleeding. The normal value averages in the vicinity of 3 to 5 minutes. In the event that the bleeding time is increased, other tests are performed in an attempt to discover the underlying cause.

Clotting time. Clotting or coagulation time is determined, according to one method, by collecting blood in a clean glass tube and then clocking the interval between the time it is withdrawn and the time it starts to clot. The average value is about 10 minutes. The clotting time is used clinically to gauge the dose of heparin.

Prothrombin time. To ascertain the concentration of prothrombin in the blood, a test called the prothrombin time is used. This test is performed by precipitating out the calcium ion, thus rendering the blood incoagulable, and then quickly adding an excess of calcium and thromboplastin. Since all the factors needed for coagulation are added except prothrombin, the time it takes for a clot to form bears an *inverse* relation to the concentration of the latter in the blood. The normal prothrombin time is about 12 seconds. Values over 30 signal bleeding tendencies. The prothrombin time is used clinically to gauge the dose of such anticoagulants as Dicumarol and Coumadin.

Thrombosis. A common cause of death is thrombosis, or the formation of an intravascular clot. Such a clot, or *thrombus,* may remain where it is, or it may be swept away by the blood. In the latter event the clot is called an *embolus,* and the condition is termed *embolism.* Death, of course, results from the obstruction of blood to a vital organ or area. The classic example is coronary thrombosis.

Thrombosis of the peripheral vessels is most often traceable to sluggish blood flow, particularly in the legs. Since some of the platelets have a tendency to adhere to the walls of the veins anyway, they are even more likely to do so in areas of poor circulation. In so doing the cells rupture and release thromboplastin, thereby triggering a clot. Any situation, therefore, accompanied by a slowly moving bloodstream is potentially dangerous. This explains the common occurrence of thromboembolism in the bedridden geriatric patient. Other causes are atherosclerosis, phlebitis, and phlebectasia.

Anticoagulants. Anticoagulants, or drugs that inhibit coagulation of the blood, act by blocking one or more of the participants in the clotting mechanism. Such drugs as heparin and Dicumarol may be lifesaving in thrombosis or embolism. Although these agents do not dissolve clots, they do prevent them from growing larger, and meanwhile the clots are destroyed by fibrinolysin (p. 256). Equally significant, anticoagulants are employed prophylactically in disorders that predispose to thromboembolism.

In the last few years certain enzymes (for example, fibrinolysin derived from blood) have proved of value in the treatment of certain thromboembolic conditions. These agents have the advantage of actually dissolving the clot.

Hemophilia. Hemophilia, the classic defect of coagulation marked by delayed clotting and hemorrhage, is inherited by the male through the female as a sex-linked characteristic. In this bizarre malady even the smallest scratch may prove a threat to life. The genetic defect is now known to be the absence of a so-called *antihemophilic factor* (factor VIII) involved in the formation of thromboplastin. There is no cure for the disease and treatment centers on the use of blood transfusions and "factor VIII concentrates."

BLOOD GROUPS

It is common knowledge that the blood of one person may prove fatal if transfused into the bloodstream of another person. The reason for this is of the utmost importance and is essential to any study having to do with the blood.

Major groups. The blood of all human beings falls into four major groups—A, B, AB, and O.* These groups are named according to two protein factors *(agglutinogens),* which may or may not appear in the red cells. Group A blood contains agglutinogen A; group B blood contains agglutinogen B; group AB blood contains both agglutinogens; and group O contains neither agglutinogen.

In addition to the two agglutinogens, three of the blood groups contain agglutinating antibodies, or *agglutinins,* in the plasma. Group A blood contains beta (β) agglutinins; group B blood contains alpha (α) agglutinins; group AB blood contains neither agglutinin; and group O blood contains both agglutinins.

This distribution of agglutinogens and agglutinins becomes understandable once it is appreciated that *alpha* agglutinins agglutinate, or clump, red cells containing agglutinogen A, and that *beta* agglutinins agglutinate red cells containing agglutinogen B. Thus, group A blood, for example, cannot contain alpha agglutinins in its plasma, for all its red cells would clump together and plug the vessels. It can and does contain *beta* agglutinins, however, because these do not react with agglutinogen A.

Now we see without difficulty why one type of blood may destroy another type. For instance, if type A blood is transfused into a person with type B blood, the plasmas will cross agglutinate the red cells and thereby cause a transfusion reaction (p. 259).

Typing. Typing of an unknown blood is a very simple procedure. Two drops of the blood are placed on a clean glass slide, one on each end, and a drop of anti-A serum (derived from type B blood) added to one and a drop of anti-B serum (derived from type A blood) added to the other. There are four possible results. If

*Group AB, about 3 percent of the population; group A, 42 percent; group B, 10 percent; group O, 45 percent.

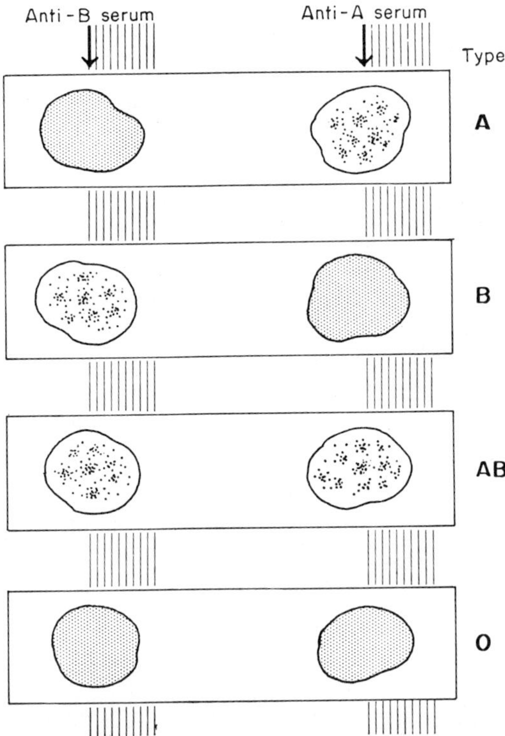

Fig. 12-7. Typing of blood. (See text.) (From Brooks, S. M.: Basic facts of medical microbiology, ed. 2, Philadelphia, 1962, W. B. Saunders Co.)

agglutination occurs in both drops (Fig. 12-7), the red cells contain *both* agglutinogens and the blood is obviously type AB. Conversely, if neither drop agglutinates, *both* agglutinogens are *absent,* and the blood is type O. Type A and type B will agglutinate only in the drop treated with anti-A serum and anti-B serum, respectively.

Rh factor. In addition to the four major groups just discussed, there is the Rh factor, a special substance present in the red cells of about 85 percent of the population. Blood that contains the factor is said to be Rh positive, and blood that does not have it is Rh negative.

If Rh-positive blood is administered to an Rh-negative person, the latter starts building up anti-Rh antibodies. Although no reaction occurs at this time, a second infusion of Rh-positive blood will result in agglutination and a severe response (p. 259).

Another well-known disorder caused by Rh incompatibility is *erythroblastosis fetalis* of the newborn.* This serious derangement occurs in about one out of every fifty children born to Rh-negative mothers and Rh-positive fathers. What happens is briefly as follows: The fetus inherits the Rh factor from the father and becomes Rh-positive. Thus, if these cells enter the mother's circulation, they provoke the production of anti-Rh antibodies, and this is very likely to happen *at the time of delivery.* What is more, each pregnancy will serve to boost the antibody titer higher and higher until the upshot is *erythroblastosis fetalis,* in some instances severe enough to result in stillbirth. Recently, a way was found around this dilemma by giving the mother a shot of anti-Rh *antibody* at the time of delivery. And the reason why this works is not difficult to understand; that is, antibody reacts with the Rh factor and in so doing prevents the latter from "immunizing" the mother. It appears that erythroblastosis fetalis will soon become a thing of the past.

Other factors. The agglutinogens mentioned are by no means all of the protein factors in the red cell. Some of the other factors include M, N, P, and Hr and the factors of Lewis and Kell. Although these factors are generally not of clinical importance, they are of great value in legal medicine in the identification of blood and the *disproving* of fatherhood. Also, red cell profiles give the anthropologist a powerful tool with which to probe the complex interrelationships among the races.

---

*The reason the disease is called erythroblastosis stems from the strenuous attempt of the fetal hemopoietic system to remedy the situation. Red cells are produced with such fervor that most of them enter the circulation in the immature erythroblastic stage.

BLOOD TRANSFUSIONS

Unless there is a grave emergency, a contemplated transfusion demands that the recipient's and the donor's bloods be cross matched to establish their compatability. Cross matching is carried out by centrifuging the bloods and then mixing the donor's diluted cells with the recipient's plasma on one slide and the donor's plasma with the recipient's diluted cells on another slide. If agglutination occurs on either slide, the bloods are mismatched and therefore incompatible.

In emergency situations, and at the physician's discretion, a person with type O blood may be used as a "universal donor." This is because type O red cells are not agglutinated by the other blood groups. Although it is certainly true that type O blood contains antibodies that agglutinate the red cells of types A, B, and AB blood, they are so greatly diluted by the recipient's relatively large blood volume that any agglutination which occurs is generally not extensive or serious. By the same token, a person with type AB blood is a "universal recipient." In this instance transfused red cells are not agglutinated because type AB blood contains no agglutinins.

Formerly, blood transfusions were carried out routinely, but not undramatically, by connecting an artery of the donor to a vein of the recipient with a cannulated rubber tube. The cross flow was continued until either the recipient showed improvement or the poor donor fainted. Today, transfusions are usually made through the blood bank. Blood is collected from the donor in sterile pint bottles containing a small amount of sodium citrate and glucose. The citrate prevents clotting, and the glucose serves as a source of nourishment during storage. The blood so collected can be transfused immediately or can be stored for a period of up to 3 weeks at a temperature of 4° C.

Transfusion reactions. Interestingly, a transfusion reaction resulting from mismatched blood is, for the most part, only indirectly related to agglutination, for in fatal cases death is generally due to kidney failure. The pathogenesis, in brief, is as follows. The agglutinated cells become trapped in the smaller vessels and shortly thereafter disintegrate, thereby releasing hemoglobin to the plasma. As a result, hemoglobin now appears in the glomerular filtrate (Chapter 17) and soon begins to crystallize out in the renal tubules. (This happens because most of the water is reabsorbed from the filtrate during its sojourn through the tubules.) The tubules now become plugged, and renal shutdown ensues in a week or so.

Treatment centers about administration of large volumes of alkaline solutions and diuretics to prevent further crystallization. This technique is often lifesaving, even in extreme reactions.

Plasma. When whole blood is not available, plasma is the substitute of choice. Indeed, in hemorrhagic shock, plasma alone will ordinarily save a life. Though plasma does not supply vital red cells, it maintains the circulation, and circulatory collapse is the usual cause of death in hemorrhage. Moreover, plasma possesses two great advantages over whole blood: (1) it may be stored indefinitely in the powdered form and (2) it may be given without regard to blood type. The use of plasma on the battlefield represents one of the great advancements in military medicine.

Plasma substitutes. Prepared plasma is by no means plentiful, and in the event of an atomic holocaust our supply would prove pathetically inadequate. Although the chemist has ransacked the laboratory for a substitute, the perfect substance has yet to be discovered.

INTRAVENOUS FLUIDS

A variety of commercially available solutions are given intravenously to supplement the oral route in seriously ill patients.

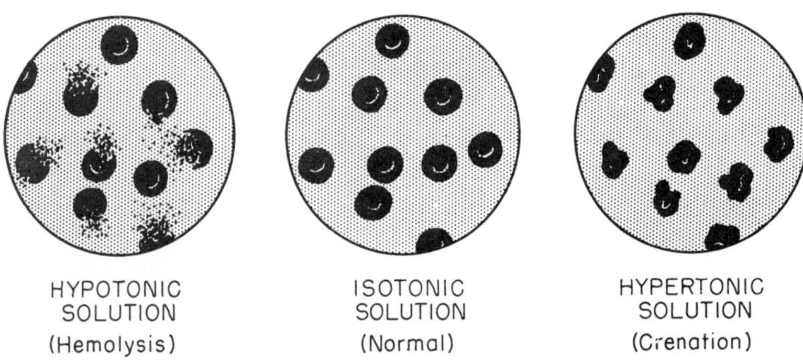

Fig. 12-8. Effect ot hypotonic and hypertonic solutions on the red cell.

Too, intravenous solutions are used to bolster the blood volume and enhance the circulation in shock.

Glucose. Glucose solutions are administered in strengths ranging from 5 to 50 percent. The 5 percent solution is *isotonic* and is the one usually used in the hospital. Glucose solutions not only supply on-the-spot energy but also are the best vehicles for supplying water. Plain water, of course, cannot be injected into the bloodstream because it would cause rupture of the red cells, or hemolysis (Fig. 12-8).

Levulose. In recent years levulose, an isomer of glucose, has gained clinical acceptance. A 10 percent levulose solution can be administered at the same rate as 5 percent glucose solutions without ill effects. In emergency situations this is obviously an advantage.

Amino acids. As the backbone of protein and protoplasm, amino acids have greatly enhanced the importance of intravenous nourishment. By stimulating the repair of damaged tissue, amino acid solutions are often lifesaving in severe debilitation, burns, malnutrition, radical surgery, and other situations characterized by a negative nitrogen balance.

Amino acid solutions are prepared by in vitro digestion of proteins such as casein that yield the essential amino acids (Chapter 16). These solutions are marketed and used at a concentration of 5 percent.

Electrolyte solutions. Electrolyte solutions contain two or more of the essential ions (namely, Na^+, K^+, Cl^-, and HCO_3^-) and are used to remedy fluid and acid-base imbalances (Chapter 18). Two popular preparations are normal saline solution and lactated Ringer's solution.

Dextran. Dextrans are polysaccharides produced by the action of the microorganism *Leuconostoc mesenteroides* on sucrose. So-called "dextran 40" (molecular weight 40,000), in a 10 percent solution, is used in shock to bolster blood volume and correct *cell aggregation* ("sludging") in the capillaries. The overall effect is the restoration of effective circulating volume, especially in the *microcirculation.*

BLOOD IN DIAGNOSIS

The physicochemical profile of the blood is without question the most valuable diagnostic tool in medicine. It is, indeed, a rare and evasive malady that does not in some way alter the cellular elements of plasma. In addition to the hematocrit (p. 249) and coagulation tests (p. 256), there are an ever-increasing number of laboratory procedures dealing with the blood.

Cell count. A complete examination of the cellular elements of the blood includes the counting of red cells and the various white cells mentioned earlier. The first step is carried out by adding a small, but accurately measured, volume of whole blood to a calibrated glass slide and, by means of the microscope, counting the cells in a

Table 12-1. Blood chemistry (normal values)*

Constituent	Material†	mg./100 ml. (mg.%) or as noted
Electrolytes		
Calcium	S	9-11 (4.5-5.5 mEq./L.)
Chloride	S	350-390 (100-110 mEq./L.)
Magnesium	S	1.8-3.6 (1.5-30 mEq./L.)
Phosphorus		
Children	S	4-6.5 (2.3-3.8 mEq./L.)
Adults	S	3-4.5 (1.8-2.3 mEq./L.)
Potassium	S	18-22 (3.5-5.5 mEq./L.)
Sodium	S	310-340 (135-147 mEq./L.)
Enzymes		
Amylase	P, S	70-200 units (Somogyi)
Cholinesterase	S	0.5-1.5 pH units
Lipase	S	0.2-1.5 units/c.mm. (N/20 NaOH)
LDH	S	25-100 units
Phosphatase, acid	S	0.5-3.5 units (King-Armstrong)
Phosphatase, alkaline		
Children	S	5-14 units (Bodansky)
Adults	S	2-4.5 units (Bodansky)
SGOT	S	Up to 40 units
Steroids		
17-Hydroxycorticosteroids		
Male	P	13 ± 6 μg/100 ml.
Female	P	15 ± 6 μg/100 ml.
17-Ketosteroids	P	60 μg/100 ml.
Vitamins		
Ascorbic acid	P	0.4-1.0
Nicotinic acid	P	0.1-0.3
Riboflavin	B	35-45 μg/100 ml.
Thiamine	S	3.5-4.2 μg/100 ml.
Vitamin A	S	40-60 μg/100 ml.
Vitamin E	P	0.8-1.2
Miscellaneous		
Albumen	S	3.5-5.5 gm./100 ml.
Cholesterol, total	S	110-300
Creatine	B	3-7
Creatinine	B	1-2
Fibrinogen	P	150-300
Globulin	P	2 gm./100 ml.
Glucose	B	80-120
Iodine, protein-bound	S	4-8 μg/100 ml.
Iron	P	50-80 μg/100 ml.
Nonprotein nitrogen	B, S	25-40
Proteins, total	P, S	6.3-8.0 gm./100 ml.
Urea	B	20-40
Uric acid	S	2-4

*From Smith, Kline & French Laboratories: Pocketbook of normal laboratory values, Philadelphia, 1960.

†S = serum; B = blood; P = plasma.

specified number of squares selected at random. The second step merely involves substitution of this count in the appropriate formula. The result is expressed as cells *per cubic millimeter.*

Sedimentation rate. When fresh citrated blood is allowed to stand, the red cells settle to the bottom, leaving the clear plasma above. The rate at which this settling, or sedimentation, occurs is altered by a number of physiologic and pathologic conditions. Although this test is far from specific, it is a simple way to obtain corroborative information.

Blood chemistry. The term *blood chemistry* refers to the various laboratory procedures used to ascertain the concentration of hemoglobin and the constituents of the plasma. The normal values for the main constituents of clinical concern are presented in Table 12-1.

An outstanding development in diagnostic medicine was the disclosure of the relationship between certain diseases and the appearancc of certain intracellular enzymes in the blood; that is, damaged tissue releases enzymes—and sometimes in a characteristic telltale fashion. In the wake of a myocardial infarction, for instance, the enzyme *serum glutamic oxalacetic transaminase* (SGOT) is sometimes more informative than an electrocardiogram. Other enzymes of diagnostic value, in addition to those cited in Table 12-1, are *serum guanase* (hepatitis) and *lactic dehydrogenase,* or LDH (kidney and heart disease).

Microbiology. Blood sent to the microbiology laboratory for the diagnosis of infection is examined bacteriologically for the presence of pathogens or serologically for the presence of antibodies. Since antibodies are provoked in response to infection, their appearance in the blood is often as significant as the presence of the microbes themselves, and in some instances, notably syphilis, serology often affords the only avenue of diagnosis.

INFECTIONS

Malaria. Malaria, the number one infection of man, is a protozoiasis associated with the blood. The precise nature of malaria depends upon which of the four species of the genus *Plasmodium* is involved. Benign tertian, the most common form of the disease, is caused by *Plasmodium vivax.* The other three forms are malignant tertian *(Plasmodium falciparum),* quartan malaria *(Plasmodium malariae),* and an uncommon form confined to East Africa and South America caused by *Plasmodium ovale.* In benign tertian and quartan malaria the paroxysms of fever (which occur every third and fourth day, respectively) are followed by chills; in malignant tertian malaria, chills may or may not occur. In each instance the fever and anemia are due to destruction of the red cells.

The plasmodium spends its life in man, monkeys, and female *Anopheles* mosquitoes, the insect being the biologic vector that injects the sporozoite, or infective stage, into the circulation (Fig. 12-9). The gametocyte (present in the blood of man and monkeys) is the infective stage for the mosquito.

The control of malaria centers about eradication of the *Anopheles* mosquito and tracking down of infected monkey populations. The latter problem has only recently been appreciated. Concerning treatment, some of the newer drugs, particularly chloroquine, have proved highly successful. Quinine is used in resistant cases.

Kala-azar. Kala-azar (black fever), a vicious tropical **protozoiasis** endemic in

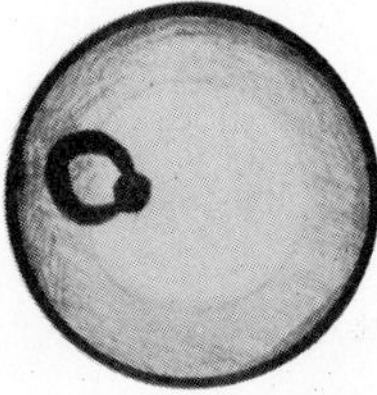

Fig. 12-9. Red cell with the so-called ring stage of *Plasmodium vivax.* (Idealized drawing.)

Africa, Asia, South America, and the Mediterranean area, is caused by *Leishmania donovani*. Once in the blood, the pathogen, which is transmitted via the sand fly, rapidly multiples and then sets out to invade other tissues, particularly the spleen and liver. There is severe anemia, enlargement of the spleen and liver, edema, and general emaciation. Diagnosis is made by demonstration of the parasite in blood films or smears of specimens taken from the spleen of sternal bone marrow. If untreated, the disease is over 90 percent fatal. Drug therapy (for example, ethyl stibamidine and pentamidine) is successful, provided that it is started early, but the best approach to kala-azar centers on eradication of the sand fly.

Schistosomiasis. Schistosomiasis, or *bilharziasis,* is a helminthiasis caused by three species of blood fluke trematodes: *Schistosoma haematobium, Schistosoma mansoni,* and *Schistosoma japonicum.* The disease is endemic in Africa, Asia, the Caribbean area, and South America.

As indicated, these worms (which measure ½ to 1 inch in length) inhabit the bloodstream. The pregnant female migrates to the mesenteric veins or terminal capillaries of the rectum and bladder to lay her eggs, an event that incites tumorous growths in these areas. Other disturbances include diarrhea, cystitis, and hematuria. Schistosomiasis may be diagnosed by a flocculation test (similar to the Kline test for syphilis). The treatment centers on administration of such specific anti-infectives as tartar emetic, stibophen (Fuadin), and lucanthone (Miracil D; Nilodin).

Questions

1. Distinguish between plasma and serum.
2. Discuss the plasma proteins.
3. Explain how a decrease in concentration of plasma proteins leads to edema.
4. Describe the maturation of the red cell.
5. Discuss the various causes of edema.
6. What is meant by hemoconcentration?
7. Discuss the etiology of pernicious anemia.
8. Describe the white cells.
9. What is meant by a differential count?
10. Describe diapedesis and phagocytosis.
11. What are the functions of the eosinophils and basophils?
12. What is the difference between leukemia and leukocytosis?
13. Compare the monocytes and the lymphocytes.
14. Compare fibrin and fibrogen.
15. Compare heparin and fibrinolysin.
16. Explain how liver damage might interfere with clotting.
17. Distinguish between bleeding time and clotting time.
18. Describe the prothrombin time test.
19. Compare the terms embolus, thrombus, thrombosis, and embolism.
20. Do anticoagulants dissolve clots?
21. Discuss hemophilia.
22. Describe the procedure you would use to identify blood of an unknown type, using samples of type A whole blood and type B whole blood.
23. Explain why erythroblastosis fetalis does not occur unless the mother is Rh negative and the father Rh positive.
24. What happens in a transfusion reaction?
25. The blood has been called the "fingerprint of disease." Explain.
26. What does a hematocrit of "40" mean?
27. Describe how the sedimentation rate is determined.
28. What happens to the hematocrit in polycythemia?
29. What is the purpose of giving amino acids intravenously?
30. What happens to red cells when they are suspended in a 2 percent sodium chloride solution?
31. Describe the general procedure for making a blood cell count.
32. Many times the physician will order a white cell count to confirm the diagnosis of appendicitis. Explain.
33. Is it possible to have anemia and still have a normal red cell count? Explain.
34. Describe the Widal test in typhoid fever.
35. How does sodium citrate prevent clotting?
36. Define the following terms: endemic, protozoiasis, splenomegaly, sternal puncture, helminthiasis, trematode, host, "milligrams percent," nonprotein nitrogen, hemolysis, erythrocytopenia, polymerization, biologic vector, enzyme, hydrogenase, electrolyte, isotonic, dextran, agranulocytosis, and neutrophilia.

Chapter 13

The respiratory system

Respiration includes the exchange of gases in the lungs between the blood and the air, the exchange of gases between the blood and the tissues, and the transport of gases (by the blood) between the lungs and the tissues. The exchange that occurs in the lungs is called *external* respiration, and that which occurs in the tissues is termed *internal* respiration.

As ordinarily used, the designation *respiratory system* concerns external respiration or, less formally, simple breathing. Although the transport of gases by the blood and their exchange in the tissues are obviously functions of the circulatory system, the entire picture is discussed in this chapter.

The respiratory system proper includes the nose, pharynx, larynx, trachea, bronchi, and lungs. We shall first discuss the structure and function of these organs before passing on to the actual mechanics of breathing and the exchange and transport of gases.

NOSE

The nose is divided into left and right cavities by the bony partition *(septum)* that arises perpendicularly from the roof of the mouth (hard palate). Each nasal cavity is further divided into three passageways by the *conchae (turbinates)* that arise from the lateral walls of the internal nose (Fig. 13-1). The superior and middle conchae, it will be recalled, are processes of the ethmoid bone, whereas the inferior conchae are separate bones. The passageways lead from the nostrils, or *anterior nares,* to the nasopharynx and enter the latter structure through the *posterior nares.* These passageways, or *meati,* take their names from the conchae, that is, superior meatus, middle meatus, and inferior meatus.

The nasal cavities (and most other structures along the respiratory tract) are lined with pseudostratified ciliated columnar epithelium (p. 166). This tissue not only secretes mucus but also propels it along, in one direction ("upward"), by the lashlike motion of the microscopic cilia (not to be confused with the macroscopic hairs of the nose). In this manner foreign particles trapped on the sticky surface are removed to the outside. Taken en masse, the cilia are unbelievably forceful.

Function. As indicated, the nose leads the air to the nasopharynx, and in so doing, filters, warms, and moistens it by means of the extensive mucosal surface. Perhaps the most obvious function of the nose is that

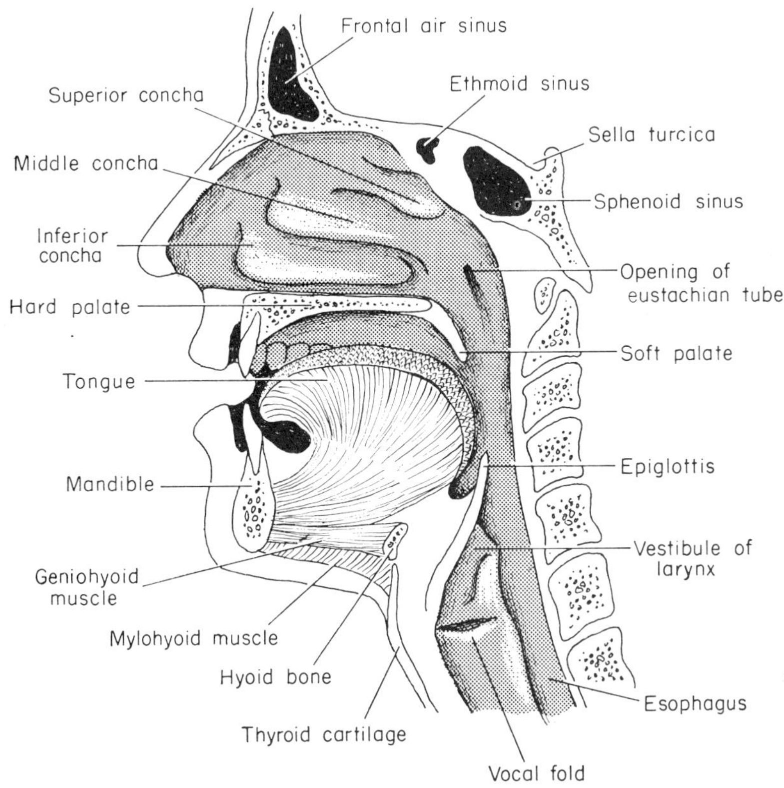

Fig. 13-1. Sagittal section of the head and neck. (Modified from Francis, C. C: Introduction to human anatomy, ed. 5, St. Louis, 1968, The C. V. Mosby Co.)

it serves as the organ of smell. This is by virtue of the fact that olfactory receptors are embedded in the mucosa that lines the roof of the nasal cavities. The nose also aids in speaking, or phonation. When the vocal cords vibrate, the air within the nasal cavities (as in the other cavities and sinuses of the head) is caused to vibrate, or resonate, in unison, an effect that imparts quality to the voice. This dramatically explains the change in voice that accompanies a "stuffy nose."

PHARYNX

The pharynx is the throat. Precisely, it is a tubelike structure, about 5 inches in length, which passes immediately before the cervical vertebrae from the base of the skull to the esophagus (Fig. 13-1). Its walls are well supplied with skeletal muscle, and with the exception of the *oropharynx* (the part behind the fauces), the pharynx is lined with ciliated epithelium. The area behind the nose is referred to as the *nasopharynx,* and that behind the larynx the *laryngopharynx.*

The pharynx bears extensive traffic (air and food) via the nose, mouth, larynx, and esophagus. Food, of course, has no place in the nasopharynx. Often forgotten are the two *eustachian* tubes which open into the nasopharynx from the middle ear. In all, then, there are seven openings of the pharynx: two from the eustachian tubes, two from the nose (posterior nares), one from the mouth (the inner fauces), one into the larynx, and one into the esophagus.

The pharynx is also characterized by the presence of lymphoid structures called tonsils. The *pharyngeal* tonsils (*adenoids*) are located on the posterior wall of the nasopharynx, opposite the posterior nares, and the *faucial* or *palatine* tonsils are located in the oropharynx (see Fig. 14-2). The *lingual* tonsils are located at the base of the tongue.

Function. The pharynx serves as a passageway for air and for food and plays an important part in phonation. Since the pharynx can change its shape in a split second, the sound waves produced in the larynx are "acted upon" to give pitch and quality to the voice. Learning to speak lies in great part in training the pharyngeal muscles.

The eustachian tubes are nature's unique way of protecting the eardrums against rupture from the impact of powerful sound waves; that is, they serve to equalize the air pressure on either side of the eardrum. The snapping and crackling sensation in the ears as one ascends in an elevator or an airplane is due to the relatively greater air pressure in the middle ear forcing out against the eardrum. Swallowing relieves the condition because air from the middle ear is sucked through the eustachian tubes. The tubes remain closed except during yawning, swallowing, and yelling.

LARYNX

The larynx (Fig. 13-2), aptly called the voice box, is situated at the top of the trachea, thus serving to communicate that structure with the pharynx. It is composed of nine pieces of cartilage and abundant skeletal muscle woven together by connective tissue into a tough, wedge-shaped box. The thyroid cartilage forms the anterior portion of the larynx and gives that organ its characteristic shape (*Adam's apple*). Generally, it is larger in men than in women.

The *epiglottis,* a tonguelike structure attached along one edge of the thyroid cartilage, serves to prevent food and drink from going down the "wrong way." The cricoid cartilage, which forms the bottom border of the larynx, is attached to the trachea by means of connective tissue.

The larynx is lined with ciliated mu-

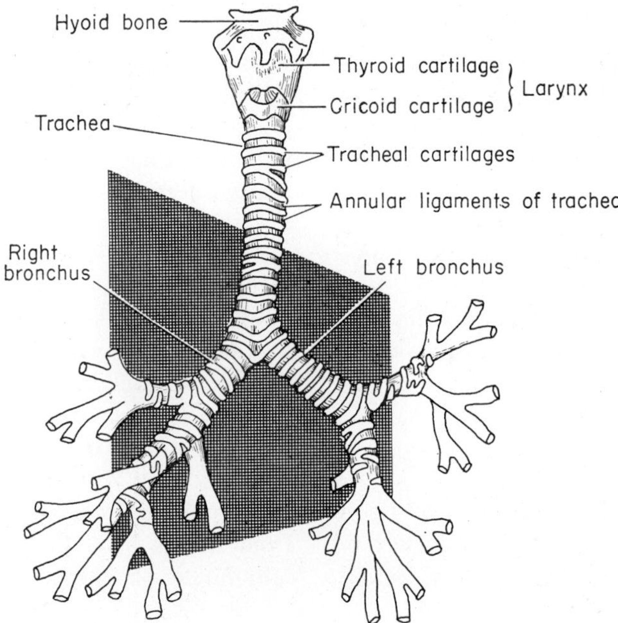

Fig. 13-2. The larynx and trachea. (Modified from Francis, C. C: Introduction to human anatomy, ed. 5, St. Louis, 1968, The C. V. Mosby Co.)

cosa thrown up in two prominent horizontal folds—the so-called *false* vocal cords. The *true* vocal cords, situated below these, are composed of two fibrous bands strung horizontally across the inside (Fig. 13-3). The opening between is called the glottis.

Physics of phonation. As explained earlier, sound is produced by a substance in vibration. In the case of the human voice it is made by ejecting bursts of air from the lungs through the glottis, thereby causing the vocal cords to vibrate. The vibrating cords, in turn, cause the air throughout the respiratory passageways, cavities, and sinuses of the head to resonate and emit sound.

Like other sounds, the human voice is characterized by loudness, pitch, and quality. The loudness, or amplitude (p. 30), of a sound wave depends upon the force of vibration. In other words, it depends upon the force employed to cause vibration; thus, it takes a more forceful blast of air to yell than to whisper.

The pitch of a sound depends upon frequency, or the number of vibrations per second (p. 30). For example, a tuning fork marked 256 means that when struck it will vibrate 256 times per second and produce sound waves with a frequency of 256.

The pitch of the human voice is controlled by the tension placed on the vocal cords by the laryngeal muscles. Tense cords yield high-pitched notes, whereas relaxed cords yield low-pitched notes. This may be demonstrated simply by plucking a rubber band under varying degrees of tension. Formally stated, the pitch of a musical string varies directly with tension and inversely with its length and diameter.

The quality of the human voice, like that of music, depends upon the number and nature of the overtones (that is, tones

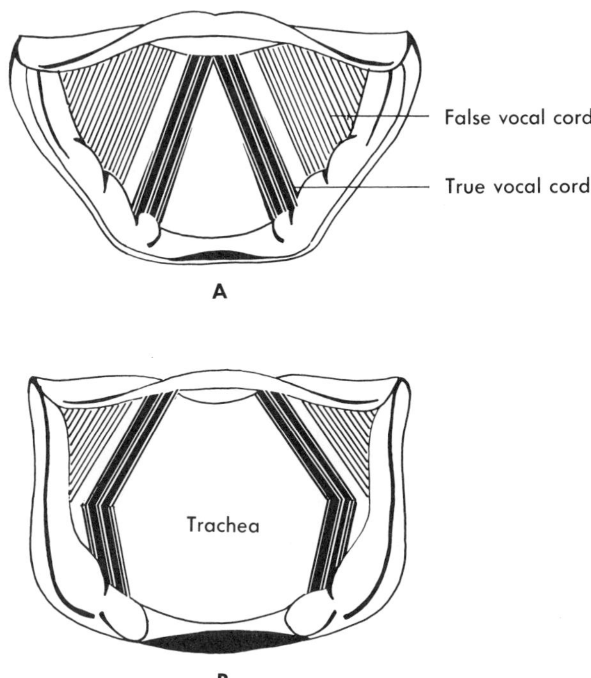

Fig. 13-3. Laryngoscopic view of the vocal cords during quiet, **A,** and deep, **B,** breathing. (Adapted from Kimber, D. C., Gray, C. E., Stackpole, M. A., and Leavell, C. E.: Anatomy and physiology, New York, 1961, The Macmillan Co. By permission.)

of a higher pitch than the fundamental) that combine with the latter to produce a more complex musical sound. For example, when a musical string vibrates, it may vibrate in isolated sections as well as a whole, and what we hear is the combined effect.

Voice quality depends upon the nose, mouth, pharynx, and sinuses as well as upon the position of the tongue. The role that the nose alone plays in affecting the quality of the voice is dramatically illustrated by severe nasal congestion, an effect analogous to pouring water into a pipe organ.

Most persons are disappointed in their recorded voice because it seems to lack "something." There is a very real reason for this, for when we speak the sound we hear is carried to the ear by bone conduction as well as by air waves. Our recorded voice, of course, hits our ears exclusively "by air."

TRACHEA

The trachea, or windpipe, is a 5-inch cartilaginous and membranous cylindrical tube descending in front of the esophagus from the larynx to the bronchi (Fig. 13-2). It averages about 1 inch in diameter. Like the other respiratory passageways, the trachea is lined with ciliated epithelium.

The cartilage is arranged in C-shaped rings embedded at equal intervals in fibrous tissue. The open ends of the rings, which face the posterior surface, are filled in with bands of smooth muscle. As one might easily guess, the purpose of these rings is to prevent the trachea from collapsing and thereby shutting off vital air.

Function. The trachea serves to lead the air into the lungs and in the process filters, warms, and moistens it via ciliated mucous lining. If for any reason the trachea should become obstructed, either an incision must be made into it (and fitted with a metal tube leading to the outside through the neck) or a tube must be passed into it through the mouth.

BRONCHI

At the level of the fifth thoracic vertebra the trachea divides, or bifurcates, into the bronchi (Fig. 13-2), the *right* bronchus being shorter, wider, and more vertical than the left. Both bronchi resemble the trachea in structure. As the bronchial tubes divide and subdivide into smaller and smaller structures, they gradually lose their cartilage and fibrous tissue until finally all that remains is a microscopic tube (the *bronchiole*) composed of only a thin layer of smooth muscle and elastic fibers. It is most important to remember that the entire bronchial tree (from the primary bronchi to the bronchioles) is lined with ciliated epithelium.

Pulmonary unit. The place at which the bronchioles finally terminate is shown in Fig. 13-4. A respiratory bronchiole enters an alveolar *duct,* which, in turn, leads into an alveolar *sac,* a structure closely resembling a bunch of hollow grapes. Each "grape" of the sac, if we may use the analogy, is called an *alveolus,* and because the alveolar wall is only one cell thick, gases easily diffuse (across it) between the air within and the blood in the surrounding capillaries.

Function. The bronchial tubes, like the trachea, conduct air and gases into and out of the lung. Of course, we must appreciate also the vital role that the extensive bronchial surface plays in filtering, warming, and moistening the air.

LUNGS

The lungs are light, spongy, cone-shaped organs (Fig. 13-5) that fill the lateral cavities of the chest; they are separated from each other by the heart and the mediastinal structures. Their bases rest on the diaphragm, and their apices extend slightly above the clavicles. To accommodate the heart and other structures, the medial aspect of each lung has a concave surface, the left lung having a greater concavity, or "notch," than the right. Histologically, the lungs are composed of an astronomical

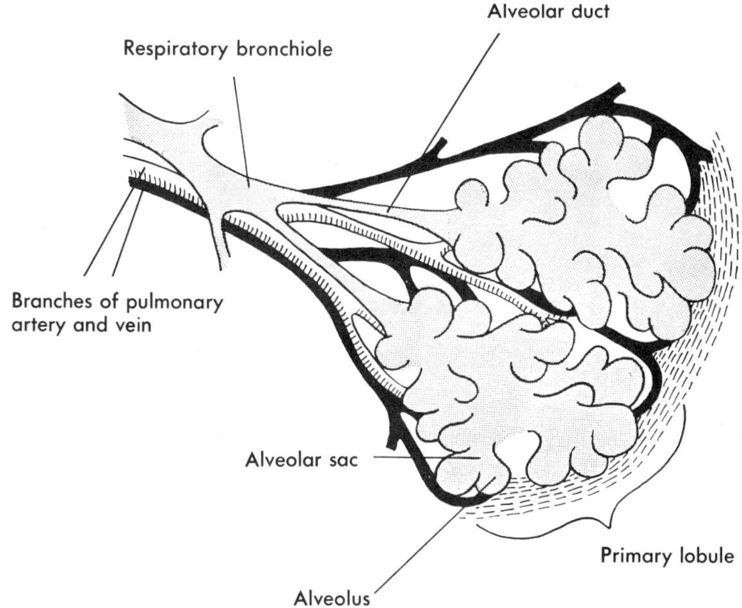

Fig. 13-4. The pulmonary unit. (Modified from Tuttle, W. W., and Schottelius, B. A.: Textbook of physiology, ed. 15, St. Louis, 1965, The C. V. Mosby Co.)

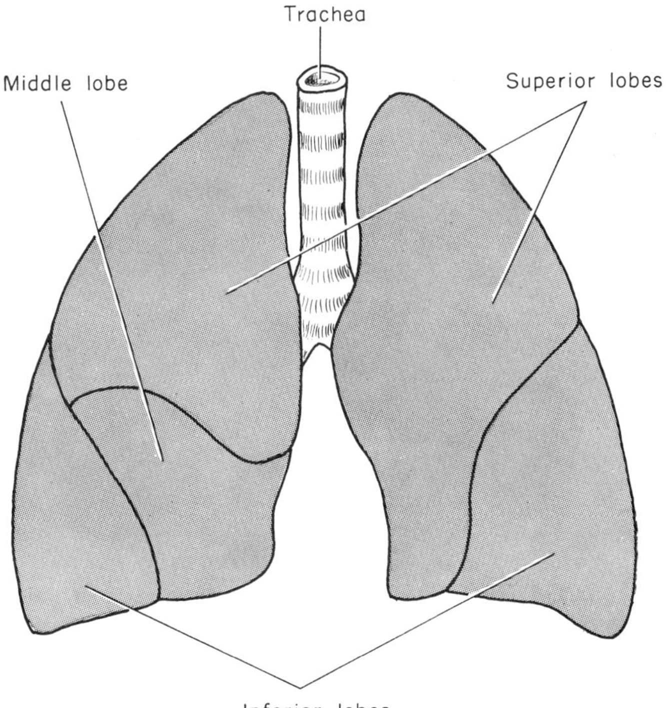

Fig. 13-5. Lobes of the lung (anterior view).

number of the pulmonary units just described (Fig. 13-4).

Other significant gross features include the hilus, the lobes, and the pleura. The *hilus* (or *hilum*) is a slit in the medial surface through which the primary bronchus and the pulmonary blood vessels, wrapped in a sheath of connective tissue, penetrate the lung. The *lobes* are the sections of the lung formed by fissuring; the left lung is partially divided into two lobes and the right lung into three.

The *visceral* pleura is a thin serous membrane that envelops the lungs and the *parietal* pleura is a similar membrane that lines the chest wall (p. 160). The two are always in immediate contact and move against each other when we breathe. To facilitate this movement and to reduce friction, they are moistened with a serous fluid.

Function. As indicated, the lungs—via the pulmonary unit—permit the exchange of gases between the air and the blood. The physical details of the process are described in the discussion of external respiration.

THORAX

The chest, or thorax, is defined by the sternum, ribs, thoracic vertebrae, and diaphragm. Inside, the pleurae describe the *mediastinal* cavity and *two pleural* cavities (p. 160). The parietal pleura proper covers the diaphragm and lines the anterior surface of the chest. As pointed out before, the parietal and visceral pleurae are in direct apposition, separated only by a film of serous fluid to act as a physiologic lubricant.

Function. The thorax is a marvelous piece of biologic architecture and engineering. When the diaphragm and the external intercostal muscles between the ribs contract, the bony cage is increased in all dimensions, thereby *increasing the volume* of the cavity almost beyond expectation. In this manner the intrathoracic pressure is *lowered* and the lungs are "sucked out," causing air to be inspired through the trachea and bronchi. To perform a normal expiration, the body merely relaxes these muscles; that is, the diaphragm goes from a stretched-out horizontal condition back to a rounded dome shape and the intercostal muscles "drop" the ribs. This causes the cavity to decrease in all dimensions, the *intrathoracic* pressure to *increase*, and thereby the lungs to deflate by elastic recoil.

In forced breathing other muscles are called into play. To take in the greatest possible volume of air, the sternocleidomastoids, rhomboids, and levator scapulae muscles, among others, aid the external intercostals in stretching the thoracic cage. Forced expiration involves the inner intercostals and abdominal muscles.

PHYSICS OF EXTERNAL AND INTERNAL RESPIRATION

Gaseous exchange takes place in the lungs and in the tissues.

In the lungs. The exchange of gases in the lungs between the air and the blood, that is, external respiration, is best approached by first analyzing the sequence of events leading to the intake of air (inspiration).

As the volume of the thoracic cavity increases as a consequence of diaphragmatic and intercostal contraction, the intrathoracic (*intrapleural*) pressure *decreases* in accordance with Boyle's law (p. 27). The drop in pressure averages about 4 mm. Hg, going from a value of about 756 mm. at the end of expiration to 752 mm. at the end of inspiration. This reduced pressure causes the lungs to *expand*, with the concomitant result that the *intrapulmonic pressure*—pressure within the lung—*decreases*, going from atmospheric (760 mm.) to about 757 mm. Hg. As a result of this negative pressure of 3 mm., air from the respiratory passageways moves into the alveoli, and, in

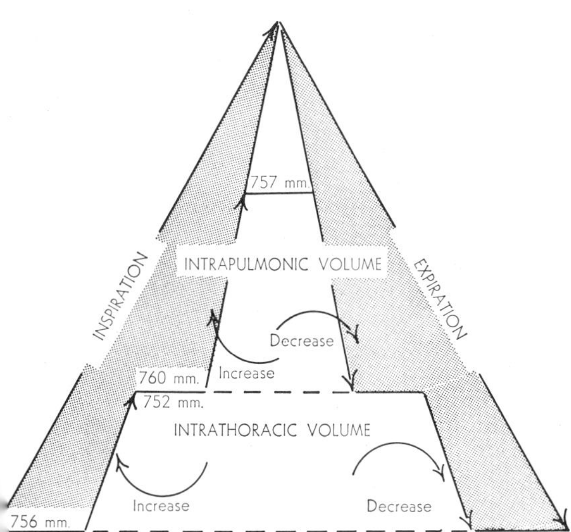

Fig. 13-6. Diagrammatic summary of the pressure changes that occur during normal breathing. (See text.)

turn, fresh air enters through the nose (Fig. 13-6).

At the end of inspiration the air pressure within the alveoli is atmospheric, that is, 760 mm. Hg. Of this pressure, 100 mm. is due to oxygen or, according to Dalton's law, we say that oxygen has a *partial* pressure (Po_2) of 100 mm. Hg. Now, since the Po_2 of venous blood entering the pulmonary capillaries is only about 40 mm. Hg, oxygen diffuses from the alveoli into the capillaries.

And the same applies to carbon dioxide. As venous blood moves into the lung, carbon dioxide, at a Pco_2 of 46 mm. Hg, diffuses into the alveoli, where the Pco_2 averages about 40 mm. Hg.

Thus, in the lungs, oxygen *enters* the blood and carbon dioxide *leaves* the blood.

In the tissues. The events in the tissues are the opposite of those in the lungs; that is, blood oxygen, at a Po_2 of 97 mm. Hg, diffuses into the tissue fluid, where the gas is present at a pressure of only about 30 mm. Conversely, tissue carbon dioxide, at a Pco_2 of 46 mm. Hg, passes into the capillaries, where the Pco_2 averages about 40 mm. Hg. Thus, the blood returns to the lung with the partial pressures cited above.

CHEMISTRY OF OXYGEN AND CARBON DIOXIDE TRANSPORT

The manner in which oxygen and carbon dioxide are transported by the blood is not exactly simple, but it certainly is biochemically fascinating.

In the lungs. As the blood spills into the vast expanse of the pulmonary capillaries, *reduced* hemoglobin (here abbreviated HHb) combines with oxygen to form oxyhemoglobin ($HHbO_2$) (Fig. 13-7). Since $HHbO_2$ is acidic, it reacts with potassium bicarbonate (also present in the red cell) to form potassium oxyhemoglobin ($KHbO_2$) and carbonic acid (H_2CO_3); thus,

$$HHbO_2 + KHCO_3 \longrightarrow KHbO_2 + H_2CO_3$$

Thereupon, H_2CO_3 (in the presence of the enzyme *carbonic anhydrase*) splits up to form CO_2 and H_2O, which subsequently escape from the red cell and enter the alveolar air:

$$H_2CO_3 \longrightarrow CO_2 + H_2O$$

The loss of $KHCO_3$ now causes an imbalance between the bicarbonate ion (HCO_3^-) in the red cell and plasma, and as a result, Cl^- diffuses out of the cell into the plasma, where it reacts with $NaHCO_3$ to release HCO_3^-. Thus,

$$NaHCO_3 + Cl^- \longrightarrow NaCl + HCO_3^-$$

Plasma HCO_3^- now diffuses into the red cell—to replace Cl^-—and reacts with KHb to form $KHCO_3$, which, as explained before, reacts with $HHbO_2$ to form H_2CO_3, and so on. This exchange of Cl^- for HCO_3^- continues until the "charge" of CO_2 (carried as $NaHCO_3$) is blown off.

What about the oxygen? As shown, oxygen has gone through two steps to become $KHbO_2$, in which form it is carried to the tissues. A very small amount of oxygen is carried in simple solution. It has been de-

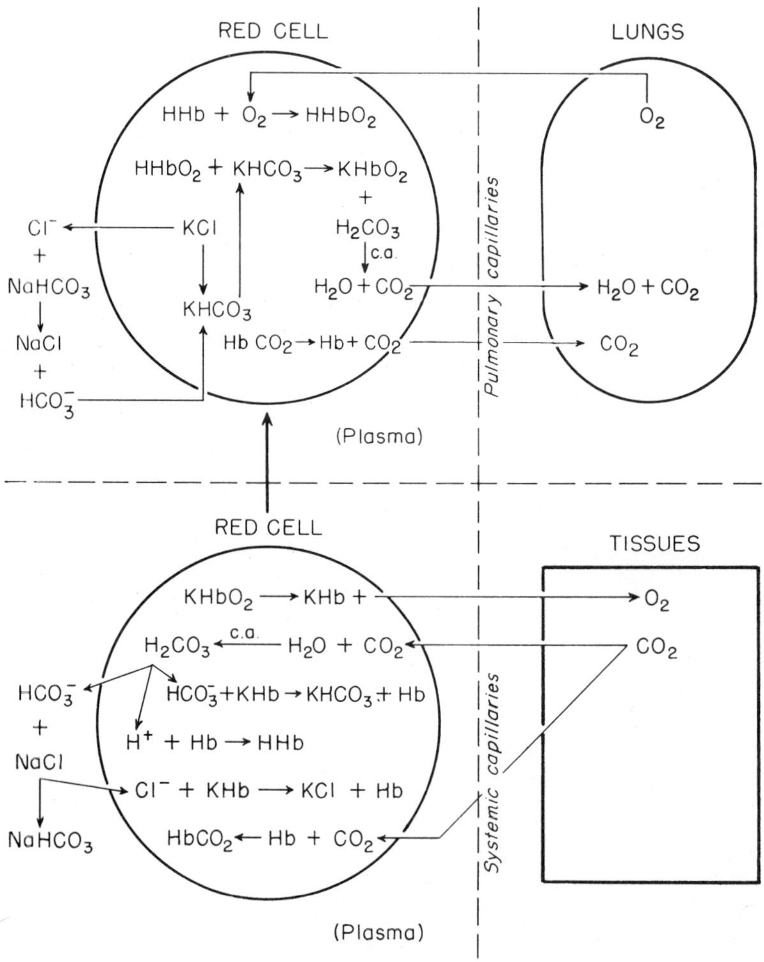

Fig. 13-7. Diagrammatic summary of the chemical events in oxygen and carbon dioxide transport by the blood. (See text.) (From Brooks, S. M.: Basic facts of general chemistry, Philadelphia, 1956, W. B. Saunders Co.)

termined that 100 ml. of normal blood (14 to 16 gm. of hemoglobin) transports 20 ml. of oxygen—19.5 ml. as $KHbO_2$ and 0.5 ml. in simple solution.

It is interesting to note that the red cell is freely permeable to HCO_3^- and Cl^- ions but not to K^+ and Na^+ ions. Indeed, this makes possible the various reactions just described.

The air expired from the lungs is about 4 percent CO_2 and 16 percent O_2, as compared to atmospheric air of 21 percent O_2 and 0.04 percent CO_2. Alveolar air contains 5.5 percent CO_2 and 14 percent O_2.

In the tissues. The chemical events that take place in the tissues go hand in hand with the reactions just described. As a matter of fact, the former aid in understanding the latter and vice versa.

When blood passes through the capillaries, O_2 is released from the unstable compound potassium oxyhemoglobin ($KHbO_2$):

$$KHbO_2 \longrightarrow KHb + O_2$$

At the same time, CO_2 diffuses into the red cells, where most of it reacts with

H_2O, in the presence of the enzyme carbonic anhydrase, to form carbonic acid:

$$CO_2 + H_2O \xrightarrow{\text{Carbonic anhydrase}} H_2CO_3$$

The carbonic acid then ionizes to H^+ ions and HCO_3^- ions. Now most of these HCO_3^- ions diffuse into the plasma, where they react with NaCl to form $NaHCO_3$ and Cl^-. The H^+ ions, which are left behind, react with hemoglobin (Hb) to produce HHb (reduced Hb). These reactions may be represented as follows:

$$H_2CO_3 \longrightarrow H^+ + HCO_3^-$$
$$HCO_3^- + Na^+Cl^- \longrightarrow NaHCO_3 + Cl^-$$
$$H^+ + Hb^- \longrightarrow HHb$$

The Cl^- formed in the plasma diffuses into the red cell, balancing the loss of HCO_3^-, and reacts with KHb:

$$Cl^- + KHb \longrightarrow KCl + Hb$$

Actually, it is the shift of Cl^- ions *(chloride shift)* that permits the plasma to carry CO_2 as $NaHCO_3$.

All of the HCO_3^- ions do not leave the cell. Some react with KHb to form $KHCO_3$ and Hb:

$$HCO_3^- + KHb \longrightarrow KHCO_3 + Hb$$

Of the original CO_2 that enters the red cells, some combines directly with hemoglobin, forming carbaminohemoglobin ($HbCO_2$):

$$CO_2 + Hb \longrightarrow HbCO_2$$

Thus, CO_2 is carried by the blood in three ways: as $NaHCO_3$, $HbCO_2$, and $KHCO_3$. Most (two thirds) of the total blood CO_2 is carried in the plasma as $NaHCO_3$ and one third is carried in the red cells (as $HbCO_2$ and $KHCO_3$).

RESPIRATORY CONTROL

As we know, breathing depends upon the alternate contraction and relaxation of the inspiratory muscles, namely, the diaphragm and external intercostals. In order for these muscles to contract, they must receive impulses via the appropriate nerves, especially the *phrenic* nerve which supplies the diaphragm. The question now arises: What mechanism controls these impulses? Put in a more practical way: What controls the depth and frequency of respiration? (Refer to Fig. 13-8 throughout the discussion.)

Respiratory center. The respiratory center, located in the *medulla oblongata* of the brain, is believed to wield the most influence over the depth and frequency of respiration. Although the *pneumotaxic* center in the *pons* of the brain also shares in this regulation, in this discussion we shall speak only of medullary control.

Obviously, in order for the respiratory center to judge the frequency and intensity of nerve impulses to be sent to the muscles of respiration, it must receive peripheral information regarding the oxygen requirements of the body at any given moment. For example, if we breathe harder during exercise than at rest, it is because the respiratory center has been apprised of the body's need and has reacted accordingly.

Hering-Breuer reflex. The frequency of normal breathing depends upon the presence of stretch receptors among the alveoli. These receptors, as the term implies, are stimulated by expansion of the alveoli during inspiration, sending impulses to the medulla via sensory nerves. This causes *inhibition* of the center and reflex relaxation of the inspiratory muscles. Now, as the lungs deflate, thereby reducing pressure upon the receptors, the inhibitory impulses flowing to the medulla cease, this time causing the respiratory center to release impulses to the muscles of inspiration. Once again, the lungs inflate, the stretch receptors are stimulated, and so on. This *feedback* series of events is known as the Hering-Breuer reflex.

Carbon dioxide. A *moderate increase* in carbon dioxide—or *decrease* in pH—is the most potent stimulant of respiration. As its

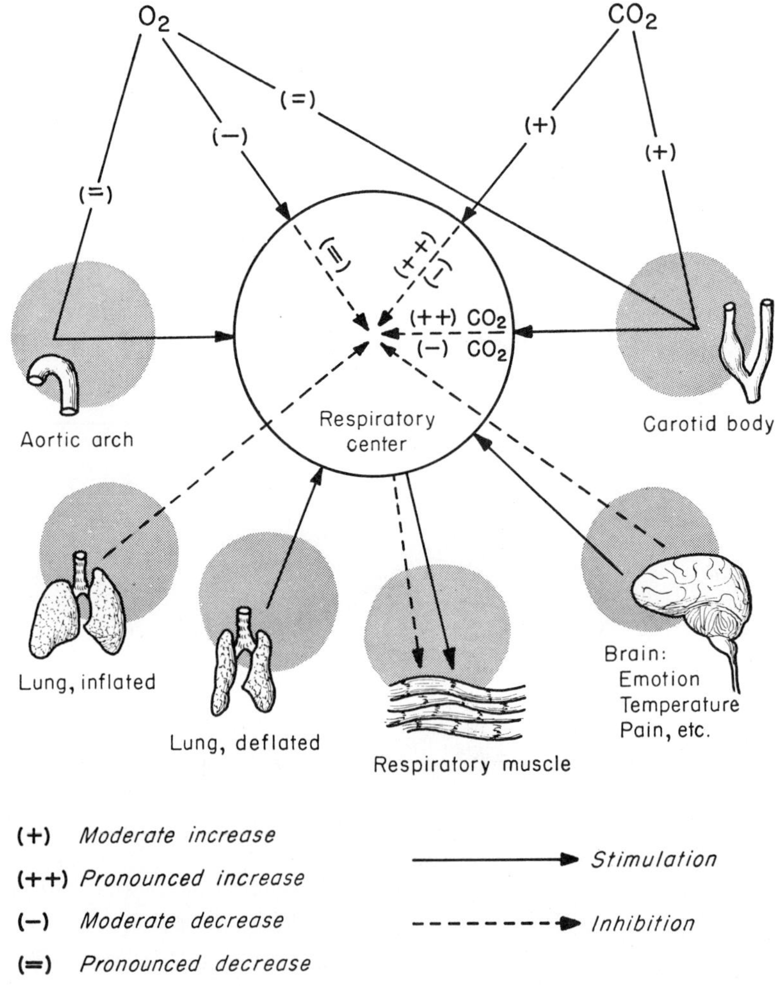

Fig. 13-8. Summary of the mechanisms involved in the control of the respiratory rate. Note that CO_2 and O_2 act on the respiratory center directly and indirectly. (See text.)

partial pressure in the blood rises above 40 mm., the gas (free or as H_2CO_3) stimulates the respiratory center directly. Indirectly, but to a much less degree, carbon dioxide steps up respiration by stimulating the chemoreceptors in the *carotid body.* At *high* concentrations, however, carbon dioxide depresses these areas. Fortunately, this does not occur under ordinary conditions.

Oxygen. A moderate decrease in blood Po_2 stimulates the respiratory center directly. This is not true in *severe* hypoxic situations, however, because nervous tissue cannot function properly when starved for oxygen. Indeed, the nervous system is the most sensitive of all tissues to oxygen deprivation. A pronounced decrease in arterial Po_2—via *chemoreceptors in the carotid body* and *aortic arch*—reflexly stimulates respiration. However, since the oxygen concentration of the blood never falls to such a level under normal conditions, this particular regulatory mechanism operates only in hypoxic emergencies.

Other factors affecting respiration. It is quite possible that the respiratory center is subject to more outside control than any other nerve center in the body. Aside from the Hering-Breuer reflex and the influence of oxygen and carbon dioxide, respiration is altered by countless stimuli. The physician takes advantage of this fact when he spanks the newborn infant to induce breathing. Irritant chemicals, strong light, sudden pain, and cold are other examples well known to everyone. Few of us can forget the distressing experience of having our breath "shut off" following a plunge into cold water. No doubt, many of us recall the dramatic response that attends administration of smelling salts to a victim of fainting. What happens here is that the whiff of ammonia stimulates the respiratory center via the myriad sensory endings in the nose.

Also, we must not forget the influence of psychic factors. It is common experience, for instance, that when one is spellbound or frightened he "forgets" to breathe. Indeed, the sigh following such an experience is quite real; that is, the period of apnea produces enough carbon dioxide to trigger an audible respiratory sound. Other emotional varieties of respiration include laughing, crying, and yawning.

AIR VOLUMES EXCHANGED DURING BREATHING

Using a simple instrument called a spirometer (Fig. 13-9), we can easily measure the intake and output of the lungs.

Tidal air. Tidal air is the volume of air that is carried to and fro in normal respiration. In most persons it averages about 500 ml.

Inspiratory capacity and expiratory reserve. Inspiratory capacity is that volume of air in excess of tidal air which can be drawn into the lungs by forced inspiration; conversely, expiratory reserve volume is that volume which can be expelled from the lungs in excess of the tidal air. The former is normally about 3000 ml. and the latter about 1100 ml.

Vital capacity. Vital capacity may be defined as the greatest volume of air that one is able to expel after the greatest possible inhalation. The student will readily see that this is equal to the combined volumes of tidal air, inspiratory capacity, and expiratory reserve—about 4600 ml.

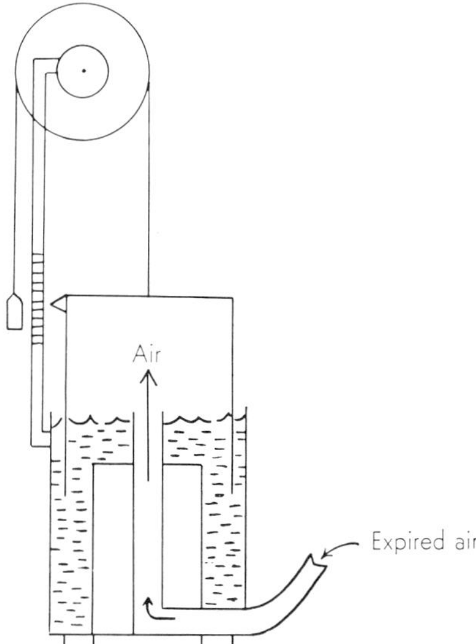

Fig. 13-9. Spirometer. The volume of air entering or leaving the bell is recorded on the scale.

Residual and minimal air. Regardless of how hard one tries, he cannot expel *all* the air from the lungs. That amount which remains trapped in the alveoli after the greatest possible expiration is called residual air (about 1200 ml).

When the thorax is opened, the lungs collapse and the residual air is forced out —but not all of it. The tiny bronchioles collapse and in so doing cut off the escape of a small amount of air from the alveoli. This permanently trapped air is referred to as minimal air. This explains why the lungs, unlike other soft tissue, do not sink when placed in water. The exception is in stillborn infants when the lungs contain no air. Advantage is taken of this fact in medicolegal work.

NORMAL BREATHING

Normal quiet breathing, called *eupnea,* may be *costal, diaphragmatic,* or a combination of both. In the costal type the upper ribs move first and the abdomen second, with the elevation of the ribs being the more noticeable of the two movements. In the diaphragmatic type the abdomen bulges outward first, followed by a less energetic movement of the thorax. Diaphragmatic respirations are deeper than those of the costal type. Costal breathing may be caused by tight clothing that obstructs diaphragmatic action.

Respiratory rate. Eupnea in the adult runs from 14 to 20 respirations per minute, but during exercise and emotional tension the rate in healthy persons will increase substantially *(polypnea).* Age has an important bearing on respiration. During the first year of life the respiratory rate averages about 50 per minute, and by the age of 5 years the rate has dropped to 25. The rate continues to drop, reaching the adult normal sometime during the late teens or early twenties.

ABNORMAL BREATHING

There are a number of breathing abnormalities. Some of the principal forms include the following:

apnea temporary cessation of respirations.

dyspnea difficult or labored breathing due to conditions that interfere with the free passage of air into and out of the lungs.

Cheyne-Stokes respiration a type of respiration characterized by rhythmical variations in intensity, occurring in cycles; each cycle consists of a dyspneic phase followed by an apneic period lasting from 5 to 30 seconds (Fig. 13-10); Cheyne-Stokes respiration is usually seen in coma.

orthopnea inability to breathe in the horizontal position.

tachypnea excessive rapidity of respiration.

WATER BALANCE

Since water is lost from the body in exhaled air (as water vapor), the lungs obviously play an important role in water balance (Chapter 18). In a 24-hour period the tissues are deprived of about 400 ml. of water in this manner. The exhalation of warm water vapor tends to cool the body, thus constituting a temperature-regulating mechanism. This is dramatically shown by the panting dog on a hot summer day.

Of clinical significance is the fact that the water lost from the lungs and skin must be replaced, a consideration of no little importance in the hospital. In the event that the patient cannot take fluid by mouth, for instance, close to 900 ml. is given intravenously to replace that lost via *insensible* perspiration (400 ml. via the lungs and 500 ml. via the skin). To this, of course, must be added the volume of water lost as urine (generally about 1500 ml.).

ACID-BASE BALANCE

The pH of the blood hovers ever so closely to 7.4, and a variation of a few tenths in either direction may spell death if not corrected. A decrease in pH is referred to as acidemia *(acidosis)* and an increase as alkalemia *(alkalosis).*

The reason why the blood normally has

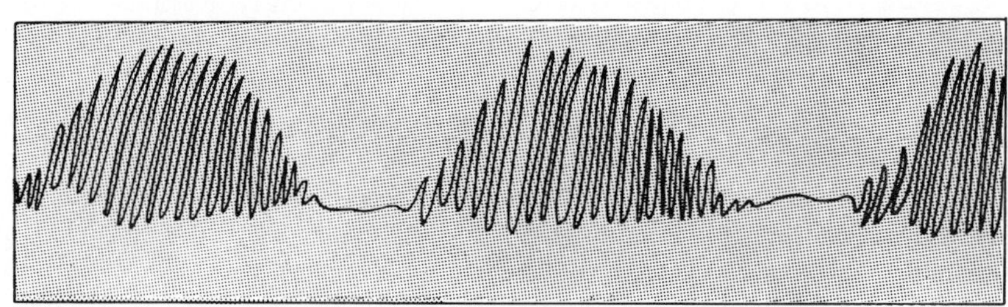

Fig. 13-10. Stethographic tracing of Cheyne-Stokes breathing. (From Halliburton, W. D.: Handbook of physiology, ed. 16, Philadelphia, 1923, P. Blakiston's Son & Co.)

a pH of 7.4 stems chiefly from the fact that the ratio of the concentration of HCO_3^- *(base)* to H_2CO_3 *(acid)* remains 20 to 1. Thus,

$$\frac{[HCO_3^-]^*}{[H_2CO_3]} = \frac{20}{1} \text{ (pH 7.4)}$$

For example, if the $[HCO_3^-]$ rises, the $[H_2CO_3]$ rises, and so on. One of the mechanisms that aids in maintaining the ratio is the respiratory system.

Respiratory acidosis. Let us suppose that for some reason the pH of the blood starts to drop. As we know, this would stimulate respiration and thereby result in the blowing off of additional CO_2 and, in turn, a drop in $[H_2CO_3]$. Thus, the ratio is prevented from changing and the pH is maintained. It is easy to see, therefore, that any condition which restricts the exit of CO_2 from the lungs (for example, constricted bronchioles) may cause respiratory acidosis.

Respiratory alkalosis. An elevation in pH inhibits the respiratory center and thereby conserves CO_2 and H_2CO_3, the desired effect being to return the pH to the 7.4 level. Thus, the respiratory system fights alkalosis as well as acidosis. The "pH abnormality" known as respiratory alkalosis is caused by excessive pulmonary ventilation (hyperpnea and tachypnea). So much carbon dioxide is expelled from the body that the $[H_2CO_3]$ drops, increasing the 20 to 1 ratio and thereby the pH.

CLINICAL CONSIDERATIONS

In this section we shall briefly consider the chief derangements affecting the respiratory system.

Anoxia. Anoxia means a reduction of oxygen in the body tissues below physiologic levels, and from what has been said, the student will readily appreciate that there are a variety of possible causes.

Oxygen starvation due to interference with the source of oxygen or inadequate ventilation of blood is called *anoxic* anoxia. This would include high altitudes, low oxygen mixtures, respiratory depression, and mechanical obstruction (namely, tracheal tumor, asthma, foreign bodies, and pulmonary edema).

Another common form is *anemic* anoxia, which results from inadequate oxygen being carried from the lungs to the tissues. The etiologic factor may be anemia, methemoglobinemia, or carbon monoxide poisoning. Anemia speaks for itself. As for the latter situations, the hemoglobin molecule is altered in such a way that it can no longer combine with oxygen. Methemoglobinemia is caused by the reaction between certain poisons and drugs (for example, nitrates and nitrites) and hemoglobin, yielding the derivative methemoglobin. Similarly, carbon monoxide reacts with hemoglobin to yield carboxyhemoglobin.

Another important anoxic possibility is some disturbance in the cells that interferes with the utilization of oxygen. This type of anoxia, aptly termed *histotoxic* anoxia, is caused by certain poisons (for example, cyanides) and drugs (for example, narcotics).

Still other forms are *anoxia neonatorum* and *stagnant anoxia.* The former is anoxia of the newborn, and the latter results from failure of the circulation to move blood fast enough through the vessels.

The clinical management of anoxia depends upon the type. It may, for instance, involve surgery (for example, tracheotomy or removal of tumors), drugs (for example, epinephrine for asthma, vitamin B_{12} for anemia, and vasodilators for gangrene), or antidotes against histotoxic poisons. In all anoxic emergencies, of course, oxygen is administered.

Infectious diseases. Infections of the respiratory tract are the most common and potentially dangerous of any that befall the body. Those of major concern are briefly discussed herewith.

*[ ] means concentration.

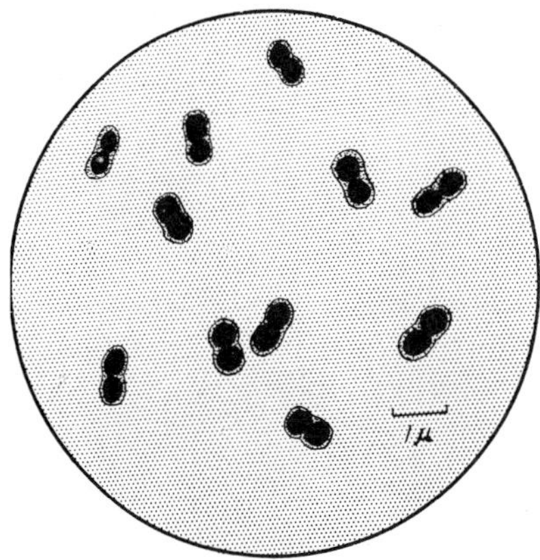

Fig. 13-11. *Diplococcus pneumoniae.* (From Brooks, S. M.: Basic facts of medical microbiology, ed. 2, Philadelphia, 1962, W. B. Saunders Co.)

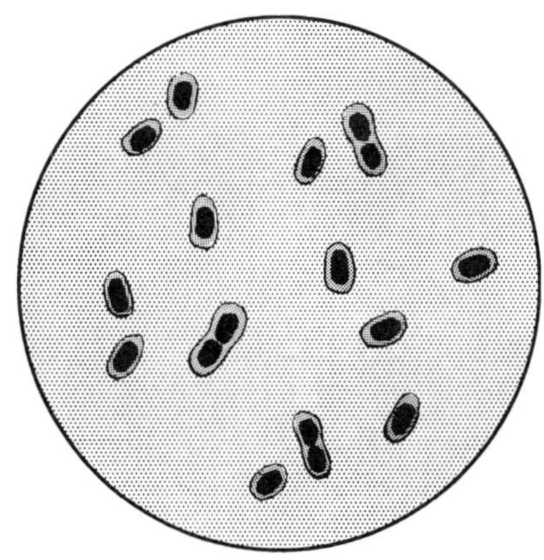

Fig. 13-12. *Klebsiella pneumoniae.* (From Brooks, S. M.: Basic facts of medical microbiology, ed. 2, Philadelphia, 1962, W. B. Saunders Co.)

Pneumonia. Pneumonia is an inflammation of the small bronchi, bronchioles, and alveoli. Since these spaces become filled with mucous exudate, not enough oxygen enters the blood to meet the requirements of the body. Indeed, death due to anoxia is not an infrequent occurrence in this ominous infection.

Pneumonia is generally characterized as *lobar* or *lobular.* Lobar pneumonia, which involves one or more lobes of the lung, is caused in most instances by *Diplococcus pneumoniae,* a gram-positive, encapsulated microorganism (Fig. 13-11) that gains entrance to the body via the nose or mouth. Although it may be transmitted indirectly by food or fomites, most cases result from droplet infection. The diagnosis is usually established by demonstration of the organism in the sputum. Even though penicillin is dramatically effective against most types of the organism, it is still occasionally necessary to make a precise determination by means of the *Neufeld* (or *quellung*) reaction, a test based upon the fact that the capsule swells in the presence of the specific immune serum. Of the seventy-odd types known, the most common are Types 1, 2, and 3.

Another pathogen that causes lobar pneumonia is *Klebsiella pneumoniae,* or *Friedländer's bacillus* (Fig. 13-12), an encapsulated, nonsporeforming, gram-negative organism. In addition, it is capable of infecting the nasal sinuses, bronchi, and middle ear. The broad-spectrum antibiotics yield good results in treatment of all these infections.

Lobular pneumonia, or bronchopneumonia, is generally a secondary infection scattered throughout the lung tissue. It may be caused by a variety of pathogens in addition to pneumococci, for example, *Haemophilus influenzae,* staphylococci, streptococci, certain viruses, and certain pathogenic fungi. Treatment centers about the use of broad-spectrum antibiotics and sulfonamides.

A rather special form of pneumonia (but apparently very common) called *primary atypical* pneumonia—heretofore believed to be caused by a virus—is now known to be due to the recently discovered microbe *Mycoplasma pneumoniae* (p. 131). The broad-spectrum antibiotics (namely, the tetracyclines) are the drugs of choice here.

Pneumotropic viruses. The common cold and influenza are *viral* infections of the respiratory passageways (Fig. 13-13).

The common cold, man's number one

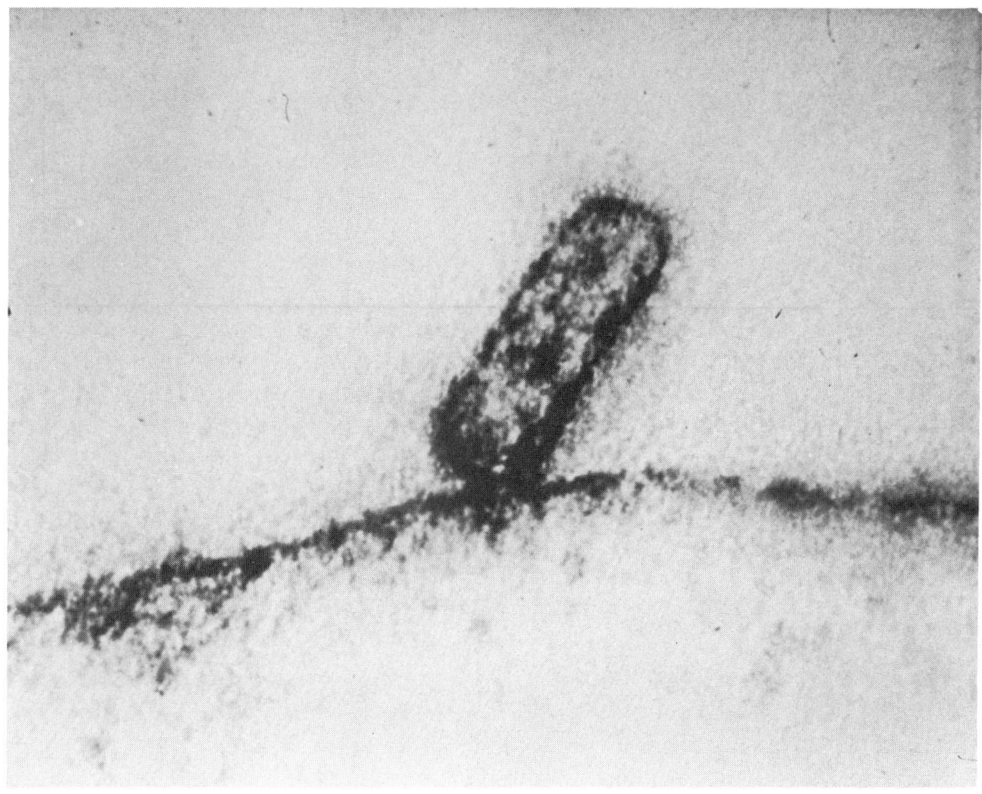

Fig. 13-13. Influenza virus showing a single virion attached to the cell membrane. (×90,000.) (Courtesy Eli Lilly & Co.)

infectious disease, is apparently caused by a score or more strains of the so-called cold virus (p. 133). Since these organisms are present in nasal discharges and saliva, the infection is easily spread via coughing, sneezing, kissing, and handling of objects contaminated thereby. Except for secondary bacterial infections, treatment is entirely symptomatic. Prophylaxis is unsatisfactory.

Contrary to popular opinion, the common cold is potentially serious. The inflammation that is set up along the respiratory passageways greatly reduces the resistance of the mucosa to secondary invaders such as staphylococci and streptococci.

Influenza is similar to a severe cold, but it is generally much more serious. Once again, the danger that accompanies the disease is due to the likelihood of secondary complications. In the great epidemic of 1918 the death toll was close to twenty million! In 1957 the so-called Asian flu sent thousands to the grave.

There is no specific therapeutic agent useful against the viruses that cause influenza. When bacterial complications appear, however, the sulfonamides and antibiotics are lifesaving. Rest and good nursing care are also essential features in treatment. As for prevention of the malady, vaccines prepared from killed strains of A and B viruses are now available. The duration of immunity produced by such vaccines is relatively short, usually ranging from 2 to 12 months.

Tuberculosis. Although the advent of streptomycin and other antibiotics has drastically reduced the death rate, tuberculosis still remains a major threat to man's welfare, particularly in underprivileged areas.

Tuberculosis is caused by the actinomycete *Mycobacterium tuberculosis,* a slender, nonmotile, nonsporing, *acid-fast* bacillus (Fig. 13-14). Like other members of the genus *Mycobacterium,* this species is often observed in the branching and filamentous state. Of the four varieties of the species, only *Mycobacterium tuberculosis hominis* and *Mycobacterium tuberculosis bovis* (from cattle) attack man. The infection usually results from contact with "open cases" through coughing, sneezing, and kissing. The organism may also enter the body via milk or other contaminated foods. The removal of infected cattle and pasteurization, however, have practically eliminated (in the United States as least) milk-borne tuberculosis.

The clinical picture of tuberculosis depends upon the tissue involved and the host's resistance. The principal lesions occur in the kidney, bone, meninges, and lungs, especially the lungs. From the primary infection the tubercle bacilli migrate throughout the body and, if unchecked, may overrun the defenses of the body. If it goes untreated, tuberculosis is fatal.

The treatment of tuberculosis centers about the use of drugs and surgery. The principal chemotherapeutic agents presently employed include streptomycin, isoniazid (INH), and para-aminosalicylic acid (PAS). Surgical resection or mechanical collapse of the diseased lung is sometimes necessary. Mental and physical rest, fresh air, nutritous food, and good nursing care are also helpful.

Prevention of tuberculosis is predicated upon early diagnosis, good sanitation, and elimination of overcrowding. Diagnosis is made by x-ray examination, isolation of the organism, and the *tuberculin test.* The tuberculin test is based upon the fact that a person infected with the tubercle bacillus (either in the past or at present) becomes *sensitized* to tuberculin (an extract derived from the tubercle bacillus). Since a positive reaction can mean an inactive as well as an active focus of infection, it can never be interpreted as unequivocal evidence of clinical tuberculosis *except* in infants and young children.

A considerable body of information now suggests that BCG vaccine *(bacille Calmette Guérin),* prepared from attenuated bovine tubercle bacilli, is safe and somewhat effective. It is given only to those with a *negative* tuberculin test.

Diphtheria. Diphtheria is a severe acute

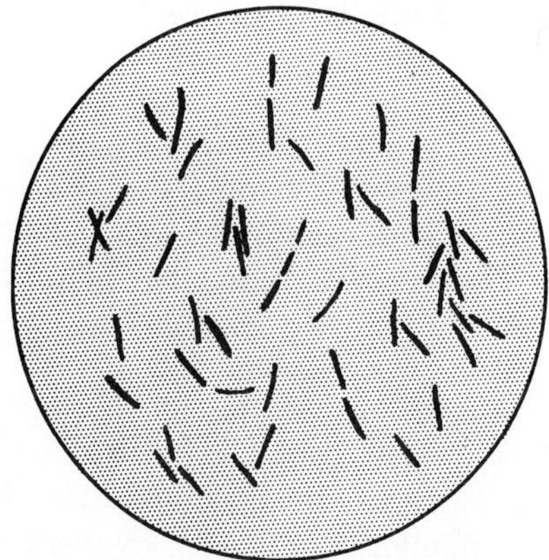

Fig. 13-14. *Mycobacterium tuberculosis.* (From Brooks, S. M.: Basic facts of medical microbiology, ed. 2, Philadelphia, 1962, W. B. Saunders Co.)

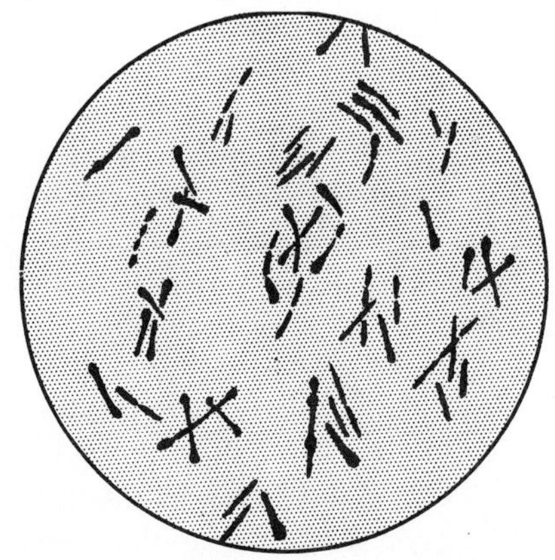

Fig. 13-15. *Corynebacterium diphtheriae.* (From Brooks, S. M.: Basic facts of medical microbiology, ed. 2, Philadelphia, 1962, W. B. Saunders Co.)

infection, generally of young children, marked locally by inflammation of the upper respiratory tract and systemically by damage to the heart, kidney, and nerves. The pathogen *Corynebacterium diphtheriae* (often called the *Klebs-Löffler bacillus* after its discoverers) is a pleomorphic, nonsporeforming, nonmotile, nonencapsulated, gram-positive bacillus. Characteristically, the bacilli stain irregularly and frequently are banded or beaded with metachromatic granules (Fig. 13-15). The principal threat to life stems from the powerful exotoxin released by the organism.

To fully establish a diagnosis of diphtheria, the bacillus must be isolated and its toxigenicity demonstrated in animals (Fig. 13-16). The specimen is taken on a swab and streaked on sterile plates of Löffler's serum agar or chocolate tellurite agar. If, after incubation, typical bacilli are found, the growth from a Löffler slant is suspended in saline solution and injected into two guinea pigs, one of which has been passively immunized with diphtheria antitoxin 24 hours previously. Death of the unprotected animal constitutes a positive test.

Therapeutically, concomitant use of the *antitoxin* and *penicillin* affords a good prognosis if given early. The antitoxin neutralizes the toxin and the penicillin attacks the bacilli. Prophylactically, active immunization with the *toxoid* is the most important measure, for when vaccinated in infancy, practically all persons are endowed with potent immunity that lasts from 2 to 5 years. It is recommended that the first shot be given at the age of 4 to 6 months and that a booster be given before the child enters school.

The *Schick* test, used to determine whether a person is *susceptible* to diphtheria, is performed by injection of a very small quantity of the toxin into the skin (intracutaneously). Susceptible persons develop a pink to red wheal at the site of the injection, but immune persons show no reaction.

Psittacosis. This disease of the respira-

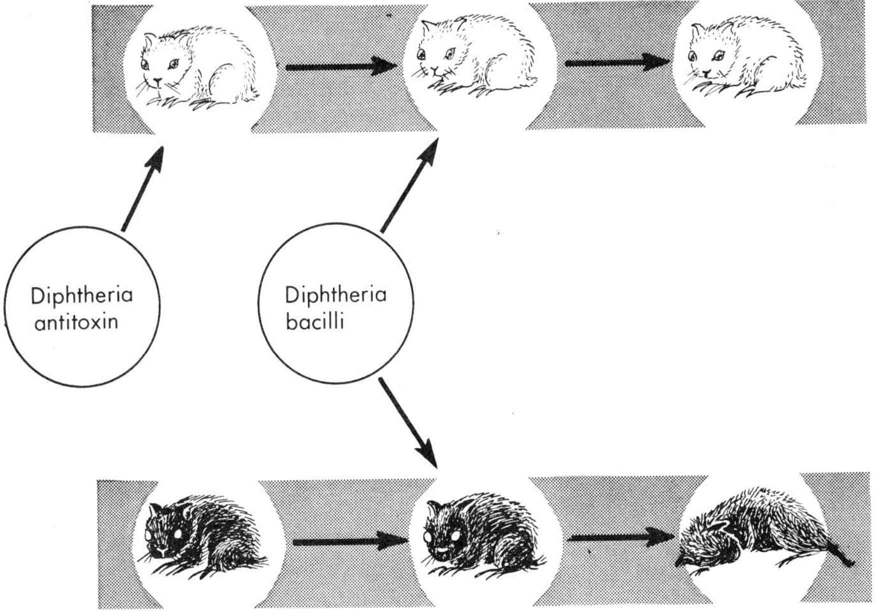

Fig. 13-16. Using guinea pig to prove identity and virulence of *Corynebacterium diphtheriae.* The illustration depicts a "positive test." (From Brooks, S. M.: Basic facts of medical microbiology, ed. 2, Philadelphia, 1962, W. B. Saunders Co.)

tory tract is marked by fever, chills, headache, sore throat, nausea, and vomiting. A severe type of pneumonia and involvement of the central nervous system are the main danger points. Up until rather recently the etiologic agent was classed as a virus, but the facts now point to a rickettsial category. The reservoir of infection embraces, among others, pigeons, sea birds, ducks, chickens, turkeys, and psittacine birds (parrots, parakeets, and the like), especially the latter. Most cases are contracted by the handling of sick birds and the inhalation of dust charged with bird feces. Treatment centers on the use of antibiotics, namely the tetracyclines, and prevention entails the destruction of diseased birds and the avoidance of undue handling of birds.

Histoplasmosis. Histoplasmosis, a severe and often fatal systemic fungal infection caused by the pathogenic yeast *Histoplasma capsulatum* (Fig. 13-17), is characterized by emaciation, leukopenia, anemia, fever, and ulceration of the nasopharynx, intestine, liver, and spleen. A mild form of the disease that attacks the lungs (common along the Mississippi basin) closely parallels early tuberculosis. As a matter of fact, cases of histoplasmosis have often been misdiagnosed as the latter infection. The histoplasmin test (a skin test) is now a valuable aid in diagnosis. Treatment centers about the administration of antifungal agents (namely, amphotericin B).

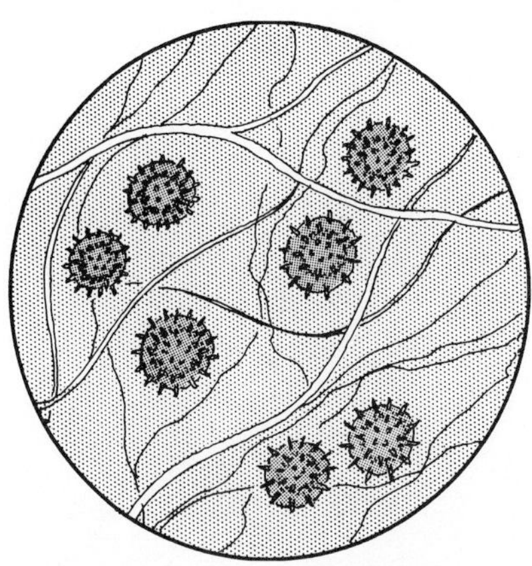

Fig. 13-17. *Histoplasma capsulatum* (in spore stage). (From Brooks, S. M.: Basic facts of medical microbiology, ed. 2, Philadelphia, 1962, W. B. Saunders Co.)

Other fungous infections of note that attack the respiratory tract and lungs include *moniliasis, coccidioidomycosis,* and *aspergillosis.*

Noninfectious diseases. In addition to infection, the lungs and air passageways are subject to a number of other disorders. Some of the more important will be briefly outlined.

*Emphysema.** Pulmonary emphysema is a disease of the lungs characterized by abnormal enlargement of the air spaces and by destructive changes in the alveolar walls. Histologically, the alveoli are distended and disrupted, with a decrease in the amount of elastic tissue and in the number and size of vascular channels. The resulting functional disturbances are increased airflow resistance and decreased ventilation.

The magnitude of pulmonary emphysema as a health problem is reflected by the increasing number of deaths reported from this cause. In the United States the incidence of emphysema has increased almost 200 percent. According to one survey, 26.5 percent of men over 40 years of age demonstrate evidence of chronic obstructive disease of the airway. And most alarming, emphysema was the second most frequent single disease for which disability benefits were granted by the Bureau of Old-Age and Survivors Insurance in 1960. Of interest, too, is the fact that incidence of the disease is four to five times greater among men than among women.

Emphysema probably develops as a result of factors that cause partial bronchial obstruction and increased resistance to airflow. Infection, bronchial muscular constriction, and mucosal congestion all may

*This discussion was adapted from Pulmonary emphysema, Therapeutic Notes, vol. 28, No. 2, 1963.

lead to increased airflow resistance and development of pulmonary distention. Repeated or prolonged pulmonary distention leads to destruction of alveolar walls and loss of pulmonary elasticity. It is also possible, however, that initial loss of elasticity is basic rather than secondary to the distention.

Destruction of the alveolar walls causes obliteration of the pulmonary capillaries, which leads to increased pulmonary vascular resistance and elevated pulmonary arterial pressure. The increased pulmonary vascular resistance places a heavy strain on the right ventricle, so that it eventually hypertrophies. One fourth to one third of patients eventually develop right-sided heart failure, or *cor pulmonale* (that is, heart disease secondary to disease of the lungs).

Symptomatic benefit and measurable improvement in pulmonary function usually follow intensive therapy for airway obstruction. This is best accomplished by the use of bronchodilators and intermittent positive pressure breathing. Above all, the patient should avoid smoking and other respiratory irritants.

Asthma. Asthma is a distressing disease marked by recurrent attacks of paroxysmal dyspnea, wheezing, and cough caused by spasmodic contraction of the bronchi and bronchioles; an acute attack leads to anoxic anoxia and often sudden death. It is believed that many cases are allergic manifestations in sensitized persons. In addition, the role of emotional factors can never be underestimated. Treatment involves the use of drugs such as epinephrine (*Adrenalin*) and aminophylline to relax the muscles in the bronchi and bronchioles as well as measures to remedy the underlying etiologic factors.

Atelectasis. Atelectasis is the collapse, or failure of expansion, of a part or all of the lung. The condition may be acquired or congenital. Acquired atelectasis may result from intrapulmonary obstruction by accumulated secretions postoperatively or by tumors of the bronchi. Also, outside pressure (as from pleural infusions or pneumothorax) may cause atelectasis. The signs and symptoms, of course, depend upon the rapidity of onset. In acute episodes, dyspnea and cyanosis are cardinal signs. Treatment centers about administration of oxygen and correction of the underlying cause.

Pleurisy. Pleurisy is inflammation of the pleura. In the acute form the membranes become reddened and covered with a serous exudate, and the inflamed surfaces tend to unite by adhesions. The symptoms are a "stitch" in the side, chills, and fever followed by a dry cough. Chronic pleurisy is long continued and characterized by dry surfaces, purulent exudation, adhesions, and even calcification. The treatment is chiefly symptomatic.

Pneumoconiosis. Pneumoconiosis is a chronic fibrous reaction in the lung provoked by inhalation of dust. Characteristically, the lungs become hard and pigmented, but the precise clinical picture depends upon the nature of the dust. Some of the more important forms include *anthracosis, silicosis,* and *berylliosis.* Anthracosis is caused by coal dust. The lungs and regional lymph glands become dark and even black in color. Silicosis is a pneumoconiosis caused by the inhalation of stone, sand, or flint dust containing silicon dioxide. Berylliosis, perhaps the most morbid pneumoconiosis, is caused by the inhalation of fumes or powders tainted with beryllium salts. The condition is characterized by formation of granulomas in the lung tissue and occasionally in the lymph nodes and liver.

Lung tumors. Carcinoma of the lung may be primary or secondary to metastasis. The early signs are cough, hemoptysis, and shadows in the x-ray film. It is certainly disturbing to learn that primary carcinoma, particularly in the male, has been on the rise throughout the present century and is now the most common cause of cancer death in the male. Ardent smokers and tobacco manufacturers to the contrary, most statistical studies disclose a causal relationship with smoking, especially cigarette smoking. Those who do not go along with this conclusion point to other factors, particularly the ever-increasing concentrations of noxious chemicals in the atmosphere released by industry and engine exhausts—a recognized health problem in its own right.

Cough. Except perhaps for a runny nose, coughing is the most common complaint of the respiratory system. Coughing, a sudden noisy expulsion of air from the lungs, is initiated by any form of irritation anywhere along the respiratory passageways. Such irritation, by provoking the discharge of sensory stimuli from the mucosal lining, triggers the so-called cough center in the medulla to release volleys of motor impulses over the nerves leading to the muscles of expiration.

In the cough reflex, nature has provided the body with a unique device for cleaning out the respiratory tree, as dramatically shown by the fitful cough that attends swallowing something the "wrong way." Also, in respiratory infections, coughing plays a vital role in removing copious amounts of troublesome mucus.

When coughing brings up mucus or foreign particles, it is obviously playing a useful role. This is a *productive* cough. In contrast, an unproductive cough serves no function other than harassment. Indeed, a dry unproductive cough, particularly in very young, elderly, and debilitated persons, can prove a serious strain upon the general strength and resistance of the body. It is the unproductive cough, then, that the physician strives to check, using one of the many synthetic antitussive drugs now available. Such drugs act by inhibiting the cough center in the medulla.

A chronic cough almost always means that all is not well along the respiratory passageways. Since it indicates some form of irritation, the physician must make a careful search for possible causes.

Questions

1. Describe the nasal septum and passageways.
2. Discuss the function of the nose.
3. Describe the structure of the pharynx.
4. What determines the pitch of the human voice?
5. Distinguish between the fundamental and overtones.
6. What is meant by a harmonic?
7. Describe the structure and function of the trachea.
8. Why is an object swallowed into the trachea more likely to lodge in the right lung than in the left?
9. Describe the gross anatomy of the lungs.
10. Describe the pulmonary unit.
11. Name and describe the cavities of the thorax.
12. On the basis of Boyle's law, explain the drop in intrapleural pressure occasioned by the contraction of the diaphragm and external intercostal muscles.
13. Why does the lung collapse in pneumothorax?
14. In the lung, oxygen diffuses from the air into the blood. Why?
15. In the tissues why does carbon dioxide diffuse from the interstitial fluid into the blood?
16. Translate the expression "753 mm. Hg."
17. When is the intrapulmonic pressure greatest?
18. Describe the chloride shift.
19. Discuss the role of carbonic anhydrase.
20. If the red cell were not permeable to HCO_3^- and Cl^- and *were* permeable to K^+ and Na^+ ions, the blood *could not* transport O_2 and CO_2 in sufficient quantities to sustain life. Explain.
21. Compare the composition of inspired and expired air.
22. What is the pneumotaxic center?
23. Describe the Hering-Breuer reflex.
24. Discuss the influence of CO_2 upon the rate and depth of respiration.
25. Discuss the influence of O_2 upon the rate and depth of respiration.
26. Distinguish between residual and minimal air.
27. What is meant by the vital capacity? How can this be determined?
28. Discuss the respiratory rate from infancy to adulthood.
29. The usual cause of death in poisonings due to depressant drugs such as narcotics and barbiturates is respiratory failure. Explain the mechanism of toxicity.

30. Distinguish between costal and diaphragmatic breathing.
31. In Cheyne-Stokes breathing why is the dyspneic phase followed by an apneic phase?
32. Discuss the role of the lungs in water balance.
33. What is the role of respiration in maintaining the pH of the blood?
34. Breathing the same air in and out of a paper bag will increase the respiratory rate. Explain.
35. Why is the respiratory rate decreased during alkalosis?
36. Distinguish among the terms *anoxic anoxia, anemic anoxia,* and *histotoxic anoxia.*
37. What is anoxia neonatorum?
38. A sudden plunge into cold water drastically alters the respiratory rhythm. Explain.
39. What is the immediate cause of death in pneumonia?
40. Distinguish between lobar and lobular pneumonia.
41. Compare the pathogens *Diplococcus pneumoniae* and *Klebsiella pneumoniae.*
42. Discuss the pneumotropic viruses.
43. Why is a "bad cold" potentially dangerous?
44. Describe the Neufeld reaction.
45. What is an actinomycete?
46. Describe the pathogen of tuberculosis.
47. Describe the principal signs and symptoms of tuberculosis.
48. Discuss the prevention and treatment of tuberculosis.
49. What is the significance of a positive tuberculin test?
50. Compare the Salk and the oral vaccines against poliomyelitis.
51. Describe the pathogen of histoplasmosis.
52. Name three other systemic mycoses that involve the lung.
53. Discuss the etiology of asthma.
54. Distinguish between atelectasis and emphysema.
55. Discuss the pneumoconioses.
56. What are the latest developments relative to smoking and lung cancer?
57. Discuss coughing relative to purpose, etiology, and control.
58. What is hyaline membrane disease?
59. How is diphtheria toxoid prepared?
60. Define the following terms: acid fast, methemoglobinemia, tracheotomy, tachypnea, hyperpnea, stretch receptors, carotid body, and hypercapnia.

Chapter 14

The digestive system

As food enters the mouth, the twenty-odd feet of gastrointestinal tract—and a score of accessory organs (Fig. 14-1)—brace themselves for a major physiologic task. During the course of its long journey through the body, the swallowed meal must be moistened, chewed, churned, mixed, digested, and absorbed into the blood. Indigestible material, of course, is not absorbed but discarded as waste, or feces. Of the six nutrients—water, minerals, vitamins, carbohydrates, fats, and proteins—only the last three must be chemically broken down, or digested, into simpler substances. Mineral and vitamin molecules largely diffuse into the blood as a consequence of "simple solution."

The purpose of the present chapter is twofold: (1) to present the structure and function of the organs comprising the digestive system and (2) to describe the chemical events in the digestive process. This will be followed by a consideration of the major diseases and disorders to which the system is heir.

MOUTH

The mouth (Fig. 14-2) begins the gastrointestinal tract. It is bounded on the sides by the cheeks, above by the hard and soft palates, and below by a sheet of muscle. In front it is opened and closed by the lips, and in the back it opens into the pharynx. Characteristically, the soft palate ends behind medially as a free projection called the *uvula.* On the outside the lips and cheeks are covered with skin, and on the inside they are lined with mucous membranes.

As shown in the illustration, the *palatine tonsils* are situated laterally in crypts formed by the glossopalatine and pharyngopalatine arches, muscular folds continuous with the soft palate. The arches aid the soft palate in closing off the mouth from the pharynx during mastication. (The tonsils, as part of the lymphatic system, were discussed earlier on p. 240.)

Tongue. The tongue, a highly agile muscular organ located at the floor of the mouth, is attached in back to the hyoid bone and epiglottis and underneath to the floor of the mouth by an anteroposterior mucosal fold called the *frenulum linguae.* The tongue is covered by a mucous membrane, continuous with the lining of the mouth, which on the upper surface is thrown up into a number of *papillae.* Most of these are slender threadlike projections called *filiform* papillae. Some are knob-

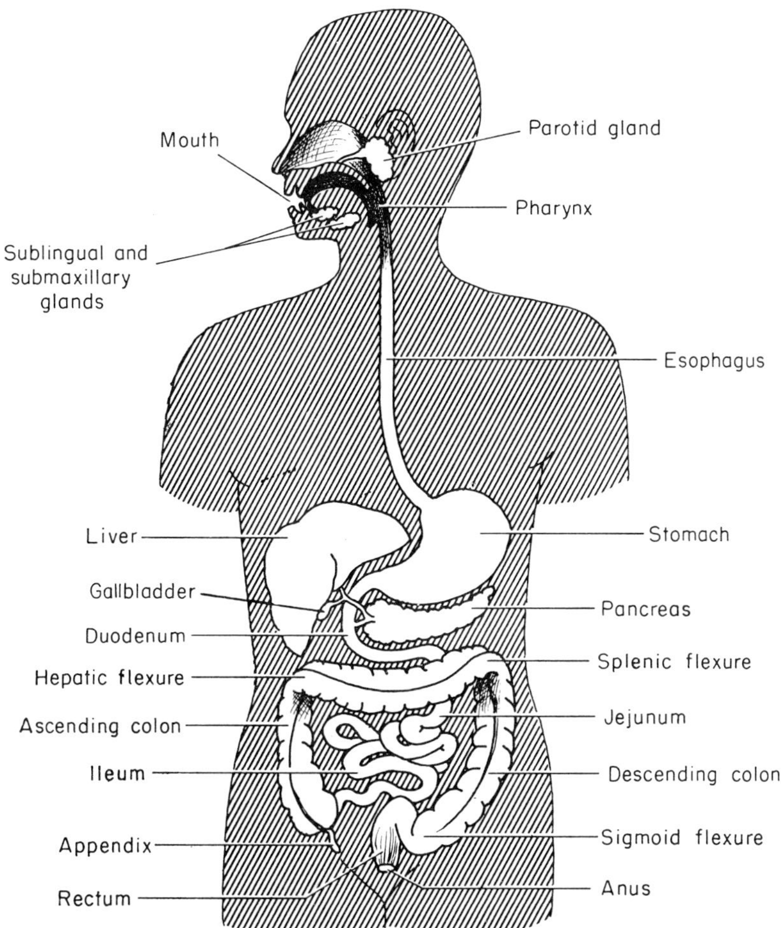

Fig. 14-1. Digestive system.

like, or *fungiform,* and the eight or so arranged on the back part of the tongue in a V-shaped line are called *vallate* papillae.

Taste. Distributed among the papillae are microscopic barrel-shaped structures called *taste buds* that serve as the receptors of taste. The nerve fibers supplying the buds carry sensory impulses to the taste areas in the brain via the seventh and ninth cranial nerves. In order for a substance to trigger a taste bud, it must diffuse through the taste pore in solution, which explains in part why such readily soluble foods as sugar and salt produce a most profound effect.

Each taste bud is sensitive to one of the

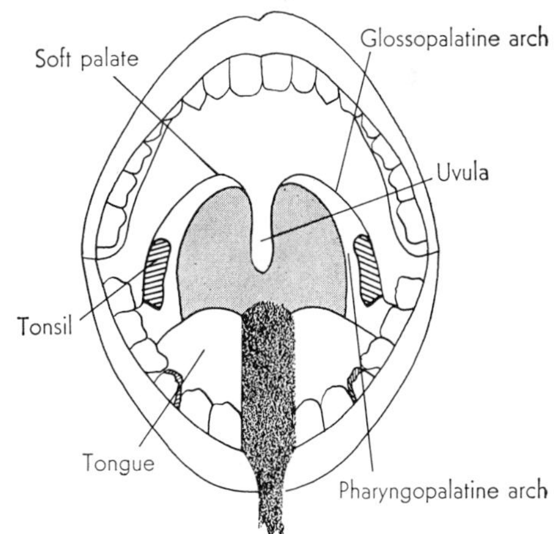

Fig. 14-2. The mouth. (Adapted from Kimber, D. C., Gray, C. E., Stackpole, M. A., and Leavell, C. E.: Anatomy and physiology, New York, 1961, The Macmillan Co. By permission.)

Table 14-1. Time of eruption of teeth*

Deciduous teeth	Months	Permanent teeth	Years
Lower central incisors	6- 8	First molars	6
Upper central incisors	9-12	Central incisors	7
Upper lateral incisors	12-14	Lateral incisors	8
Lower lateral incisors	14-15	First premolars	9-10
First molars	15-16	Second premolars	10
Canines	20-24	Canines	11
Second molars	30-32	Second molars	12
		Third molars	17-18

*From Francis, C. C.: Introduction to human anatomy, ed. 5, St. Louis, 1968, The C. V. Mosby Co.

four primary tastes—bitter, sweet, sour, and salty. The more sophisticated taste sensations, provoked by such items as a juicy steak smothered with mushrooms or a vintage wine, apparently result from a cerebral interplay of the primary tastes. Also not to be forgotten is the role played by the olfactory receptors in the nose, a fact that is underscored when we "lose our taste" during a bad cold.

Teeth. The teeth are the bony structures of mastication. The *deciduous* or milk dentition consists of twenty teeth (ten in each jaw), and the *permanent* dentition contains thirty-two teeth (sixteen in each jaw). Table 14-1 shows the number and average eruption time of the four types of teeth in the two dentitions.

Anatomy. The basic anatomy of a tooth is shown in Fig. 14-3. The *crown,* or the portion above the gum, is coated with *enamel*—the hardest substance in the body. Beneath this, and constituting the bulk of the tooth, is the *dentin,* a dense, yellow-white, hard, striated material. The cavity within the dentin, the pulp chamber, contains connective tissue, nerve endings, and blood vessels.

The *root,* or the portion of the tooth below the gum, is anchored to the *alveolar* process of the jawbone by the alveolar periosteum, or periodontal membrane. The *cementum* (Fig. 14-3) is a layer of modified bone forming a sheath for the root.

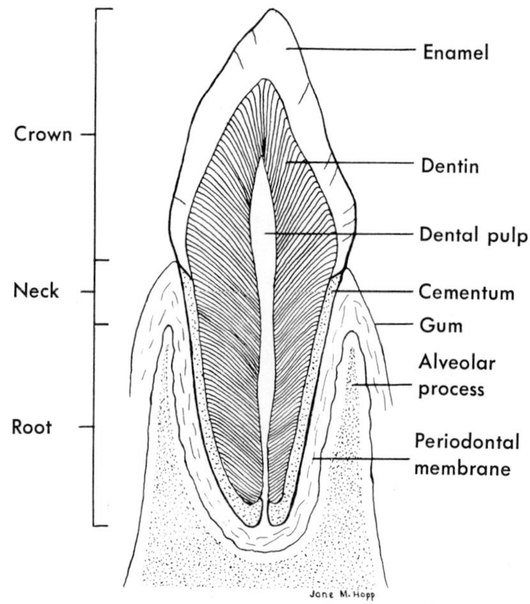

Fig. 14-3. Basic anatomy of the tooth. (From Francis, C. C.: Introduction to human anatomy, ed. 5, St. Louis, 1968, The C. V. Mosby Co.)

The teeth are divided into four groups —*incisors, canines, premolars,* and *molars.* The incisors, with their sharp chisel-shaped crowns, are the cutting teeth. The aptly named canines, with their sharp, pointed crowns, are used in tearing, and the premolars and molars are the grinders of food. Whereas the incisors and canines each have a single root, the molars have two or three. The premolars usually have but one root.

Composition. Like bone, the teeth are composed of calcium carbonate and calcium phosphate bound together into a hard crystalline substance. The deposition and reabsorption of this chemical complex occur almost exclusively in the dentin and cementum. The mineral turnover in the enamel is almost nil.

Formation. The speed of growth and the rate of eruption of the teeth are stimulated by the thyroid and growth hormones (Chapter 22). Also, deposition of the calcium salts in the dentin depends upon the supply of calcium, phosphorus, fluorine, vitamin D, and the parathyroid hormone. A deficiency of one or more of these factors leads to defective ossification and poor teeth.

Fluorine. Of considerable interest and importance was the finding that the fluoride ion plays a vital role in the prevention of dental caries. In communities where fluoridation has been adopted, tooth decay has been reduced as much as 70 percent!

Nevertheless, fluoridation has stirred up more controversy than any other public health measure of the present century, a singularly strange view when we consider that the general public readily accepts new drugs that have received but a small fraction of the rigorous testing accorded fluoridation. Both the American Medical Association and the American Dental Association recommend fluoridation without reservation. A good deal of all this controversy no doubt relates to the fact that fluorides are poisonous—but so is water itself if we ingest too much of it! And some natural water supplies do have "excess" fluoride, a situation resulting in endemic fluorosis, a condition characterized by mottled teeth.

The optimum concentration of fluoride in drinking water is somewhere in the vicinity of 1 part fluoride to 1 million parts water. If a water supply is below this concentration, fluoridation is accomplished simply by adding the calculated amount of sodium fluoride.

The mechanism of action of fluorine relates, it is believed, to *bacterial* enzymes. One view is that the fluoride ion in the teeth combines with various trace metals necessary for activation of bacterial enzymes, and because the enzymes are thus deprived of these metals, they remain inactive and cause no caries.

Salivary glands. The salivary glands are exocrine glands arranged in pairs about the face (Fig. 14-1). They include the *parotid, sublingual,* and *submaxillary* glands. The parotid lies immediately below and in front of the ear. Its duct, known as *Stensen's duct,* pierces the buccinator muscle and opens in the mouth at the level of the upper second molar. The submaxillary, a smaller gland than the parotid, is situated below the mandible about midway between the angle and the end of the lower jaw. Its secretions enter the mouth via *Wharton's duct,* which opens in the floor of the mouth near the midline. The sublingual glands lie in the floor of the mouth on either side of the tongue. Each gland communicates with the mouth via several small ducts that open into the floor behind Wharton's ducts.

Saliva. Saliva, the clear, colorless, sticky juice secreted by the salivary glands, facilitates mastication and swallowing by its moistening and lubrication effects; saliva also commences the digestion of carbohydrate.

Saliva is composed of water, mucin, ptyalin, and certain inorganic salts. Its pH averages between 6 and 7. Mucin, the characteristic constituent of mucus and digestive juices, is an amazing substance, for it not only serves as an excellent lubricant but also protects the gastrointestinal mucosa against the eroding action of the potent digestive enzymes. Ptyalin, or *salivary amylase,* is the only enzyme present in saliva. Its action will be discussed in connection with digestion.

The secretion of saliva is provoked by the presence of food in the mouth (gustatory stimuli) and by seeing, smelling, and thinking about food (psychic stimuli). Such stimuli trigger the superior and inferior salivatory nuclei in the brain which, in turn, via the autonomic nervous system, stimulate the glands.

Mastication and deglutition. Mastication, or the chewing of food, is the chief function of the mouth. The purpose, of course, is to facilitate the digestive process. And because of the joy of eating, man finds this a most pleasant physiologic chore. Following mastication, the tongue pushes the bolus of food backward toward the pharynx, where special receptors in the pharyngeal wall initiate swallowing, or deglutition.

PHARYNX

The throat, or pharynx, a musculomembranous structure connecting the nose, the mouth, and the esophagus, serves as a passageway for air and food. It leads air into the larynx and food into the esophagus. Anatomy of the pharynx was presented earlier in the discussion of the respiratory system.

ESOPHAGUS

The esophagus is a muscular tube, 10 to 12 inches long, running behind the trachea from the lower pharynx (at the level of the sixth cervical vertebra) to the cardiac orifice of the stomach. On the way it passes through the posterior mediastinum and pierces the diaphragm just before the cardiac orifice.

The esophagus as well as the rest of the alimentary tract is composed of four so-called coats. From inside out these include the *mucosal, submucosal, muscular,* and *serous* coats. The muscular coat has an inner layer and an outer layer of fibers arranged in a circular and a longitudinal fashion, respectively. In the upper esophagus the muscle is of the skeletal type, and in the lower esophagus it is of the smooth type.

In cross section the lumen of the esophagus has a stellate outline as a result of the partial contraction of its musculature. During swallowing, however, the puckered wall is distended. Mucus is the only secretion of the esophagus.

STOMACH

The stomach is an ovoid musculomembranous pouch connected above to the esophagus and below to the duodenum. As shown in Fig. 14-4, the major areas include the *cardia, fundus, body,* and *pylorus.* The cardia and the pylorus lead into the esophagus and duodenum, respectively. The fundus is the dome-shaped portion above the cardia, and the body is the portion between the cardia and the pylorus.

Along the *lesser curvature* or concave margin of the stomach (Fig. 14-4) is attached the *lesser omentum,* a peritoneal fold running to the transverse fissure of the liver. The *greater omentum* is an expansive peritoneal fold that runs along the *greater curvature* and attaches its opposite border to the transverse colon.

The healthy empty stomach has a small cavity and a thick, tough wall thrown up into deep wrinkles, or *rugae,* on the inside. This telescoped surface permits great distention and accounts for the fact that the adult stomach can accommodate up to 3 or 4 quarts of food and drink. Indeed, without the stomach there never could have been a Roman banquet.

The stomach wall, as indicated earlier, has four coats: an outer peritoneal or serous coat, a muscular coat, a submucosal coat (submucosa), and a mucous coat (mucosa) that lines the inside. The muscular coat is composed of an outer layer of longitudinal fibers, a middle layer of oblique

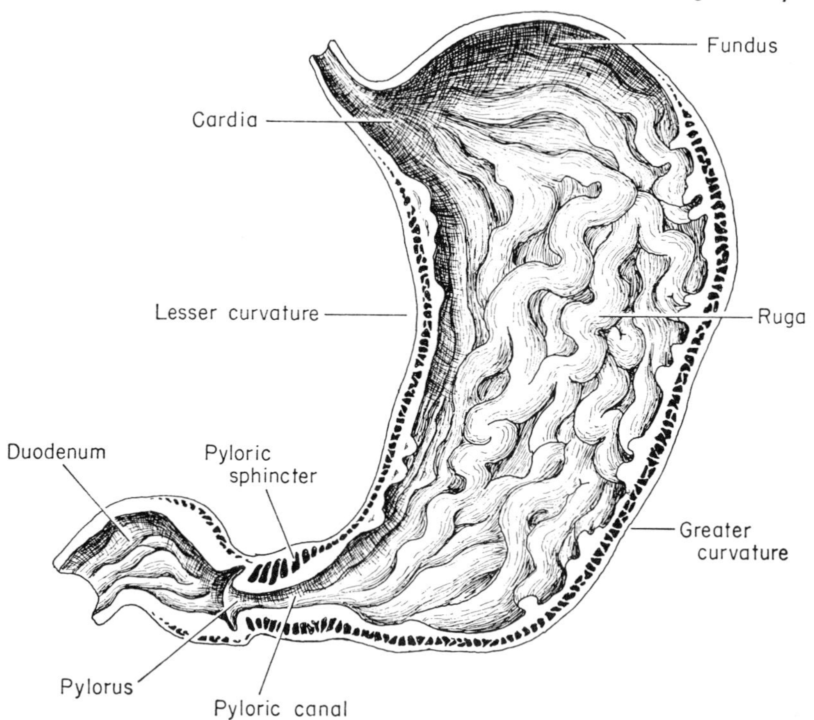

Fig. 14-4. The stomach. (Modified from Francis, C. C: Introduction to human anatomy, ed. 5, St. Louis, 1968, The C. V. Mosby Co.)

fibers, and an inner layer of circular fibers, the latter forming the *pyloric sphincter.*

Gastric juice. Gastric juice contains water, mucin, salts, enzymes, and hydrochloric acid and is secreted by three types of mucosal cells working in concert. The *parietal* cells, located in the fundus and body of the stomach, secrete hydrochloric acid; the *mucous* cells, located throughout the stomach, secrete mucin; and the zymogenic or *chief* cells (also found throughout the stomach) secrete the enzymes. During fasting the juice has a pH of about 3.5 but following stimulation of secretion by food, it has a pH of about 1.

The principal enzyme is pepsin, which in the presence of the highly acid environment of the stomach exerts a powerful digestive action upon proteins. As a matter of fact, the stomach wall would be eaten away in a matter of hours if it were not for the protective action of mucin. Pepsin is not secreted as such but in an inactive form called *pepsinogen,* and the latter becomes pepsin in the presence of hydrochloric acid.

Gastric *lipase* and *rennin,* two other gastric enzymes, are relatively unimportant. The former has a slight action upon fat, and the latter causes milk protein to *coagulate* and therefore to stay in the stomach longer. Rennin is almost absent from adult gastric juice.

Regulation. The flow of gastric juice is regulated by neurogenic and hormonal mechanisms. Secretory signals are reflexly transmitted to the gastric glands from the medulla as a consequence of both psychic and physical factors—that is thinking about a juicy steak may call forth as much juice as its actual presence in the stomach.

Meat and other protein foods in the stomach provoke the release of a hormone called *gastrin* which, in turn, stimulates the secretion of a highly acidic gastric juice. Interestingly, *histamine,* an intracellular chemical agent associated with allergy (p.

114), also stimulates the output of gastric juice.

Mixing. In stark contrast to the idealized architecture shown in Fig. 14-4, the stomach can contort itself into an endless variety of shapes in the course of mixing the swallowed meal, at any given moment its shape depending upon the contents, muscle tone, and position of the body.

Mixing is performed by closing of the pyloric sphincter in the face of forward movement of powerful peristaltic waves. And in the presence of copious amounts of gastric juice the meal is thus transformed into a semifluid mush called *chyme.*

Emptying. Chyme enters the duodenum in intermittent squirts, the frequency of which depends upon the acidity and the volume ejected. That is, as the volume of chyme builds up in the intestine, the walls become distended and the *myenteric receptors* thereby stimulated. Reflexly, this causes contraction of the pyloric sphincter and permits the intestine to accommodate what it has before receiving further charges. (The irritant action of the acidic chyme on the intestinal mucosa intensifies this reflex closing of the pylorus.) In time, when distention has subsided and the acid has become neutralized, the reflex becomes nonoperative, thus allowing the sphincter to open and more chyme to be ejected.

SMALL INTESTINE

The small intestine is the musculomembranous tube (Fig. 14-5) that extends from the pylorus to the ileocecal valve. It has three somewhat arbitrary divisions—the *duodenum,* the *jejunum,* and the *ileum.* The intestine begins with the duodenum, a C-shaped tube about 10 inches in length, which curves toward the right, and into its descending portion open the ducts from the liver and the pancreas. The jejunum and the ileum, forming the main body of the small intestine, measure about 8 and 11 feet, respectively. The jejunum occupies the upper abdominal cavity, and the ileum fills the lower right abdominal cavity and the upper pelvic cavity.

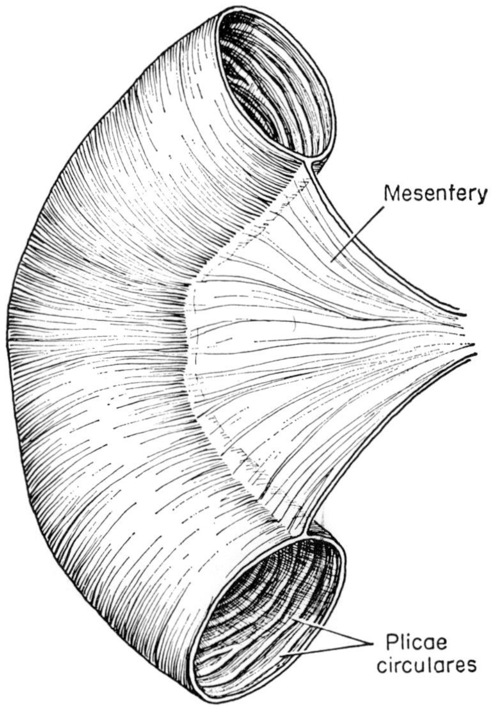

Fig. 14-5. Segment of the small intestine.

Mucosa. The small intestine, like the other portions of the digestive tract, has four basic coats. The inside coat, or mucosa (Fig. 14-6), consists of a surface layer of simple columnar epithelium supported by a thin layer of connective tissue called the *lamina propria,* and below this a very thin layer of smooth muscle called the *muscularis mucosae.* Characteristically, the mucosa sends up an astronomical number of fingerlike projections called *villi,* structures that give the inside surface its soft, velvety texture. Each villus is supplied with a capillary network and a large lymphatic vessel called a *lacteal* (Fig. 14-7).

The mucosa is thrown up into a large number of circular folds called *plicae circulares* (Fig. 14-5) which, like the villi, gradually decrease toward the end of the intestine. Thus, the intestinal lining is like a roller coaster upon a roller coaster, the

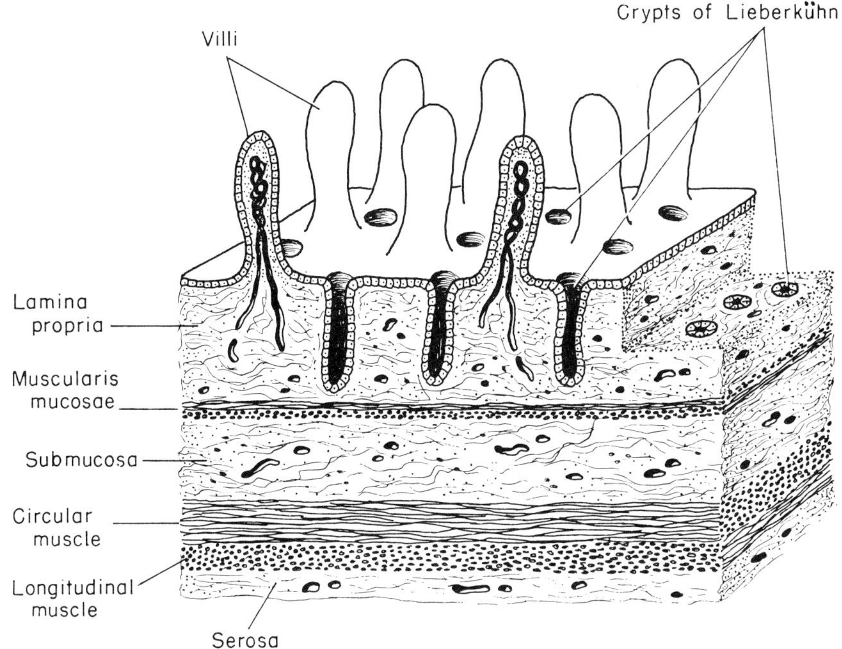

Fig. 14-6. Three-dimensional view of the wall of the small intestine.

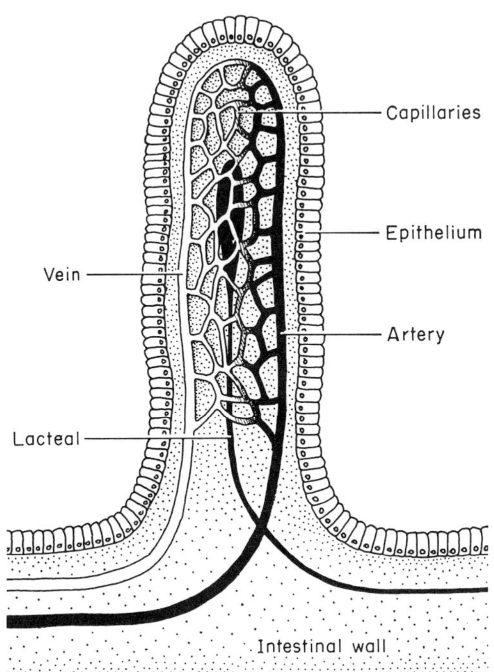

Fig. 14-7. The villus. (From Brooks, S. M.: Basic facts of general chemistry, Philadelphia, 1956, W. B. Saunders Co.)

purpose being to maximize the surface area for digestion and absorption.

Peyer's patches. Peyer's patches are oval, elevated areas in the mucosa of the lower ileum composed of *lymph nodules* closely packed together. In contrast, the nodules in the other sections of the intestine are solitary. These patches, therefore, are highly characteristic of the ilium.

Other coats. Beneath the mucosa lies the submucosa, which is composed of a layer of strong connective tissue. Next comes the muscular coat composed of an inner circular layer and an outer longitudinal layer of smooth muscle. The outermost coat, the serosa, is made up of transparent tissue continuous with the *mesentery* (Fig. 14-5), a fan-shaped fold of peritoneum that attaches the entire length of the jejunum and ileum to the posterior abdominal wall. Between the two layers of the mesentery run blood vessels, lymphatic vessels, and nerve fibers to the intestine.

Intestinal juice. Among the villi are

openings that lead into microscopic tubular structures called the *glands* (or crypts) of *Lieberkühn* (Fig. 14-6). The modified epithelium lining these glands secretes the intestinal juice, or *succus entericus.* This secretion contains water, mucin, carbohydrases, peptidases, and enterokinase. In addition, *Brunner's glands,* lying deep in the duodenal mucosa, secrete large amounts of mucus for the purpose of counteracting the highly acidic chyme. In a 24-hour period the total intestinal secretion amounts to about 3 quarts of fluid! This volume—plus an equal volume of juice contributed by the mouth, stomach, liver, and pancreas—is almost entirely reabsorbed before reaching the large intestine.

Regulation. Intestinal juice is secreted in response to a number of factors, but the myenteric reflexes, triggered by distention and acidity, are considered to be the most significant. Hormonal agents, collectively called "enterocrinin," are thought to be important in determining the character of the juice; that is, protein increases the concentration of peptidases, and carbohydrate increases the concentration of carbohydrases. Intestinal juice is also weakly stimulated by parasympathetic bombardment.

Peristalsis. Peristalsis is the wormlike movement along the gastrointestinal tract by which ingested material is propelled from the pharynx to the anal opening. This characteristic movement results chiefly from a slowly advancing circular constriction. Intestinal peristalsis is more than a propulsive force, however, for by swishing the chyme back and forth, it also brings about thorough mixing.

Regulation. Throughout the gastrointestinal tract the musculature is supplied with ganglia (groups of nerve cells) and nerve fibers. This so-called *myenteric plexus* controls practically all peristaltic movements. The effects may be local (for example, irritation along a small segment of the intestine causes contraction and secretion only in that area) or generalized due to impulses arriving at the ganglia over the autonomic nervous system. Parasympathetic stimulation *increases* peristalsis and relaxes the sphincters guarding the pyloric and ileocecal valves, whereas sympathetic stimulation *decreases* peristalsis and constricts the sphincters.

LARGE INTESTINE

The large intestine is a musculomenbranous tube, 5 feet or so in length, which runs up, across, and down the lower abdominal cavity. In order, its various sections include the cecum, ascending colon, hepatic flexure, transverse colon, splenic flexure, descending colon, sigmoid flexure, rectum, and anal canal (Fig. 14-1). In contrast to the small intestine, the large intestine has no villi and an incomplete layer of longitudinal smooth muscle arranged in three ribbonlike strips called *taeniae coli.* Characteristically, its walls are puckered into incomplete sacculations called haustra (sing., *haustrum*). These characteristic features are clearly shown in Fig. 14-8.

Cecum. The cecum is the dilated intestinal pouch into which open the ileum and the vermiform appendix (Fig. 14-8). The ileocecal valve guards the opening of the ileum, and when a peristaltic wave reaches the valve, the sphincter is reflexly relaxed and the chyme pushed on through. Conversely, the valve is constructed in such a way that fecal matter is kept in the colon where it belongs.

Appendix. The *vermiform* appendix ("appendix") is a blind wormlike tube branching from the lower cecum. It averages about ¼ inch in diameter and varies anywhere from 3 to 6 inches in length. Microscopically, the structure resembles the rest of the intestine. Presumably, it serves little useful purpose and is generally regarded as a vestigial organ.

Rectum. The terminal part of the large intestine, extending from the sigmoid flexure to the anus, is called the rectum. In

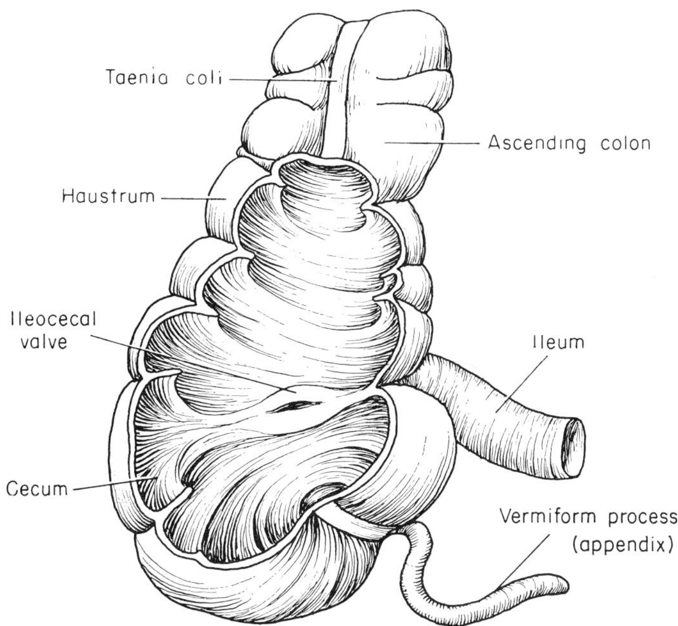

Fig. 14-8. The cecum and associated structures.

the adult it measures from 6 to 8 inches in length. In the terminal inch, referred to as the *anal canal,* the mucosa is arranged in vertical folds known as rectal columns, each supplied with an artery and a vein. The *anus,* or external opening, is guarded by two sphincters: an *internal* one composed of smooth muscle and an *external* one composed of skeletal muscle.

Feces. The major role of the large intestine is to absorb water and electrolytes from the soupy chyme. Thus, as the chyme is propelled along, it becomes progressively less watery and eventually becomes a semisolid material called feces, an excrement composed of food residues (for example, cellulose), bacteria, and intestinal secretions. Its characteristic chocolate color is due to the pigments formed by the action of the digestive enzymes on bile.

Defecation. Defecation, or discharge of feces, is initiated by the passage of fecal material into the rectum. Sensory impulses are relayed to the spinal cord and peristalsis is thereby stimulated; simultaneously the internal anal sphincter is relaxed to aid passage through the anal opening. The external sphincter is relaxed voluntarily to complete the act.

The abdominal muscles, too, play a role in defecation, for when contracted, they compress the intestinal contents downward against the rectum and stimulate the sensory endings in the rectum. In this manner defecation is both initiated and promoted.

LIVER

The liver (Fig. 14-9), the largest gland in the body, is situated beneath the diaphragm and occupies practically all the *right* hypochondrium and *upper part* of the epigastrium (Fig. 14-10). It has a characteristic dark red color and a plasticlike texture.

Lobes and lobules. The liver is divided by the *falciform ligament* into the *left* and *right lobes* (Fig. 14-9). The latter, in turn, is divided into the right lobe proper, the caudate lobe, and the quadrate lobe.

Histologically, the liver is composed of anatomic units called *hepatic lobules,* each characterized by a central or intralobular

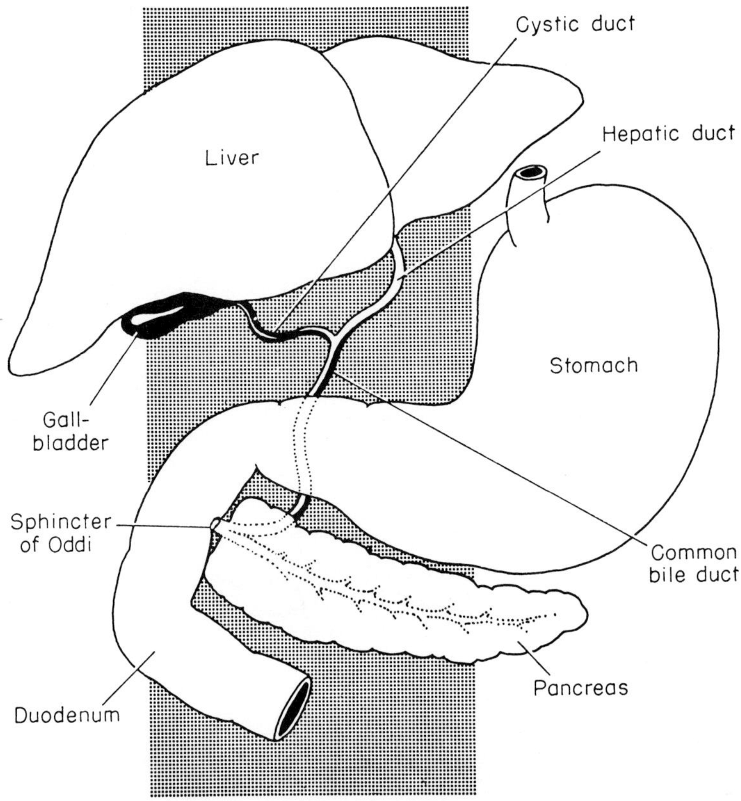

Fig. 14-9. The stomach, liver, pancreas, and associated ducts.

vein (a branch of the hepatic vein) surrounded by radiating columns of hepatic cells (Fig. 14-11). About each lobule are tiny arteries (branches of the hepatic artery), interlobular veins (branches of the portal vein), and interlobular bile ducts (branches of the hepatic bile duct). Finally, microscopic channels (or *sinusoids*) extending between the radiating columns of hepatic cells serve to connect the interlobular veins with the central vein.

Ducts. The interlobular bile ducts within the liver come together to form two large ducts that emerge from the undersurface and immediately join to form the *hepatic duct.* This duct and the *cystic duct* from the gallbladder then merge to form the *common bile duct,* which opens into the duodenum at the papilla, or *ampulla of Vater,* a small raised area about 3 inches below the pylorus. The cardinal features of this duct system are clearly shown in Fig. 14-9.

Functions. Chemically, the liver is perhaps the most amazing organ in the body. It plays a key role in the metabolism of carbohydrates, fats, and proteins; it stores vitamins and minerals; it detoxifies harmful substances; it bolsters the body's immunity; it produces large amounts of body heat (second only to skeletal muscle); and it manufactures, among other things, heparin, prothrombin, blood proteins, and bile. Since our present concern is with digestion, we shall here confine our remarks to bile; the many other hepatic activities are discussed throughout the book at the appropriate place.

Bile. Bile is a yellowish green secretion of the liver containing minerals, mucin,

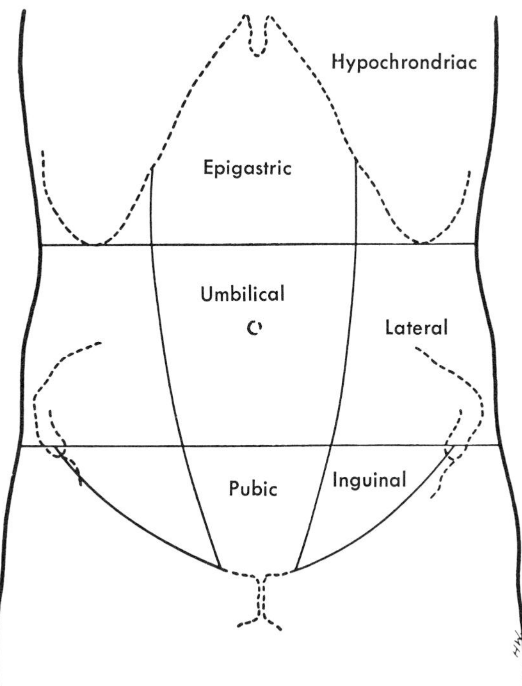

Fig. 14-10. Diagram of abdominal region. (From Francis, C. C: Introduction to human anatomy, ed. 5, St. Louis, 1968, The C. V. Mosby Co.)

cholesterol, bile salts, and bile pigments. The latter include *bilirubin* and *biliverdin.* Bilirubin, a red pigment, is actually a waste product resulting from the breakdown of hemoglobin; biliverdin (which is green in color) is a derivative of bilirubin.

The production of bile is weakly stimulated by *secretin,* a hormone released into the blood by the duodenal mucosa in response to the presence of chyme. Secretin has a more pronounced effect on the pancreas (p. 298).

The role of bile in the digestive process is to *emulsify* fat into microscopic globules. This action, due entirely to the presence of the bile salts, allows fat to be more readily acted upon by pancreatic lipase.

GALLBLADDER

The gallbladder, a pear-shaped pouch 3 to 4 inches long and 1 inch or so wide, is partially embedded in the undersurface of the liver (Fig. 14-9). Its walls are composed of smooth muscle, and it is lined on the inside with a mucosa thrown up into rugae.

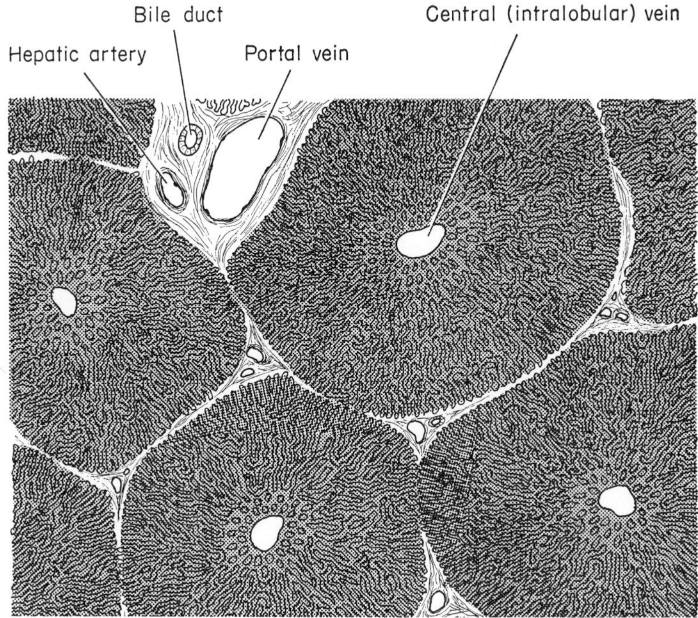

Fig. 14-11. The liver as seen under the microscope.

The bile trickles into the *common bile duct* and finally backs up into the gallbladder via the cystic duct. This happens because the common bile duct is guarded by the *sphincter of Oddi* at the neck of the ampulla of Vater. Bile is stored and concentrated in the gallbladder.

Cholecystokinin. When chyme containing fat enters the duodenum, it causes the release of a hormone called cholecystokinin, which makes its way to the gallbladder via the blood and there brings about the ejection of bile by stimulating the contraction of the muscular wall. At the same time peristalsis, enhanced by the presence of chyme, stretches the sphincter of Oddi and facilitates the passage of bile into the duodenum.

PANCREAS

The pancreas is a pinkish, fish-shaped gland running behind the stomach and horizontally across the posterior abdominal wall (Fig. 14-9). Its head and neck are nestled in the C-shaped curve of the duodenum and its tail just touches the spleen. The organ measures about 9 inches in length and weighs about 3 ounces.

Upon careful dissection and microscopic examination, the pancreas is found to be divided into lobes and lobules, the latter being composed of cells arranged about microscopic ducts. These ducts unite into larger ducts which, in turn, join the *duct of Wirsung*, the chief pancreatic duct. This duct extends the entire length of the gland and empties into the duodenum at the ampulla of Vater (Fig. 14-9). Another duct, the duct of *Santorini*, is usually found arising from the head of the pancreas and entering the duodenum about 1 inch above the papilla.

Islands of Langerhans. Scattered throughout the pancreas and among the enzyme-secreting cells are a million or so cell clusters situated about blood capillaries. These areas, aptly called the islands (or *islets*) of Langerhans, are easily seen under the microscope (Chapter 22). The so-called *beta cells* of these islets secrete the all-important hormone *insulin* (Chapter 22). The *alpha cells* are thought to secrete *glucagon*, a factor that antagonizes the action of insulin. Whereas the lobule cells secrete into ducts, the alpha and beta cells have no ducts and secrete directly into the blood. Thus, the pancreas has the distinction of being at once an *exocrine* and an *endocrine* gland.

Pancreatic juice. Each day the pancreas empties about a pint and a half of juice into the duodenum. This contains principally pancreatic amylase for digesting starches, pancreatic lipase for digesting fats, trypsin and chymotrypsin for digesting proteins, and large amounts of sodium bicarbonate for neutralizing the hydrochloric acid from the stomach. The latter action represents one of the most important functions of the pancreas.

Secretin. As previously stated, the acidic chyme causes the release of the hormone secretin from the duodenal mucosa. This is taken via the blood to the pancreas, where it stimulates a copious flow of juice containing large amounts of sodium bicarbonate.

Pancreozymin. In addition to secretin, chyme also causes the mucosa to release a hormone called pancreozymin. Unlike secretin, pancreozymin calls forth a secretion containing little bicarbonate and high concentrations of digestive enzymes.

CARBOHYDRATE DIGESTION

In order for carbohydrates to pass into the villi and enter the circulation, they must be broken down into *monosaccharides* (p. 116). Since polysaccharides (namely, starches, dextrins, and pectins) are polymers of the monosaccharide *glucose*, the latter is an end product of digestion. Moreover, since the disaccharide sucrose, the principal sugar of the diet, and lactose, the sugar in milk, also yield glucose, we see that glucose is the chief end product of carbohydrate digestion. On the average, about 80 percent of the monosaccharides produced in the digestive mill is glucose; the remaining 20 percent is made up almost entirely of *fructose* (from sucrose) and *galactose* (from lactose).

Let us now take a look at the major chemical events that occur throughout the gastrointestinal tract following ingestion of carbohydrate.

Mouth. In the mouth, food is mixed with saliva and the digestive process begins, with *salivary amylase,* or ptyalin, the only enzyme in saliva, working on the starches. Although most starches are not substantially altered during their short stay in the mouth, the continued action of the enzyme in the stomach converts about 40 percent of their molecules into the disaccharide *maltose.*

As in the hydrolytic digestion of proteins, the starch molecule is successively split apart by water (hydrolysis), the enzyme catalyzing the reaction. Before maltose is reached, however, the molecule yields intermediate products called *dextrins,* simpler polysaccharides assigned the empirical formula $(C_6H_{10}O_5)_n$. The salivary digestion of starch, therefore, may be expressed as shown at the bottom of the page.

Stomach. There are no gastric enzymes that act upon carbohydrates, but hydrochloric acid no doubt converts some starch into maltose. Like salivary amylase, it does this by catalytic action. (In the presence of high heat a few drops of hydrochloric acid are extremely adept at this job, breaking the starch molecule completely down into glucose. This can be easily shown in the laboratory.)

Intestine. The bulk of carbohydrate digestion is carried out in the intestine. Not only are starches and dextrins broken down into maltose by *pancreatic amylase,* but also all disaccharides are converted into monosaccharides by the appropriate carbohydrase. *Maltase* splits a molecule of maltose into two molecules of glucose; *sucrase* splits a molecule of sucrose into one molecule of glucose and one molecule of fructose; and *lactase* splits a molecule of lactose into one molecule of glucose and one molecule of galactose. These reactions may be summarized as follows:

$$\underset{\text{Starch}}{(C_6H_{10}O_5)_n} + H_2O \xrightarrow[\text{Amylase}]{\text{Pancreatic}} \text{Dextrins}$$

$$\underset{\text{Dextrins}}{(C_6H_{10}O_5)_n} + H_2O \xrightarrow[\text{Amylase}]{\text{Pancreatic}} \underset{\text{Maltose}}{C_{12}H_{22}O_{11}}$$

$$\underset{\substack{\text{Maltose}\\\text{Sucrose}\\\text{Lactose}}}{C_{12}H_{22}O_{11}} + H_2O \xrightarrow{\substack{\text{Maltase}\\\text{Sucrase}\\\text{Lactase}}} \underset{\substack{\text{Glucose}\\\text{Fructose}\\\text{Galactose}}}{2C_6H_{12}O_6}{}^*$$

FAT DIGESTION

Fats and oils are glyceryl esters of fatty acids (p. 109); the most important of these include stearic ($C_{17}H_{35}COOH$), palmitic ($C_{15}H_{31}COOH$), oleic ($C_{17}H_{33}COOH$), linoleic ($C_{17}H_{31}COOH$), linolenic ($C_{17}H_{29}$-$COOH$), and arachidonic ($C_{19}H_{31}COOH$). Too, the diet contains a small amount and variety of other lipids, perhaps the most important of which are the fatty acid esters of certain sterols, especially cholesterol.

Bile and lipase. Before fats and oils can be effectively acted upon by the water-soluble *pancreatic lipase* (*steapsin*), they must first be emulsified into tiny globules (to increase their surface area) by the bile salts. In the absence of these emulsifying

*It is not to be forgotten that these sugars are isomers—hence, the same formula.

$$\underset{\text{Starch}}{(C_6H_{10}O_5)_n} + H_2O \xrightarrow[\text{Amylase}]{\text{Salivary}} \text{Dextrins} \xrightarrow[\text{Amylase}]{\text{Salivary}} \underset{\text{Maltose}}{C_{12}H_{22}O_{11}}$$

agents, most of the fat leaves the body in the undigested state.

Once emulsified, the fats are split by lipase into *glycerol, fatty acids,* and *glycerides.* Althought many texts say nothing about the glycerides, it is now known that only about half the fat molecules are completely digested into glycerol and fatty acids. The glyceride, a molecule with one or two acid residues, may be considered a partial fat. Nevertheless, the glycerides are apparently absorbed with almost the same speed as glycerol and the free fatty acids.

Using glyceryl tristearate, or stearin, as a typical example, the complete digestion of fat may be expressed as shown by the equation at the bottom of the page. Note especially that *one* molecule of completely digested fat yields *one* molecule of glycerol and *three* molecules of fatty acid. Steapsin, of course, acts as the catalyst.

PROTEIN DIGESTION

During the process of digestion, proteins are broken down into amino acids, the building blocks of the protein molecule. Before these final end products are reached, however, the various enzymes successively chop off a great many intermediate products of decreasing complexity—proteoses, peptones, and polypeptides, in that order. The simplest possible molecule before the amino acid stage is the dipeptide, one molecule of which, upon digestion, yields two molecules of amino acid (see equation on p. 301).

Stomach. Protein digestion begins in the stomach. Here *pepsin,* secreted as *pepsinogen* and activated by *hydrochloric acid,* converts protein into proteoses, peptones, and some polypeptides. In addition to activating pepsinogen, hydrochloric acid also provides the proper pH for optimum digestion.

Intestine. Upon entering the small intestine, the protein intermediates are then acted upon by *trypsin* and *chymotrypsin* of the pancreatic juice and converted into polypeptides of low molecular weight. The *coupe de grâce* comes when the intestinal *peptidases** (namely, the dipeptidases and the aminopolypeptidases) split the peptides into amino acids, as shown at the top of the facing page.

Enterokinase. Like pepsin, trypsin and chymotrypsin are secreted in inactive forms called *trypsinogen* and *chymotrypsinogen,* respectively. The latter are then activated by the intestinal enzyme enterokinase.

ABSORPTION

Following digestion, the end products are absorbed into the millions of villi that line the small intestine. Water, minerals and most vitamins, in the main, passively diffuse into the blood; monosaccharides and amino acids diffuse to some extent but are mostly absorbed in an active fashion. According to one view, in active absorption the substance to be absorbed combines with some carrier agent in the epithelial cells and is transported in this form from the lumen into the villi. Once inside it breaks away from the carrier and diffuses into the capillaries.

Fats. Fats are absorbed as glycerol, fatty acids, glycerides, and to some extent undigested fat. Once through the mucosa, glyc-

*Formerly referred to as *erepsin.*

$$\begin{array}{lcl} \quad\quad 3H \;\vdots\; 3OH & & \\ C_{17}H_{35}COO\text{-}\vdots\text{-}CH_2 & & C_{17}H_{35}COOH \quad HO\text{—}CH_2 \\ \quad\quad\quad\quad\;\; | & \text{Steapsin} & \quad\quad\quad\quad\quad\quad\quad\quad\;\; | \\ C_{17}H_{35}COO\text{-}\vdots\text{-}CH + 3H_2O & \longrightarrow & C_{17}H_{35}COOH + HO\text{—}CH \\ \quad\quad\quad\quad\;\; | & & \quad\quad\quad\quad\quad\quad\quad\quad\;\; | \\ C_{17}H_{35}COO\text{-}\vdots\text{-}CH_2 & & C_{17}H_{35}COOH \quad HO\text{—}CH_2 \\ \text{Stearin} & & \text{Stearic acid} \quad \text{Glycerol} \end{array}$$

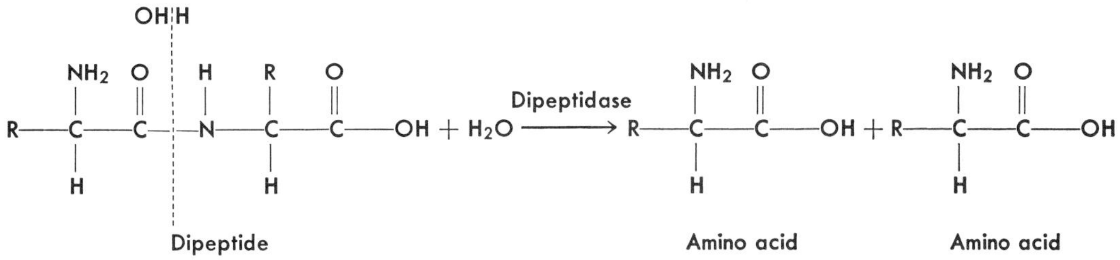

$$\underset{\text{Dipeptide}}{R-\overset{NH_2}{\underset{H}{C}}-\overset{O}{\overset{\|}{C}}-\overset{H}{N}-\overset{R}{\underset{H}{C}}-\overset{O}{\overset{\|}{C}}-OH} + H_2O \xrightarrow{\text{Dipeptidase}} \underset{\text{Amino acid}}{R-\overset{NH_2}{\underset{H}{C}}-\overset{O}{\overset{\|}{C}}-OH} + \underset{\text{Amino acid}}{R-\overset{NH_2}{\underset{H}{C}}-\overset{O}{\overset{\|}{C}}-OH}$$

(OH and H of water added at the broken peptide bond)

erol and fatty acids reunite into neutral fat, which then enters the lacteal vessels. By rhythmic contractions of the villi (stimulated by a hormone released from the intestinal mucosa called *villikinin*), the fat-laden lymph is massaged along into the lymphatic vessels and eventually enters the blood (p. 240).

Chyle. The milky, fat-laden lymph emerging from the lacteals after digestion is called chyle. When examined under the microscope, this is seen to be a fine emulsion of fat globules, or chylomicrons, dispersed in lymph. Chylomicrons are also found in the blood for about 3 hours following a fatty meal. Normally, however, they will have disappeared in 8 to 10 hours unless additional food has been taken.

INFECTIOUS DISEASES OF THE DIGESTIVE SYSTEM

Considering the fact that at any time we might unknowingly ingest contaminated food or drink, it is little wonder that the gastrointestinal canal is easy prey to infection. Too, there are a good number of pathogenic microbes that preferentially attack the other organs of the digestive machinery. The more common diseases of this nature are discussed here.

Diarrhea and food poisoning. Acute diarrhea is encountered in three general forms: (1) an epidemic of viral origin, (2) isolated cases in which no infectious agent is apparent (due to such things as dietary indiscretion, misuse of cathartics, food allergy, emotionally labile individuals, and the like), and (3) individuals or groups of persons who experience gastroenteritis of bacterial etiology following ingestion of contaminated food or water.

Because acute diarrhea associated with food or water could possibly turn out to be the initial stage of bacillary dysentery, amebic dysentery, or typhoid fever, it is essential to make a definite diagnosis in suspicious cases. The most common cause of food poisoning, however, is the *enterotoxin* produced by certain strains of *Staphylococcus aureus.* The usual events, which begin 2 to 4 hours following ingestion of food, include nausea, severe vomiting, abdominal cramps, diarrhea, and prostration. But despite the violence of the acute attack, the symptoms usually subside after about 6 hours. Symptomatic treatment, with replacement of fluids, is generally all that is required.

Inasmuch as "staph" food poisoning is due to a toxin *preformed* in the food (by the growth of the organism), many authors refer to it as a type of *food intoxication.* Another and much more deadly variety of intoxication is *botulism* (p. 303).

The most common type of food poisoning due to the living organism (so-called *food infection*) is *salmonellosis,* a gastroenteritis involving dozens of species of the genus *Salmonella*—the same genus to which belong the pathogens of typhoid and paratyphoid fever. Many of these species are natural pathogens of domestic animals and thus meats, fish, milk, eggs, and milk and egg products are the usual culprits. Also, foods may become contaminated during processing by human carriers and by infected rats and mice that inhabit food plants, warehouses, and kitchens. The treatment of salmonellosis centers on the replacement of water and electrolytes and use of antimicrobials, particularly chloramphenicol.

Typhoid fever. Typhoid fever is a severe bacterial infection that starts in the intestinal mucosa and, if untreated, progressively infiltrates the tissues throughout the body. It is characterized by severe diarrhea (often with bloody stools), fever, abdominal pain, and prostration. The most serious aspect of the infection is the possibility of intestinal perforation, for once the organism enters the abdominal cavity, a fulminating peritonitis ensues. When this occurs, the prognosis is poor indeed.

The etiologic microbe, *Salmonella typhosa,* is a motile, nonsporeforming, gram-negative bacillus that enters the body through the mouth via contaminated food or drink. Obviously, its presence in the feces, urine, or blood affords a positive diagnosis. Also, the demonstration of typhoid-specific agglutinins in the patient's blood serum is of diagnostic value. In the *Widal test* a suspension of typhoid bacilli is mixed with the patient's serum and the mixture observed microscopically (Fig. 14-12). Since persons who have had typhoid fever, who have been vaccinated against typhoid fever, or who harbor the organism (as a carrier) give a positive test (that is, agglutination of the bacilli), the results must be interpreted with these factors in mind. According to Burrows, an O agglutinin titer of 1:100 and an H agglutinin titer of 1:200 may be considered significant.* Even more significant is a rise in so-called *Vi antibodies* ("Vi" stands for *virulence*) because, unlike O and H agglutinins, they do not occur in the wake of vaccination.

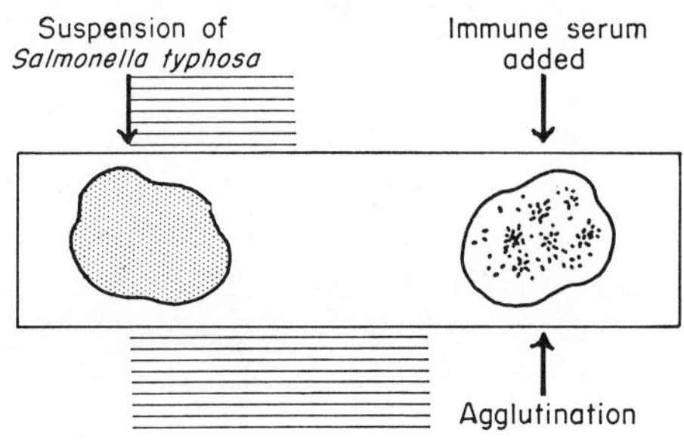

Fig. 14-12. The Widal test. (See text.)

The treatment of typhoid fever entails good nursing care and the use of antibiotics. At present chloramphenicol *(Chloromycetin)* is the drug of choice. As for prevention, vaccination (using a "killed vaccine") is a must in endemic and disaster areas. Eradication of the malady also entails paying meticulous attention to the handling of food, water, garbage, and sewage. Indeed, these measures in the United States have reduced the typhoid fever death rate from 40 per 100,000 in 1900 to less than 0.1 per 100,000 in 1960.

Paratyphoid fever. Paratyphoid fever, an enteric infection similar to typhoid but much less severe, is caused by three species of *Salmonella* that are often spoken of collectively as *Salmonella paratyphi.* The modes of infection, diagnosis, prevention, and treatment are about the same as those cited for typhoid fever.

Bacillary dysentery. The term *dysentery* is applied to a number of enteric inflammations marked by abdominal pain and severe diarrhea, often with stools streaked with blood and mucus. Bacillary dysentery is the type caused by several species of the genus *Shigella.* These microbes are nonmotile, nonsporeforming, gram-negative bacilli that are easily cultured on most ordinary laboratory media. Like the typhoid and paratyphoid organisms, the shigellae find their way into the body via contaminated food and drink. Since they appear in the feces during the first few days of the infection, stool specimens afford a means of diagnosis.

*Certain bacteria contain two kinds of agglutinogens, one in the cell (O antigens) and the other in the capsule or flagella (H antigens); O antigens provoke O agglutinins, and H antigens provoke H agglutinins.

Of the various agents used to treat bacillary dysentery, the sulfonamides (namely, sulfadiazine) generally give the best results. Prophylactically, good sanitation is the most effective way to control the infection.

Amebic dysentery. Amebic dysentery, or *amebiasis*, is caused by the protozoan *Entamoeba histolytica.* The ingested cyst develops into a trophozoite that subsequently burrows its way into the intestinal wall. (Both of these forms are shown in Fig. 14-13.) The invasion soon results in ulceration, pain, and diarrhea. In the event that the amebas enter the blood, abscesses may be produced in the liver, lungs, and brain. The student can readily appreciate then that amebic dysentery is extremely dangerous. Although one is prone to think of amebiasis as being confined to tropical and subtropical regions, the incidence of the malady in certain areas of the United States and Canada reportedly approaches 20 percent of the population.

Amebic dysentery is diagnosed by demonstration of the cyst or trophozoite in stool specimens. As for treatment, a wide variety of drugs have been used in management of the intestinal and systemic stages. The more successful agents include carbarsone, broad-spectrum antibiotics, fumagillin, emetine, and chloroquine. Persons with diagnosed cases must be kept under close surveillance to prevent carriers from contaminating food and drink. Good sanitation, of course, is of prime concern.

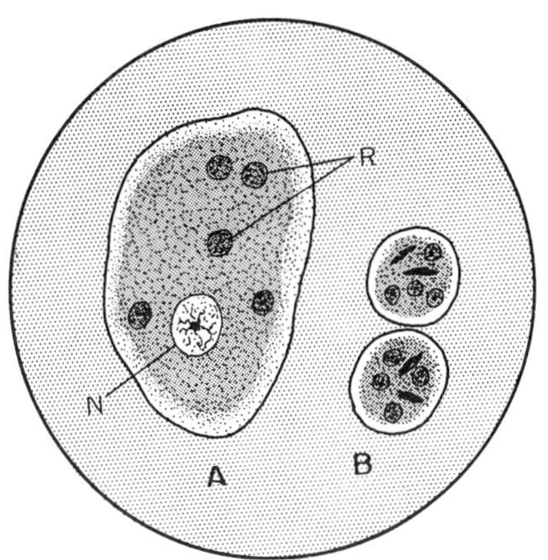

Fig. 14-13. *Entamoeba histolytica.* **A,** Trophozoite. **B,** Cyst stage. **N,** Nucleus; **R,** red cells.

Botulism. It is certainly fortunate that botulism strikes infrequently, for once the signs and symptoms appear, there is sometimes little hope for survival. The causative organism, *Clostridium botulinum,* a gram-positive, sporeforming anaerobic bacillus, releases one of the most potent biologic poisons known. It has been estimated that as little as 1/6000 of a grain can kill a man! The classic clinical picture is severe enteritis, paralysis, and sudden death.

Botulism is always contracted by eating contaminated food, especially uncooked or improperly processed sausage, ham, fish, and vegetables. Many cases have been caused by canned food prepared in the home, the food not having been cooked long enough to destroy the toxin, bacilli, and/or spores. Diagnosis is made by injecting the suspected food into mice or by isolating the pathogen from the food, feces, or vomitus.

Regarding treatment, time is of the essence, for *immediate* injection of the antitoxin may save a life. Nowhere is the old saying that "an ounce of prevention is worth a pound of cure" more apropos than here.

Cholera. Cholera is a vicious enteric infection that has plagued the peoples of Asia for centuries—hence, the term *Asiatic cholera.* The etiologic agent, *Vibrio comma,* a short spirillum with one or two polar flagella (Fig. 14-14), is a motile, nonsporeforming, gram-negative organism that grows well on most ordinary artificial media.

The classic signs of cholera are profuse rice-water stools, severe vomiting, general emaciation, prostration, and collapse. A definitive diagnosis, however, is made by isolating the pathogen from the feces of patients and carriers.

Treatment is directed against the symptoms and against the organism. The sul-

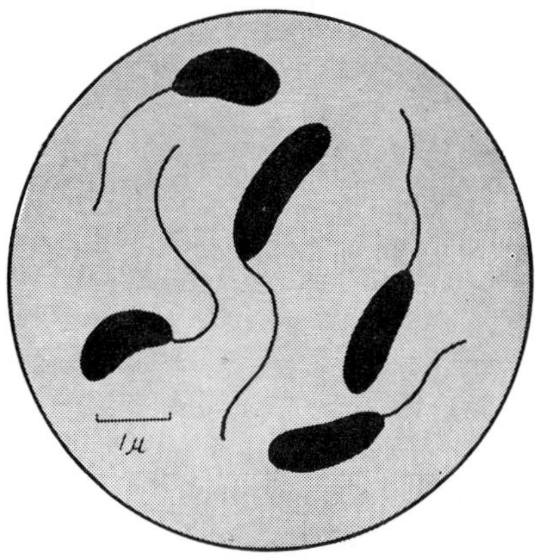

Fig. 14-14. *Vibrio comma.*

fonamides and antibiotics have produced encouraging results. For prevention, stringent sanitary codes are a must, and active immunization employing killed cholera spirilla has been shown to offer protection in most persons. All those going into cholera areas should be vaccinated.

Yellow fever. The discovery by Reed that a mosquito *(Aedes aegypti)* transmits yellow fever was one of the great moments in medicine, a discovery that led to the conquest of the disease in Panama and made possible the construction of the Panama Canal.

Yellow fever is an acute viral disease marked by high fever, pain, hemorrhage, and jaundice. The latter results from the damaging effect of the virus upon the liver. Since there is no specific therapy available, the emphasis is upon prevention, that is, eradication of mosquitoes and active immunization with a vaccine prepared from the attenuated virus. The immunity engendered by this vaccine is good for about 6 years. An actual attack of yellow fever usually confers life-long immunity.

Infectious hepatitis. Infectious hepatitis is a viral disease characterized by liver damage and jaundice. The virus occurs in the feces and is transmitted via contaminated water and food, especially shellfish. The treatment of the disease is largely symptomatic. Prophylactically, gamma globulin, if given early, will often protect susceptible persons who become exposed.

Serum hepatitis. Serum hepatitis is a viral infection indistinguishable from infectious hepatitis. The virus is present in the blood throughout the course of the disease and in some instances months afterward, which explains why it is readily transmitted by administration of infected blood plasma or serum. Means are presently being explored to eliminate the virus from the blood and plasma used in transfusions. Treatment is entirely symptomatic.

Mumps. Mumps, or *parotitis,* an acute viral infection characterized by swelling of the salivary glands, usually strikes somewhere between the ages of 5 and 15 years. The infection is not ordinarily considered serious, but if it occurs after puberty, sterility may develop in both sexes as a result of orchitis or oophoritis.

There is no specific form of therapy. Prophylactically, however, *gamma globulin* has proved of considerable value. When it is administered 7 to 10 days after exposure, a substantial proportion of susceptible persons are protected. Recently, there have appeared encouraging reports on the use of a mumps vaccine for active immunization. Typically, an attack of mumps engenders a permanent immunity.

Diseases caused by enteroviruses. In the wake of the tissue culture techniques developed by Enders, Robbins, and Weller, intensive research into the nature of the viruses of the gut (the so-called enteroviruses) has disclosed three major groups: polioviruses (Chapter 19), Coxsackie viruses, and echoviruses.

Coxsackie viruses. Named after the village in New York where the first strains were isolated in 1948, the Coxsackie viruses comprise two clinical groups (A and B). Viruses of Group A cause herpangina (an illness marked by fever and eruption of blisters) and aseptic meningitis (a nonbacterial meningitis often indistinguishable from nonparalytic poliomyelitis). All five viruses of Group B have been found to be associated with human illness, the most important being aseptic meningitis, pleurodynia (painful disease of the muscles of the chest and diaphragm), fatal inflammation of the heart in newborn infants, and certain poliolike diseases. It is now apparent that many illnesses diagnosed as nonparalytic poliomyelitis may actually be Coxsackie virus infections.

Echoviruses. The search for the poliovirus in the human gastrointestinal tract unexpectedly turned up twenty or more microbes that have been dubbed ECHO viruses (*e*nteric *c*ytopathogenic *h*uman *o*rphan). The term *orphan* refers to the fact that in many cases there has been no association with disease. Other enteric viruses of a similar nature have been isolated from monkeys (ECMO), cattle (ECBO), and swine (ECSO).

It is now recognized that certain echoviruses cause disease. Their association with outbreaks of diarrhea, particularly in hospital nurseries, has recently been proved. In one study echoviruses were isolated in 31 percent of cases. Echoviruses have also been associated with febrile infections of the respiratory and enteric tracts, paralytic aseptic meningitis, and skin eruptions.

Trench mouth. Also known as *Vincent's angina,* trench mouth is an ulcerative infection of the mouth and pharynx marked by the presence of a pseudomembrane. Stained smears from the ulcers disclose two microbes—*Borrelia vincentii,* a spirochete, and *Fusobacterium fusiforme,* a bacillus—which may or may not be the etiologic factors. No one knows. The drug of choice in treating the condition is penicillin. Patients are instructed to observe strict oral hygiene, and all dishes and other objects that might be contaminated must be sterilized.

Worm infestations. The presence of parasitic worms in the intestine is the most common form of helminthiasis. Such infestations harass the host by causing intestinal obstruction, faulty digestion, inflammation, and anemia.

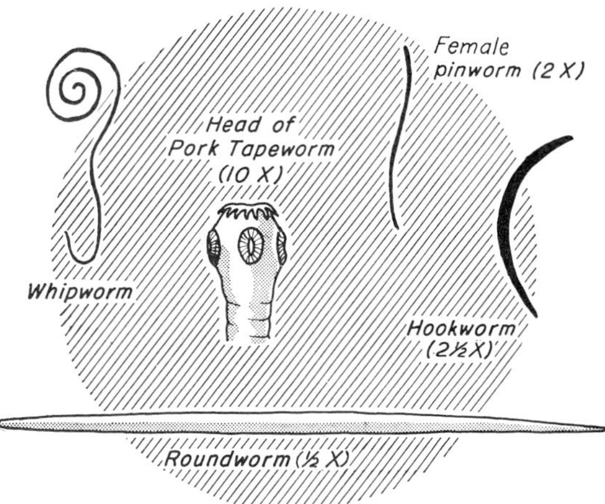

Fig. 14-15. Parasitic worms. (From Brooks, S. M.: Basic facts of pharmacology, ed. 2, Philadelphia, 1963, W. B. Saunders Co.)

Hookworm. The hookworm (Fig. 14-15) belongs to two species—*Ancylostoma duodenale* and *Necator americanus.* In the United States the latter species is the usual culprit.

The adult worm, which measures about ⅓ inch in length, is equipped with teeth and hooks its head into the mucosa, thereby deriving sustenance from the blood. Microscopic ova, released by the female, leave the body via the feces and, in the proper environment, develop into larvae. Human beings become infected with the larvae either by walking barefoot in contaminated soil or by ingesting contaminated food or drink. The former mode of infection, however, is far more common. Once the larvae have burrowed through the soft skin between the toes and have gained entrance into the blood, they proceed to enter the alveoli. From here, they begin their long journey to the small intestine via the bronchioles, bronchi, trachea, esophagus, and stomach, in that order.

Once in the intestine, the larvae develop into adults, and the cycle begins anew.

As in other intestinal helminthiases, diagnosis is made by finding ova in the stool specimens. Since ova vary considerably among the various worms, a definitive diagnosis is generally possible.

Drugs used against worms are called *anthelmintics*. The best agent of this type in the treatment of hookworm is tetrachloroethylene. Like most anthelmintics, tetrachloroethylene narcotizes the worms to the point where they lose their grip on the mucosa and thus can be easily flushed out in the stool.

Roundworm. Infestation by the roundworm (ascariasis) is caused by the nematode *Ascaris lumbricoides*. This worm, the largest nematode that attacks man, measures between 8 and 12 inches in length (Fig. 14-15). Though worldwide in distribution, it is most common in the Far East. The adult lives in the intestine, and the larvae, which enter the body in contaminated food and drink, migrate through the body much like those of the hookworm. The signs and symptoms of the infestation result from the presence of the worms in the intestine and the larvae in the tissues.

Of the various anthelmintics that have been used in treating the infestation, piperazine (Antepar) is considered by many authorities to be a drug of choice. It is given on an empty stomach and then followed by a saline cathartic to expel the dazed worms.

Pinworm. Pinworm infestation, the commonest helminthiasis in the United States, usually strikes children. The adult worm (known technically as *Enterobius vermicularis*) measures about ½ inch in length (Fig. 14-15) and resides in the colon and rectum. At night, about 9 o'clock, as a matter of fact, the pregnant female wiggles through the anal opening and deposits ova in the surrounding area. This produces itching, scratching, and contamination of fingernails—thereby ensuring infection via the oral route.

A wide variety of drugs have been employed against pinworm infestation; hexylresorcinol and piperazine (Antepar) are among the most useful.

Whipworm. The whipworm *(Trichuris trichiura)*, as its name indicates, is a whip-shaped helminth 1 inch or so in length. It lives in the cecum and large intestine, with its pointed end embedded in the mucosa. In children the infestation is usually mild, and in adults it is often asymptomatic. The anthelmintic dithiazinine (Delvex) reportedly has produced 100 percent cures in this infestation.

Tapeworm. Even the thought of having a tapeworm causes many of us to squirm with as much emotion as seeing a snake wiggling through the grass. This unsavory parasite runs anywhere from 20 to 30 feet in length and has a tiny head (scolex) equipped with suckers or hooklets (Fig. 14-15). With these structures the worm embeds its scolex into the mucosa and settles down to a comfortable life at the expense of the host.

The beef tapeworm *(Taenia saginata)* causes most taeniasis in this country. The worm has a complex life cycle requiring the cow as well as man for its survival. Infestation can be eradicated by raising cattle on land uncontaminated by human feces. Quinacrine (Atabrine) is the anthelmintic of choice.

The pork tapeworm *(Taenia solium)* closely resembles the beef tapeworm. It passes through the same stages in its life cycle in the pig and in man as the beef tapeworm and presents just about the same clinical picture. Treatment and prophylaxis are about the same as those cited for the beef tapeworm.

NONINFECTIOUS DISEASES

Because of its great bulk and expanse of tissue, the digestive system is also subject to a variety of essentially noninfectious disorders. Some of the more common conditions include gastritis, peptic ulcer, diverticulosis, intestinal obstruction, ulcerative colitis, jaundice, cirrhosis, gallstones, pancreatitis, appendicitis, and tumors. Concerning tumors, the chief sites of malignant growths (cancer) are the stomach, large intestine, and rectum.

Questions

1. Describe the anatomy of the mouth.
2. What is the function of the frenulum linguae?
3. Name the three types of papillae found on the surface of the tongue.
4. Discuss the mechanism of taste.
5. Compare the deciduous and permanent teeth.
6. Describe the anatomy of the tooth.
7. Discuss the structure and formation of the teeth and the role played by calcium, vitamin D, parathyroid hormone, and fluorine.
8. Discuss the pros and cons of fluoridation.
9. Discuss the anatomy and physiology of the salivary glands.
10. Describe the acts of mastication and deglutition.
11. Describe the structure of the esophagus.
12. Describe the stomach wall.
13. Discuss the neurogenic and hormonal stimulation of gastric juice.
14. Describe the mixing and emptying of the stomach contents.
15. Describe the gross anatomy of the small intestine.
16. Describe the gross anatomy of the large intestine.
17. Compare the walls of the small and large intestines.
18. What are Peyer's patches?
19. Give the precise location of the vermiform appendix.
20. Distinguish between the villi and plicae circulares.
21. What is the lamina propria?
22. Describe the structure and function of the mesentery.
23. Discuss the hormonal activation of the glands of Lieberkühn.
24. Describe peristalsis and its regulation.
25. Describe in detail the structure of the rectum and the anal canal.
26. Describe the mechanism of defecation and the composition of the feces.
27. What prevents passage of bile into the duodenum during fasting?
28. What are the composition and function of the bile?
29. Briefly discuss the various functions of the liver.
30. What role does secretin play in the digestive process?
31. What is the relationship of the gallbladder to the liver?
32. What is the function of cholecystokinin?
33. The pancreas is a "dual gland." Explain.
34. Locate the ducts of Wirsung and Santorini.
35. What is the function of pancreozymin?
36. When saliva is added to a dilute starch solution colored blue by the addition of a drop of iodine, the color slowly fades away. Explain.
37. What is the chief function of the mouth in the digestive process?
38. The presence of gastric juice in the stomach when food is not present is a serious matter. Explain.
39. Relatively speaking, the stomach plays a minor *chemical* role in the digestive process. Explain.
40. Write the equation for the reaction that occurs when baking soda enters the stomach.
41. What are antacids?
42. What is pepsinogen?
43. Compare the digestion of maltose, sucrose, and lactose.
44. Name the two most important amylases in the digestive process.
45. Compare the action of trypsin and erepsin.
46. Glucose, fructose, and galactose are isomers. Explain.
47. What is a polypeptide?
48. Write the balanced equation for the enzymatic hydrolysis of glyceryl tripalmitate into palmitic acid and glycerol.
49. Write the equation for the enzymatic hydrolysis of glycylglycine.
50. State the function of enterokinase.
51. State the function of villikinin.
52. Distinguish between chyle and chyme.
53. Discuss the etiology and treatment of parotitis.
54. Discuss the etiology and treatment of Vincent's angina.
55. Discuss the etiology, clinical picture, treatment, and prevention of typhoid fever.
56. What is paratyphoid fever?
57. Distinguish between bacillary and amebic dysentery.
58. Canning food at home is a serious matter. Explain.
59. Discuss the etiology, clinical picture, treatment, and prevention of Asiatic cholera.
60. What is infectious hepatitis?
61. What is yellow fever?
62. Name three common helminthiases in the United States.
63. Describe the life cycle of *Necator americanus.*
64. What are anthelmintics?
65. Discuss the cause and treatment of peptic ulcer.

Chapter 15

Metabolism

Metabolism concerns the myriad reactions among the ions, atoms, and molecules of the body. More especially, it deals with the fate of the nutrients that enter the blood incident to the digestive process.

GLUCOSE

From the standpoint of metabolism, the carbohydrate spotlight falls on glucose, for it makes up 80 percent of all absorbed monosaccharides. Thus, for all practical purposes, glucose is the sugar of the body. Its normal concentration in the blood averages about 90 mg. per 100 ml. of blood.

Glycogenesis. Following a meal, the increase in blood glucose stimulates the pancreas to release large quantities of *insulin,* a hormone that promotes the rapid transport of glucose into the cells; here the sugar is burned to provide energy or, in excess, is converted into fat. But this is not all. Liver cells convert glucose into *glycogen,* a polymer of glucose, for the purpose of storage, and when the blood sugar drops below normal, *epinephrine* causes glycogen to be split back into glucose. Thus, as shown in Fig. 15-1, insulin promotes the formation of glycogen (*glycogenesis*) and epinephrine stimulates the formation of glucose (*glycogenolysis*). In essence, then, the liver is the "glucostat" of of the body.

Gluconeogenesis. In addition to glycogenolysis, a low blood sugar stimulates, via the adrenocortical hormones (Chapter 22), gluconeogenesis, or the conversion of proteins (and to a much less extent fats) into glucose. Thus, in starvation the cells are torn apart in order to provide energy. It is little wonder, then, that the starved body is nothing but "skin and bones."

Release of energy. The cell needs energy to run its household, and the manner in which it obtains this energy is one of the great sagas of biochemistry. Because of the very complex nature of the subject, however, the present discussion will be confined to the general sequence of events.

Adenosine triphosphate. Let us understand at the outset that the body derives its energy indirectly from foods. Its *immediate* energy source is the miraculous compound adenosine triphosphate (ATP), whose structural formula is given at the bottom of the facing page.

The bonds that attach the last two phosphate radicals to the remainder of the ATP molecule may be likened to a coiled spring awaiting to be sprung—hence, the expression *high-energy phosphate bonds.*

Whenever the cell needs energy, a phosphate radical is broken off and the liberated energy put to work. Chemically, this may be expressed as follows:

$$\text{ATP} \longrightarrow \text{Adenosine diphosphate (ADP)} + PO_4^{\equiv} + \Delta$$

Glycolysis. Obviously, ATP must be replenished if life is to continue, and here is where glucose enters the picture, for the energy released in the burning of glucose (and other nutrients) is used to resynthesize ATP from ADP and $PO_4^{\equiv}$. That is, the equation just presented is reversible. Thus,

$$\text{ATP} \rightleftarrows \text{ADP} + PO_4^{\equiv} + \Delta$$

Glucose is "bio-oxidized" in a most cunning fashion. Instead of exploding with a flash and a puff, nature pulls the molecule apart in successive steps, releasing tiny spurts of energy along the way. The first several steps constitute what is known as glycolysis (Fig. 15-2). Here the six-carbon chain is split by an array of cellular enzymes into two molecules of *pyruvic acid.* Thus,

$$\underset{\text{Glucose}}{C_6H_{12}O_6} \longrightarrow \underset{\text{Pyruvic acid}}{2CH_3{-}\overset{\overset{\displaystyle O}{\|}}{C}{-}COOH} + 4H^+ + \Delta$$

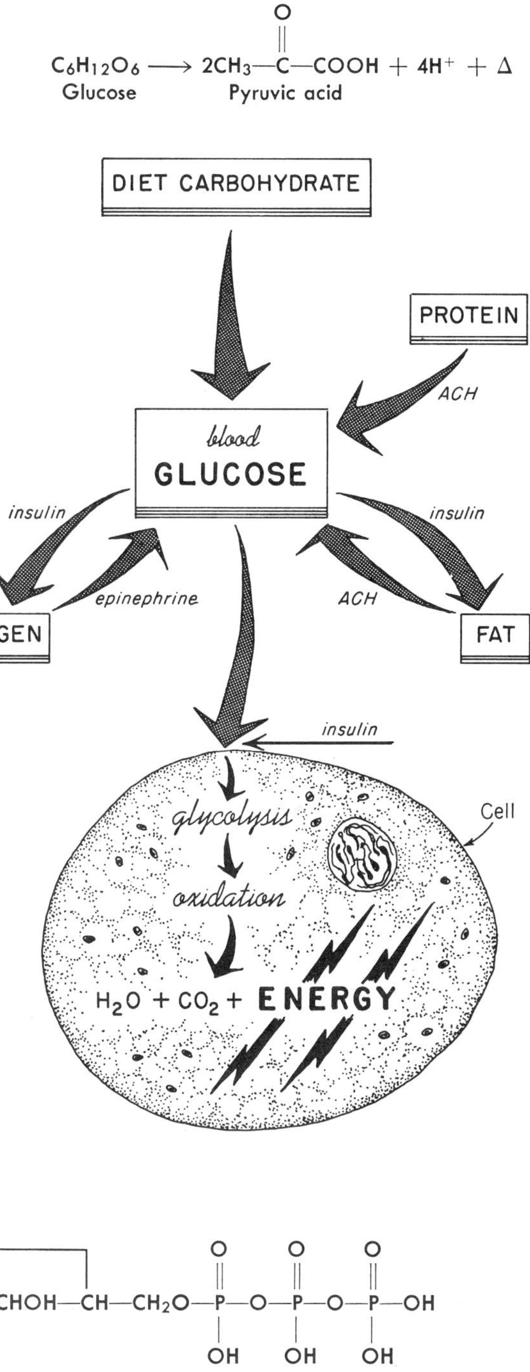

Fig. 15-1. Metabolism of glucose (ACH, adrenocortical hormones).

Adenosine triphosphate

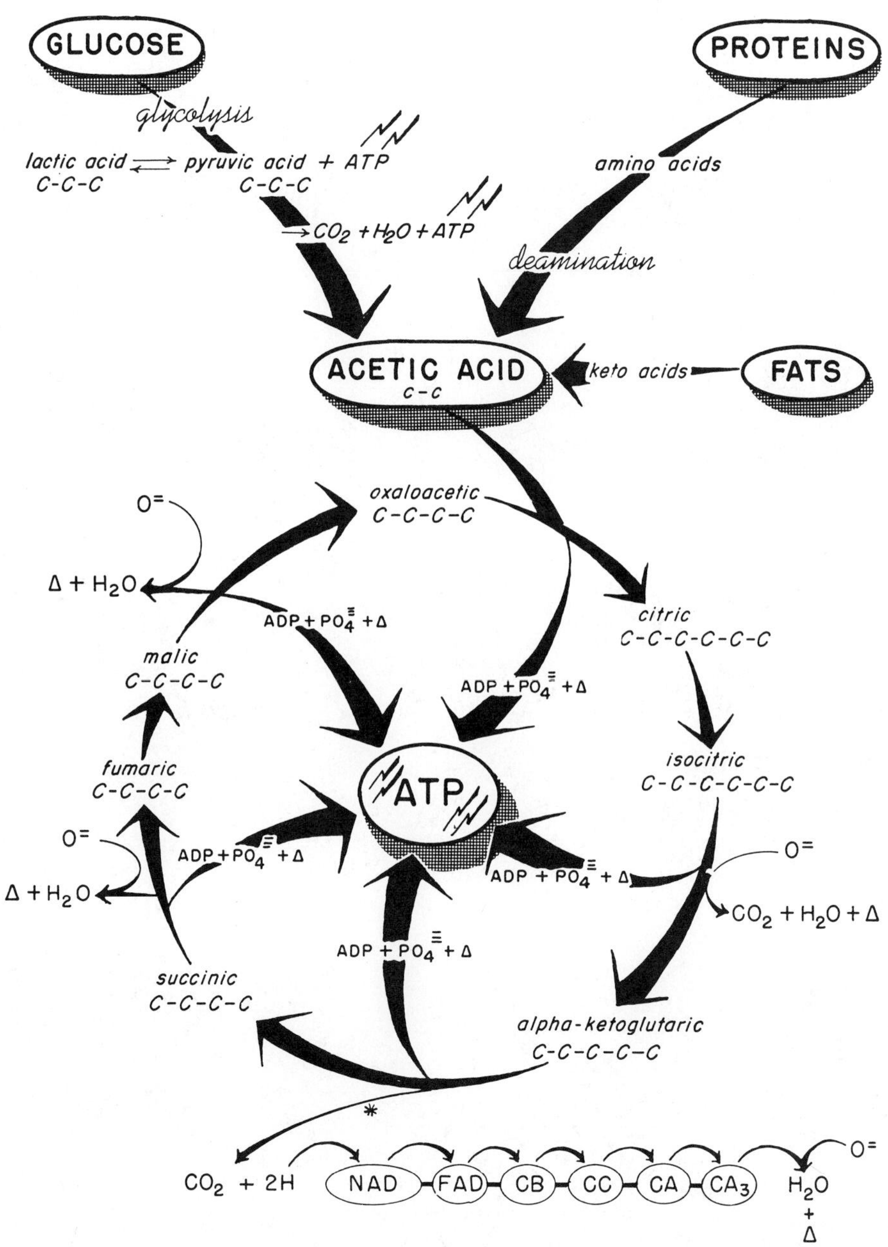

Fig. 15-2. Summary of the major events of the Krebs cycle. The arrow with an asterisk (*) beside it indicates the mechanism by which hydrogen electrons are passed and finally react with H^+ and $O^=$ to form water. **NAD** (nicotinamide adenine dinucleotide), **FAD** (flavin adenine dinucleotide), **CB** (cytochrome B), **CC** (cytochrome C), **CA** (cytochrome A), and $\mathbf{CA_3}$ (cytochrome A_3) are the coenzymes.

As indicated, this is an *oxidation* reaction because it involves the removal of hydrogen (from glucose). Put another way, glycolysis may be characterized as the *anaerobic* phase of bio-oxidation.

Krebs cycle. The steps of the second stage of bio-oxidation together release almost twenty times as much energy as glycolysis. This is the stage, therefore, chiefly responsible for the resynthesis of ATP from ADP and phosphate. The various reactions have been shown to be of a cyclical nature and are collectively referred to as the *citric acid cycle,* or Krebs cycle (Fig. 15-2) in honor of the biochemist who first proposed the scheme. Briefly, enzymes called *decarboxylases* and *dehydrogenases* chop off carbon dioxide and hydrogen, respectively, from pyruvic acid. Though this activity yields some energy, the bulk of the energy is liberated in the passing along of *electrons* released from the hydrogen. As shown in the illustration, nature has seen fit to bring hydrogen and oxygen together in a roundabout way, to say the least. That is, the freshly chopped-off hydrogen electrons are successively passed along by coenzymes, and at the cytochrome A_3 stage, the last coenzyme, hydrogen finally reacts with oxygen. The overall reaction may be expressed as follows:

$$2CH_2\overset{\overset{\displaystyle O}{\|}}{C}\text{—}COOH + 5O_2 \longrightarrow 6CO_2 + 4H_2O + \Delta$$

In *summary,* ATP provides immediate energy to the cell by breaking down into ADP and $PO_4^{\equiv}$. To replenish ATP, bio-oxidation furnishes the necessary energy for sparking the reaction between ADP and $PO_4^{\equiv}$. Once all the ADP has been converted back into ATP, the oxidative reactions cease. Thus, to a great degree, bio-oxidation is regulated by the amount of ADP. In the language of pure chemistry, one molecule of glucose—via bio-oxidation—yields thirty-eight molecules of ATP, two of which are produced during glycolysis and thirty-six of which are produced in the Krebs cycle.

Phosphocreatine. Closely related to ATP is another high-energy phosphate called phosphocreatine (or creatine phosphate). During times of minimal cellular activity, the large amounts of ATP available furnish energy for the synthesis of this substance. However, in times of acute chemical stress, when the cell needs every scrap of ATP it can get, phosphocreatine breaks down into creatine and phosphate and the energy released is used to re-form ATP. Since this reaction takes place at a much faster rate than the oxidative reactions just discussed, phosphocreatine serves as the cell's immediate reserve, especially *in muscle.*

Role of fats and proteins. Though the tissues prefer to obtain their energy from glucose, they can and do burn fats and proteins. Of particular interest in this connection is the fact that they enter the Krebs cycle right along with the end product of glycolysis (Fig. 15-2).

Oxygen debt. When energy is expended at a rate exceeding the capabilities of the Krebs cycle, the pyruvic acid that accumulates at the furnace door is converted, largely in the liver, into *lactic acid* (Fig. 15-2). Since the latter must eventually be turned back into pyruvic acid and burned, we say that the body has incurred an oxygen debt. Thus, the runner continues to breathe very hard for a few minutes after a race in order to pay this debt.

FATS

Physiologically, one is prone to think of fat as a "passive" substance that accumulates beneath the skin. However, this is decidedly not the case, for the biochemist has learned that the body's fat is not only highly mobile but also subject to countless alterations in the complex machinery of the tissues (Fig. 15-3).

Synthesis of fat. Above all, let us not forget that the bulk of the fat in the body is not derived from the diet; it is synthe-

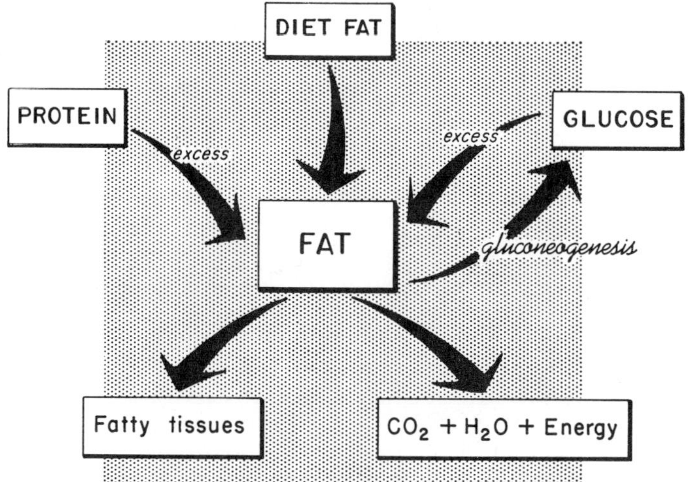

Fig. 15-3. Diagrammatic summary of fat metabolism.

sized. Indeed, any type of food, as we well know, can fatten the tissues. Although this has been known since time immemorial, only in the last few years have the chemical gymnastics been explained.

As one can easily guess, glucose is the chief raw material that the body converts into fat, for all excess sugar not immediately burned or stored as glycogen is deposited in the fatty tissues. To a much less degree, extra amounts of amino acids are handled in the same manner. These synthetic processes are performed in the liver, and the fat produced thereby is transported to the fatty tissues.

Energy. When the supply of glucose drops below the body's needs, fats are burned, which explains the shrinking waistline occasioned by a low-calorie diet.

In the burning of fats, they are first split into *glycerol* and *fatty acids* in the liver. Although glycerol fits into the Krebs cycle about as easily as glucose, the fatty acids must be further split into simpler acids. Usually, this is carried out by so-called *beta oxidation.* In the illustrative reaction shown below, note that the twelve-carbon chain fatty acid ends up as six molecules of acetic acid, which then reacts with *coenzyme A* to form *acetyl coenzyme A*—one of the most important "intermediates" in the body. Acetyl coenzyme A serves in the synthesis of acetoacetic acid and β-hydroxybutyric acid (collectively referred to as "ketone bodies"), acetylcholine, and cholesterol and, central to the discussion at hand, "starts" the Krebs cycle. In Fig. 15-2, acetyl coenzyme A is indicated as "acetic acid."

PROTEINS

The proteins and amino acids of the body are always in a state of biochemical flux. An amino acid that was free in the bloodstream yesterday may today be structured in a protein of the protoplasm, and so on. Conversely, proteins are continually being torn apart in some tissues to provide amino acids for other tissues. Although the principal chemical "flow" is toward protein, amino acids can follow other routes. As shown in Fig. 15-4, they may be converted into glucose or fat, made into special chemicals, burned, or excreted.

$$\begin{array}{l} \quad\;\; O_2 \qquad\quad\;\; O_2 \qquad\quad\;\; O_2 \qquad\quad\;\; O_2 \qquad\quad\;\; O_2 \qquad\qquad\quad O \\ \quad\;\;\downarrow \qquad\quad\;\;\downarrow \qquad\quad\;\;\downarrow \qquad\quad\;\;\downarrow \qquad\quad\;\;\downarrow \qquad\qquad\quad \| \\ CH_3{-}CH_2{-}CH_2{-}CH_2{-}CH_2{-}CH_2{-}CH_2{-}CH_2{-}CH_2{-}CH_2{-}CH_2{-}C{-}OH \end{array} \longrightarrow 6CH_3{-}\overset{\displaystyle O}{\overset{\|}{C}}{-}OH$$

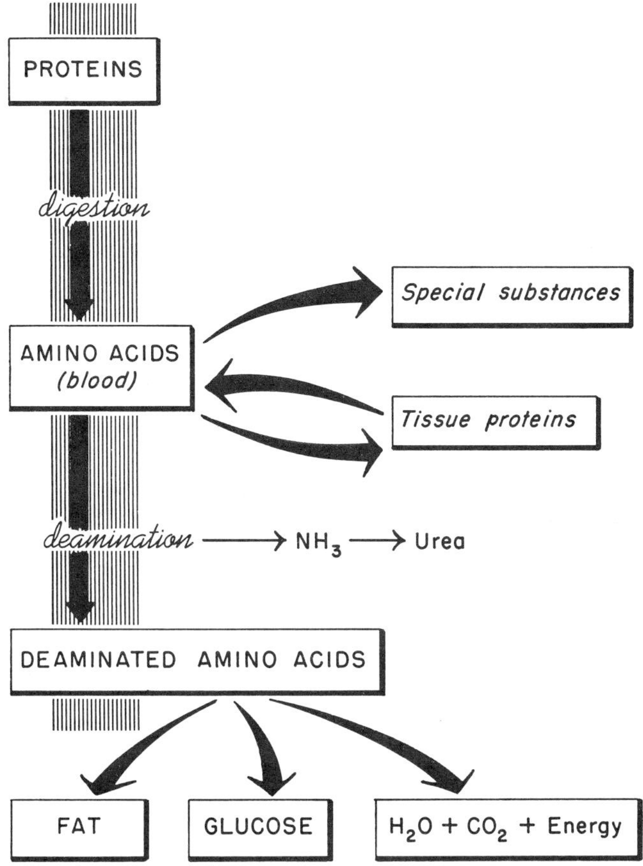

Fig. 15-4. Diagrammatic summary of protein metabolism.

Amino acids of the blood. The concentration of amino acids in the blood is about 30 mg. per 100 ml., a homeostatic state resulting from the ease by which they can be absorbed and released by the liver and the tissue cells. Specifically, when the concentration rises, the acids are absorbed and forged into protein, and when the concentration falls, proteins are degraded and the resulting acids passed back into the blood.

Adrenocortical hormones. The adrenocortical hormones secreted by the adrenal glands (Chapter 22) have a profound influence on the amino acid flux throughout the body. By some mechanism (perhaps by increasing the permeability of the cellular membrane) they promote the release of amino acids from the tissues. Since these hormones are secreted mainly in response to stress, the object of this mobilization is apparently to provide the body with the raw materials to bolster the defense and repair damaged cells.

Tissue proteins. Once amino acids enter the cell, they are synthesized into proteins and subsequently fashioned into protoplasm and enzymes. The manner in which the genes direct this work was discussed earlier in Chapter 5.

As indicated, proteins are also constantly being reconverted into amino acids for the purpose of performing some service elsewhere. Thus, the quantity of protein in a given cell is determined by the balance between synthesis and reconversion. The intracellular splitting of proteins into amino acids, incidentally, is catalyzed by special enzymes called *cathepsins.*

Plasma proteins. The proteins of the plasma—albumins, fibrinogen, and globulins (p. 123)—are formed principally in the liver and are released into the blood. When there is a drop in concentration, that organ responds by stepping up their production. In this way the blood maintains its osmotic pressure and volume (Chapter 18).

Conversion to glucose and fat. Under normal conditions the body needs about 30 gm. of new protein daily to replace the protoplasm destroyed through wear and tear and to fortify the reserves. Amounts over and above this figure are *deaminated* and converted into glucose or fat or are burned for energy. The ammonia released in deamination is converted into urea and excreted by the kidney (Chapter 17).

Special substances. Special substances of a nonprotein nature are made from amino acids. Adenine and creatine (the precursors of adenosine triphosphate and phosphocreatine), glutamine (used in forming ammonia), and the hormones epinephrine and thyroxine are outstanding examples. Some hormones, however (for example, oxytocin and insulin), are true proteins.

Energy. To supply energy, proteins are split into amino acids and the latter deaminated and oxidized in the Krebs cycle. The deaminated acids (for example, acetic acid) may enter the cycle directly, or if energy is not immediately needed, they may be converted into glucose or fat and burned later.

METABOLIC RATE

Since the energy released in the body eventually appears as heat, the rate at which the latter is produced provides the most accurate measure of metabolism—hence, the term *metabolic rate.* Depending upon the degree of physiologic activity, the metabolic rate may run from a low of about 50 Calories (Cal.) per hour all the way up to 2000 Cal. per hour.

Factors affecting rate. Obviously, any factor that increases the liberation of energy will increase the metabolic rate. The more important factors of this nature are presented here.

Exercise. We know from experience that exercise yields tremendous amounts of heat. Indeed, strenuous exercise can push the metabolic rate almost 50 percent above normal! As explained earlier (p. 311), an increase in ADP—as a result of the breakdown of ATP—is a powerful stimulant of bio-oxidation.

Thyroxine. Thyroxine, the chief hormone of the thyroid (Chapter 22), increases metabolism in all the tissues. A lack of it can lower the metabolic rate to 50 percent of normal, and excess amounts can push the rate up as high as 300 percent above normal! The mechanism of action and other particulars relating to the thyroid and thyroxine are discussed in detail in Chapter 22.

Insulin. Insulin is also a key hormone in metabolism, for it promotes the transport of glucose across the cellular membrane, thereby enabling the tissues to meet their energy requirements. If for some reason the pancreas fails to secrete the hormone in adequate amounts, or if the hormone were in some way deactivated or inhibited, metabolism suffers and diabetes ensues.

Epinephrine. Stimulation of the sympathetic nervous system causes the release of norepinephrine from the nerve endings and epinephrine from the adrenal medullae (Chapter 22). The hormone stimulates metabolism by promoting glycogenolysis and probably also by enhancing bio-oxidation, but just how the latter is effected is as yet unknown.

Although strong sympathetic stimulation can push the metabolic rate two or three times above normal, the effect is short lived. However, when we consider that the system is primarily concerned with emergency situations, this is readily understandable. In brief, epinephrine affords an effective means of turning the metabolism on and off at a moment's notice.

Body temperature. Since an increase in temperature enhances the speed of a chemical reaction, we see immediately why increased body temperature steps up the metabolic rate. A high fever may increase the rate as much as two or three times. This enhanced metabolism is dramatically evidenced by the increase in heart rate (Fig. 15-5).

Specific dynamic action. Following a meal, the metabolic rate rises and remains elevated for several hours. Though this response, referred to as specific dynamic action (SDA), undoubtedly results in part from the activities of digestion, absorption, and assimilation, it is believed that the products of digestion, namely, the amino acids, exert a special stimulating action on the metabolic processes. Fats and carbohydrates increase the rate by an average of about 20 percent, and proteins increase it by about 40 percent.

Basal metabolic rate. Because the metabolic rate is the most meaningful statistic relating to body chemistry, the student should not be surprised to learn of its diagnostic value to the physician. However, a person's metabolic rate has little or no meaning unless it is taken under *basal* conditions, that is, at complete physical and mental rest. Thus, the basal metabolic rate, or BMR, measures *inherent* cellular chemistry.

Taking the basal metabolic rate. The obvious way to take the basal metabolic rate would be to place the subject in a giant calorimeter and measure the number of calories given off in a given period of time. But this is too cumbersome and expensive for routine use.

Therefore, an indirect method, using the spirometer, is employed for routine clinical work. As shown in Fig. 15-6, this device records directly the subject's oxygen consumption, and from this data calories can be calculated. (Consumption of 1 liter of oxygen corresponds to the release of 4.825 Cal.) And since the basal metabolic rate has been shown to vary in proportion to the body surface, the latter must be found and "incorporated" into the BMR. For this purpose, use is made of the chart shown in Fig. 15-7.

Let us now illustrate what we have learned by an example: A 30-year-old man weighing 154 pounds and measuring 5 feet 8 inches in height consumed 2.5 liters of oxygen in 10 minutes. Thus, in 1 hour he uses 15 liters of oxygen and releases 15 times 4.825, or 72.38 Cal. Now, since the surface area of his body according to the chart is 1.8 sq.m., his BMR is 72.38 divided

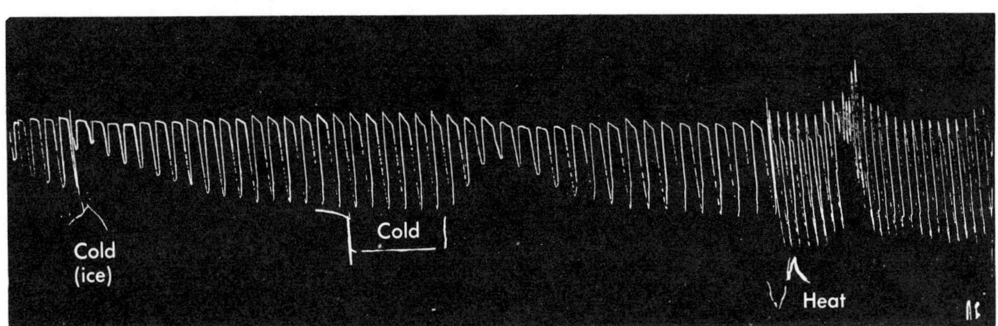

Fig. 15-5. Kymographic recording of the effects of cold (ice) and heat (warm water) upon the frog heart. Note that whereas cold slows the heart, heat causes an immediate increase in rate and strength of beat.

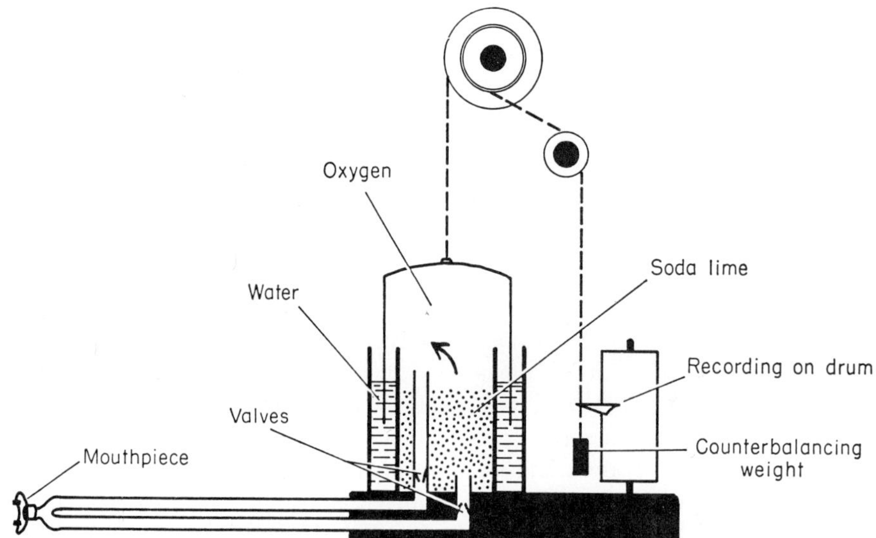

Fig. 15-6. Diagrammatic representation of the oxygen-filled spirometer used to measure basal metabolism. The subject (with nose closed) breathes in and out through the mouthpiece. As the oxygen is consumed, the metal can descends and the volume of oxygen used is thereby recorded on the drum. (After Guyton, A. C.: Function of the human body, Philadelphia, 1959, W. B. Saunders Co.)

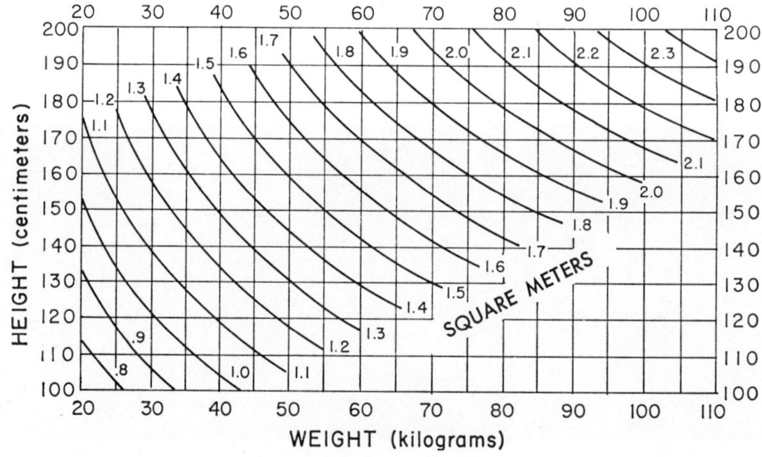

Fig. 15-7. BMR chart for determining the body surface area (in square meters) when the weight and height are known. (After Dubois; from Guyton, A. C.: Function of the human body, Philadelphia, 1959, W. B. Saunders Co.)

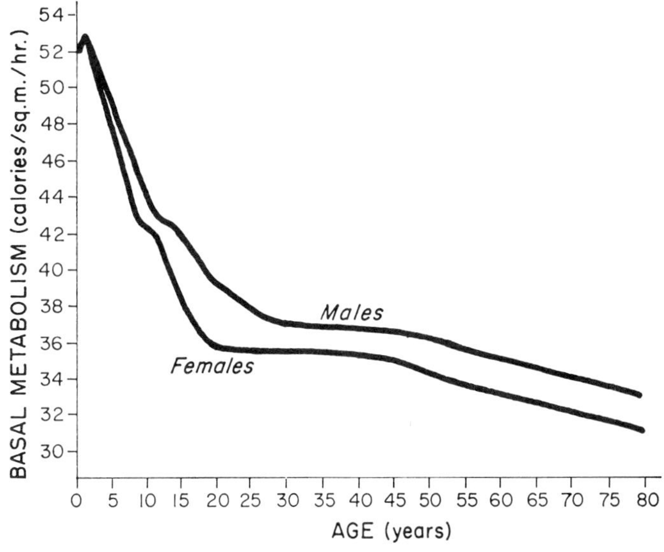

Fig. 15-8. Normal basal metabolic rates of males and females at different ages. (After Guyton, A. C.: Function of the human body, Philadelphia, 1959, W. B. Saunders Co.)

by 1.8, or 40.2 Cal. per square meter per hour (40.2 Cal./sq.m./hr.).

This value, however, is relatively useless unless we compare it with the *normal* BMR, which for this particular person is 37.2 Cal./sq.m./hr. (Fig. 15-8). This we do on a percentage basis. Thus,

$$\frac{40.2 - 37.2}{37} \times 100 = 8\%$$

Clinically, this is expressed as +8, meaning 8 percent *above* normal. On the other hand, had the subject's oxygen consumption been less than 40.2 Cal., say 34.2 Cal./sq.m./hr., his rate would be −8, or 8 percent *below* normal.

In cases of extreme hyperthyroidism the BMR may climb at high as +100, and in severe hypothyroid states the BMR may drop to a low of −50. Generally speaking, a BMR of ±15 is considered a normal range.

RESPIRATORY QUOTIENT

Another interesting metabolic statistic is the respiratory quotient (RQ), which is equal to the ratio of the volume of carbon dioxide expired to the volume of oxygen inspired in a given time. On a pure carbohydrate diet the RQ is 1, a fact that is simply explained by the following equation:

$$C_6H_{12}O_6 + 6O_2 \longrightarrow 6CO_2 + 6H_2O$$
$$RQ = 6/6, \text{ or } 1$$

In the catabolism of fats and proteins, however, proportionately less carbon dioxide is given off, making the RQ less than 1. Fats have an RQ of about 0.7 and proteins an RQ of about 0.8. On a mixed diet the RQ is in the vicinity of 0.85.

BODY TEMPERATURE

Heat is a manifestation of life. In less poetic terms, it is, as we know, a product of metabolism. The oral temperature of the human body hovers ever so closely to 98.6° F., and even when we are exposed to extreme cold or heat, the temperature rarely varies more than a degree or so. The mechanism responsible for this fine control is of great theoretical and practical importance.

Hypothalamic thermostat. Maintaining

an even temperature requires a thermostat, and that is just what the body has in the form of an elaborate nervous device situated in the hypothalamus. Like any thermostat, the hypothalamic version, in essence, turns on the heat when the body temperature starts to drop and turns it off when the temperature starts to rise.

Increasing temperature. Whenever the temperature of the blood drops below normal, the sympathetic centers in the hypothalamic thermostat are strongly stimulated. This electrifies the sympathetic nerves throughout the body, producing, among other things, vasoconstriction, increased metabolism, increased muscle tone, and piloerection.

Vasoconstriction and an increased metabolism (caused by the release of epinephrine and thyroxine) conserve and increase heat, respectively. The increased muscle tone also steps up the release of heat; indeed, in extreme cold the muscles become so excited that we shiver.

The term *piloerection* refers to the hairs standing on end. This response is a means of survival in the animal world, and it indicates that at one time man was covered with a hairy coat. Piloerection works by entrapping trillions upon trillions of air molecules in the microscopic recesses of the erected hairs (or feathers in birds), providing one of the best types of insulation known to nature. The piloerection of fright, always noticeable on the arms and rarely on the head, also results from sympathetic bombardment.

Decreasing temperature. Let us now consider what happens when the hypothalamus is bathed in overheated blood. In this case the parasympathetic centers are stimulated and the sympathetic centers are inhibited, just the opposite of what happens when the blood is "cool." This causes vasodilatation, decreased metabolism, and decreased muscle tone (the *reverse* of the effects noted previously) and one added feature—sweating. By the evaporation of water from its surface, the body cools itself, even in the heat of the Sahara. On an extremely hot day a man may perspire as much as a gallon per hour!

Lacking an adequate sweating mechanism, animals solve their cooling problem by panting. In this way they bring about the evaporation of water from the moist respiratory passageways.

Fever. Since a fever indicates that all is not well within the body, it serves as a most important diagnostic sign. A fever is more than a danger signal, however. Fevers combat infection by inhibiting the multiplication of many pathogens (p. 139) and facilitate tissue repair by increasing metabolism. It is for these reasons that many authorities believe that *mild* fevers are best left alone. High fevers, however, must be controlled by antipyretic drugs such as aspirin. At a temperature of about 108° F. or so the cells begin to "burn up," and at about 112° F. the body succumbs. The principal insult from elevated temperature is sustained by the heart and brain.

Cause. It is now believed most fevers are caused by proteins released from microbes or damaged tissue cells. In some way these agents reset the hypothalamic thermostat to a higher temperature level. At the beginning of a fever the preponderant sympathetic activity is manifested in chills. When the fever breaks, parasympathetic activity prevails, resulting in vasodilatation and sweating. In the first instance the body is adjusting to the higher "setting," and in the second, it is readjusting to its normal level.

Questions

1. Write the structural formulas for glucose, fructose, and galactose.
2. Distinguish between glycogenesis and glycogenolysis.
3. What is meant by gluconeogenesis?
4. Discuss the role of adenosine triphosphate in the release of energy.
5. Describe the highlights of glycolysis.
6. Describe the highlights of the citric acid cycle.
7. What is a coenzyme?

8. Discuss the role of phosphocreatine in the release of energy.
9. Carbohydrates, fats, and proteins are burned in the same "furnace." Explain.
10. What do we mean by "oxygen debt"?
11. Discuss the synthesis of fat.
12. Describe the process of beta oxidation in the burning of fats.
13. Discuss the formation and fate of acetoacetic acid.
14. In a brief paragraph summarize the metabolism of proteins.
15. Briefly discuss the effects of exercise, thyroxine, insulin, epinephrine, and food upon the metabolic rate.
16. What is meant by the basal metabolic rate?
17. Briefly describe the technique for taking the BMR.
18. A man, 40 years of age, weighing 160 pounds and measuring 5 feet 9 inches in height, consumed 3 liters of oxygen in 15 minutes. Calculate his BMR.
19. Briefly discuss the action of the hypothalamic thermostat.
20. Discuss the cause and treatment of fever.

Chapter 16

Nutrition

Many of the great triumphs in human welfare have been in the art and science of nutrition. We are what we eat, and time may well show that many, if not most, disorders of the body are in one way or another associated with our diet.

ENERGY REQUIREMENT

The daily needs of the body for energy depend upon its total activities. To see how this works, let us assume that in a 24-hour period a metabolically normal 154-pound man sleeps for 10 hours, saws wood for 2 hours, walks for 4 hours, sits for 6 hours, and stands for 2 hours. Consulting Table 16-1, we see that for these activities he expends about 3220 Cal. And to this we must add roughly 10 percent of the total, or 322 Cal., to cover the specific dynamic action (SDA) expenditure. Thus, his energy requirement for the 24-hour period is 3542 Cal.

Whether we gain, lose, or maintain our weight depends upon the balance between our energy output and our caloric intake. If we eat too little, the caloric deficit must come from the tissues, and weight is lost. If we eat too much, the food not burned is turned into fat, and weight is gained. The war of the waistline, then, is fought on the battlefield of metabolism, and in almost all cases victory depends chiefly upon one exercise—pushing oneself away from the table.

Energy, however, is only one phase of nutrition, for in addition to providing fuel to run the machinery of the body, food must also build and maintain healthy tissues. Thus, though both a glass of milk and a lollipop supply energy, the former is more nutritious than the latter. In the sections that follow are presented the basic facts relating to "food and the body."

PROTEIN REQUIREMENT

Each day about 30 gm. of protein are torn from the tissues and catabolized. Unless it is replaced, the body begins to lose its flesh! In the language of biochemistry, a negative *nitrogen balance* is said to exist; that is, more nitrogen is being excreted as urea and other nitrogenous waste products than is being ingested as protein. To ensure against this possibility, therefore, and to provide a sound metabolic environment, the daily protein intake should be in the vicinity of 75 gm., or roughly 15 percent of the daily caloric intake (1 gm. of protein yields 4 Cal.).

But this is not all. If the body is to re-

Table 16-1. Energy expenditure per hour during various types of activity for a man weighing 70 kg. (M. S. Rose)*

Form of activity	Calories†
Sleeping	65
Awake, lying still	77
Sitting at rest	100
Standing relaxed	105
Dressing and undressing	118
Tailoring	135
Typewriting rapidly	140
Light exercise	170
Walking slowly (2.6 mph)	200
Carpentry, metal working, and industrial painting	240
Active exercise	290
Severe exercise	450
Sawing wood	480
Swimming	500
Running (5.3 mph)	570
Very severe exercise	600
Walking very fast (5.3 mph)	650
Climbing stairs	1100

*From Guyton, A. C.: Functions of the human body, Philadelphia, 1959, W. B. Saunders Co.
†Large Calories, or kilocalories.

main healthy, we must pay as much attention to quality as to quantity. A protein, to be of real nutritional value, must supply all the *essential* amino acids (see accompanying formulas), that is, those which the body is unable to synthesize. Such proteins, referred to as biologically *complete* proteins, occur principally in meat. In contrast, the proteins of vegetables and grains are generally *incomplete;* that is, they lack one or more essential amino acids.

Kwashiorkor. One of the most important problems in areas where diets are substandard, namely, Africa, Asia, and parts of Latin America, is kwashiorkor, a fatal childhood disease caused by a shortage of high-quality protein. The cardinal signs of kwashiorkor include enlargement of the

Arginine*

```
           NH H   H   H   H   H
           ||  |   |   |   |   |
     H2N—C—N—C—C—C—C—COOH
                   |   |   |   |
                   H   H   H   NH2
```

Histidine*

```
        HC—N
        ||   \\
        ||    CH
        ||   /
        C—N—H
        |
     H—C—H
        |
     H—C—NH2
        |
       COOH
```

Isoleucine

```
      H   H   H       H
      |   |   |       |
   H—C—C—C———C—COOH
      |   |   |       |
      H   H   CH3     NH2
```

Leucine

```
      H
      |
   H—C
      | \    H   H   H
      H   \  |   |   |
            C—C—C—COOH
      H   /      |   |
      | /        H   NH2
   H—C
      |
      H
```

Lysine

```
      H       H   H   H   H
      |       |   |   |   |
   H—C———C—C—C—C—COOH
      |       |   |   |   |
      NH2     H   H   H   NH2
```

Methionine

```
              H   H   H
              |   |   |
   CH3—S—C—C—C—COOH
              |   |   |
              H   H   NH2
```

*Essential in young rats but not man.

Phenylalanine

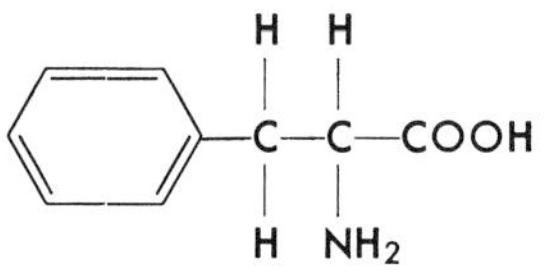

```
            H  H
            |  |
 (benzene)—C—C—COOH
            |  |
            H  NH2
```

Threonine

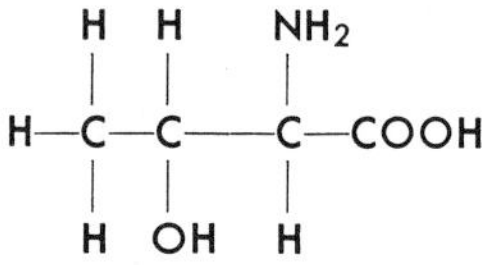

```
     H   H    NH2
     |   |    |
  H—C—C—————C—COOH
     |   |    |
     H   OH   H
```

Tryptophan

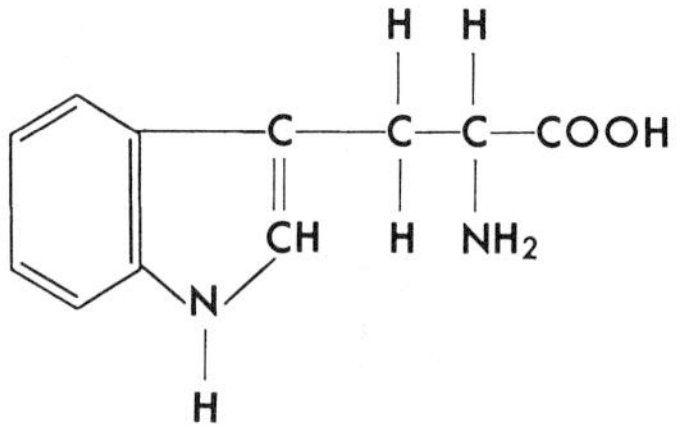

```
                  H  H
                  |  |
 (benzene)—C———C—C—COOH
            ||    |  |
            CH    H  NH2
       N
       |
       H
```

Valine

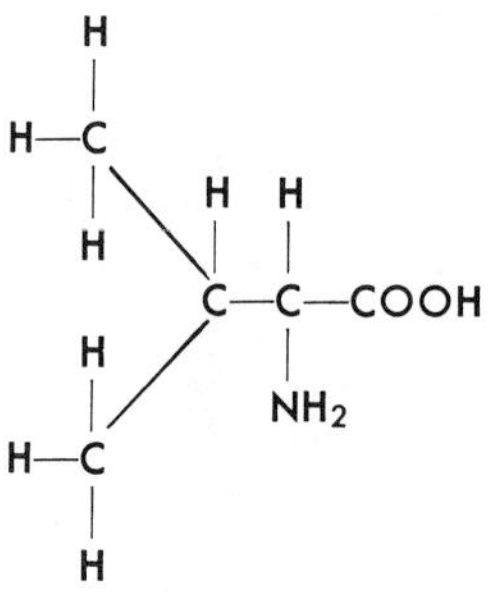

```
     H
     |
  H—C
     |\    H  H
     H \   |  |
         C—C—COOH
     H  /     |
     | /      NH2
  H—C
     |
     H
```

liver, changes in the pigmentation of skin and hair, restlessness, and lethargy.

FAT REQUIREMENT

About 40 percent of the daily calories of a typical American diet are usually in the form of fat. Although it was originally believed that "fat is fat," recent work has established the essential nature of certain *unsaturated* fats, namely, those that supply *linoleic, linolenic,* and *arachidonic* acids (p. 109). Animals raised on diets deficient in these unsaturated acids present a picture of general physical and mental deterioration. Fortunately, since such small amounts of these are needed, deficiency states do not appear likely. It is thought by some authorities that a reduction in fat so that it provides approximately 30 percent of the total daily calories would be desirable.

Cholesterol. Any discussion of fat would be incomplete without reference to a somewhat controversial fatty *alcohol* called cholesterol. For several years researchers have become increasingly aware of the association between cholesterol and cardiovascular disease. Rabbits and certain other animals fed cholesterol for an extended period of time develop arterial lesions somewhat resembling human atherosclerosis, and patients with atherosclerosis commonly possess high amounts of cholesterol in the blood. Cholesterol is a conspicuous constituent of all animal and plant tissues and is present in most foods. Egg yolk, for instance, is especially rich, one yolk containing about 0.25 gm. This explains why eggs are taboo on a diet designed to lower blood cholesterol.

Another interesting facet is the role played by certain oils and drugs in inhibiting the synthesis of cholesterol. Currently, these agents are being employed as an adjunct to the dietary management of atherosclerosis, hypertension, and similar disorders.

CARBOHYDRATE REQUIREMENT

As stated previously, the protein and fat in the diet together average about 55 percent of the total daily caloric intake, and carbohydrate contributes the remaining 45 percent. In planning meals, the dietitian distributes the daily calories more or less in this fashion. To supply 2000 Cal., for example, 0.15×2000, or 300 Cal., is allotted to protein; 0.40×2000, or 800 Cal., to fat; and the remainder, or 900 Cal., to carbohydrate. In terms of weight this turns out to be $300 \div 4.0$, or 75 gm. of protein; $800 \div 9.0$, or 89 gm. of fat; and $900 \div 4.0$, or 225 gm. of carbohydrate.

VITAMINS

In 1906 Hopkins proved the existence in normal foods of certain accessory factors essential to the diet, and 5 years later, in 1911, Funk, believing these factors to be chemical amines, coined the term *vitamine*. When further work disclosed that the amino group was not characteristic, Drummund saved the day by proposing that the *e* be dropped, giving us our present word *vitamin*.

Vitamins sustain life, promote growth, and maintain health. It is hardly an exaggeration to say that the discovery of the vitamin and the various *avitaminoses* represents the highest achievement in nutrition. Although the *precise* mechanisms by which most vitamins perform their miracles are still not completely understood, the biochemist has apparently succeeded in unraveling the essential facts.

All the known vitamins have been isolated in the pure state and synthesized in the laboratory. Generally, they are categorized according to their solubility in *water* or *fat*. The water-soluble vitamins include vitamin C and the members of the B complex group, and the fat-soluble vitamins include vitamins A, D, K, and E (Table 16-2).

Table 16-2. Recommended daily vitamin requirements

Vitamin	Requirement: Children	Adults
A	50 units/lb. of body weight	5000 units
D	400 units	400 units
K	Not known	Not known
E	Not known	Not known
C	30-80 mg.*	70 mg.
Thiamine	Infants 0.5 mg. Children 1.5 mg.	1.5 mg.
Riboflavin	1-2.0 mg.*	1.8 mg.
Nicotinic acid	8-25 mg.*	20 mg.
Pantothenic acid	Not known	Not known
Pyridoxine	Not known	1.5 mg.
B_{12}	2.0 μg (?)	4.0 μg (?)
Folic acid	0.5 μg (?)	0.2 mg.

*Amount depends on age.

Vitamin A. Vitamin A and its precursors (*alpha* and *beta carotenes*) occur most abundantly in liver, egg yolk, dairy products, and green and yellow vegetables. Deficiences result not only from an inadequate intake of the vitamin but also from poor absorption in such conditions as diarrhea and lack of bile.

Vitamin A is needed for the proper development of the epithelium, bones, and eyes (Chapter 20), and the chief signs of deficiency relate to these structures. One of the first signs of vitamin A deficiency is *nyctalopia*, or night blindness. More severe manifestations include keratomalacia, ulceration of the cornea, dental defects, and retarded bone growth.

Vitamin D. The designation *vitamin D* is given to several fat-soluble sterols (p. 299) possessing antirachitic properties, the most important being vitamin D_2 (calciferol) and vitamin D_3. The former results from the action of ultraviolet rays on *ergosterol*, a vegetable sterol, and the latter from the action of ultraviolet rays on *7-dehydrocholesterol*, a constituent of the skin (hence, the expression *sunshine vitamin*). Provided that there is adequate sunlight, a considerable part of the daily requirement can be met by a trip to the beach. The principal sources are fish liver oils, fats, eggs, and dairy products.

Vitamin D stimulates the absorption of calcium and phosphate from the gastrointestinal tract and thereby promotes the formation of bone and teeth. A deficiency leads to rickets in children (Fig. 16-1) and softening of the bones (osteomalacia) in adults. Unlike most vitamins, the daily requirement (Table 16-2) bears little relationship to age.

Vitamin E. The name *vitamin E* is applied to three closely related substances

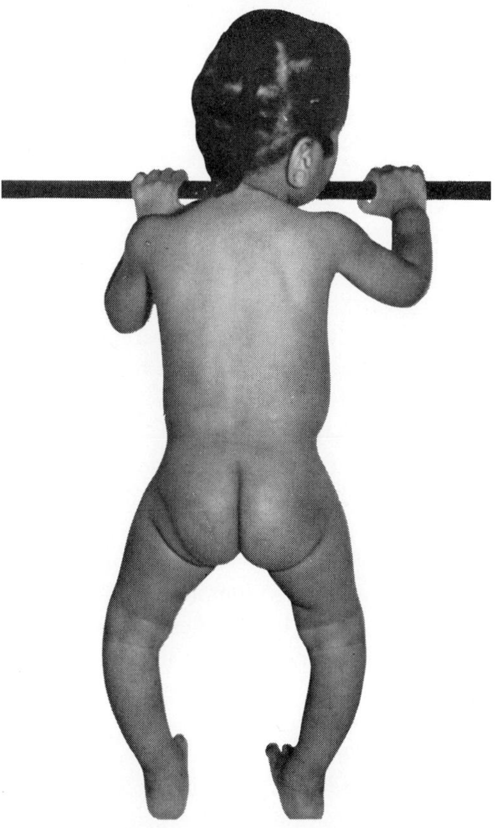

Fig. 16-1. Rickets in a young child. (Courtesy Rosa L. Nemire, M.D., The Upjohn Co.)

called *tocopherols*—alpha, beta, and gamma—the former being the most abundant and the most potent. Alll three are soluble in oil and are readily absorbed from the digestive tract. Vitamin E occurs in wheat-germ oil, fresh vegetables, fruits, liver, and muscle.

Deficiency phenomena differ considerably in various species. It has been demonstrated without question that vitamin E is essential to the fertility of both male and female rats and mice, but in larger animals and in man this has yet to be proved. Also of significance is the fact that vitamin E deficiency in rats, guinea pigs, and rabbits results in muscular dystrophy and lesions of the spinal cord. The administration of vitamin E in human beings with similar dysfunctions, however, has yielded equivocal results. The precise role of this vitamin in human nutrition remains to be found. Essentially, then, vitamin E enjoys about the same status as biotin, choline, and inositol.

Vitamin K. The name *vitamin K* is applied to a variety of derivatives of naphthoquinone (p. 109) that aid in the formation of *prothrombin* (p. 256). Because these substances are plentifully supplied in food and synthesized by bacteria in the colon, deficiencies (evidenced by delayed clotting and hemorrhage) are seldom of dietary origin. Most deficiencies are caused by antibiotics (which kill off the intestinal bacteria) and poor absorption resulting from obstructive jaundice or diarrhea. The absence of bile in obstructive jaundice prevents the absorption of fat and fat-soluble vitamin K.

In medicine, vitamin K preparations are used in the prevention and treatment of bleeding due to lack of prothrombin, and as antidotes against an overdosage of Dicumarol and other oral anticoagulants.

Vitamin C. Vitamin C, or *ascorbic acid,* is found in citrus fruits, berries, and certain vegetables. Among its many biochemical roles, it is first and foremost essential to the formation of connective tissue. The classic deficiency syndrome, scurvy, is marked by degenerative changes in the bones, cartilage, dentin, and blood vessels. Because of the weakened capillary walls, hemorrhages occur in the skin, mucous membranes, bones, joints, gingiva, and muscles. Also (and this is most significant), there is slow healing of wounds, decreased resistance to infection, and tendency toward anemia. For these very good reasons, it is almost routine today to give large doses of vitamin C to surgical patients.

Vitamin P. The expression *vitamin P* is applied to a variety of complex compounds that characteristically occur along with vitamin C (for example, hesperidin, citrin, rutin, and esculin). Although the vitamin has not been proved essential to human beings, there is clinical evidence that it does increase capillary strength and reduce

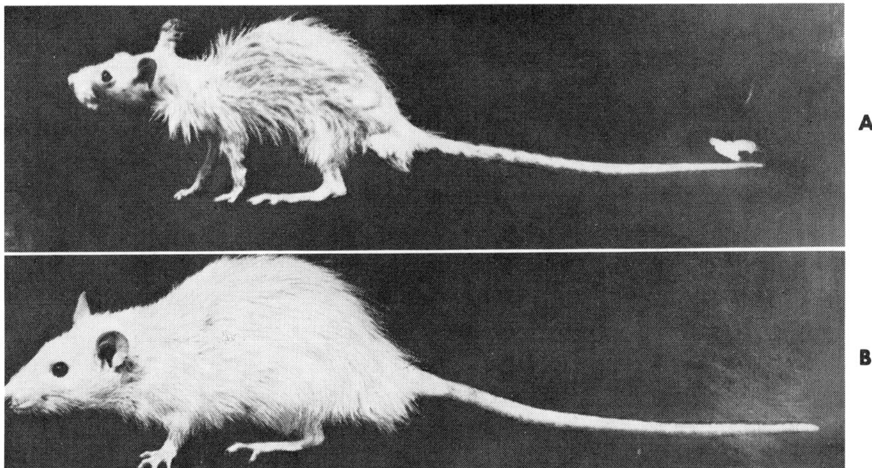

Fig. 16-2. A, White rat with ariboflavinosis. **B,** Same rat 6 weeks later after being placed on diet rich in riboflavin. (United States Department of Agriculture photograph.)

bleeding tendencies. Most especially, vitamin P inhibits the destructive effects of radiation on the capillaries.

Thiamine. Thiamine, or vitamin B_1, occurs in enriched bread, nuts, pork, whole grains, legumes, and liver. Since it functions as a coenzyme in bio-oxidation, a deficiency leads to a general metabolic disturbance.

The major deficiency signs include *polyneuritis* and *enlargement* of the heart. When these derangements occur at the same time, the syndrome is referred to as beriberi. It is wrong to assume, however, that a thiamine avitaminosis and beriberi are synonymous, because lesser deficiencies lead to a variety of vague and "unimportant" symptoms. Indeed, the deficiencies that the physician sees—*and this applies to all the vitamins*—are usually not the picture painted by the high school biology text. Moreover, it is not common to come across a patient with a single avitaminosis, for a poor diet—the usual etiology—leads to a multiple deficiency.

Riboflavin. Also known as vitamin B_2, riboflavin is present in milk, liver, yeast, kidneys, eggs, nuts, seafoods, meats, cheese, and green leafy vegetables. Like thiamine, riboflavin also serves as a coenzyme in oxidative metabolism. The chief deficiency signs include a purplish red tongue (glossitis), redding of the lips, fissuring of the angles of the mouth (cheilosis), and cornification of the skin. The repercussions of riboflavin deficiency in the rat are dramatically evidenced in Fig. 16-2.

Niacin. Niacin (nicotinic acid) or its amide (nicotinamide) is a B complex vitamin abundantly present in rice, bran, liver, yeast, meat, peanuts, and fish. It functions as part of the coenzyme NAD, and a deficiency results in metabolic chaos. The major clinical signs and symptoms are referable to the skin, gastrointestinal tract, and nervous system. *Pellagra,* the classic syndrome, characterized by muscular weakness, discoloration of the skin, and mental derangement, is actually a multiple deficiency involving thiamine and riboflavin as well as niacin.

Vitamin B_{12} and folic acid. Two members of the B complex group, vitamin B_{12} and folic acid, are required for the formation of new protoplasm. This is borne out by the fact that areas of rapid turnover, such as bone marrow, are the first to reflect a deficiency. Lack of vitamin B_{12}, usually the result of inadequate *intrinsic factor*, leads to *pernicious* anemia (p. 252). Lack of folic acid leads to the so-called *megaloblastic* anemias of infancy and pregnancy (p. 251). In addition, there is general retardation in growth and body development, especially in children.

Vitamin B_{12} occurs principally in liver, muscle tissue, milk, and cheese; folic acid occurs principally in green leafy vegetables, yeast, soybeans, and wheat.

Pyridoxine. Pyridoxine, which acts as a coenzyme in the metabolism of amino acids, is present in egg yolk, nuts, whole grains, legumes, kidneys, muscle, liver, and fish. Though the importance of this B complex vitamin in animals has been known for some time, its essential role in human nutrition was not appreciated until an unfortunate but nevertheless excusable and instructive incident occurred a few years ago. This related to widely scattered reports of a nervous syndrome (increased excitability, convulsions, and the like) of unknown origin among infants receiving a commercial milk substitute. An investigation soon demonstrated that the condition resulted from the absence of pyridoxine in the formula. Other deficiency disorders arising from this avitaminosis are seborrheic dermatitis, impaired growth in infants, and vomiting in pregnancy.

Pantothenic acid. Pantothenic acid is a B complex vitamin used by the body in the synthesis of coenzyme A, a cellular agent vital to normal metabolism. Since the vitamin is present in such a wide variety of foods, a deficiency in man has not as yet been described except in experimental situations. In animals the artificially created avitaminosis results in retarded growth, gray hair, dermatitis, and liver damage.

Biotin, choline, and inositol. The three vitamins known as biotin, choline, and inositol, all members of the B complex group, are essential to both man and animals. Both biotin and choline play essential roles in the metabolism of fats. A deficiency of biotin is characterized by a dry, scaly dermatitis, and a deficiency of choline is considered to be a contributing factor in the development of cirrhosis of the liver. Inositol also plays a role in fat metabolism (serving as a *lipotropic* factor) and, additionally, is thought to be necessary for maintaining gastrointestinal motility.

MINERALS

Life without mineral matter is just as impossible as life without water. Indeed, just a "pinch" either way often spells the difference between health and disease. In a biologic and nutritional sense, minerals refer to the inorganic components of food that supply the essential anions and cations. In the present section a few words will be said about those elements not discussed elsewhere.

Iron. Approximately 70 percent of the total body iron resides in the hemoglobin; the bulk of the remainder is stored in the liver as *ferritin* and in muscle as *myoglobulin.* The recommended daily allowance is 10 to 12 mg. Quite understandably, a deficiency of dietary iron leads to lack of hemoglobin and thus to anemia. Iron-deficiency anemia responds dramatically to such iron salts as ferrous sulfate and ferrous fumarate.

Iodine. It seems fantastic, but the thyroid gland requires only about 0.25 mg. of iodine daily to manufacture sufficient thyroxine for normal metabolism. An iodine deficiency leads to endemic goiter (Chapter 22), a classic condition that use to be common in the Great Lakes region, Alps, Pyrenees and other such areas where there is lack of the element in the soil. Through the use of iodized salt (salt containing a pinch of sodium or potassium iodide), these so-called goiter belts have become a thing of the past.

Fluorine and chlorine. In the form of their anions the halogens fluorine and chlorine are essential mineral nutrients. Fluorine protects against tooth decay (p. 289) and chlorine (generally along with sodium) is associated with countless biochemical mechanisms. The fluoride content is frequently low in foods and water, but this can be easily remedied by fluoridation (p. 289).

Copper and cobalt. Copper and cobalt are referred to as trace metals; that is, the daily requirements, although unknown, are infinitesimally small. Under normal conditions, therefore, it is almost impossible to develop a deficiency.

Both metals play a role in blood building. Copper catalyzes the synthesis of hemoglobin, and cobalt, as the key element in vitamin B_{12}, stimulates maturation of red blood cells.

Zinc. Zinc is also a trace mineral and, like copper and cobalt, does not present a deficiency problem. It constitutes part of the enzyme carbonic acid anhydrase (p. 271) and plays a role in the storage and release of insulin.

Manganese. Manganese is a trace metal essential for proper growth of animals, and we can assume that it is likewise essential for human growth. It is present in all animal tissues as a part of the prosthetic group of many enzymes.

Questions

1. Distinguish between the terms *small* calorie and *large* Calorie.
2. Discuss obesity relative to cause, pathologic implications, and treatment.
3. What is meant by specific dynamic action?
4. Discuss the expression nitrogen balance.
5. Discuss the daily protein requirements.
6. What are "biologically complete" proteins?
7. What is kwashiorkor?
8. Discuss the daily fat requirement.
9. Discuss cholesterol relative to its association with cardiovascular disease.
10. Since both proteins and fats supply energy, why is it necessary to eat carbohydrates?
11. On the average, how is a 3000 Cal. diet apportioned on a basis of grams?
12. Why was the *e* on the word *vitamine* dropped?
13. What is the relationship between vitamins and enzymes?
14. What are tocopherols?
15. What is the biochemical role of pantothenic acid?
16. Explain how lack of bile could lead to vitamin A deficiency.
17. Explain how certain antibiotics might bring about a vitamin K deficiency.
18. It is common practice to administer vitamin K to the mother just prior to delivery. Why?
19. Explain how liver damage might interfere with clotting.
20. Discuss the physiologic role of vitamin C.
21. What is the biochemical role of thiamine?
22. What is ariboflavinosis?
23. What is the difference between niacin and niacinamide?
24. Distinguish between the roles of vitamin B_{12} and folic acid in hemopoiesis.
25. Discuss the importance of minerals in the diet.

Chapter 17

The urinary system

The kidney (Fig. 17-1) is the prime guardian of homeostasis, for by excreting unwanted materials—and retaining others—it rids the internal environment of wastes and at the same time maintains acid-base balance and fluid and electrolyte balance (Chapter 18).

KIDNEYS

The kidneys are bean-shaped organs embedded in the posterior abdominal wall, one on either side of the vertebral column. Since they are located behind the peritoneum, they are said to be *retroperitoneally* situated. Technically, therefore, they lie outside the peritoneal cavity. Each kidney is about 4 inches long, 2½ inches wide, and 1½ inches thick and weighs somewhere between ¼ and ½ pound. Characteristically, the organ is covered with a smooth and tough fibrous membrane. Through the hilum on the medial aspect pass the ureter, blood vessels, nerves, and lymphatics.

When cut longitudinally, the kidney is seen to be composed of two regions—an outer *cortex* and an inner *medulla* (Fig. 17-2). It will be seen also that the ureter dilates into the *pelvis* and that the latter branches into a number of cup-shaped structures called *calyces*. As shown in the illustration, leading into the calyces are the apices, or papillae, of triangular structures called *pyramids*. Each pyramid is actually a bundle of collecting tubules that open at the papilla and serve to carry urine into the calyx.

Nephron. The nephron is the *unit* of the kidney. There are approximately one million nephrons in each organ. The basic anatomy of the unit is shown in somewhat idealized form in Fig. 17-3. Its chief fea-

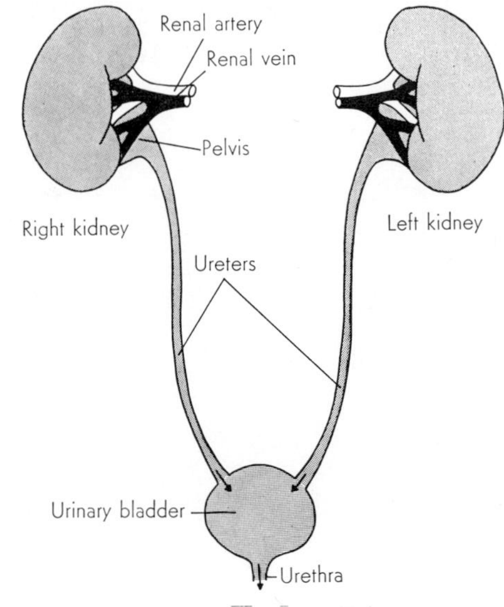

Fig. 17-1. Urinary system.

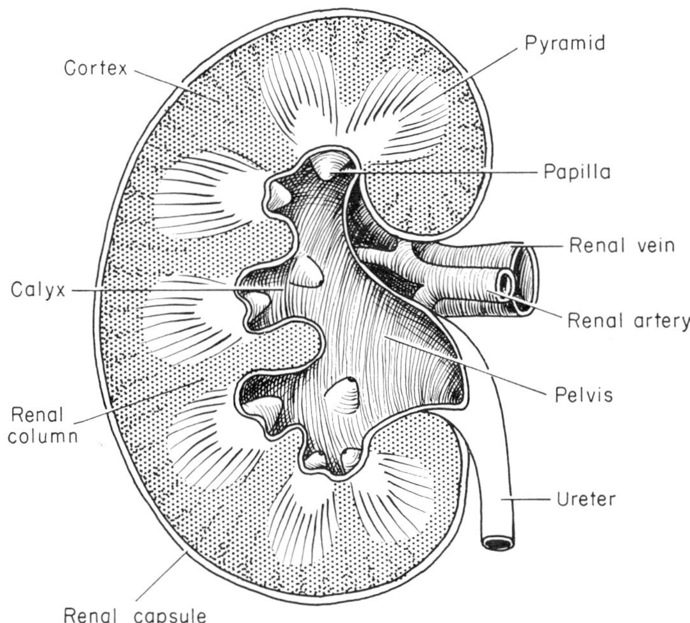

Fig. 17-2. The kidney. (Modified from Anthony, C. P.: Anatomy and physiology, ed. 7, St. Louis, 1967, The C. V. Mosby Co.)

tures are the *renal corpuscle* (or malpighian body) and the *renal tubule.* The corpuscle is composed of a tuft of capillaries, called the *glomerulus,* enclosed within a double-walled membrane called *Bowman's capsule.* The latter is actually the dilated and invaginated blind end of the proximal convoluted tubule; the distal convoluted tubule enters a *collecting* duct.

In order to understand renal function, it is especially important to understand the blood supply: Once the renal artery enters the kidney, it branches into the interlobar arteries and the latter branch into the arcuate arteries, interlobular arteries, and afferent arterioles, in that order. The *afferent* arterioles lead the blood *into* the glomeruli; the *efferent* arterioles lead the blood *out of* the glomeruli and then go on to form the capillary networks that surround the tubules. After working its way through these networks, the blood then returns to the general circulation via the interlobular vein, the arcuate vein, the interlobar vein, and the renal vein, in that order.

Formation of urine. The formation of urine by the nephron entails three basic processes: *filtration, reabsorption,* and *secretion.* In the normal function of the human kidney, however, secretion (that is, tubular secretion) is of little importance. We shall now discuss each mechanism in some detail.

Glomerular filtration. The disparity in size between the diameters of the glomerular arterioles, the *efferent being the smaller,* produces a very high pressure within the glomerular capillaries (somewhere in the vicinity of 57 mm. Hg), which forces fluid out of the glomerulus—a fluid that eventually becomes urine. Counterpressures, that is, the osmotic pressure of the blood (28 mm. Hg) and the pressure in Bowman's capsule (10 mm. Hg), however, tend to keep fluid in the glomerulus. The overall effect, therefore, is that fluid from the glomerulus is squeezed out by the so-called *filtration pressure,* or the *difference* between the glomerular blood pressure on the one hand and the osmotic and capsular

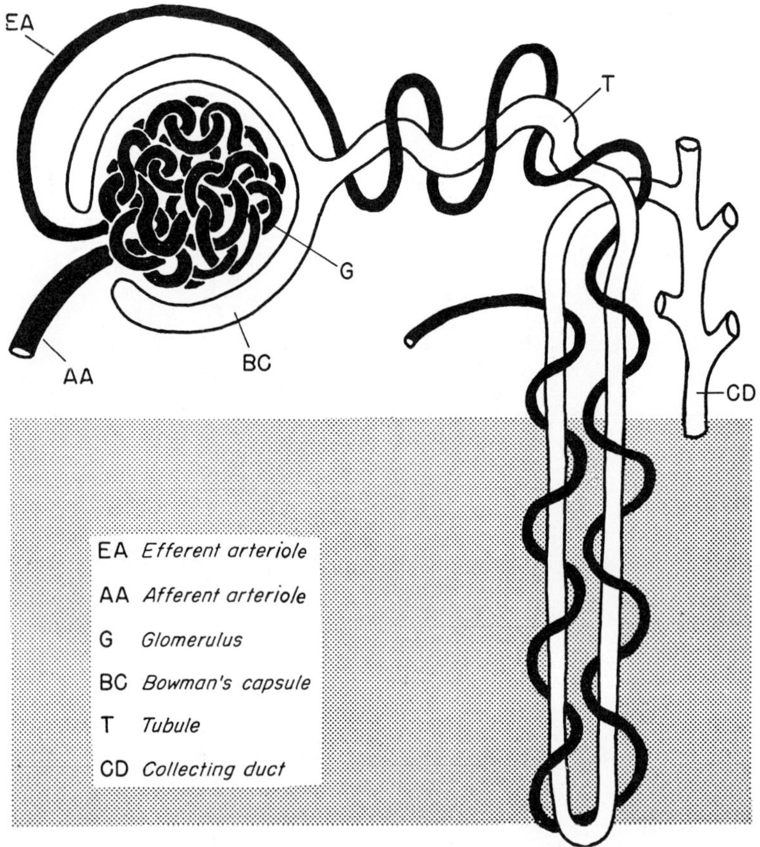

Fig. 17-3. The nephron. The U-shaped turn of the tubule is called the *loop of Henle.* (From Brooks, S. M.: Basic facts of body water and ions, ed. 2, New York, 1968, Springer Publishing Co., Inc.)

pressures on the other. Taking the figures just cited, the filtration pressure is 57 − (28 + 10), or 19 mm. Hg.

Obviously, a significant drop in glomerular blood pressure will severely curb the output of glomerular filtrate—and urine. Constriction of the afferent arterioles (via sympathetic nerves), for instance, drastically lowers the pressure by impeding the blood flow into the glomerulus. Conversely, afferent arteriolar dilatation enhances the flow of blood, thereby elevating the pressure and stepping up the output of glomerular filtrate and urine. The systemic arterial pressure, too, plays a key role, for when it rises, the increased quantity of blood flowing into the glomeruli increases the pressure and thereby the output of urine. Conversely, a drop in systemic pressure decreases the output of urine. In short, blood pressure plays a key role in the output of urine.

The glomerular filtrate that passes into Bowman's capsule is essentially a cell-free, protein-free, aqueous solution of the constituents present in the plasma. The filtrate is formed at a rate of about 125 ml. per minute, and during a 24-hour period this amounts to a volume close to 200 quarts! Obviously, most of this fantastic volume must be returned to the blood, and herein lies the role of the tubules. As the filtrate moves along, practically all the water and most of the dissolved substances are reabsorbed, thereby reducing the 200 quarts to about 1½ quarts of urine.

Passive reabsorption. By passive reabsorption is meant the diffusion of molecules through the pores in the tubular epithelium, thence through the capillary walls and into the blood. Certain substances vital to the blood such as water and electrolytes diffuse with relative ease, whereas some substances, mainly those that need to be eliminated (for example, urea, uric acid, creatinine, phosphates, and sulfates), diffuse with difficulty. Essentially, then, the tubular walls pick out the good things for the blood and leave the bad things for the urine.

Active reabsorption. Passive reabsorption, however, falls far short of an adequate renal performance, which means that electrolytes, glucose, amino acids, and protein must also be taken back into the blood via active reabsorption. Nutrients are actively reabsorbed principally in the proximal convoluted tubule, whereas water and electrolytes are actively reabsorbed principally in the distal convoluted tubule.

In contrast to passive reabsorption, or diffusion, active reabsorption removes materials *from a lesser* concentration to a greater concentration. That is, whereas diffusion stops when the molecules have become equally distributed on either side of the tubular epithelium, active reabsorption continues to pump vital constituents out of the glomerular filtrate long after the concentration in the tubule has fallen below that in the interstitial fluid. This, of course, requires work and energy and explains why the tubular wall is a metabolic powerhouse.

One theory as to the mechanism of active reabsorption holds that the substance to be reabsorbed combines at the epithelial surface with a so-called *carrier.* The resulting complex then diffuses through the tubular wall to the other side, where it releases the reabsorbed substance to the interstitial fluid, leaving the carrier free to form a new complex.

Tubular secretion. Interestingly, the tubular epithelium actively secretes certain substances into the glomerular filtrate. Creatinine and potassium, for example, are partially excreted in this fashion. Also, a number of drugs (penicillin, for instance) are secreted rather than filtered.

Acid-base balance. Considering the fact that a drop in pH below 6 or a rise above 8 can mean sudden death, the topic of acid-base balance is of no little interest. Stripped to the essentials, it concerns the *hydrogen ion*—that is, to get rid of it (to prevent *acidosis*) or to retain it (to prevent *alkalosis*). The body does this via three mechanisms working in concert: respiratory regulation (p. 276), chemical buffers (Chapter 18), and renal regulation.

The kidneys regulate acid-base balance by three avenues: hydrogen ion secretion, ammonia formation, and bicarbonate ion excretion. Hydrogen ion secretion is effected principally in the distal tubules, where the free ions (secreted by the tubular epithelium) react with disodium phosphate (Na_2HPO_4), in the glomerular filtrate, to form monosodium phosphate (NaH_2PO_4) and sodium, the latter being reabsorbed into the tubular epithelium. Thus, this mechanism in effect entails the exchange of a hydrogen ion for a sodium ion.

But in the event that the aforementioned mechanism is overtaxed, the tubular cells come to the rescue by the synthesis of ammonia (NH_3)—chiefly from glutamine—which thereupon combines with hydrogen ions to form ammonium ions (NH_4^+), the latter being excreted in the urine as ammonium salts.

These mechanisms effect removal of hydrogen ions and operate to prevent a decrease in pH, the most usual tendency since metabolic wastes are, in the main, acids (namely, phosphoric, sulfuric, uric, carbonic, and keto acids). However, alkalosis is always a possibility, particularly as a result of taking alkaline drugs; in this case hydrogen ions are *retained* by the tubules and bicarbonate ions (basic ions) are *excreted*. More will be said about these acid-base mechanisms in Chapter 18.

Extrarenal control. The kidney is subject to outside influence. *Aldosterone,* a hormone secreted by the adrenal cortex (Chapter 22), causes the tubules to *increase* their uptake of *sodium* and their rejection of *potassium,* and the *antidiuretic hormone* secreted by the posterior pituitary gland (Chapter 22) stimulates the reabsorption of *water.* Also, drugs called *diuretics* cause the kidney to drastically step up its production of urine by inhibiting the reabsorption of sodium and, with it, water.* These drugs are lifesaving in severe edema.

Renal clearance. The ability of the kidney to clear the blood and the intercellular fluid of unwanted substances is referred to as renal clearance. Knowing the renal clearance, therefore, is of great diagnostic significance in dealing with diseases of the kidney. One simple and widely used technique for ascertaining renal clearance is the *PSP test,* which is performed by injecting a dye called phenolsulfonphthalein into a vein and clocking the time that it takes for the dye to appear in the urine. A normal kidney clears most of the dye in an hour's time and all of it within 2 hours. If it takes significantly longer for the dye to be cleared from the blood, one or both kidneys are probably damaged. In this event other more definitive tests are employed to determine whether the impairment is glomerular or tubular.

URETERS

The ureters are cylindrical fibromuscular tubules that convey urine from the renal pelvis to the bladder (Fig. 17-1). They average about 11 inches in length and ⅕ inch in diameter. Each is composed of three coats—inner mucous, middle muscular, and outer fibrous coats. Commencing at the kidney, peristaltic waves force the urine along into the bladder, where it is held until voided.

*The sodium ion has an affinity for water.

BLADDER

The urinary bladder is a tough, muscular storage sac located in the pelvic cavity, immediately before the vagina in the female and immediately before the rectum in the male. Though held in place by folds of peritoneum and fascia, it is subject to considerable movement.

The bladder wall is composed of four coats. Beginning with the inside, these include the mucous, submucous, muscular, and serous coats. The muscular coat has three layers—the inner longitudinal, middle circular, and outer longitudinal layers. The mucous lining consists of transitional epithelium that is thrown into folds, or rugae, when the bladder is empty.

The bladder has three openings at the neck—two through which the ureters deliver urine and one through which urine enters the urethra. The ureters open into the posterior angles of a triangular depression called the *trigone,* and the urethral opening is at the anterior and lower angle.

As indicated, the bladder serves as a reservoir for urine. Its capacity varies widely, but in most cases the adult bladder can accommodate a volume of about 1 liter. The urge to urinate, however, is experienced long before this volume is attained, usually when the bladder contains somewhere around 400 ml. of urine.

URETHRA

The female urethra is a membranous tube about 1½ inches in length that extends from the bladder to the urinary meatus, or external orifice, situated between the clitoris and the vaginal opening (Chapter 23). Its walls are composed of three coats—an inner mucous coat, a middle spongy coat containing a plexus of veins, and an outer muscular coat.

The male urethra is about 8 inches long and is divided into three parts: the *prostatic,* which runs through the prostate gland; the *membranous,* which pierces the body wall; and the *cavernous,* which extends the length of the penis (Chapter 23). The urethral wall has two coats—an inner mucous lining and an outer coat composed of connective tissue; the latter serves as a means of attachment to the structures through which the urethra passes.

Table 17-1. Average values for normal urine (24-hour sample)*

Volume: 1200 ml.	
Color: pale yellow	
Transparency: clear	
Odor: characteristic	
Acidity: pH 6 (4.7-8.0)	
Specific gravity: 1.020	
Total solids	60 gm.
Ammonia	0.7 gm.
Calcium	0.2 gm.
Chlorides, as NaCl	12 gm.
Creatine	0.03 gm.
Creatinine	1.4 gm.
Magnesium	0.1 gm.
Potassium	2 gm.
Sodium	4 gm.
Urea	30 gm.
Other	9.6 gm.

*From Brooks, S. M.: Basic facts of body water and ions, ed. 2, New York, 1968, Springer Publishing Co., Inc.

MICTURITION

As just stated, the urge to urinate, or micturate, comes when the volume of urine in the bladder reaches about 400 ml., at which volume the intrabladder pressure becomes of sufficient intensity to excite the stretch receptors in the bladder wall and send sensory stimuli on their way to the spinal cord. The parasympathetic nerves supplying the musculature are now triggered and the bladder wall starts to contract. Simultaneously, the *internal* sphincter guarding the opening between the bladder and the urethra is opened. However, if it is not convenient to urinate, the *external* sphincter around the urethra is voluntarily closed and held closed until such time as it is convenient, and then it is *relaxed.* Micturition, then, is both voluntary and involuntary.

The reason that infants have micturition problems is that it takes a while to develop control over the external sphincter. Adults with spinal injuries lose control of the act because the message from the brain to the external sphincter is not able to get through.

URINE

Freshly voided normal urine is a clear pale yellow and has a faint, somewhat aromatic odor. Upon standing, it becomes cloudy and develops an *ammoniacal* odor as a result of the conversion of urea into ammonia. The pH varies from about 4.6 to 8, and the specific gravity ranges from 1.003 to 1.030. In a 24-hour period the total volume of urine expelled from the body averages around 1200 ml., with a range anywhere from 600 to 2500 ml.

Urine is a dilute aqueous solution containing about 60 gm. of solids in a 24-hour sample. Approximately one half of the amount is *urea,* the chief waste product, and the remainder creatinine, sodium chloride, and an assortment of other organic and inorganic constituents (Table 17-1). The characteristic color of urine is due to *urochrome,* a pigment derived from bile.

Abnormal constituents. Among the abnormal urine constituents of diagnostic importance are blood (hematuria), glucose (glycosuria or glucosuria), albumin (albuminuria), pus (pyuria), and casts. In brief, hematuria indicates bleeding somewhere along the urinary tract, glycosuria generally points to diabetes mellitus, albuminuria is a feature of nephrosis, and pus indicates infection. Urine *normally* contains a *trace* of glucose and, interestingly, its complete absence indicates the presence of bacteria (*bacteriuria*). This is because bacteria metabolize and use up glucose. Special tests have been devised for the detection of trace glucose and these are now being used in the diagnosis of urinary tract infections. The physical attributes of urine are also helpful in diagnosis since a great many pathologic conditions cause a change in the color, volume, and specific gravity of urine (Fig. 17-4). In diabetes insipidus, for instance, the volume increases and the specific gravity decreases.

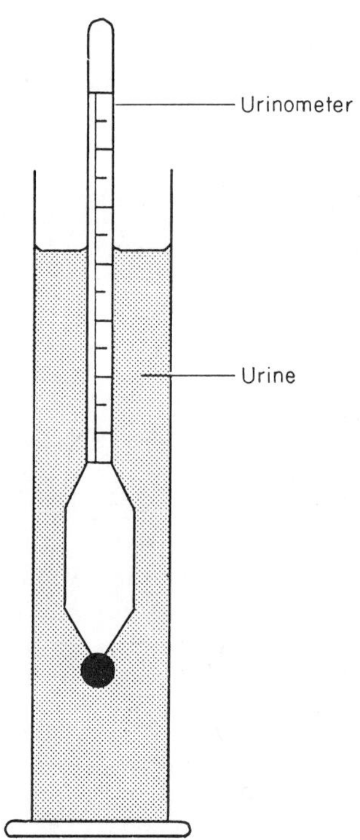

Fig. 17-4. Taking the specific gravity of urine.

URINARY DISEASES

The urinary system is subject to a wide variety of degenerative changes and infections, the kidney being especially prone to damage. Very roughly, disease of the kidney may be categorized as nephritis or nephrosis. By *nephritis* is meant an inflammation of the kidney marked by diffuse and progressive lesions. In glomerulonephritis, for example, the damage spreads through the glomeruli.

Though the expression *nephrosis* can be and is applied to any disease of the kidney, it is usually reserved for renal derangements characterized by lesions of the glomeruli and tubules, particularly the latter. In the so-called *nephrotic syndrome* these lesions lead to edema and albuminuria, classic signs of renal insufficiency. A rather special type of kidney disorder is *nephrolithiasis,* or stones in the kidney. These abnormal concretions, technically referred to as *calculi,* are composed of mineral salts that have precipitated from the urine. In most instances they are easily removed by surgical means.

Acute kidney failure. Acute kidney failure, also referred to as acute renal insufficiency, is an ominous condition marked by a drastic cut in the output of urine

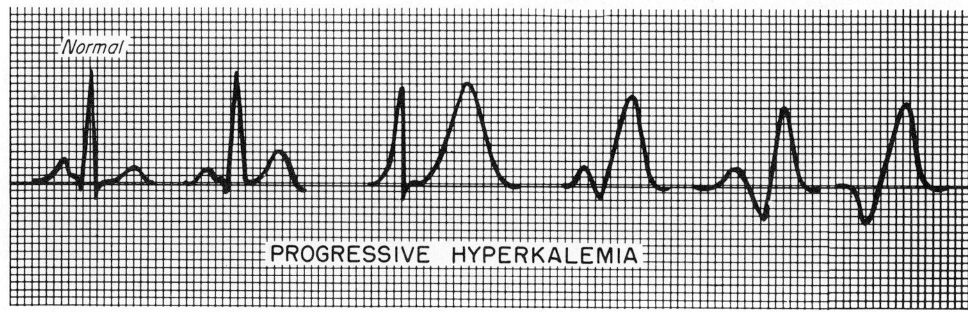

Fig. 17-5. Effect of hyperkalemia upon the electrocardiogram.

(*oliguria*); and sometimes no urine is formed at all (*anuria*). The underlying cause is now generally believed to be severe tubular nephrosis, which follows in the wake of nephrotoxic poisons (for example, carbon tetrachloride and mercury salts), burns, shock, trauma, and transfusion reactions. In poisoning, for example, the damaged tubular epithelium becomes nonfunctional and permits the glomerular filtrate to seep right back into the circulation (hence, the oliguria).

The anuric patient is in delicate balance between life and death. The cause of death is due to the accumulation of waste products (uremic poisoning), aided and abetted by excess fluid and acidosis. Laboratory and clinical data show that *potassium* intoxication is one of the major hazards (Fig. 17-5).

Dialysis. In severe but reversible kidney failure the artificial kidney may save the patient's life. This device operates on the principle of dialysis (p. 84) and essentially employs the setup shown in Fig. 17-6. It is placed in operation by allowing the patient's blood to pass through the long, narrow cellophane tube shown wound about the rotating horizontal cylinder. As the blood courses through, the cells and protein remain within while the waste products diffuse into the bath. Since the bath contains glucose and the essential electrolytes at the same concentration as in normal blood, only the *wastes* are removed. The figures shown in Table 17-2 are those of an actual case of renal shutdown in which the artificial kidney was used.

Another therapeutic approach in renal failure is *peritoneal dialysis.* In this tech-

Table 17-2. Results of dialysis in a patient with renal failure*†

Blood constituent	Initial	Final
K (mEq./L.)	7.3	5.1
Na (mEq./L.)	108	130
Cl (mEq./L.)	76	106
Ca (mEq./L.)	3.7	5.1
NPN (mg.%)‡	162	106
BUN (mg.%)‡	72	48

*After Merrill; from Brooks, S. M.: Basic facts of body water and ions, ed. 2, New York, 1968, Springer Publishing Co., Inc.
†Results obtained after 6 hours of dialysis in a 35-year-old patient with renal insufficiency.
‡NPN, Nonprotein nitrogen; BUN, blood urea nitrogen.

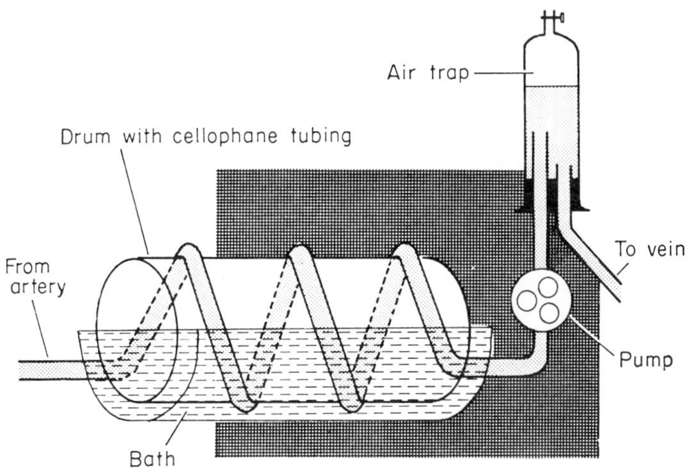

Fig. 17-6. Basic features of the artificial kidney. As the blood flows through the tubing, waste products diffuse into the bath. (Modified from Maclean, J. T.: Acute renal failure, Springfield, Ill., 1952, Charles C Thomas, Publisher.)

nique the peritoneum serves as the dialyzing membrane; that is, when solutions of the proper composition are introduced into the abdominal cavity (via closed-drainage paracentesis), diffusable wastes, electrolytes, poisons, and the like pass from the blood into the solution. The "spent" solution is thereupon withdrawn and replaced with a fresh solution.

Kidney transplantation. One of the great achievements of modern surgery has been kidney transplantation. Thousands of successful transplants have already been carried out both here and abroad. For the future, however, most authorities predict an artificial device small enough to be placed within the body.

Renal hypertension. Just about any damage or injury to the kidneys can cause hypertension. As to why this happens, the best explanation centers on the poor elimination of water and salt which, in turn, elevates the blood volume—and thereby the blood pressure. Formerly, the culprit was considered to be a substance secreted by the ischemic kidney called *renin.* The latter converts an alpha globulin (of the plasma) into angiotensin I which, in turn, is converted by some other plasma factor into angiotensin II, a potent *vasoconstrictor.* However, renin is present for only a day or two following the onset of ischemia and therefore could not account for hypertension of long standing.

Infection. Infections of the urinary tract are common and often highly resistant to treatment; the more troublesome cases are caused by *Escherichia coli, Proteus vulgaris,* and *Pseudomonas aeruginosa.* Treatment centers on the use of sulfonamides, antibiotics, and such anti-infective agents as naladixic acid and nitrofurantoin.

Questions

1. Briefly describe the gross anatomy of the kidney.
2. Describe the nephron.
3. Describe in detail how the nephron manufactures urine.
4. What is the role of aldosterone in kidney function?
5. What is the role of ADH in kidney function?
6. What is meant by renal clearance?
7. What is the urea clearance test?
8. Describe the structure of the ureters.
9. Describe the structure of the bladder.
10. Compare the male and female urethras.
11. Describe the physiologic events of micturition.
12. Describe the physical and chemical characteristics of normal urine.
13. Discuss the etiology and treatment of diabetes insipidus.
14. What is the medical significance of hematuria, albuminuria, and glycosuria?
15. Distinguish between nephritis and nephrosis.
16. What is the relationship of albuminuria to edema?
17. Discuss the etiology and treatment of acute kidney failure.
18. Discuss the etiology and treatment of nephrolithiasis.
19. Discuss the basic function of the artificial kidney.
20. Distinguish between active and passive reabsorption.
21. Differentiate between renal hypertension and essential hypertension.
22. What is the origin of urochrome?
23. In kidney transplantation why are drugs used to inhibit the reticuloendothelial system?
24. What is the relationship between NPN and BUN?
25. According to the Brönsted theory, ammonia and bicarbonate are bases. Explain.

Chapter 18

Inorganic metabolism

As used here, inorganic metabolism means the sum total of all physicochemical activities involving body water and ions. The purpose of the present chapter is to acquaint the student with the cardinal facts and figures as they apply to health and disease.

WATER

It seems fantastic, but protoplasm (the "stuff of life") is mostly water! The adult body is about 60 percent water, the newborn baby 77 percent water, and the embryo 97 percent water. In a very real sense, then, all life is aquatic!

Though there is a degree of fiction to e idea, especially since water is always ı the move, physiologists consider the water of the body to be "compartmentalized." According to this concept, there are two types of water within the body—the *intra*cellular water, or water *with*in the cells, and the *extra*cellular water, or water *outside* the cells. As shown on p. 172, the latter is further compartmentalized into *plasma* water and *inter*cellular water. (Intercellular water is also commonly referred to as *interstitial* fluid and *tissue* fluid.)

Of the 60 percent figure just cited, 40 percent is *intra*cellular and 20 percent *extra*cellular water; intercellular water and plasma water, in turn, account for 15 and 5 percent, respectively. According to this breakdown, a man weighing 70 kg. (154 pounds) is composed of about 0.60 × 70, or 42 kg. of water. Since 1 kg. of water is equal to 1 liter, this amounts to about 42 liters of water—28 liters (0.40 × 70) within the cells and 14 liters (0.20 × 70) without. Of the latter volume, 3.5 liters (0.05 × 70) is plasma water, and 10.5 liters (0.15 × 70) is intercellular water.

Compartmental balance. As indicated, we must not for a moment look upon the water in the body as being locked up in this or that compartment. On the contrary, water is continually seeping back and forth between the compartments. How is it, then, that the percentage of water in a given compartment remains essentially the same, day in and day out?

The answer to this question is the backbone of water balance (also referred to as *fluid* balance) and deserves the utmost appreciation. Balance is maintained because, in health, the water that leaves a compartment is offset by the water that enters the compartment and vice versa. In formal language, it is a pure case of dynamic equilibrium. This expression is especially apropos, because it carries the idea not only of balance but also of movement.

The mechanisms by which water balance is effected must be clearly understood if one is to acquire a sound view of the body as a whole. Moreover, since many diseases are in one way or another related to water disturbances, such an understanding assumes great practical value. The principal forces regulating body water are discussed herewith in some detail.

Protein. Plasma protein—namely "serum albumin"—is the chief factor regulating the exchange of water between the plasma and the intercellular compartment, the essential mechanism of which is depicted in Fig. 18-1. In brief, as blood enters the capillaries from the arterioles, its (hydrostatic) pressure (B.P.) forces water through the permeable walls into the tissue fluid. Water continues to leave until this pressure is offset by the osmotic pull of the protein molecules, which largely remain within the capillaries. Indeed, at the venular end where the blood pressure drops below the *colloidal osmotic pressure* (C.O.P.), water will be drawn into the circulation from the intercellular compartment.

More precisely, the amount of water that leaves the capillaries at the arteriolar end is determined by the so-called *filtration pressure* (F.P.), or the difference between B.P. and C.O.P.; that is, F.P. = B.P. − C.O.P. But note that at the venular end the F.P. value will be *negative,* explaining why water is sucked in rather than squeezed out. Thus, the water lost at one end is balanced by a gain at the other. This to-and-fro flow of water throughout the tissues is referred to as *Starling's principle.*

From the foregoing, we can readily see

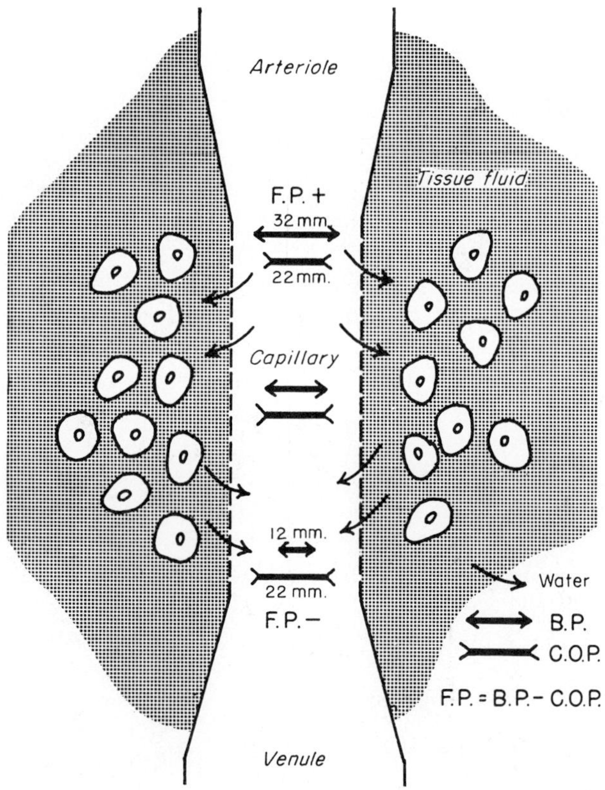

Fig. 18-1. Fluid balance in the tissues. (See text.) (From Brooks, S. M.: Basic facts of body water and ions, ed. 2, New York, 1968, Springer Publishing Co., Inc.)

why *hypoproteinemia,* or a drop in blood protein, leads to edema, for a drop in protein means a drop in C.O.P. which, in turn, means an increase in F.P. This explains the edema of malnutrition and why the best remedy is beefsteak. For patients unable to take food by mouth, amino acid solutions may be given intravenously.

Sodium. The key regulator of water balance between the *intra*cellular and the *inter*cellular compartments is sodium. "Forced" by the cell membrane to remain outside, this cation acts as a brake on the water entering the cells. "Water, water everywhere nor any drop to drink" bears striking testimony to the role of sodium in compartmental balance. When a person drinks seawater, the kidney is unable to remove the incoming salt fast enough to prevent an abnormal buildup in the intercellular compartment. As a consequence, the osmotic pressure of the latter compartment intensifies and overpowers the pull of the protein within the cell. Thus, cellular water is lost and dehydration ensues. Indeed, for each quart of seawater the castaway drinks, he eliminates 1½ quarts of urine, with the difference coming from the cells. In essence, then, excess salt serves to pump the cells dry.

Lymph vessels. During times of increased metabolic activity, intercellular fluid is produced faster than it can be removed by the capillaries. And were it not for the drainage system afforded by the lymphatic system, severe edema would be the rule and not the exception. Under normal conditions, increased intercellular pressure forces tissue fluid into the lymph capillaries (Fig. 18-2), then into the lymph vessels, and finally back into the blood. The importance of this escape route is grotesquely epitomized in elephantiasis, a disease in which filarial worms get into the lymph vessels and obstruct the flow of lymph. Here the edema is especially pronounced in the lower extremities.

Gastrointestinal secretions. In a 24-hour period the total volume of juices secreted by the gastrointestinal mucosa and accessory digestive organs amounts to about 8 liters, over twice the volume of the plasma! Phenomenally, all but 200 ml. or so is *reabsorbed* by the intestine, particularly by the large intestine. The importance of this reabsorption becomes immediately ap-

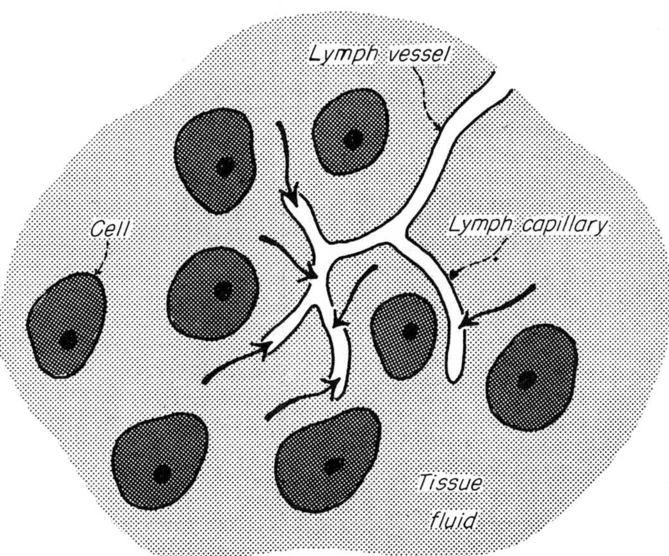

Fig. 18-2. Movement of tissue fluid into the lymph capillaries.

parent in severe vomiting and diarrhea. These situations lead not only to water imbalances and dehydration but also to electrolyte disturbances.

Intake vs. output. Plants and animals vary tremendously in their water requirements. The intake increases with size and, interestingly enough, in a mathematical way. Also of interest is the time required for a given species to imbibe a quantity of water equal to its own weight. A mouse takes 5 days, a cow 2 weeks, a camel 3 months, a tortoise 1 year, and a man 1 month. But the cactus beats them all—29 years!

Regardless of the intake, however, the body normally balances the gain with an equivalent loss. Conversely, the body balances the loss with an equivalent gain. Either way, the central idea is balance. And we human beings possess phenomenal balance, for in a 24-hour period, man's weight may vary less than ½ pound.

Intake. On a typical day a man's intake of water is close to 3 liters. This comes not only from imbibed fluids but also from *preformed* water (water trapped in food) and *oxidative* water (water formed as a by-product of oxidation). The respective volumes from these sources are shown in Fig. 18-3.

Obviously, the food intake has a great bearing on the need for imbibed fluid. As a matter of fact, the kangaroo rat of the desert never takes a drink as long as it lives, deriving its water solely from solid food! Indeed, we could do the same thing if we lived on cucumbers and lettuce.

Output. As noted, the daily output balances the daily intake (Fig. 18-3). Naturally, the kidneys carry the heaviest load, excreting up to 1.7 liters. The other channels, though not as apparent, are no less vital. From the skin and lungs, about 0.5 and 0.4 liter of water are lost, respectively. About 0.2 liter leaves the body in the feces.

Water escapes from the lungs as vapor. That lost from the skin is usually vapor

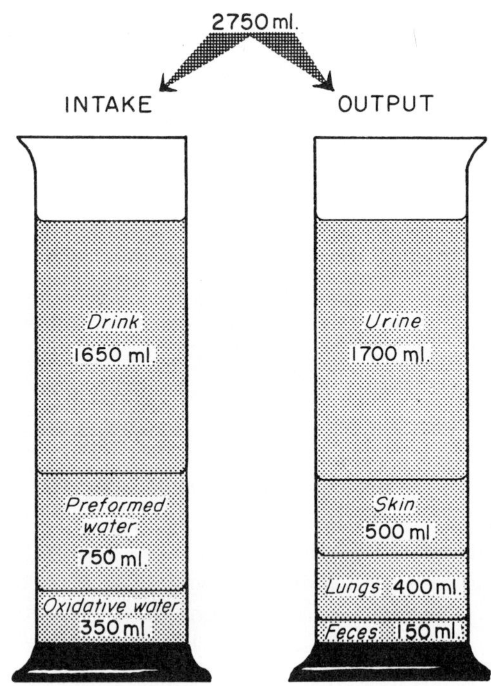

Fig. 18-3. A typical daily intake and output of water. (From Brooks, S. M.: Basic facts of body water and ions, ed. 2, New York, 1968, Springer Publishing Co., Inc.)

(*insensible* perspiration), but, as we know, builds up into sweat when the body becomes overheated. Perspiration is about 99 percent water, with traces of salts (NaCl) and urea. In certain diseases other constituents may appear, such as bile pigments, albumin, and sugar.

From the foregoing, then, we can see that body water is a matter of both compartmental balance and intake-output balance. This is succinctly shown in Fig. 18-4.

ELECTROLYTES

Physiologically, the word *electrolyte* refers to the ions present in body water. Since these charged particles play an essential role in the workings of the cell, we can readily understand why an upset in water balance is invariably associated with an upset in electrolyte balance. Indeed, water balance and electrolyte balance, in practice anyway, are generally

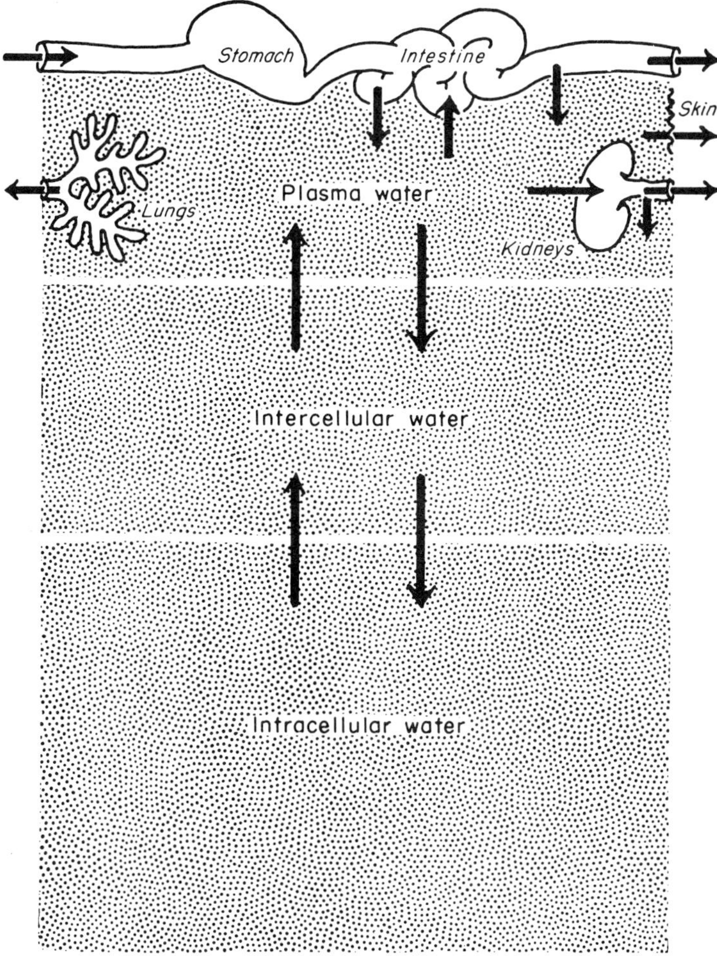

Fig. 18-4. Distribution and movement of body water. (After Gamble; from Brooks, S. M.: Basic facts of body water and ions, ed. 2, New York, 1968, Springer Publishing Co., Inc.)

looked upon as "one and the same." Commonly, the expression *fluid balance* is used to ensure the concept of both ideas.

Expressing concentration. Because the slightest alteration in electrolytes can often cause havoc—and even death—it is imperative that we have the best possible means for expressing ionic concentration. This turns out to be the *milliequivalent weight* (mEq.), which is equal to the atomic or ionic weight divided by 1000 times the valence. Thus,

$$\text{mEq.} = \frac{\text{Atomic weight (gm.)}}{1000 \times \text{Valence}}$$

Table 18-1. Milliequivalent weights of the body's chief ions

Ion	Symbol	At. wt.	Valence	mEq.
Sodium	Na^{+}	23	1	0.023
Potassium	K^{+}	39	1	0.039
Calcium	Ca^{++}	40	2	0.020
Magnesium	Mg^{++}	24	2	0.012
Chloride	Cl^{-}	35	1	0.035
Bicarbonate	HCO_3^{-}	61	1	0.061
Phosphate	$HPO_3^{=}$	96	2	0.048
Sulfate	$SO_4^{=}$	96	2	0.048

The milliequivalent weight for the sodium ion, for example, is as follows:

$$\frac{23}{1000 \times 1} \text{ or } 0.023 \text{ gm.}$$

For the calcium ion, it is as follows:

$$\frac{40}{1000 \times 2} \text{ or } 0.020 \text{ gm.}$$

Table 18-1 gives the milliequivalent weights for the body's chief ions.

Now in actual use the electrolyte concentration of a given compartment is expressed as the *number of milliequivalents* per liter (abbreviated mEq./L.). Thus, when it is said that the concentration of calcium in blood serum is 5 mEq./L., this means that in each liter of serum there is 5 × 0.02 gm., or 0.10 gm., of this electrolyte. On the basis of milligrams per 100 ml., or *milligrams percent* (mg.%), another method of expressing blood serum concentrations, this would be 10 mg.%.

Extracellular electrolytes. For all practical purposes, the electrolyte profile of the

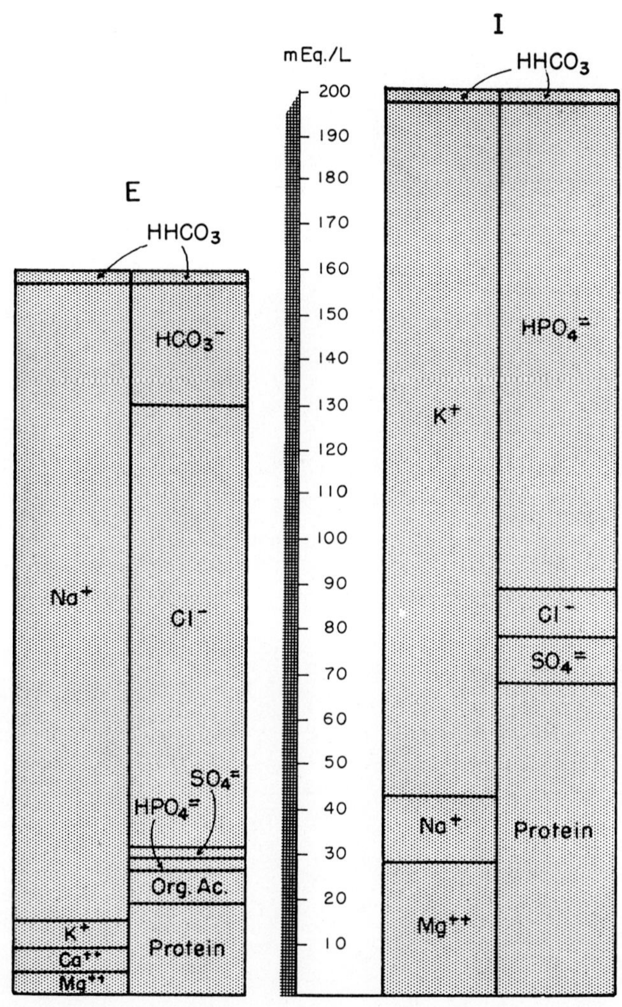

Fig. 18-5. Chemical composition of the body fluids. **E**, Extracellular compartment (plasma and tissue fluids). **I**, Intracellular compartment. (After Gamble; from Brooks, S. M.: Basic facts of body water and ions, ed. 2, New York, 1968, Springer Publishing Co., Inc.)

plasma and intercellular compartments are the same and are so recognized in Fig. 18-5. The positive ions, or *cations,* of the extracellular compartment include Na^+, K^+, Ca^{++}, and Mg^{++}. Sodium, with a concentration of 142 mEq./L., accounts for the bulk of the ions and, as stated previously, plays the most influential role in the distribution of body water. Though the other three ions are of little significance in water balance, they are an integral part of the metabolic machinery of the cell.

Just a glance at Fig. 18-5 shows that the predominating extracellular *anions* are Cl^- and HCO_3^-. The remaining anions include protein, organic acids, biphosphate ($HPO_4^=$), and sulfate ($SO_4^=$).

Since an electrolyte solution is always electrically neutral, the *total* milliequivalents of *cation* are always equal to the *total* milliequivalents of *anion.* This is quite interesting physiologically, for regardless of the degree of electrolyte imbalance occasioned by disease, the ions are adjusted to comply with the laws of chemistry. A loss of chloride, for instance, is compensated chemically by a gain in bicarbonate.

Intracellular electrolytes. The electrolyte profile of the intracellular compartment is just about the reverse of that of the extracellular compartment, particularly in relation to concentrations of Na^+ and K^+. Whereas the extracellular $[K^+]$ is only 4 to 5 mEq./L., the intracellular runs about 150 mEq./L. Intracellular sodium runs about 12 mEq./L.

The intracellular ratio of $[Na^+]$ to $[K^+]$ is critical; that is, an increase in one brings about a speedy decrease in the other. This is not peculiar to just this situation, however, for all tissues of the body demand a balanced ionic environment.

Sodium. As the chief cation, sodium is perhaps the "star" of inorganic metabolism, for aside from the part that it plays in water balance, it also reacts with HCO_3^- to form $NaHCO_3$, the main source of alkali for the body. Also, sodium per se is needed for the proper function of the muscles, nerves, and heart. Thus, a severe depletion of the ion bears an ominous prognosis. The converse situation, an excess, may also do great harm.

Potassium. In contrast to their striking chemical similarity, sodium and potassium are more often than not physiologically antagonistic. Potassium is part of the fabric of protoplasm, aids in the transport of CO_2 and O_2, and is associated with acid-base balance. In the heart it antagonizes the action of calcium and allows the muscle to get its proper rest during diastole. In acute kidney failure, excess potassium may be the cause of death (p. 245).

Calcium. Though 99 percent of the calcium of the body is deposited in the bones, the small amount present as the ion in the extracellular compartment is nonetheless essential for normal physiology. The calcium ion is an integral part of the clotting mechanism (p. 255) and of muscle metabolism (p. 207). The relation of vitamin D and the parathyroid hormone to calcium metabolism is discussed in Chapter 22 and on p. 192, respectively.

Magnesium. Laboratory and clinical studies have proved that magnesium is an essential ion. Animals raised on a magnesium-free diet are subject to convulsions. On the other hand, an excess of the ion acts as a depressant. But clinically, the signs and symptoms of hypomagnesemia and hypermagnesemia are ill defined. In hypomagnesemia the syndrome may be marked by nausea, tremors, twitching of the face, anxiety, and delirium, whereas in hypermagnesemia, respiratory depression, lethargy, and coma have been reported.

ACID-BASE BALANCE

Considering the galaxy of diverse materials entering and leaving the interstitial fluid and blood at any given moment, it is indeed remarkable that the pH of the extracellular compartment remains between

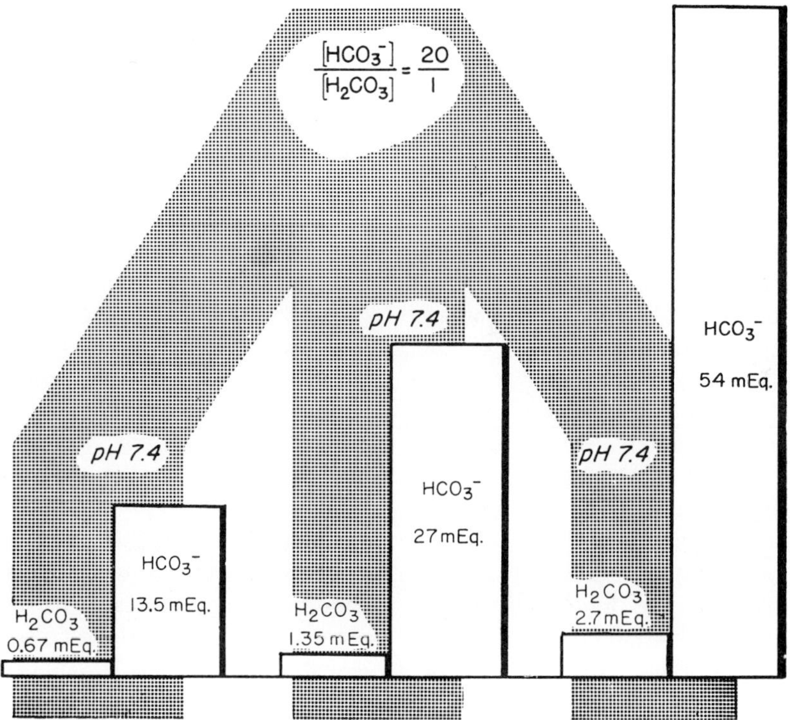

Fig. 18-6. The pH and buffer mechanism of the blood. As long as the $[HCO_3^-]$ to $[H_2CO_3]$ ratio is 20 to 1, the pH remains at 7.4. (From Brooks, S. M.: Basic facts of body water and ions, ed. 2, New York, 1968, Springer Publishing Co., Inc.)

7.35 and 7.45. This is most fortunate, for a pH below 6 or above 8 generally proves fatal. The factors responsible for the maintenance of this pH—or acid-base balance—include a variety of chemical buffers in addition to the respiratory (p. 276) and renal (p. 331) mechanisms already discussed.

Buffers. The ability of a solution such as blood serum to resist a change in pH depends upon the presence of a so-called buffer system, that is, a combination of a *weak acid and one of its salts.* The principal buffer system in the body—carbonic acid (H_2CO_3) and bicarbonate (HCO_3^-)—works, like all buffers, in the following way: If strong acid enters the system, the H^+ ions are grabbed up by the HCO_3^- ions and converted to H_2CO_3, a *weak* acid. Thus,

$$HCO_3^- + H^+ \longrightarrow H_2CO_3$$

Conversely, if base is added, it is immediately *neutralized* by H_2CO_3. The OH^- ion, for example, a *strong* base, reacts to form water and HCO_3^-, a *weak* base*:

$$OH^- + H_2CO_3 \longrightarrow HCO_3^- + H_2O$$

Now, by using the proper concentrations of acid and salt, the chemist can produce a buffer system of the desired pH. The body, the master chemist, maintains a pH of 7.4 by keeping the ratio of $[HCO_3^-]$ to $[H_2CO_3]$ at 20 to 1 (Fig. 18-6). The term *ratio* cannot be overemphasized, for it is the proportion and not the absolute amounts of HCO_3^- and H_2CO_3 that must remain constant to keep the pH at 7.4. Nonetheless, the body does strive toward normal concentrations, in this instance 1.35 mEq. for H_2CO_3 and 27 mEq. for HCO_3^-.

*HCO_3^- is a base because it accepts H^+ ions (Brönsted's theory).

Other important buffers include phosphate and protein, which are particularly important in control of intracellular acid-base balance.

Acidosis. A decreased pH of the blood, or *acidemia,* is generally referred to as acidosis. In the event that the altered pH is soon restored by the buffer system just described, we speak of it as *compensated* acidosis. On the other hand, if the restoration falls short of the normal pH, we speak of the acidosis as being *uncompensated.*

Let us consider a specific case of acidosis and see how the body in general and the buffer system in particular cope with this dangerous situation. In diabetic acidosis, for example, ketonic acids (Chapter 22) accumulate in the blood at the expense of HCO_3^-, thereby reducing the $[HCO_3^-]$ to $[H_2CO_3]$ ratio and lowering the pH. But concomitantly, the respiratory center in the medulla is stimulated (by the lowered pH), and the lungs are prodded into blowing off more CO_2. Since CO_2 comes from H_2CO_3, the concentration of the latter starts to drop and the altered ratio is thereby turned toward normal.

Alkalosis. Alkalosis refers to an *alkalemia,* or increased pH. Once again, an example is the best way to demonstrate the buffer system in action. In severe vomiting, enough hydrochloric acid may be lost to cause a *relative* increase in base (HCO_3^-) and an altered ratio. To compensate, respiration is diminished, thereby increasing the $[H_2CO_3]$, and the kidney steps up the excretion of HCO_3^-. In this way both mechanisms, working together, bring the ratio back toward 20 to 1 and a normal pH.

Another interesting case of alkalosis results from hyperventilation, or excessive breathing. Here the body is plunged into a state of alkalosis because H_2CO_3 (as CO_2) is blown off, resulting, as in the example just cited, in a *relative* increase in HCO_3^-.

FLUID IMBALANCES

The loss or retention of abnormal amounts of fluid (water and ions) is, as indicated in the foregoing discussion, a cardinal pathologic feature of many disorders of the body. The more commonly encountered imbalances are touched upon here.

Hemorrhage. The blood, being the smallest of the water compartments, can obviously not sustain a great loss. Hemorrhage, therefore, is an emergency of the first order and demands speedy treatment if a life is to be saved. Since the immediate threat is shock (due to circulatory collapse), plasma, plasma expanders, or even normal saline solution will suffice if whole blood is not available. Though it is quite true that salt and water readily leave the circulation, cardiac output can often be maintained until proper replacement becomes available.

Burns. Aside from unbelievable agony, the burn victim is beset by an upheaval of inorganic metabolism. Plasma escapes into the intercellular compartment, producing shock and edema; *hemoconcentration* (due to loss of plasma) withdraws intracellular water and produces dehydration; the accumulation of salt in the edematous area robs the body as a whole of sodium; and the damaged cells release their considerable amounts of toxic potassium. As a matter of fact, recent data suggest quite strongly that the displacement of sodium and the excess extracellular potassium (hyperkalemia) could very well be the main cause of so-called *burn shock.*

Burns covering less than 50 percent of the body offer a favorable prognosis, provided that proper treatment is instituted immediately. In addition to giving drugs to relieve pain and antibiotics to fight infection, the physician must restore the displaced and lost fluid. This entails accurate computation of the amount of fluid lost (p. 188) and selection of the appropriate solutions, namely, plasma, 5 percent glucose, and electrolyte. Whenever possible, saline solution is given orally.

Vomiting. Severe vomiting results in loss of fluid from the extracellular compartment, producing dehydration and usually alkalosis due to the loss of gastric acid. Treatment centers about the use of water to correct dehydration and the appropriate salt to restore the acid-base balance. If the alkalosis is not pronounced, these objectives can be met by administration of normal saline or Ringer's solution. In severe cases, however, ammonium chloride, an "acid" salt, may be needed.

Diarrhea. Fluid and acid-base imbalance is a common feature in diarrhea, particularly in infants. Since the ion-rich gastrointestinal secretions are swept away before the intestinal wall has a chance to reabsorb them back into the circulation, the body is deprived of water and electrolytes, especially potassium. Because these secretions contain more base than acid, the syndrome is generally accompanied by *acidosis.* Treatment entails replacement of water, salt, and potassium and use of sodium bicarbonate or sodium lactate to correct the acidosis. The latter salt is metabolized in the liver into HCO_3^-, the chief source of alkali in the body.

Low-salt syndrome. Perhaps the most frequently encountered fluid imbalance is a self-inflicted variety referred to technically as the low-salt syndrome and popularly as "heat cramps." This condition, marked by nausea, fatigue, and muscle cramps, is caused by excessive sweating.

In brief, what happens is as follows: The water that one drinks in response to the incited thirst lowers the $[Na^+]$ of the extracellular fluid and renders that compartment hypotonic. Consequently, fluid now seeps into the more hypertonic intracellular comparement. In other words, the signs and symptoms cited result from a drop in $[Na^+]$, extracellular dehydration, and intracellular hydration. The condition is simply treated and prevented by taking plain salt.

Acute kidney failure. Acute kidney failure, or renal shutdown, though still an ominous condition, today often yields to the modern principles of electrolyte balance. Its treatment and the use of the artificial kidney were discussed on p. 335.

Edema. We have mentioned edema, or the accumulation of fluid in the tissues, several times before. Actually, there are a variety of etiologic factors. One, hypoproteinemia, was discussed on p. 338. Others include an increased capillary permeability (for example, the edema seen in inflammation and allergies), an increased hydrostatic pressure (for example, in standing), "clogged" lymphatics (filariasis), and a failing heart. In the latter condition, or *cardiac* edema, the heart fails to pump out the returning blood fast enough. As a result, the venous pressure becomes elevated and fluid is forced out into the intercellular compartment.

The treatment of edema is directed against the underlying cause (for example, giving digitalis to strengthen the heart) and against the water-logged tissues. The latter is accomplished through the use of diuretics (p. 332).

Questions

1. Discuss the manner in which the water of the body is "compartmentalized."
2. Distinguish between the terms *plasma water* and *interstitial water.*
3. What is meant by the term *fluid?*
4. What is meant by water balance?
5. What effect does hypoproteinemia have upon the filtration pressure in the capillaries?
6. Why is the term *colloidal* (for example, colloidal osmotic pressure) used in reference to protein solutions?
7. Explain the sequence of events by which the drinking of salt water leads to dehydration.
8. Distinguish between preformed water and oxidative water.
9. What effect does excessive peristalsis have upon water absorption?
10. What is meant by insensible perspiration?
11. Compare the meanings of the terms *water balance, electrolyte balance,* and *fluid balance.*
12. What events are called into play following the ingestion of excess fluid?

13. What is the mg.% concentration of sodium in blood serum?
14. Compute the mEq. for Mg^{++} (show arithmetic).
15. What is the difference between an atom and ion?
16. Why are electrolyte solutions neutral?
17. Compare the cations of the extracellular and intracellular compartments.
18. Tissue injury not infrequently leads to hyperkalemia. Explain.
19. Compare the physiologic effects of calcium and magnesium.
20. What is the relationship of $[Ca^{++}]$ to the parathyroids?
21. Explain how a solution containing citric acid and sodium citrate resists a change in pH.
22. Why is HCO_3^- called a base?
23. Explain how apnea can lead to acidosis.
24. Venous blood has a slightly lower pH than arterial blood. Explain.
25. Discuss the effect of a severe burn upon body water and electrolytes.

Chapter 19

The nervous system

"The nervous system is an extensive and complicated organization of structures by which the internal reactions of the individual are correlated and integrated and by which his adjustments with his environment are controlled."* In the present chapter an attempt has been made to treat this great system in a manner that reflects the foregoing definition, always keeping in mind, of course, that the trees should not obstruct our view of the forest.

For convenience of study the nervous system may be considered to fall into two major divisions—the *central* nervous system and the *peripheral* nervous system. The former includes the *brain* and *spinal cord* and the latter the *nerves, ganglia,* and *receptors* (Fig. 19-1). Before we take up these various parts, however, it is essential that we first consider the general microscopic structure and function of nervous tissue.

NEURONS

Nervous tissue is essentially made up of two kinds of cells—neurons, the functional units, and neuroglia, special connective tissue cells that serve to support the neurons.

The neuron is characterized especially by its intricately branched extensions or processes, which radiate out from the cell body, or *perikaryon* (Fig. 19-2). The processes that conduct nervous impulses toward the perikaryon are called *dendrites;* those that carry impulses away from it are called *axons.* While the dendrites of most neurons are short and extensively branched, axons are single. The latter may, however, send out one or two side branches called collateral axons.

Returning to the perikaryon, we note, as shown in Fig. 19-2, delicate fibers, or *neurofibrils,* and chromatophilic granules called *Nissl bodies.* The latter, which can be seen only via staining techniques employing basic dyes, are present in addition to the usual cytoplasmic furnishings (p. 161) and are unique to nervous tissue. Following injury, Nissl bodies undergo *chromatolysis;* that is, they break up and disappear. In research this phenomenon has enabled the physiologist to trace nerve pathways in the brain and cord; that is, different nerves are cut to see where the area or areas of chromatolysis will occur. Nissl bodies contain large amounts of RNA and play a key role in the synthesis of proteins.

*From Goss, C. M., editor: Gray's anatomy of the human body, ed. 27, Philadelphia, 1959, Lea & Febiger.

Nerve fibers. A nerve fiber is a dendrite or axon that extends from the central nervous system or ganglion out into the body, sometimes for several feet. Except for certain autonomic fibers, most nerve fibers are myelinated; that is, they are enveloped by a white fatty material called *myelin.* Characteristically, this myelin sheath indents itself along the way, forming the *nodes of Ranvier* (Fig. 19-2). The myelin sheath has a thin, multinucleated outer covering called the *neurilemma.* The neurilemma is more than just another coat, however, for it serves in regeneration of the fiber. When a fiber is cut, the distal end degenerates, whereupon, after a few days, the neurilemma extends itself to the distal stump and thereby initiates the regeneration of the axon and myelin. If all goes well, in a couple of months or so the severed fiber or nerve becomes operational again and the affected part returned to normal.

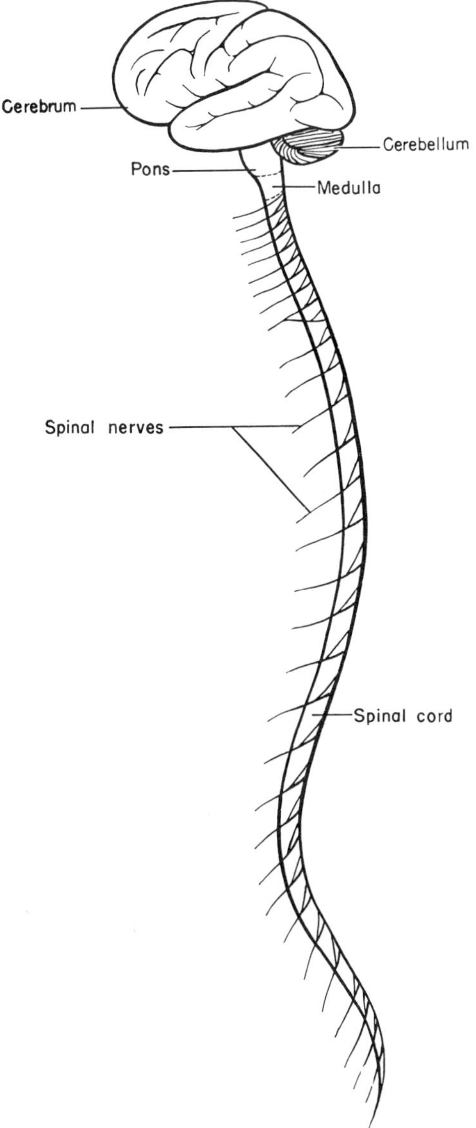

Fig. 19-1. The brain and spinal cord. (From Brooks, S. M.: Basic facts of pharmacology, ed. 2, Philadelphia, 1963, W. B. Saunders Co.)

Classification of neurons. Neurons are classified according to both architecture and function. The former scheme recognizes three types of cells—*unipolar, dipolar,* and *multipolar,* depending upon the number of processes projecting from the perikaryon. With respect to function, there are also three types of neurons—*afferent, efferent,* and *internuncial.* Afferent or *sensory* neurons conduct impulses toward the central nervous system; efferent or *motor* neurons conduct impulses away from the central nervous system; and internuncial or *connective* neurons conduct impulses from sensory to motor neurons. An afferent neuron is unipolar, with a long dendrite and a relatively short axon (Fig. 19-2). In contrast, a motor neuron has a long axon and short dendrites. Internuncial neurons, situated as they are within the central nervous system, generally have relatively short dendrites and axons. They are multipolar.

Gray and white matter. The gray areas of the central nervous system are composed essentially of cell bodies and unmyelinated fibers. White matter, on the other hand, is composed of myelinated fibers. The outside of the brain is gray, and the inside is white with islands of gray. In contrast, the spinal cord is white on the outside and gray on the inside.

The nerve. A nerve is an anatomic cable

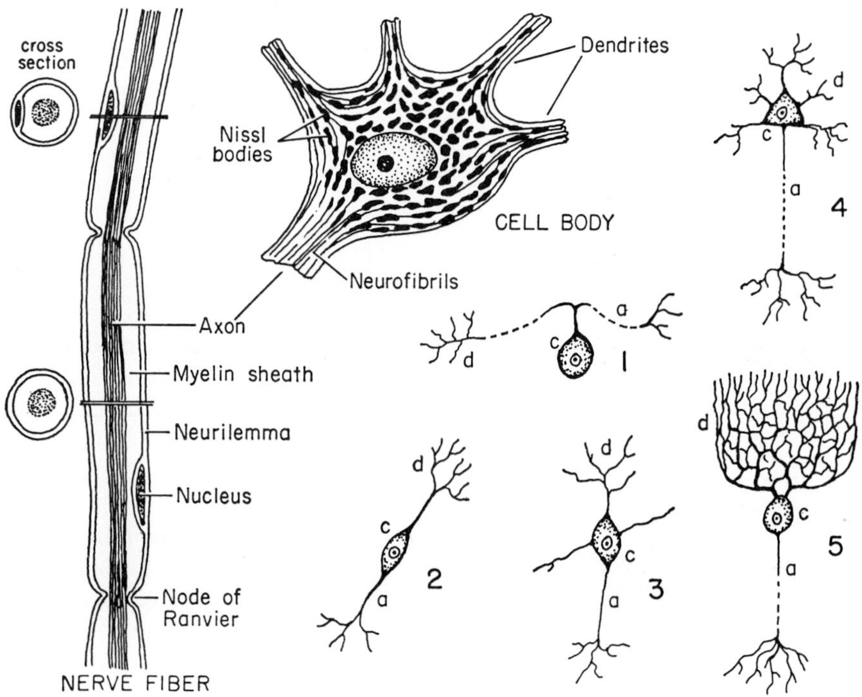

Fig. 19-2. The neuron. Microscopic details of the cell body and nerve fiber and the basic types are shown. **1,** Unipolar cell. **2,** Bipolar cell. **3,** Cell of cerebral cortex. **4,** Motor cell. **5,** Purkinje cell of cerebellar cortex. **a,** Axon; **c,** cell body; **d,** dendrites.

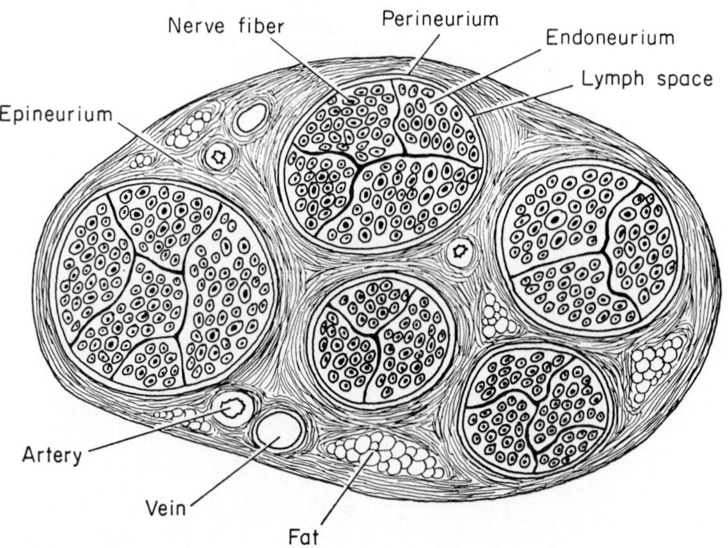

Fig. 19-3. Cross section of a nerve. This particular nerve trunk is made up of five bundles *(funiculi)* of nerve fibers. (After Harris; modified from Tuttle, W. W., and Schottelius, B. A.: Textbook of physiology, ed. 16, St. Louis, 1969, The C. V. Mosby Co.)

composed of nerve fibers, blood vessels, and lymphatics wrapped together by connective tissue (Fig. 19-3). Afferent fibers carry impulses from the receptors to the cord and brain, and efferent fibers carry impulses to the effectors (muscles and glands). Most nerves are mixed; that is, they contain both afferent and efferent fibers. Autonomic nerves, however, are considered to be exclusively efferent (or motor) fibers, and the olfactory, optic, and acoustic nerves are purely afferent (or sensory).

A bundle of fibers *within* the central nervous system is referred to as a *tract.* We shall have more to say about tracts later in the present chapter.

THE NERVE IMPULSE

Most authorities seem to be in essential agreement on the so-called *membrane theory* of nerve impulse transmission. According to this view, the outside membrane (the neurilemma) is permeable to anions and impermeable to cations. As a result, the fiber is charged, or *polarized;* that is, the outside is *positive* and the inside is *negative.* That there is such a charge can be shown quite easily by placing one delicate electrode on the surface of a nerve and another into the cut end and then connecting both electrodes to an ultrasensitive galvanometer. As shown in Fig. 19-4, the instrument demonstrates that a charge, or potential, does exist between the outside and the inside. Commonly, this is referred to as the *resting potential.*

Referring to Fig. 19-4, let us see what happens when a nerve is stimulated. If an electric shock is applied to the nerve fiber, it is believed, according to the membrane

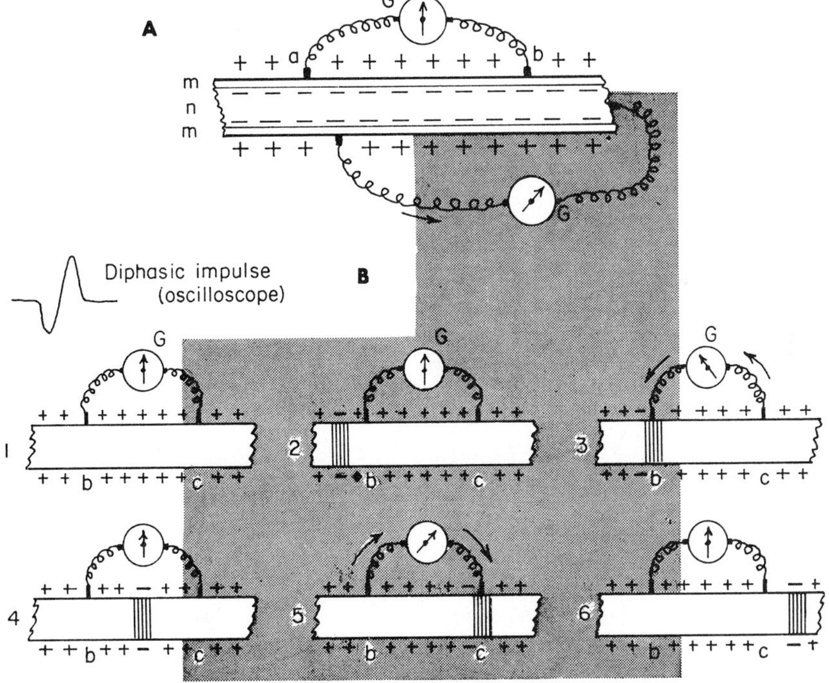

Fig. 19-4. Electrical character of the resting nerve fiber, **A,** and the transmission of the nerve impulse, **B.** The setup in **A** demonstrates that the outside membrane, **m,** bears no charge between points **a** and **b** on the surface but is charged relative to the interior of the fiber, **n.** In **B** we see that when the resting fiber, **1,** is stimulated, **2,** a negative wave of excitation (the impulse) is propagated. This is evidenced by the swing of the galvanometer needle, **G,** first one way and then the other; hence, the expression diphasic impulse.

theory, that the membrane in the immediate area becomes permeable to the surface cations (namely, sodium) and permits them to enter the fiber. As a result, this area is *depolarized* and, relative to the adjacent area, *negative.* As a consequence, a tiny current jumps from − to +, neutralizing the latter and in the process rendering the positive area negative. This continues on and on down the fiber.

This electrical disturbance has been variously referred to as the *nerve impulse, action current, wave of depolarization,* and *action potential.* In general terms, nerve impulse seems to be the preferred designation; in more definitive terms, action potential seems to be preferred, particularly since the expression *resting potential* is quite apropos to the unexcited fiber. The oscilloscope captures the action potential in visible form (Fig. 19-4).

Stimulus. There are, among others, two especially amazing features of the nerve impulse. In the first place the stimulus that initiates the impulse may be just about anything. Although we use an electric shock in the laboratory, because of its convenience, fibers can be excited by any physical or chemical stimulus. But, and this is the key point, the impulse that travels down the fiber is always of the same character—electrical. Second, since the fiber is charged all along its length, the action potential does not diminish as it passes away from the stimulus. In a crude but striking analogy, these features can be dramatized by laying down a line of gunpowder on the sidewalk and igniting one end. Stimulated by a spark, match, blowtorch, friction, oxidizer, or what have you, the line of gunpowder catches fire and burns with undiminished fury along its entire length.

Threshold stimulus. The weakest possible stimulus that can trigger an action potential is referred to as the threshold stimulus. Also, and this is most important, a nerve fiber reacts maximally to such a stimulus. Thus, the nerve fiber obeys the *all-or-none law,* just the same as does the muscle fiber (p. 208). This law is in no way invalidated by the fact that a nerve, which is a bundle of fibers, shows a graded response to an increase in the strength of a stimulus, for this simply means that more fibers are being called into play. Indeed, after all fibers have been called into play, the response cannot be intensified by increasing the strength of the stimulus.

Summation. As one would expect, the effect of a stimulus depends to a degree upon the irritability of the nerve fiber. This probably explains why a series of *subthreshold* stimuli delivered at intervals of about 0.001 second can provoke a nerve impulse. Apparently, the first few stimuli of the series excite the membrane to a point where it can be triggered by subthreshold strength. This phenomenon is called summation or, more formally, *subliminal* summation.

Duration. Though it is true that all stimuli above the threshold level provoke the same response, it is also true that a stronger stimulus usually provokes the response in a shorter period of time. In other words, the length of time an impulse must be applied to be effective is inversely related to its strength. The time involved, however, is always fantastically short (generally one thousandth or so of a second).

Refractory period. After the action potential has passed along the nerve fiber, the latter requires about one thousandth of a second to *repolarize* itself, because, as explained previously, the membrane must be polarized in order to propagate a new impulse. This restorative intermission is called the refractory period. Of interest to us is the fact that all stimuli received during this period cannot be acted upon. In other words, the rate at which stimuli are delivered to a nerve fiber will enhance the response only up to a point.

Impulse velocity. In this day and age when decisions have to be made and acted upon in a split second (by a jet pilot, for instance), the velocity, or speed, at which an impulse travels is of no little concern. The latest figures show that the velocity varies anywhere from 1 to 300 mph.

Velocity depends upon the *diameter* of the fiber and upon whether it is *myelinated.* Fibers of large diameter transmit an impulse faster than fibers of small diameter, and myelinated fibers transmit an impulse faster than unmyelinated ones. Generally speaking, voluntary (somatic) nerve fibers are larger than the autonomic fibers. Also, voluntary fibers have myelin, whereas autonomic fibers usually do not. Sensations and skeletal muscle responses therefore are much faster than autonomic responses. Thus, whereas sound travels to the brain with the speed of a bullet, one can actually witness the closing and opening of the pupil of the eye.

REFLEXES

A reflex is an automatic, involuntary, often unconscious response to a stimulus. In its essential form it entails a *receptor,* an *afferen*t neuron, an *internuncial* neuron, an *efferent* neuron, and an *effector.* Upon stimulation the receptor initiates an impulse that runs along the afferent dendrite, thence through the cell body and along the afferent axon to the terminal endings at the *synapse,* the latter referring to the region of contact between adjacent neurons. Here, by some neurohormonal mechanism, the impulse is relayed to the dendrites of the internuncial neuron, then across the second synapse to the efferent dendrites, and finally to the efferent terminal endings at the *myoneural junction.* As a consequence, the endings release a neurohormone, and the effector (muscle or gland) responds. It is of considerable interest that an impulse can pass across a synapse in only one direction—that is, from the afferent to the efferent. The reverse does not occur. As a matter of fact, this and other synaptic phenomena are a keystone in nervous physiology.

The complete pathway over which the impulse must travel from receptor to effector is called the *reflex arc.* Though only one reflex in man (the knee jerk) is as simple as described (most arcs involve hundreds or even thousands of neurons), the general idea is always the same. In just a moment we shall discuss a more complex reflex arc.

Let us now consider the basic anatomy of the reflex arc. As we know, receptors are widely distributed throughout the body in the skin, mucosa, muscles, tendons, and special sense organs. The afferent dendrites attached to these receptors are found in the spinal nerves and generally run long distances before they reach the cell bodies housed in the *spinal ganglia* on the *posterior roots* (Fig. 19-5). From here the afferent axons make their way into the *posterior gray horns* of the cord, where they synapse with one or more internuncial neurons and sometimes directly with efferent neurons. The dendrites and cell bodies of the efferent neurons are confined to the *anterior gray horns,* and their axons extend into the *anterior roots.*

In *summary,* sensory impulses are relayed to the spinal cord via afferent neurons. Here, in the simplest instance, they synapse directly with efferent neurons or, as is usually the case, with internuncial neurons which, in turn, synapse with efferent neurons. The efferent axons now relay the impulse to the effector via the spinal nerves. One should note especially that a spinal nerve proper is mixed; that is, it carries both sensory and motor fibers. Equally significant, the posterior roots of the spinal nerves carry *only* sensory fibers, and the *anterior* roots carry only *motor* fibers. Finally, the cell bodies of the afferent, internuncial, and efferent neurons are located in the spinal ganglia, posterior gray horns, and anterior gray horns, respectively.

Another point to keep in mind is also vividly revealed in Fig. 19-5; that is, an

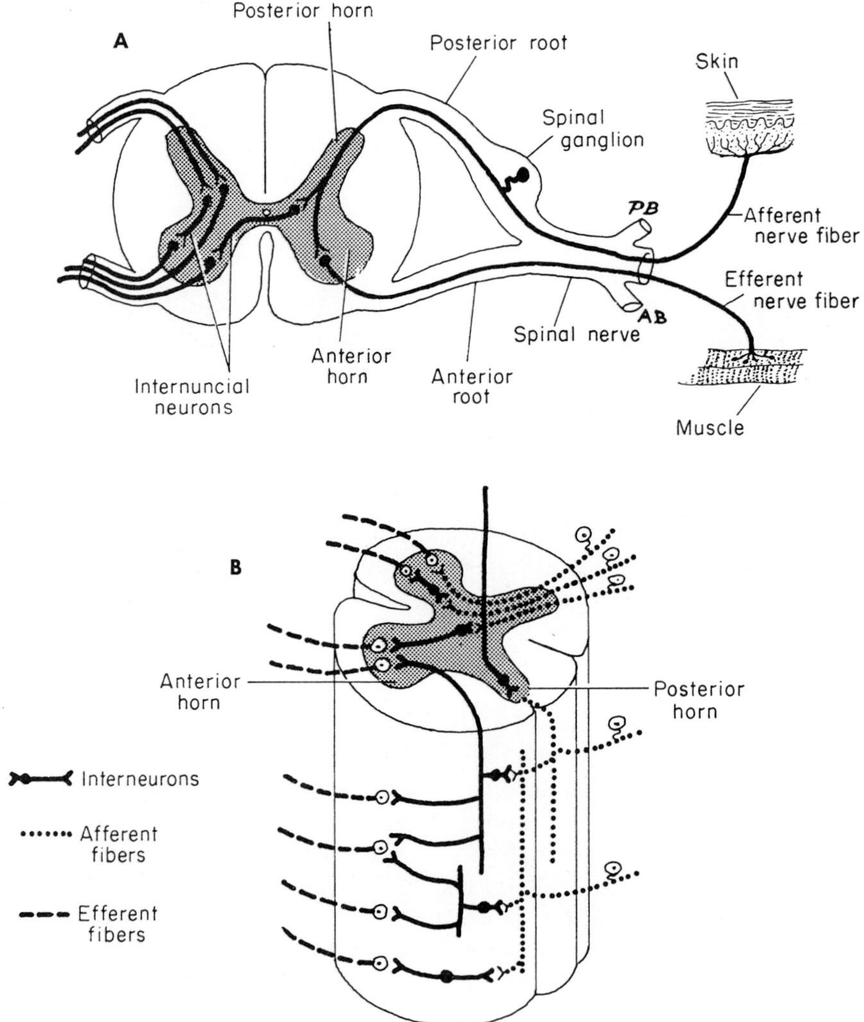

Fig. 19-5. Idealized diagram showing the basic features of afferent and efferent fibers as they relate to each other, the cord, and the reflex. **A,** Details of a spinal nerve. **B,** A few simple ramifications of fibers passing to higher and lower levels within the cord. **PB,** Posterior branch, or ramus, of spinal nerve; **AB,** anterior branch, or ramus, of spinal nerve.

afferent neuron may trigger an efferent neuron on the same side of the cord, on the opposite side of the cord, or on both sides. (The first situation constitutes a so-called ipsilateral reflex arc.) Also, an afferent axon usually triggers internuncial and efferent neurons not only at one level of the cord, producing a *segmental* reflex, but also at other levels, producing what is called an *intersegmental* reflex arc. Thus, a single sensory neuron can call into action an almost infinite number of motor neurons, an effect referred to as *divergence.* Conversely, a number of sensory neurons may synapse, or focus, upon a single motor neuron, an effect called *convergence.*

Regardless of the complexity of the reflex arc, the basic mechanism and purpose are always the same; that is, sensory impulses, through the agency of synaptic relays, are turned into motor impulses which, in turn, effect the response.

Inhibition and facilitation. In our discussion so far it has been implied that an incoming impulse always triggers an internuncial or motor neuron with which it forms a synapse. Actually, the cord and brain, especially, the latter, have quite a bit to say about what will pass and what will not pass across the synapses. Indeed, if this were not true, the astronomical number of incoming impulses would keep the central nervous system in a continuous electrical frenzy. Just how this *central inhibitory state* is effected still remains largely unknown, but that it centers largely about the synapse is quite well established. A dramatic example of reflex inhibition is shown when one stems a sneeze by applying pressure to the upper lip.

Sometimes, however, a sensory impulse is reinforced, or facilitated, via a corollary phenomenon referred to as the *central excitatory state.* In some way, as yet not known, synaptic resistance is decreased, thereby permitting a weak stimulus to evoke a strong response. This, too, can be easily demonstrated by pulling the clasped hands at the same time the patellar tendon is tapped. The resulting knee jerk is greatly intensified even though the tap is made ever so lightly.

Types. Since reflexes are named in various ways, it is important for the beginning student to understand the basis of classification. The types that follow are those usually recognized in standard works. Note especially that a given reflex can usually be designated by two or three expressions.

Reflexes classed according to receptor. Reflexes triggered by stimulated exteroceptors, that is, receptors located in the skin and surface membranes, are referred to as *exteroceptive* reflexes. Coughing, winking, tearing, sneezing, and response to pain, touch, and heat applied to the surface are all reflexes of this character.

Interoceptive (visceroceptive) reflexes, on the other hand, result from the stimulation of interoceptive receptors located in the viscera. The CO_2 stimulation of respiration, the cardiac reflexes, and micturition are examples.

The third type of reflex named according to the nature of the receptor is the *proprioceptive* reflex. Proprioceptors, which are located in the muscles, tendons, and semicircular canals, are sensitive to stretch, pressure, and movement and serve generally to maintain muscle tone and body balance. The knee jark is a classic example.

Reflexes classed according to response. The usual procedure here is to label a reflex a "flexor" or an "extensor." As the term implies, a flexor reflex is a response marked by the flexion of a muscle. Since such a reflex usually appears to indicate that the body is protecting itself against a harmful stimulus (for example, flexing at the knee in response to stepping on a nail or at the elbow when the finger is burned), these responses are sometimes referred to as *nociceptive* reflexes.

Extensor reflexes are responses effected by contraction of the extensor muscles. Because they oppose the force of gravity, they are always operating to keep the body in balance. When one steps on a nail, for instance, the extensors in the opposite leg are convulsed so as to enhance that leg's support.

Reflexes classed according to part affected. In clinical work the physician generally refers to a reflex according to the most obvious manifestation, the part affected. Some of the more classic reflexes of this type include the knee jerk, the corneal reflex (winking), the pupil reflex (constricting of the pupil in response to light), and the Babinski big toe reflex. The latter reflex, which involves extension of the big toe and fanning of the others, is elicited only during the first few months of infancy by tickling the sole of the foot. However, this reflex is also given by persons who have sustained lesions of the upper motor neurons (p. 349). Similarly, the other reflexes mentioned are also of diagnostic value.

Conditioned reflexes. At birth we are endowed with a certain number of natural reflexes. When the nipple is placed in the baby's mouth, he sucks away without hesitancy; when his foot is tickled, the toes move; and when his eye is touched, he winks. As the baby grows, however, he begins to acquire learned or *conditioned* reflexes and he continues to do so throughout life.

Whereas a natural or *unconditioned* reflex is mediated through the spinal cord or lower levels of the brain, a conditioned reflex involves the higher centers of the brain as well. For example, when an infant is shown a piece of strawberry shortcake, he probably will make no response other than to put his finger into the whipped cream. The older child, on the other hand, may feel his mouth water upon just hearing the words *strawberry shortcake.* And so it is with the gourmet who experiences a flow of saliva from just thinking about a juicy steak, let alone smelling it. Thus, in the conditioned reflex, stimuli that do not at first evoke a response (in this instance, salivation) are *conditioned* into action by cerebral association gained through experience and training. In the case of the juicy steak, the cortical areas of sight and smell have established pathways with the salivary centers at the lower levels.

At maturity, then, the brain has a vast repertoire of conditioned reflexes relating not only to salivation but also to many other processes important to the welfare of the body. Since these functions are psychic in nature and stem from experience, they are of cardinal interest to the psychologist. In experimental psychology, for example, the conditioned reflex affords a valuable tool for studying animal behavior.

SPINAL CORD

The spinal cord serves as a reflex center and two-way avenue between the brain and the peripheral nervous system. It carries motor impulses from the brain to the neurons of the anterior horns and sensory impulses from the spinal ganglia to the brain (Fig. 19-5). In essence, then, the cord is the functional "backbone" of the entire nervous system. Let us now direct our attention to its anatomy.

The spinal cord is a fairly soft, white, ovoid structure, measuring about 17 inches in length and ½ inch in diameter, that occupies the spinal canal from the foramen magnum to the first lumbar vertebra. Aside from two bulges in the cervical and lumbar regions, it tapers slightly, finally terminating as the *conus medullaris* (Fig. 19-6). The *filum terminale,* a nonfunctional filament that brings the cord to a point, is really not nervous tissue but a continuation of the *pia mater* (see below).

In cross section the spinal cord has an H-shaped area of gray matter surrounded by white matter (Fig. 19-5). The forward projections of the H are called *anterior* or *ventral horns* and the backward projections are called *posterior* or *dorsal horns.* The slight protrusions on either end of the cross of the H, or the *central gray,* are called the *lateral horns.* As indicated before, the anterior horns are composed of *motor* neurons and the lateral and posterior horns of *internuncial* neurons. The latter neurons receive sensory impulses from the nerve fibers housed in the *posterior roots* of the spinal nerves. (The *anterior roots* are composed of motor fibers sent out by the motor neurons located in the anterior horns.)

Meninges. The spinal cord does not lie naked in its bony vault, for it is ensheathed by three membranes continuous with those of the same name covering the brain. These membranes are called meninges. From without inward, they include the dura *mater,* the *arachnoid,* and the *pia mater* (Fig. 19-6). The dura mater, a relatively thick fibrous membrane lining the spinal canal, is slightly separated from the arachnoid. The latter is a more delicate structure composed of fibrous and elastic tissue. Be-

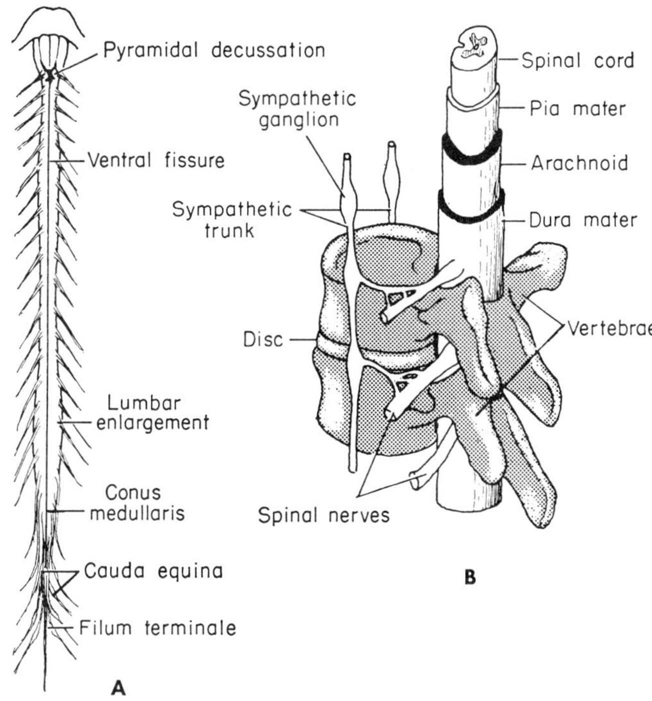

Fig. 19-6. Spinal cord, **A,** and its relation to the meninges and vertebral canal, **B.** (Redrawn from Anthony, C. P.: Textbook of anatomy and physiology, ed. 6, St. Louis, 1963, The C. V. Mosby Co.)

tween the arachnoid and the pia mater, the most delicate membrane of the three, there is a considerable interval called the *subarachnoid space.* Since the pia mater (which adheres closely to the surface of the cord) terminates as the filum terminale while the other two membranes continue on beyond the cord, a needle can be inserted into the subarachnoid space at the level of the fourth or fifth lumbar vertebra without damage to the cord. Indeed, if it were not for this anatomic feature, lumbar punctures and spinal anesthesia would not be feasible.

Cerebrospinal fluid. The *subarachnoid space, ventricles* (spaces within the brain, p. 371), and *central canal* are filled with a watery liquid called the cerebrospinal fluid. Produced by networks of capillaries in the ventricles called *choroid plexuses,* the total volume in a full-grown man is about 130 ml. Qualitatively, but not quantitatively, cerebrospinal fluid resembles plasma and tissue fluid. There are fewer cells and less protein, calcium, potassium, and glucose, for example, than in tissue fluid. However, the concentration of sodium chloride is appreciably greater.

Cerebrospinal fluid, removed by lumbar puncture, is of considerable diagnostic value in diseases of the central nervous system, especially in meningitis, tumors, and syphilis. In these conditions the protein and cell count are elevated. Also, a bacteriologic examination of the fluid may disclose pathogenic microbes.

Spinal tracts. The white matter of the cord is divided by the anterior *fissure,* the posterior *sulcus,* and the *gray* matter into three *columns* (in each half)—the anterior, posterior, and lateral. (Incidentally, it should be noted that the fissure and the sulcus almost "sever" the cord into equal parts.) The fibers that compose these columns are grouped together into tracts, or *fasciculi,* which are named according to their origin and destination. Those carrying impulses *upward* to the brain are called *ascending* tracts, and those carrying impulses *downward* from the brain are called *descending* tracts. Obviously, the former tracts are sensory and the latter motor.

The principal tracts and the nature of the impulses they transmit are presented in Fig. 19-7 and Table 19-1. The student should appreciate that these tracts cannot be seen in cross section; that is, their location and function have been ascertained by experimental procedures in animals and by the study of clinical conditions in human beings.

Spinal nerves. Along its length the spinal cord gives birth to *thirty-one* pairs of nerves (Fig. 19-6) that emerge from the spinal canal via the *intervertebral* foramina (see Fig. 9-8, p. 198). Named according to the

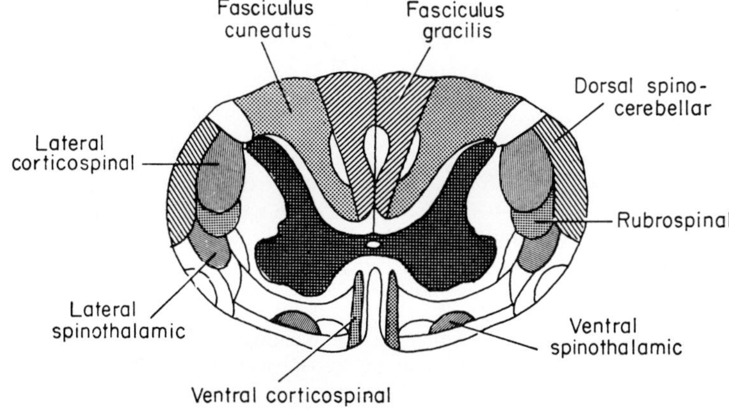

Fig. 19-7. General location of some of the major spinal tracts. Note that the anterior fissure (not labeled) lies between the ventral corticospinal tracts and that the posterior sulcus lies between the right fasciculus gracilis and left fasciculus gracilis. Also, note the central canal in the "central gray" and the slight protrusion of the lateral horns.

Table 19-1. Major tracts of the spinal cord

Tract	General nature of impulse
Ascending	
Dorsal spinocerebellar	Subconscious kinesthesia
Ventral spinocerebellar	Subconscious kinesthesia
Lateral spinothalamic	Pain and temperature
Ventral spinothalamic	Touch
Fasciculus gracilis	Conscious kinesthesia
Fasciculus cuneatus	Conscious kinesthesia
Descending	
Lateral corticospinal	Skeletal muscle contraction
Ventral corticospinal	Skeletal muscle contraction
Rubrospinal	Unconscious muscle coordination
Vestibulospinal	Muscle tone and equilibrium

vertebrae from which they exit, there are eight pairs of cervical, twelve pairs of thoracic, five pairs of lumbar, five pairs of sacral, and one pair of coccygeal nerves. Whereas the cervical and thoracic nerves emerge immediately from the vertebral canal, the others pass down the canal a distance before they enter the foramina. Thus, the lower spinal nerves bring to mind a horse's tail and are appropriately called the *cauda equina* (Fig. 19-6).

It is very important to understand the structure of a spinal nerve and particularly its association with the spinal cord. To this end, let us refer to the somewhat idealized drawing shown in Fig. 19-5. Starting at the cord, we note that the posterior and anterior roots of the nerve arise from the gray matter of the respective horns. Also, as mentioned several times previously, let us not forget that the anterior roots and the posterior roots are composed of motor and sensory fibers, respectively. Just before these roots pass through the intervertebral foramina, however, they join—forming a mixed nerve trunk (the spinal nerve), which then splits into two mixed branches called the *anterior* and *posterior primary rami.* Whereas the posterior rami run uninterrupted to the muscles and skin of the back, most of the anterior rami fuse into complex networks called *plexuses* (Fig. 19-8). And here (at the plexus) there is a rearrangement of fibers so that the nerves or branches that finally emerge possess fiber groupings different from those in the primary rami. The four main plexuses include the cervical, brachial, lumbar, and sacral.

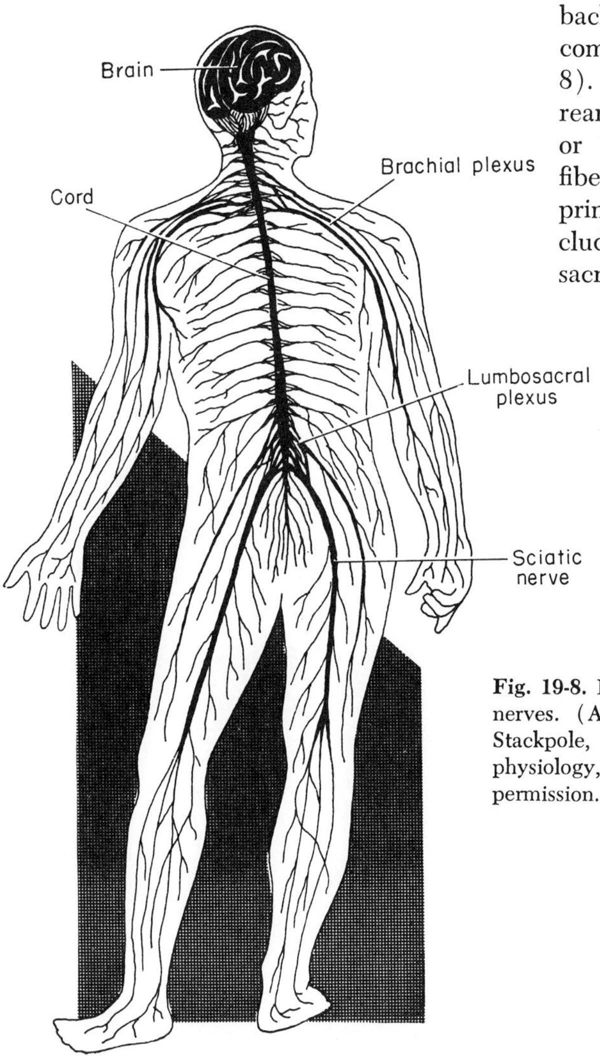

Fig. 19-8. Plexuses and general distribution of the major nerves. (Adapted from Kimber, D. C., Gray, C. E., Stackpole, M. A., and Leavell, C. E.: Anatomy and physiology, New York, 1961, The Macmillan Co. By permission.)

Cervical plexus. The cervical plexus, formed by the anterior rami of the cervical spinal nerves, lies deep in the neck in the area of the upper four cervical vertebrae. Its branches supply the diaphragm *(phrenic nerve)*, the muscles and skin of the neck, and the back portion of the skull.

Brachial plexus. The brachial plexus, formed by the anterior rami of the lower four cervical nerves and first thoracic nerve, lies in the lower neck and axillary region. Its branches supply the skin and the majority of muscles in the neck, chest, and upper extremities.

Thoracic anterior rami. The thoracic anterior rami do not form a plexus. They run along the lower borders of the ribs and are referred to as the *intercostal nerves.* Their terminal endings supply the intercostal muscles, the skin of the thorax, and the skin and muscles of the abdominal wall.

Lumbar plexus. The lumbar plexus, which lies within the psoas major muscle, is formed by the anterior primary rami of the first, second, and third lumbar nerves and most of the fibers of the anterior primary ramus of the fourth lumbar nerve. Its branches supply the skin over the anterior part of the buttocks, external genitals, and thighs.

Sacral plexus. The sacral plexus lies in the vicinity of the piriformis muscle and the internal iliac vessels. It is formed by the fusion of the lumbosacral trunk, the first three sacral nerves, and part of the fibers of the fourth sacral nerve. The lumbosacral trunk, incidentally, is made up of part of the fibers of the fourth lumbar anterior ramus and all the fibers of the fifth anterior lumbar ramus. The branches emerging from the sacral plexus innervate mainly the skin over the gluteal and perianal regions and the muscles of the legs. It is of interest to note that the *sciatic nerve* of the sacral plexus is the largest nerve in the body.

Dermatomes. The nerves entering or leaving the spinal cord at each level innervate segments of the body relating to that level of the spinal cord, and these segments are referred to as dermatomes. More specifically, a dermatome is the area of skin supplied with afferent nerve fibers by a single posterior spinal root. Of considerable diagnostic significance is the fact that loss of feeling in a given dermatomic segment is pathognomonic of the corresponding spinal nerve or cord segment.

BRAIN

It hardly need be repeated here that the human brain is the last word in biologic ingenuity. As the nervous system climbs the evolutionary ladder from the lowly vertebrate to man, the brain is transformed

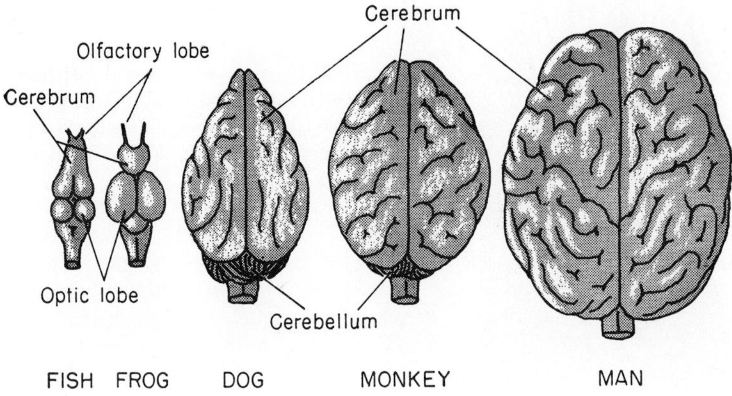

Fig. 19-9. Comparison of the brains of different vertebrates. (Viewed from above.)

from a rudimentary structure to a viscus of grandeur (Fig. 19-9).

The brain, or *encephalon,* is a 3-pound mass of nervous tissue composed of about twelve billion neurons organized and interconnected in a manner that defies description. Mathematicians estimate that an electronic computer with even a fraction of its ability would have to be as large as the Empire State Building.

In the most severe, but perhaps the best, anatomic classification the brain is divided into three *primordial* parts—the prosencephalon (forebrain), the mesencephalon (midbrain), and the rhombencephalon (hindbrain). In turn, the prosencephalon is divided into the telencephalon (cerebrum) and the diencephalon ('tweenbrain), and the rhombencephalon is divided into the metencephalon and the myelencephalon (Fig. 19-10).

Telencephalon. The telencephalon, or *cerebrum,* is the largest and most spectacular part of the brain. Its outer gray surface, or *cortex,* is thrown into convolutions called *gyri,* and it is divided lengthwise into *hemispheres* by the *longitudinal fissure.* Two other fissures—the fissure of Rolando (*central fissure*) and the fissure of Sylvius (*lateral fissure*)—divide each hemisphere into so-called *lobes.* As indicated, the deep grooves between the gyri are the fissures; the shallow grooves are called *sulci.*

Lobes. Each of the two cerebral hemispheres has five lobes. These include the *frontal* lobe, the *parietal* lobe, the *temporal* lobe, the *occipital* lobe, and the *insula,* or the *island of Reil.* As shown in Fig. 19-11, the frontal lobe is before and the parietal lobe immediately behind the fissure of Rolando, and the fissure of Sylvius serves to separate these two lobes from the temporal lobe below. The occipital lobe is the pyra-

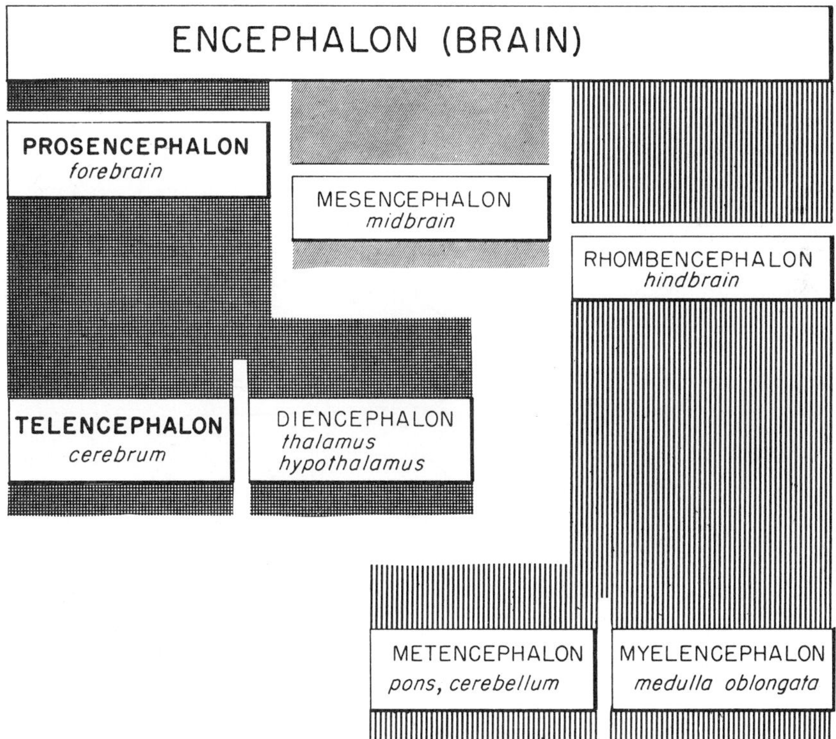

Fig. 19-10. Basic divisions of the brain.

midal portion of the hemisphere lying behind the parietal and temporal lobes.

The insula is located below the lateral fissure and cannot be seen unless the adjacent portions of the frontal and temporal lobes are raised.

Tracts. Whereas the cerebral cortex is made up of gray matter exclusively, the interior contains both gray and white matter. The white matter is composed of countless nerve fibers that run in tracts (Fig. 19-12) in countless directions. Regardless of their great number, however, these tracts may be conveniently grouped into three categories—*associational* tracts, *commissural* tracts, and *projection* tracts. Associational tracts connect different areas of the cortex of the same hemisphere, whereas commissural tracts run from one hemisphere to the other, principally via the *corpus callosum* (Fig. 19-12).

The projection tracts, the longest of the three types, extend from the cerebrum to other parts of the brain and the spinal cord. Depending upon the character of the impulses carried, they are designated as either *ascending* or *descending;* that is, the former tracts convey impulses to the brain, and the latter carry impulses from the cortex to the lower portions of the brain and to the spinal cord. Further, those projection tracts that extend into the cord now become *spinal* tracts. For example, the corticospinal, a descending tract, extends from the cerebral cortex through the brainstem and down into the spinal cord, where it synapses with neurons in the anterior horns; again, the spinothalamic, an ascending

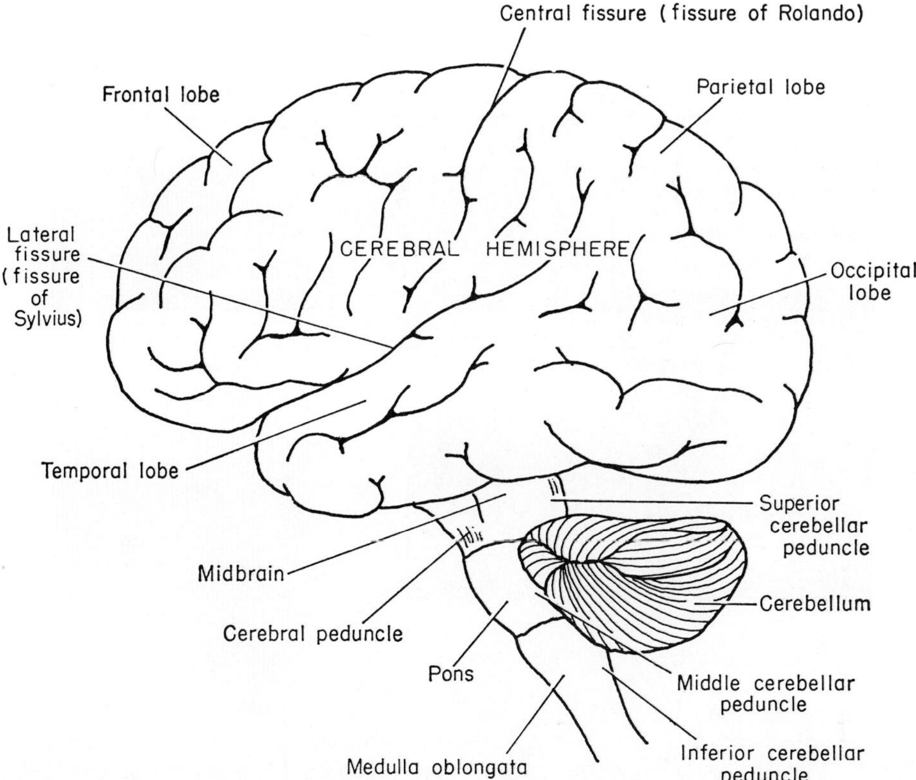

Fig. 19-11. General lateral view of the brain showing the lobes, fissures, and major divisions. (After Quain; from Tuttle, W. W., and Schottelius, B. A.: Textbook of physiology, ed. 16, St. Louis, 1969, The C. V. Mosby Co.)

tract, originates at the posterior horn, runs up the spinal cord, and finally synapses at the thalamus.

Corpus striatum. The collection of gray matter embedded in the white matter of each cerebral hemisphere is called the corpus striatum; this, in turn, is composed of two nuclear masses (or *basal ganglia*) called the *caudate nucleus* and the *lentiform nucleus.* As shown in Fig. 19-13, the former lies medial to the internal capsule, and the latter lies lateral to the *internal capsule.* Though we have a great deal more to learn about these areas, there is consid-

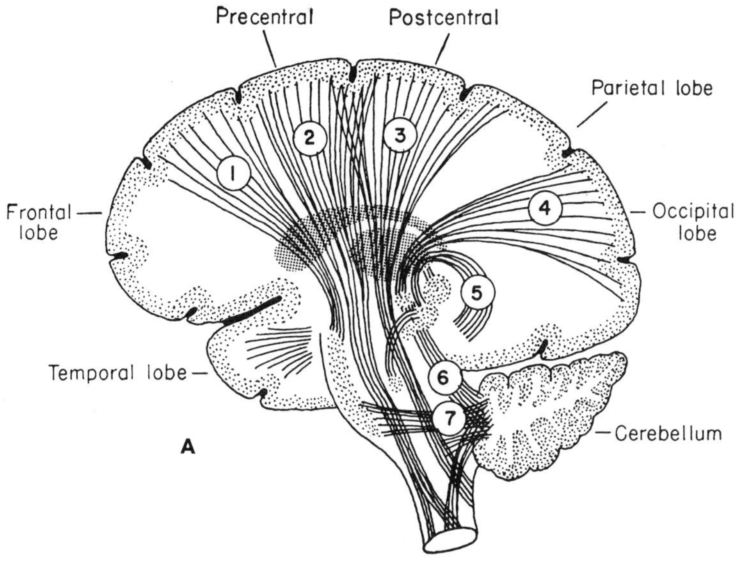

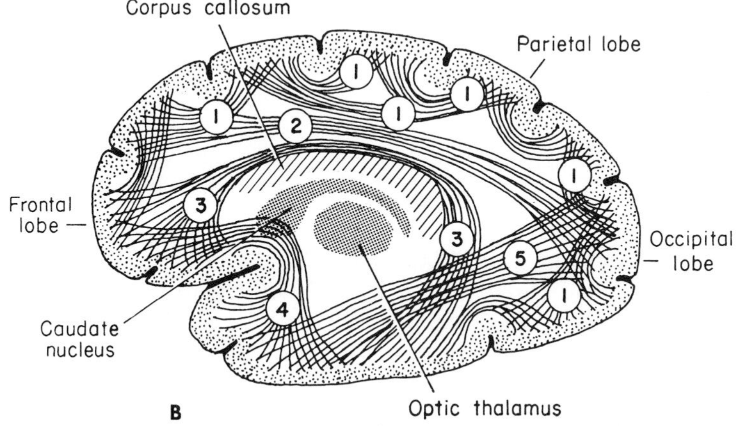

Fig. 19-12. Diagrams illustrating the projection, **A**, and association, **B**, tracts of the brain. **A: 1**, A tract connecting the frontal convolutions with the cells lying in the pons; **2**, a tract descending into the cord after decussating in the medulla; **3**, a sensory tract carrying impulses to the postcentral gyri; **4**, the visual tract; **5**, the auditory tract; **6**, the superior cerebellar peduncle; **7**, the middle cerebellar peduncle. **B: 1**, Tracts between adjacent convolutions; **2**, a tract between the frontal and occipital areas; **3** and **4**, the tracts between the frontal and temporal areas; **5**, the tract between the occipital and temporal areas. In **B** also note the corpus callosum, through which pass the commissural tracts between the hemispheres.

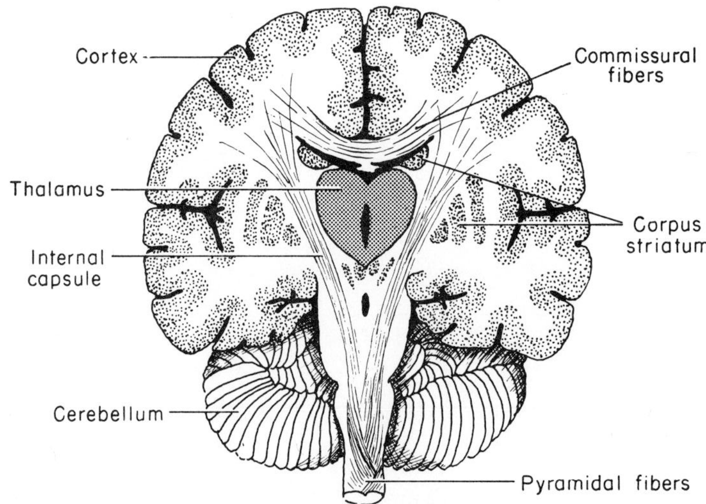

Fig. 19-13. Coronal section through the brain showing the internal structure. The corpus striatum is composed of the caudate nucleus and the lentiform nucleus, which are medial and lateral to the internal capsule, respectively. (Adapted from Best, C. H., and Taylor, N. B.: The human body, ed. 3, New York, 1956, Holt, Rinehart & Winston, Inc. By permission.)

erable evidence to indicate that in some way they are associated with muscle tone.

As shown in Fig. 19-13, the internal capsule is a strip of white matter that passes between the lentiform nucleus and thalamus. Since its tracts (both types) are compressed into such a narrow space, a lesion in this region can cause pronounced damage to the impulses going to and from the brain.

Functions of cerebrum. There can be little doubt that the cerebrum is the seat of that evasive thing we call the mind. Thought, intelligence, memory, reason, and all other mental attributes are fabricated in this mysterious and awesome structure. In contrast to earlier views which held that these attributes were peculiar to the frontal lobes, today most physiologists believe that no one region can be singled out as the most significant. This seems only logical, for mental and intellectual performance is associated with impressions that have been electrically imprinted in all cerebral areas. In short, one may consider the cerebrum a galaxy of sophisticated tape recordings that are integrated and fashioned into intellectual behavior. How this is done, of course, is one of the great secrets of life.

However, the brain has yielded some of its secrets. Animal experiments, especially experiments on apes and monkeys, clinical findings in cases of brain damage, and instrumentation of the exposed cortex in patients under local anesthesia have enabled the researcher to define certain areas of the brain with great accuracy (Fig. 19-14). Mainly, these include the *motor* area, the *somesthetic* area, and the centers of *taste, hearing, smell,* and *vision.* The motor area, situated in the gyrus immediately anterior to the fissure of Rolando, contains characteristic motor neurons, or pyramidal cells (Fig. 19-2), which give rise to the corticospinal (or *pyramidal*) tracts. As we know, these are descending tracts that transmit motor impulses to the muscles and make possible voluntary movement.

The somesthetic area resides in the gyrus immediately behind the fissure of Rolando. Here are received and experienced the sensations of touch, pain, heat, cold, and

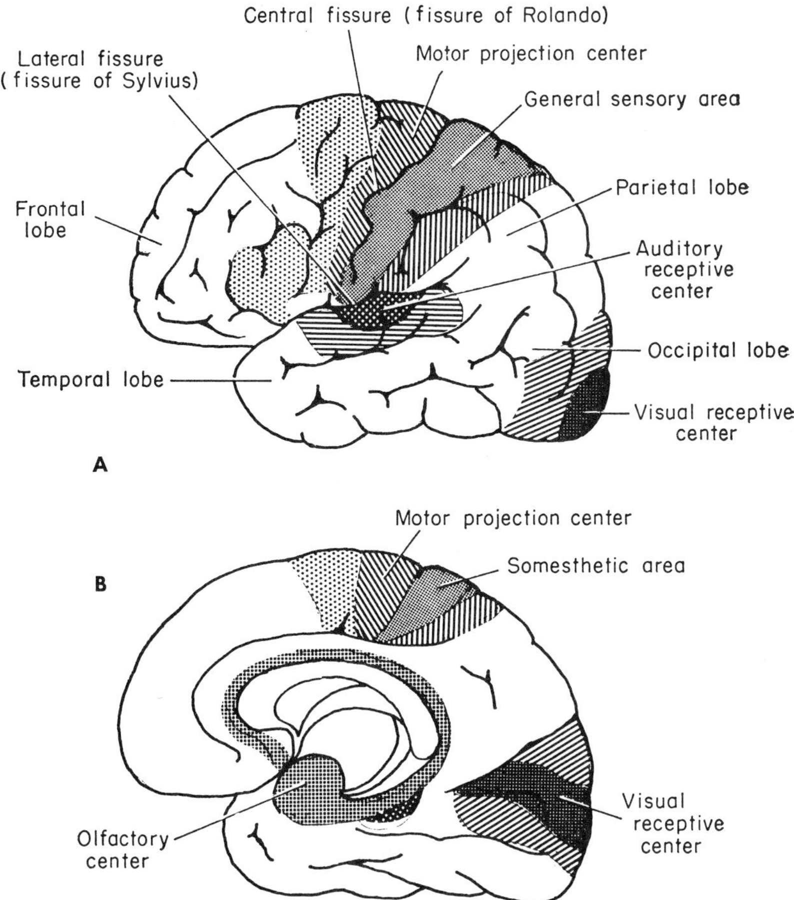

Fig. 19-14. Diagram of the brain showing the various functional areas. **A**, Lateral view. **B**, Medial view.

body movement (kinesthetic sense). At the lower end of the gyrus is situated the *taste* center. The auditory (hearing) center lies in the upper part of the temporal lobe, and the visual receptive center is located on the medial aspect of the occipital lobe. The olfactory (smell) center lies deeper within the brain, in a region roughly adjacent to the anterior pole of the temporal lobe.

Motor pathways. As mentioned previously, the motor impulses that govern skeletal muscle are generated by the pyramidal cells in the cerebral cortex and are carried to their destination via the corticospinal tracts and peripheral nerves. For clinical reasons one should be able to follow such impulses from start to finish.

Motor impulses leave the cerebral cortex via the axons of the pyramidal cells. Such fibers make up the corticospinal tracts of the internal capsule, the cerebral peduncles, the pons, and the medulla oblongata, in that order (Fig. 19-15). At the level of the latter structure these tracts appear on the anterior surface as two well-defined columns called *pyramids* (Fig. 19-13), each of which divides into the anterior corticospinal tract and the lateral corticospinal tract. And significantly, whereas the anterior tracts descend directly down the cord, the lateral tracts cross over, or *decussate.*

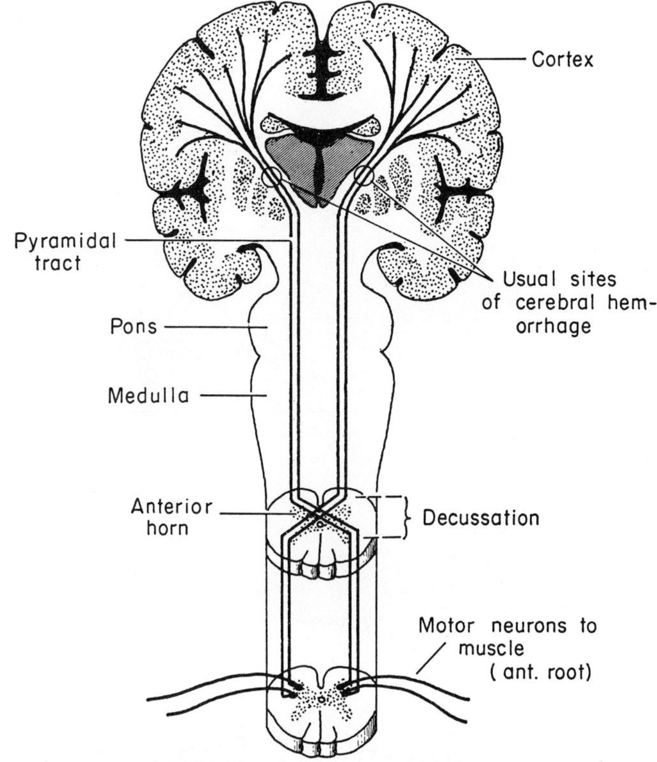

Fig. 19-15. Lateral corticospinal motor tracts.

Finally, the corticospinal fibers synapse with neurons in the anterior horns which, in turn, innervate the skeletal muscles via the spinal nerves. In summary, then, an impulse travels from the cortex to muscle via two neurons—one whose cell body resides in the *cortex* and the other whose cell body resides in the *anterior horn* of the cord. The former is known as an *upper* motor neuron and the latter as a *lower* motor neuron.

From the foregoing it should be quite clear that injury or damage along the motor pathway will result in paralysis. There are four etiologic possibilities: (1) cortical damage, (2) tract damage, (3) anterior horn damage, and (4) peripheral nerve damage. In upper motor neuron damage (cortical or tract damage) the muscles are stiff, or *spastic,* and the knee jerk or tendon reflex is exaggerated. On the other hand, lower neuron damage (anterior horn or peripheral nerve damage) leads to a *flaccid* paralysis; that is, the muscles are flabby and the limbs are uncontrollably loose. Too, the tendon reflexes cannot be demonstrated, and there is extreme wasting of muscle tissue.

Sensory pathways. Sensory axons that travel up the spinal cord via the posterior columns synapse with dendrites in the *nucleus gracilis* and the *nucleus cuneatus,* situated in the lower medulla (Fig. 19-16). The former receives the axons of the *fasciculus gracilis,* and the latter receives the axons of the *fasciculus cuneatus.* The axons that emerge from the nuclear neurons then decussate and ascend to the thalamus through the pons and midbrain as a tract called the *lateral lemniscus.* At the thalamus there is another synaptic connection, and finally the axons from the thalamic

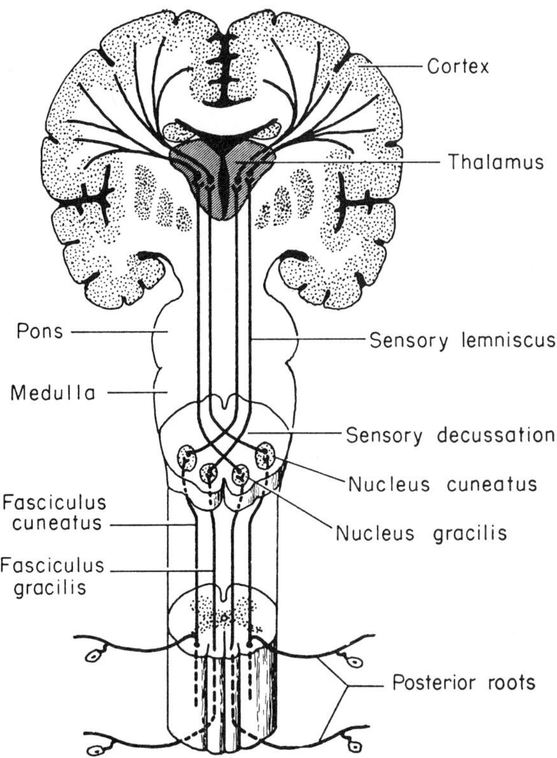

Fig. 19-16. Sensory pathways from the cord to the brain. (Adapted from Best, C. H., and Taylor, N. B.: The human body, ed. 3, New York, 1956, Holt, Rinehart & Winston, Inc. By permission.)

neurons terminate in the cortical *somesthetic area.* In brief, then, the impulse is carried from receptor to cortex via three sensory neurons—the first with its cell body located in the *posterior root ganglion,* the second with its cell body in the *medullary nucleus,* and the third with its cell body in the *thalamus.*

On the other hand, sensory impulses carried up the cord via the anterior and lateral spinothalamic tracts pass through the medulla without interruption. They travel through the sensory lemniscus and then reach the cortex via synaptic connections in the thalamus.

Diencephalon. The diencephalon, or *'tween-brain,* is that part of the prosencephalon situated between the cerebrum and the midbrain and surrounds the third ventricle (p. 371). It is composed of the thalamus and the hypothalamus (Fig. 19-17).

Thalamus. A large mass of gray matter between the epithalamus and the hypothalamus, the thalamus forms part of the lateral wall of the third ventricle. As indicated previously, it is the principal relay center for sensory impulses going to the cerebral cortex.

Hypothalamus. The hypothalamus is a small region of the diencephalon lying immediately behind the *optic chiasm* (p. 395) and beneath the floor of the third ventricle. It is an area that plays a key role in directing the nonmental activities of the body. Apparently, the array of nuclei spread throughout its substance is in one way or other associated with just about every major impulse thoroughfare in the brain. One pathway of established function, the

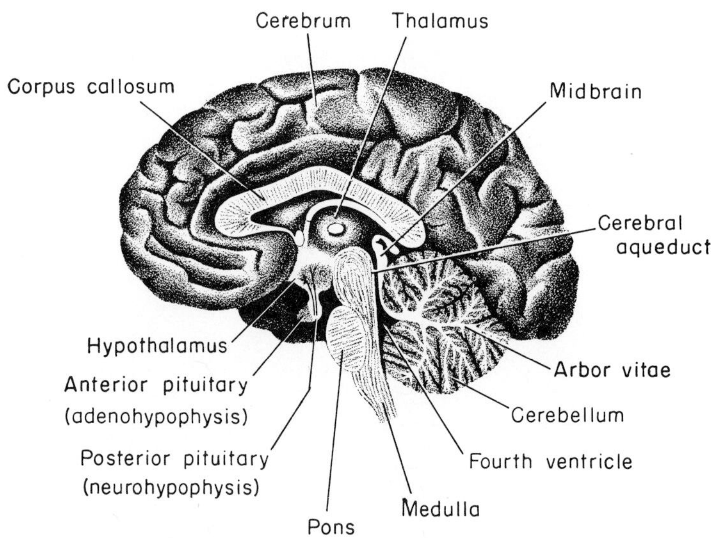

Fig. 19-17. Sagittal view of the right side of the brain. (Modified from Rogers, T. A.: Elementary human physiology, New York, 1961, John Wiley & Sons, Inc.)

hypothalamicohypophyseal tract, governs the neural lobe of the pituitary gland (Chapter 22).

According to recent research data, the hypothalamus is now believed to be the central control area for autonomic activity (p. 372), temperature regulation, fat metabolism, carbohydrate metabolism, and inorganic metabolism. It has also been postulated that this nervous keystone is the appetite-regulating center (or appestat) and wake center.

Another intriguing facet concerns the possible role played by the hypothalamus as the seat of primitive emotions. This can be demonstrated in experimental animals by decortication, or the removal of the entire cerebral cortex. Without the restraint of the higher centers situated in the cortex, the tranquil, friendly cat now spits, arches its back, and bares its claws.

Mesencephalon. The mesencephalon, or *midbrain,* is situated beneath the diencephalon (Fig. 19-17). Its ventral portion is formed by the two *cerebral peduncles* and its dorsal portion, or tectum, by the *corpora quadrigemina.* The cerebral aqueduct (or aqueduct of Sylvius), which connects the third and fourth ventricles, serves to mark off the ventral and dorsal aspects. Although the bulk of the midbrain is composed of white matter, vital areas of gray matter are present in its interior around the cerebral aqueduct and in the region ventral to the superior corpora quadrigemina.

The peduncles, which are composed of both ascending and descending tracts, plunge into the undersurface of the cerebral hemispheres. Functionally, then, as well as anatomically, the midbrain is the main link between the higher and lower parts of the brain. The corpora quadrigemina (the four hemispherical eminences) are reflex centers for muscular movements (for example, turning of the head and eyes) provoked by visual and auditory stimuli. The gray area about the cerebral aqueduct gives rise to the *third* and *fourth cranial nerves,* and the two gray areas (*red nuclei*) in the tectum give rise to the *rubrospinal tracts.* Because the red nuclei receive information from the cerebellum, these tracts carry impulses effecting muscle coordination.

Metencephalon. The metencephalon is composed of the pons and the cerebellum (Fig. 19-17).

Pons. The pons, or pons varolii, is an egg-shaped mass immediately above the medulla (Fig. 19-17) and in front of the fourth ventricle. Its white matter is made up of projection tracts that travel between the cerebrum and the cerebellum; its several small internal nuclei of gray matter give rise to the *fifth, sixth, seventh,* and *eighth* cranial nerves (p. 370).

Cerebellum. The cerebellum, or "little brain," is a large mass of nervous tissue that lies beneath the back part of the cerebrum (Fig. 19-17). Its two lateral halves, or hemispheres, are joined together centrally by a wormlike bridge aptly called the *vermis.* The surface of the cerebellum, or cerebellar cortex, composed of gray matter fashioned into shallow, parallel grooves and ridges, differs markedly from the large irregular convolutions that so vividly characterize the cerebral cortex. Within the cerebellum we find white matter and islands of gray matter, the most important of which are the *dentate nuclei.* These nuclei give rise to axons that travel to the cerebrum, red nucleus, and midbrain.

The sole paths of communication between the cerebellum and the rest of the brain reside in three pairs of tracts called *cerebellar peduncles.* The superior peduncles, composed chiefly of axons that make connections with neurons in the midbrain, relay impulses upward to the cerebrum and downward to the *pontine nuclei* (gray areas within the pons). The middle peduncles are made up of transverse fibers connecting the cerebellum to the pons. Finally, the inferior peduncles, which serve to connect the cerebellum with the spinal cord, carry impulses from the muscles, tendons, joints, and semicircular canals (Chapter 21).

The cerebellum performs its duties below the level of consciousness. These functions include maintenance of proper muscle tension and reinforcement and refinement of impulses transmitted by the motor area of the cerebral cortex. In brief, then, the cerebellum ensures the strength, precision, and smoothness of muscular movements. The truth of this statement is borne out by cerebellar damage. For example, a hemorrhage in this structure usually results in loss of muscle tone, tremors, difficulty in walking, and poor equilibrium or balance.

Myelencephalon. The myelencephalon, or *medulla oblongata,* is actually an enlargement of the spinal cord just below the pons (Fig. 19-17). Since it contains the centers regulating the heart, blood vessels, respiration, vomiting, sneezing, coughing, micturition, and defecation, it is perhaps the most vital part of the brain physiologically. These centers reside in small gray nuclei distributed throughout the interior among the projection tracts. The motor, or pyramidal, tracts, it will be recalled, decussate on the anterior aspect of the medulla. We should also recall that the *nucleus gracilis* and the *nucleus cuneatus* in this structure serve as relay centers for sensory impulses on their way up to the thalamus. Last, but in no sense least, the medulla gives rise to the *ninth, tenth, eleventh,* and *twelfth* cranial nerves.

Reticular formation. In recent years an area of the medulla called the reticular or *bulboreticular* formation has aroused considerable neurophysiologic interest. Composed of a maze of neurons and interlacing fibers that run in all directions from the level of the upper spinal cord to the diencephalon, its chief function seems to be to coordinate muscular activity and to arouse the cerebral cortex via the "wake center" in the hypothalamus.

Sleep. One of the most logical explanations of wakefulness and sleep—a true mystery of the brain—holds that the wake center stimulates the reticular formation, with the latter, in turn, causing an increase in muscle tone throughout the body. As a consequence, the proprioceptors in the

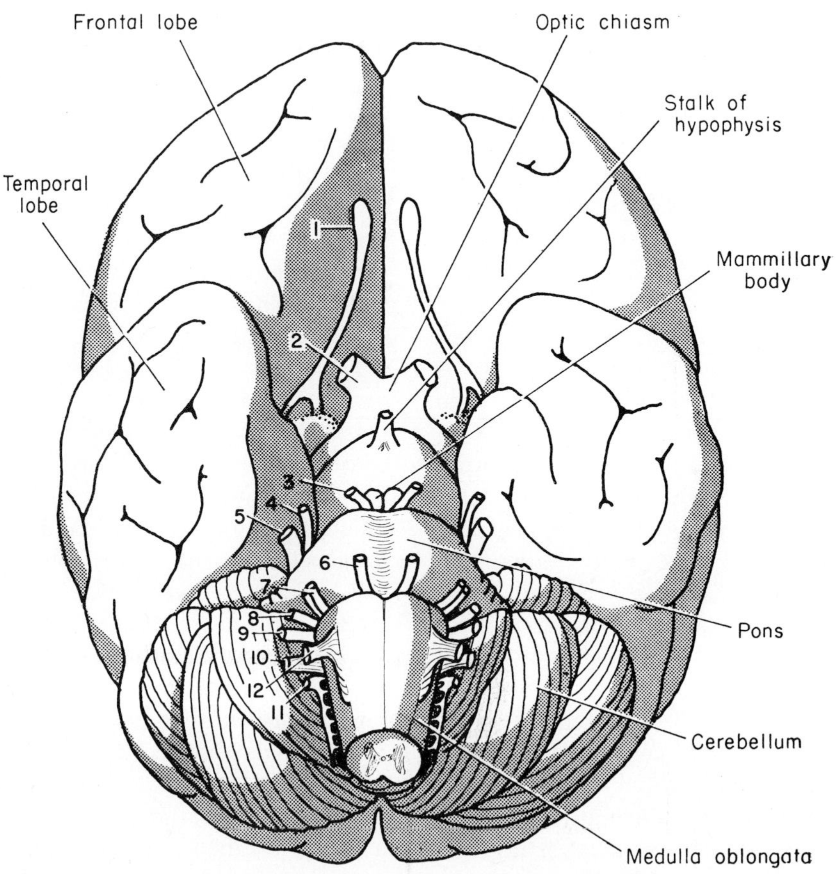

Fig. 19-18. Undersurface of the brain showing the origin of the cranial nerves: **1,** Olfactory; **2,** optic; **3,** oculomotor; **4,** trochlear; **5,** trigeminal; **6,** abducens; **7,** facial; **8,** acoustic; **9,** glossopharyngeal; **10,** vagus; **11,** accessory; **12,** hypoglossal.

muscle respond to the increased tone and transmit sensory impulses to the wake center (via the thalamus), causing the latter to be reexcited. The theory holds that as long as this oscillatory effect (and others like it) continues, we remain awake by virtue of the high degree of neural activity. Conversely, when the oscillatory system becomes sluggish, for example, as a result of fatigue, we fall asleep. Even when we are not fatigued, we can fall asleep if our body is relaxed; that is, if there are fewer sensory impulses feeding into the reticular formation. Indeed, certain other facts about sleep may be explained on the basis of the foregoing theory. For instance, recent work has shown that depressant drugs such as hypnotics and tranquilizers owe their pharmacologic action to their ability to inhibit the reticular system.

Cranial nerves. The twelve pairs of cranial nerves that emerge from the undersurface of the brain (Fig. 19-18) are numbered from front to back according to their function or to the structure or structures that they innervate. In looking over a list of these nerves (Table 19-2), it is of interest to note that the first, second, and eighth are purely *sensory;* the others are mixed—that is, they contain both afferent and efferent fibers. Whereas the cell bodies of the efferent fibers are located *within* the

Table 19-2. Cranial nerves

Nerve	Function
I. Olfactory	Smell
II. Optic	Vision
III. Oculomotor	Eye movements; regulation of size of pupil
IV. Trochlear	Eye movements; proprioception
V. Trigeminal	Mastication; sensations of head and face
VI. Abducens	Abduction of eye; proprioception
VII. Facial	Facial expressions; salivary secretion; taste
VIII. Acoustic	
A. Cochlear or auditory branch	Hearing
B. Vestibular branch	Equilibrium
IX. Glossopharyngeal	Swallowing; secretion of saliva; taste
X. Vagus	Sensory and parasympathetic fibers to major abdominal viscera
XI. Spinal accessory	Motor fibers to shoulder and head
XII. Hypoglossal	Tongue movements

brainstem (that is, midbrain, pons, and medulla), most of the afferent cell bodies are situated in ganglia *outside* the brain.

MENINGES

The three membranes, or meninges, that cover the spinal cord (p. 357) continue upward and envelop the brain. The *dura mater,* the outermost membrane, is a double-layered membrane that serves both as a covering for the brain and as a periosteal lining for the skull. Its inner layer extends between the parts of the brain, forming septa. Two of these, the *falx cerebri* and the *tentorium cerebelli,* are especially prominent. The former is a sickle-shaped fold that runs vertically between the cerebral hemispheres, and the latter runs between the cerebellum and the occipital lobes above. Also, between its two layers the dura mater forms blood sinuses that drain into the jugular veins. The larger of these, the *superior sagittal sinus,* forms the top border of the falx cerebri, and the *inferior sagittal sinus* forms the bottom border.

The arachnoid membrane forms a rather loose investment about the brain and is separated from the dura mater by the *subdural space,* the latter being crisscrossed by a fine network of connective tissue fibers. In turn, the arachnoid membrane is separated from the pia mater by a greater interval called the *subarachnoid space.* In the areas where this space is expanded, the term *subarachnoid cisterna* is used. The largest of these spaces, the *cisterna magna,* is located between the undersurface of the cerebellum and the posterior surface of the medulla oblongata.

VENTRICLES

Within the brain itself are four interconnecting spaces, or ventricles, that communicate with the central canal of the spinal cord and subarachnoid space about both the brain and the cord. The largest are the two *lateral* ventricles, one in each cerebral hemisphere. As shown in Fig. 19-19, the central portion of the lateral ventricle extends into three horns—anterior, inferior, and posterior—which invade the frontal, temporal, and occipital lobes, respectively. The *third* ventricle is a single irregular

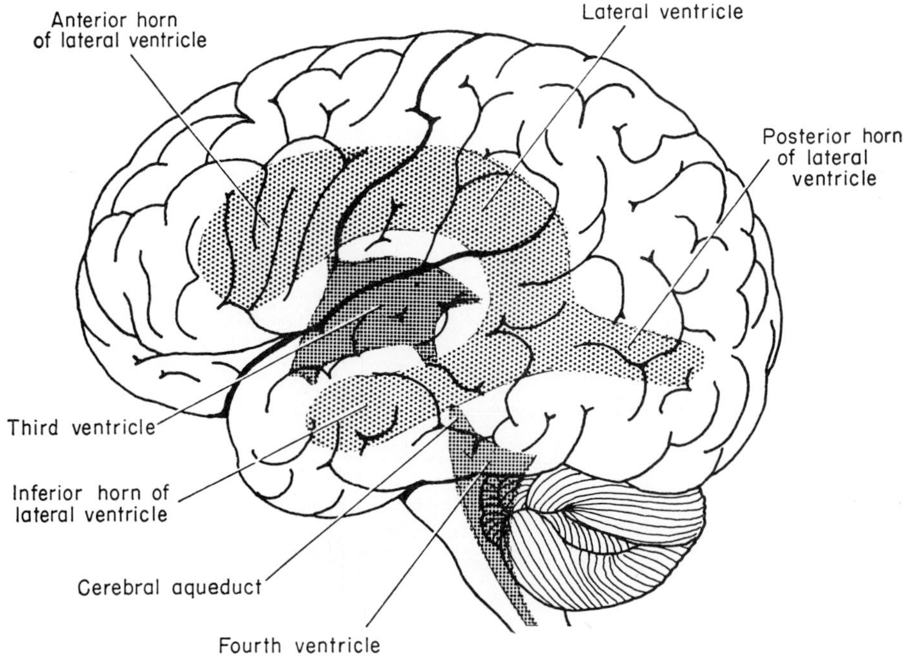

Fig. 19-19. Ventricles of the brain.

space lying below the lateral ventricles and between the two thalami. The *fourth* ventricle (also single) is a diamond-shaped space immediately before the cerebellum.

The *cerebrospinal fluid* (p. 357) collects in each lateral ventricle and then makes its way into the third ventricle via the *interventricular foramen,* or *foramen of Monro.* In turn, the fluid enters the fourth ventricle via the *aqueduct of Sylvius,* and through the three openings in the latter ventricle—the *foramina of Luschka* and the *foramen of Magendie*—the fluid escapes into the subarachnoid space.

AUTONOMIC NERVOUS SYSTEM

The autonomic nervous system (Fig. 19-20) concerns those *efferent* nerve fibers of the peripheral nervous system that transmit motor impulses to the *glands* and *smooth muscles.* In contrast to the nerves that innervate skeletal muscle, autonomic nerves act automatically and *involuntarily.* In short, the autonomic nervous system governs the internal environment of the body. But let us not for a moment assume that the autonomic system is an independent unit, for its higher centers—all situated in the hypothalamus (p. 367)—are right in the path of the impulse traffic to and from the brain and cord. For example, while it is quite true that the presence of food in the mouth provokes salivation automatically, it is also true that merely thinking about lemon juice will often have the same effect. It is well established that peptic ulcer can result from excessive secretion of gastric juice which, in turn, stems from excessive cortical stimulation (from overwork, worry, and the like) of the autonomic centers. The same is true of nervous hypertension and a variety of other disorders.

Thus, the nervous system is all one, and it is wrong to consider one part as functioning independently of another. Provided that we appreciate this fact, it is acceptable, convenient, and helpful to dis-

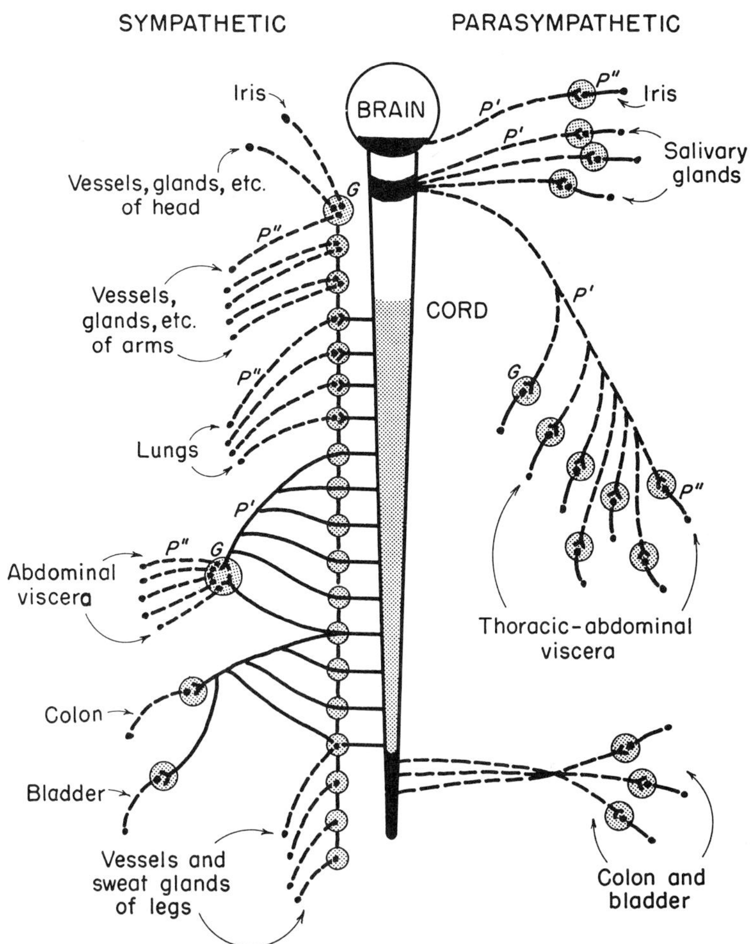

Fig. 19-20. Autonomic nervous system. The gray portion of the spinal cord represents the thoracolumbar region, and the dark portion at the bottom represents the sacral region. Dark areas of the brain represent the midbrain (upper) and medulla (lower). **P′**, Preganglionic fiber; **P″**, postganglionic fiber; **G**, ganglion. (From Brooks, S. M.: Basic facts of pharmacology, ed. 2, Philadelphia, 1963, W. B. Saunders Co.)

cuss the autonomic system as a "separate entity."

The autonomic nervous system may be divided both anatomically and physiologically into the parasympathetic division and the sympathetic division. In general, the viscera receive impulses from both divisions, and with but one or two exceptions their effects are *antagonistic*. For example, sympathetic stimulation speeds the heart, whereas parasympathetic stimulation slows the heart. (Throughout the discussion that follows the student should refer to Fig. 19-20.)

Parasympathetic division. An autonomic impulse originates within the central nervous system and travels to the periphery over two neurons. The "central" neurons of the parasympathetic division lie in the midbrain, pons, medulla, and sacral portions of the spinal cord. (For this reason, the parasympathetic is sometimes referred to as the *craniosacral* division.) The axon of a central neuron runs in a certain cranial

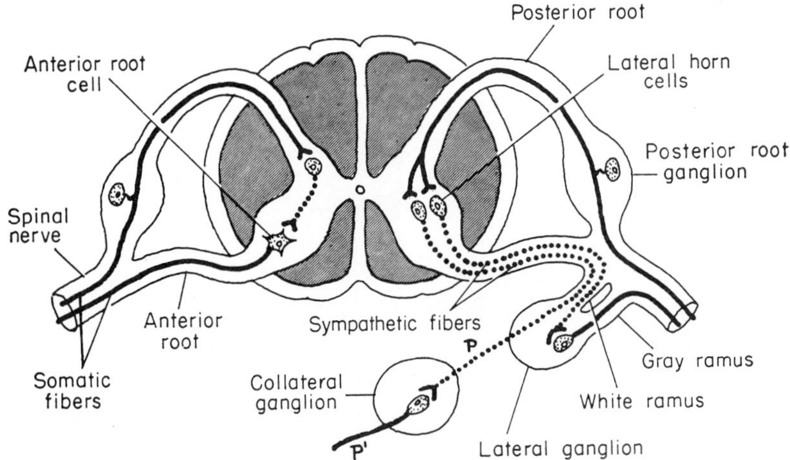

Fig. 19-21. Diagram showing the relationship between the somatic and sympathetic nerves. **P**, Preganglionic fiber; **P'**, postganglionic fiber. (After Gaskell; modified from Mountcastle, V. B., editor: Medical physiology, ed. 12, St. Louis, 1968, The C. V. Mosby Co.)

or pelvic nerve and finally synapses with a *second* neuron whose cell body is located in a *ganglion close to or upon the structure innervated.* The comparatively short axon of the latter neuron finally terminates at the myoneural junction (p. 207). By convention, the axon of the central neuron is called the *preganglionic fiber,* and the axon of the second neuron is the *postganglionic fiber.*

Sympathetic division. In contrast to the parasympathetic division, the cell bodies of the preganglionic sympathetic fibers originate in the lateral gray columns of the thoracic and first four lumbar segments of the cord—hence, the expression *thoracolumbar* division. From these sites the fibers issue through the anterior roots of the corresponding spinal nerves and then via side branches called *white rami* enter the two *sympathetic chains of ganglia* that parallel the spinal cord (Fig. 19-21). Here they synapse with the postganglionic fibers at the same level, pass up or down the chain and then synapse, or extend through the sympathetic chain and become *splanchnic nerves* (that is, purely autonomic nerves) that synapse with postganglionic fibers at the *collateral ganglia.* However, regardless of the path a preganglionic fiber takes, it generally synapses with several postganglionic fibers, thereby provoking a widespread response. This is in contrast to the parasympathetic system in which a single preganglionic fiber makes but a single synapse.

Action. Though the parasympathetic system, like the sympathetic, is always in operation, it prevails in times of quietude; that is, it "concentrates" on such things as resting the heart (Fig. 19-22), keeping down the blood pressure, and digesting food. A summary of the effects upon specific organs and structures is presented in Table 19-3. In looking over these effects, it is to be remembered that a given response is due to *either* stimulation or inhibition

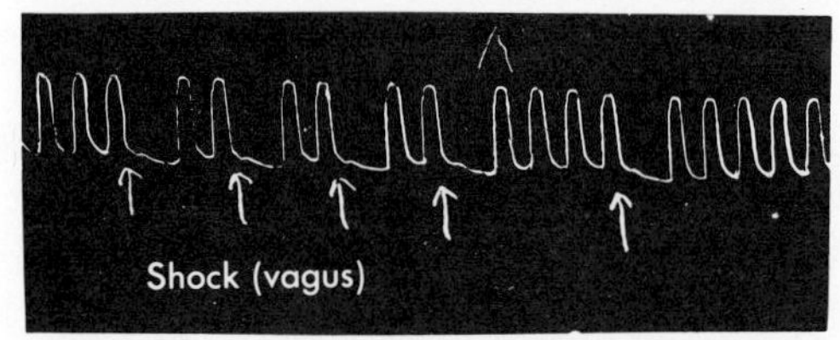

Fig. 19-22. Effect upon the frog heart of electrical stimulation of the vagus nerve. (From Brooks, S. M.: Basic facts of pharmacology, ed. 2, Philadelphia, 1963, W. B. Saunders Co.)

Table 19-3. Autonomic nervous system*

Organ	Sympathetic effects	Parasympathetic effects
Heart	Acceleration	Inhibition
Vessels		
Cutaneous	Constriction	—
Muscular	Dilatation	—
Coronary	Dilatation	Constriction
Salivary glands	Constriction	Dilatation
Pulmonary	Constriction and dilatation	Constriction
Cerebral	Constriction	Dilatation
Abdominal and pelvic viscera	Constriction	Dilatation
External genitals	Constriction	Dilatation
Eye		
Iris	Dilatation	Constriction
Ciliary muscle	Relaxation	Contraction
Smooth muscle of orbit and upper lid	Contraction	—
Bronchi	Dilatation	Constriction
Glands		
Sweat	Secretion	—
Salivary	Secretion	Secretion
Gastric	Inhibition; secretion of mucus	Secretion
Pancreas		
Acini	—	Secretion
Islets	—	Secretion
Liver	Glycogenolysis	—
Adrenal medulla	Secretion	—
Smooth muscle		
Of skin	Contraction	—
Of stomach wall	Contraction or inhibition	Contraction or inhibition
Of small intestine	Inhibition	Increased tone and motility
Of large intestine	Inhibition	Increased tone and motility
Of bladder wall (detrusor muscle)	Inhibition	Contraction
Of trigone and sphincter	Contraction	Inhibition

*Adapted from Best, C. H., and Taylor, N. B.: The human body, ed. 3, New York, 1956, Holt, Rinehart & Winston, Inc. By permission.

of glandular secretion or the contraction or relaxation of smooth muscle. For instance, the reason parasympathetic stimulation causes the bronchioles to constrict is that the smooth muscle in their walls is made to contract. On the other hand, parasympathetic stimulation causes certain blood vessels to dilate because the smooth muscle in their walls is made to relax. The student will just have to accept the fact that the system causes smooth muscle to contract in one structure and to relax in another.

The sympathetic division prevails in times of stress and emergencies. As has been so aptly stated, it prepares the body for "fight or flight." Among other effects, it dilates the pupils, facilitates breathing, steps up the blood pressure, and stimulates the release of *epinephrine.* Interestingly, however, these responses (at least in modern man) are not essential to life. Indeed, in malignant hypertension, sympathetic fibers are sometimes cut (sympathectomy) to relieve the pressure. Completely sympathectomized animals, provided they are properly cared for, live to a "ripe old age." On the other hand, the body cannot get along without its parasympathetic division.

Chemical transmission. One of the most ingenious experiments known to physiology was first performed in 1921 by Otto Loewi. Using a very simple setup (shown diagrammatically in Fig. 19-23), Loewi demonstrated that some chemical substance was the mediator of nerve impulses at the myoneural junction. Not knowing its identity, he called the agent *vagusstoff*. Thus began the era of neurohumoral transmission, one of the most fruitful areas in nervous physiology and pharmacology.

Through the efforts of the chemist, Loewi's *vagusstoff* turned out to be a comparatively simple chemical called *acetylcholine*. Further, it is now known that acetylcholine transmits the impulse across the ganglionic synapses of *both* autonomic divisions and across the myoneural junction at the endings of all nerves *except* the sympathetic nerves (Fig. 19-24). The neurohumoral transmission in the latter case is effected by the release of both *epinephrine* and *norepinephrine*, the latter being the most important.

As explained elsewhere (p. 207), acetylcholine is deactivated by the enzyme *cholinesterase* once the impulse has been passed on to the effector cell. A similar enzyme or group of enzymes perhaps operates at sympathetic endings.

Cholinergic and adrenergic fibers. The English physiologist Dale was the first to employ the terms *cholinergic* and *adren-*

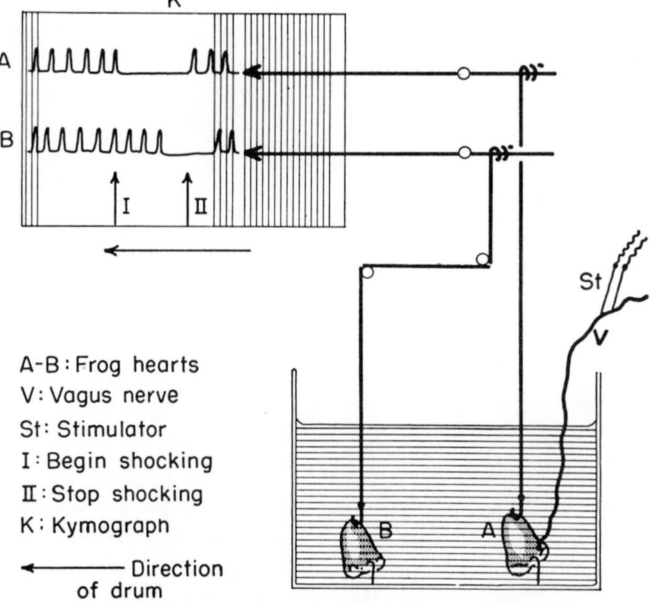

Fig. 19-23. Famous tandem heart experiment. A schematic representation of Loewi's original experiment demonstrating that acetylcholine (called *vagusstoff* by Loewi) is released at the ends of parasympathetic nerve fibers when these fibers are stimulated. Note that stopping of heart **A**, caused by shocking the vagus nerve, is followed shortly by stopping of heart **B**. Thus, acetylcholine formed at the myoneural junctions of heart **A** is carried via the solution to heart **B**. (From Brooks, S. M.: Basic facts of pharmacology, ed. 2, Philadelphia, 1963, W. B. Saunders Co.)

ergic. According to this scheme, *all voluntary* motor fibers, *all preganglionic autonomic* fibers, and *all postganglionic parasympathetic* fibers are said to be cholinergic because they release acetylcholine at their endings. *Postganglionic sympathetic fibers* are said to be adrenergic because they release adrenaline (epinephrine) and noradrenaline (norepinephrine).

Autonomic drugs. The alert student has no doubt been wondering what would happen if acetylcholine or epinephrine were injected into the body. Well, this is easily done, and the effects fit in nicely with the facts just presented. Acetylcholine mimics parasympathetic stimulation (for example, miosis, slow heart, and salivation), and epinephrine mimics sympathetic stimulation) for example, mydriasis, fast heart, and dry mouth). The mechanism of action in both cases is believed to be a direct stimulation of the effector cells at the myoneural junction.

Though acetylcholine is not used in medicine (its action is too short), a great number of related drugs (Fig. 19-25) are em-

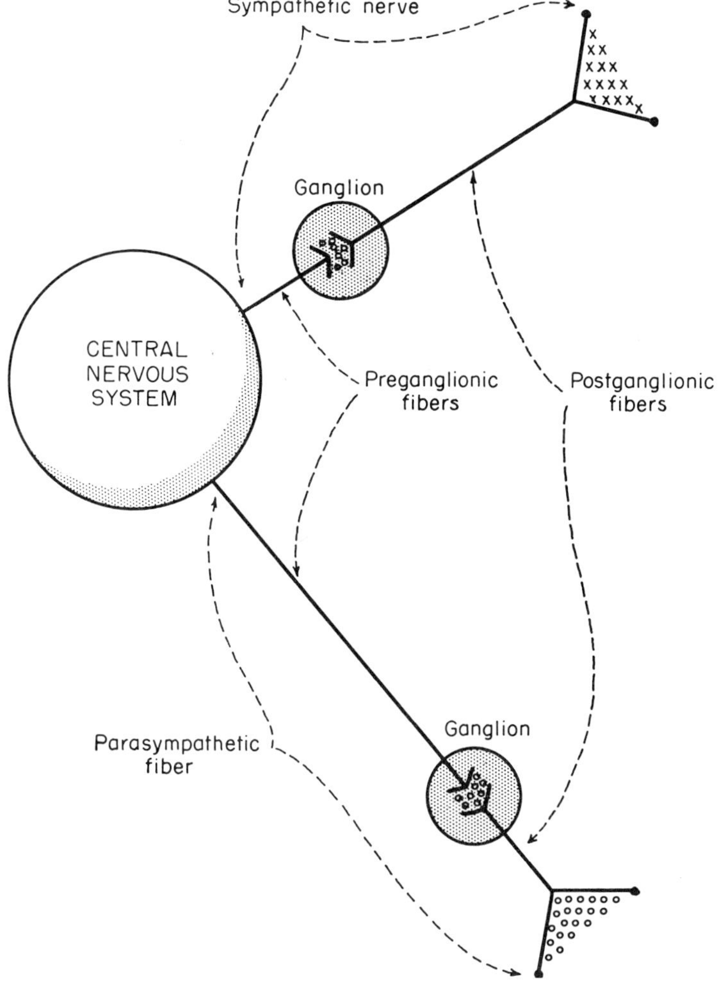

Fig. 19-24. Neurohumoral transmission of autonomic nerve impulses. (See text.) **x**, Epinephrine and norepinephrine; **o**, acetylcholine. (From Brooks, S. M.: Basic facts of general chemistry, Philadelphia, 1956, W. B. Saunders Co.)

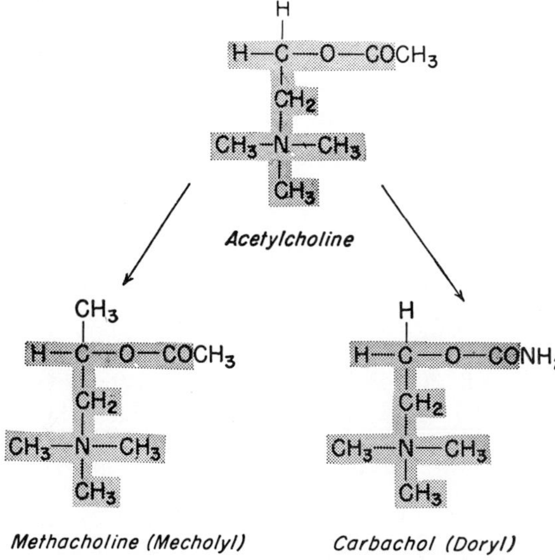

Fig. 19-25. Structural formulas of acetylcholine and two parasympathomimetic derivatives.

ployed for a variety of disorders in which parasympathetic stimulation yields salutary effects. In urinary retention following surgery such drugs as Prostigmin and Urecholine stimulate the atonic bladder. Epinephrine (Fig. 19-26) is used therapeutically in asthma to dilate the bronchioles, norepinephrine is used in shock to raise blood pressure, and so on.

Autonomic drugs that mimic the parasympathetic system are aptly called *parasympathomimetics,* or *cholinergics.* Their sympathetic counterparts are *sympathomimetics,* or *adrenergics.* It is of considerable interest to learn that there are also autonomic *blocking agents,* that is, drugs that inhibit the autonomic system. Drugs that block parasympathetic action are called *parasympatholytics,* and those

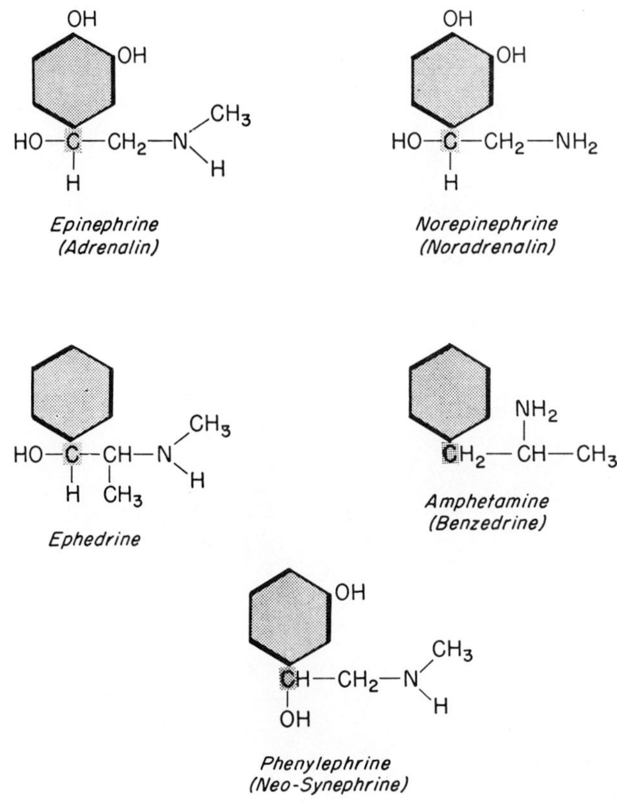

Fig. 19-26. Structural formulas of five sympathomimetic drugs. Note the close similarity.

that block sympathetic action *sympatholytics.* In general, and in a way consistent with what has been said, parasympathomimetic and sympatholytic agents often provoke similar pharmacologic effects, and the *same* is true of sympathomimetics and parasympatholytics. Just a little thought will readily disclose why this is true.

DISEASES OF THE NERVOUS SYSTEM

Any functional or organic disorder of nervous tissue, especially that of the brain and cord, may prove to be extremely serious if it is not corrected. Many times there is little to do other than treat the symptoms and hope for the best. This is always true in pathologic situations in which the damage or injury proves irreversible. In the present section we shall touch upon the highlights of the more important disorders of the nervous system.

Unconsciousness. Unconsciousness is a state of insensibility that is normal only during sleep. It may range in depth from stupor or semiunconsciousness to coma, a profound unconsciousness from which the victim cannot be aroused even by powerful stimulants. Because unconsciousness is a manifestation of an underlying injury or disease, its duration and intensity will naturally depend upon the cause. Among the many and varied causes are simple fainting, acute alcoholism, head injury, cerebrovascular accidents, depressant poisoning, epilepsy, and diabetic acidosis.

Unconsciousness, of course, is an emergency situation. Pending diagnosis of the underlying disorder, and this is obviously essential, the physician must direct his skills toward maintenance of respiration and circulation. This includes such measures as controlling hemorrhage, giving oxygen, and applying artificial respiration. Stimulants are contraindicated unless the etiologic factor is depressant poisoning (opiates, barbiturates, and the like).

Epilepsy. Epilepsy is a chronic disorder of cerebral function characterized by recurrent attacks of altered consciousness, often accompanied by convulsions in which the patient falls involuntarily. Although in most cases no significant underlying cause is revealed, it is believed that a cerebral lesion of some magnitude is always present. This may have resulted from injury or from other morbid processes.

There are five types of epileptic seizure, each with a specific pattern: *grand mal, petit mal, psychomotor, focal,* and *minor motor.* In approximately 70 percent of the patients only one type of seizure occurs; the remaining 30 percent have two or more types. It is most important to understand that most epileptics are normal between attacks. Indeed, three fourths of the noninstitutionalized epileptic patients are mentally competent, and when there is mental deterioration, it generally is related to accompanying brain damage.

The treatment of epilepsy is multidimensional. It includes correction of the causative or precipitating factor, physical and mental hygiene, and drug therapy. The last method of treatment centers about the use of chemical agents that serve to control and prevent seizures. It is of interest to note that drugs which are effective in one type of seizure often fail in the others. Dilantin, for instance, yields good results in grand mal epilepsy but fails to control the petit mal form. This, of course, indicates —and justly so—that the forms of epilepsy just mentioned are of diverse etiology.

Cerebral palsy. Cerebral palsy is a nonprogressive disturbance of the motor system resulting from injury at birth or from intrauterine cerebral degeneration. The most common manifestation is spastic weakness of the extremities, characterized by scissor gait and exaggerated tendon reflexes. In the most severe cases the extremities are stiff and there is great difficulty in swallowing. Though most patients afflicted with cerebral palsy exhibit some degree of mental retardation, this poor showing could well result from difficulty in self-expression.

In addition to drugs to relieve spasticity and control convulsions, if and when they occur, special courses and vocational guidance are essential if the patient is to live out his years in a meaningful way. This is especially true in the milder cases, in which the potential exists for a normal way of life. As indicated, many cerebral palsy victims are much brighter than they appear.

Multiple sclerosis. Multiple sclerosis is marked histologically by disseminated sclerosed or demyelinated patches in the brain and spinal cord; clinically, it is characterized by progressive weakness, incoordination, jerking movements, abnormal mental exhilaration, and disturbances of speech and vision. The cause remains unknown.

The duration of the disease averages between 10 and 15 years following onset. However, the course is highly variable. In some cases attacks are frequent; in others there may be remissions of as long as 20 years or more. At present, there is no specific therapy. The patient is made as comfortable as possible, and the physician may recommend such measures as physiotherapy and psychotherapy. Also, moving to a warmer climate may help. Multiple sclerosis is relatively uncommon in the tropics.

Paralysis agitans. Paralysis agitans, also variously referred to as *Parkinson's syndrome, parkinsonism,* and *shaking palsy,* is a chronic disorder marked by tremor, muscular rigidity, and slowness of movement. The cause is unknown. In addition to the use of skeletal muscle relaxants (for example, Benadryl, Artane, and Pagitane) to relieve tremor and rigidity, every effort should be made to cultivate a cheerful mental outlook and to keep the patient active and busy. The latter approach is especially important, for in most instances the patient possesses considerable potential for many years after the onset of the illness.

Cerebral apoplexy. Cerebral apoplexy, commonly referred to as "stroke," results from one of three possible cerebrovascular accidents—hemorrhage, thrombosis, or embolism. In each instance there is injury to the substance of the brain. The general symptoms, which are immediate, include headache, vomiting, convulsions, and coma (p. 379). The specific symptoms will naturally depend upon the site of the lesion. In cerebral hemorrhage, for example, in which the lesion is usually well within the brain substance, the characteristic manifestations are hemiplegia and hemianesthesia (paralysis and loss of sensation, respectively, of one side of the body).

The specific treatment will depend upon the cause. If the diagnosis is thrombosis or embolism, anticoagulants are indicated in the hope of preventing further enlargement of the clot. General measures include skillful nursing care, chemotherapy, and physiotherapy. In the event that a small vessel is involved, almost complete recovery can be expected sometime within a year, but massive brain damage generally results in death a week or so following the attack.

Tumors. Brain tumors, or intracranial neoplasms, are understandably a serious threat to life. The *primary* growths, that is, those that *originate* intracranially, include tumors of the skull (for example, osteoma), tumors of the meninges (for example, meningioma), tumors of the cranial nerves (for example, neurofibroma of the auditory nerve), tumors of the pituitary gland (for example, adenoma), and congenital tumors (for example, dermoid cyst). *Secondary* (or *metastatic*) tumors generally arise from a malignant growth of the kidney, breast, lung, or adrenal gland.

Because of increased intracranial pressure, most brain tumors have certain symptoms in common, namely headache, nausea, and vomiting. Other manifestations naturally depend upon the site of the lesion. In the main, treatment centers on surgery and radiation.

Infection. The brain, cord, and meninges

are subject to a number of infections. Generally, the causative agent arises from foci elsewhere in the body.

Meningitis. Meningitis, or inflammation of the meninges, is usually caused by meningococci, pneumococci, streptococci, staphylococci, and influenza or tubercle bacilli. The classic signs and symptoms include severe headache, fever, and stiffness in the neck and back. At autopsy there is often a layer of yellowish green pus in the subarachnoid space over the brain as well as a thin layer of exudation over the cord when the disease extends down from the brain.

The most common form of meningitis—referred to as *meningococcal* or *epidemic* meningitis—is caused by the gram-negative diplococcus *Neisseria meningitidis.* Spread via droplet spray from the nose and mouth of carriers and persons with upper respiratory meningococcal infection, this form of the disease has struck one fourth of the population during an epidemic. Diagnosis is based upon the clinical picture and the presence of the pathogen in the cerebrospinal fluid. However, the physician may not wait for a laboratory diagnosis if he suspects meningitis. Provided that the patient is given sulfadiazine or penicillin in the very early stages of the infection, the prognosis is generally good. Also, during epidemics the spread of the infection may be greatly reduced by the prophylactic administration of these agents to persons in the affected area.

Encephalitis. The various forms of encephalitis, or inflammation of the brain, almost defy enumeration. Fortunately, they are *relatively* uncommon in the United States. The chief forms of the disease of an infectious nature include *St. Louis* encephalitis, *eastern* equine encephalomyelitis, *western* equine encephalomyelitis *Venezuelan* equine encephalomyelitis, and *Japanese B* encephalitis. Each is caused by a virus, and the mosquito serves as the vector; for the most part, wild birds serve as the reservoir.

The specific signs and symptoms of encephalitis depend upon the particular type. In general, however, there is usually some degree of headache, fever, muscle pain, stiffness, and delirium. In severe cases there may be convulsions and coma. At this time there is no specific treatment.

Poliomyelitis. Poliomyelitis (also called acute anterior poliomyelitis and infantile paralysis) is an acute viral (Fig. 19-27) infection characterized by fever, headache, stiffness, and flaccid paralysis. However, these signs and symptoms apply only to the full-blown infection. In most instances an attack goes unnoticed, the patient merely complaining of slight malaise, headache, sore throat, and gastrointestinal upset. Contrary to the consensus, less than one fourth of the patients who do develop paralysis sustain *permanent* disability. Although poliomyelitis still strikes chiefly at the younger segments of the population (Fig. 19-28), over the years it has definitely broadened its attack. Whereas 90 percent of the cases in an epidemic that hit New York City in 1916 were in children under 5 years of age, in a more recent outbreak in New England 35 percent of the victims were over 15 years of age.

The poliopathogen is an enterovirus (p. 134) that exists in three immunologic types: Type I (Brunhilde), Type II (Lansing), and Type III (Leon). Authorities now believe that the virus enters the body via the oral route and, having multiplied in the gastrointestinal mucosa, invades the blood and ultimately the central nervous system, where it attacks the cord and/or medulla (Fig. 19-29). It now seems quite reasonable to assume that in a mild case of poliomyelitis the virus either does not pass beyond the mucosa or, if it does, fails to invade nervous tissue.

The introduction of an effective vaccine against poliomyelitis represents one of the great medical conquests of the present century. The Salk vaccine (a formalin-*killed* preparation containing a strain of each of the three types of virus) is any-

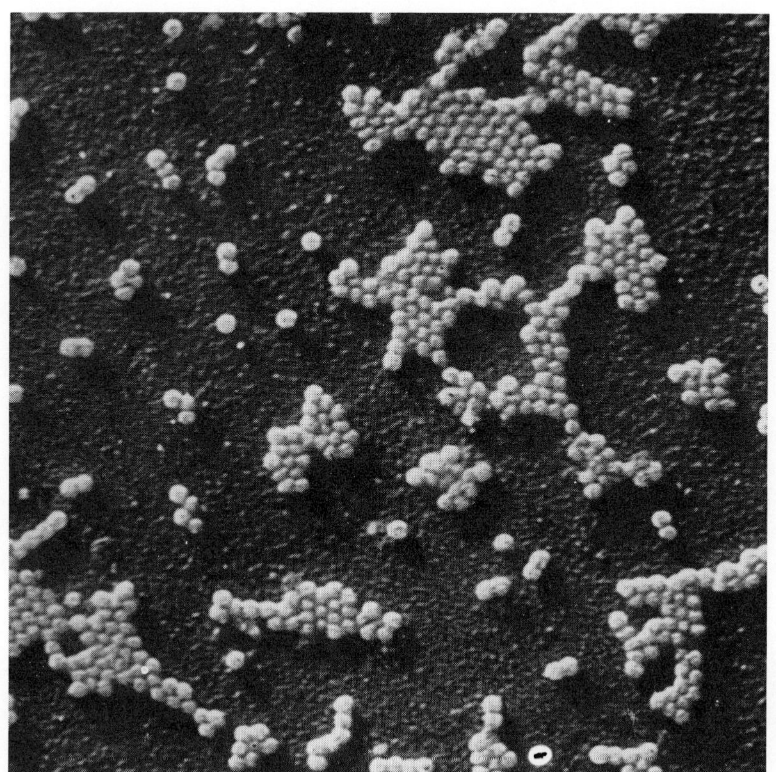

Fig. 19-27. Type 2 poliovirus. (×79,000.) (Courtesy Parke, Davis & Co.)

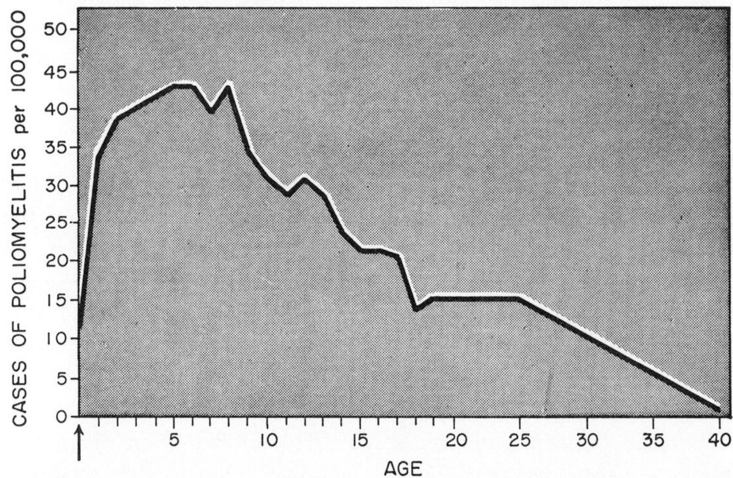

Fig. 19-28. Incidence of poliomyelitis among the various age groups, ranging from under 1 year (at arrow) to 40 years. (From Brooks, S. M.: Basic facts of medical microbiology, ed. 2, Philadelphia, 1962, W. B. Saunders Co.)

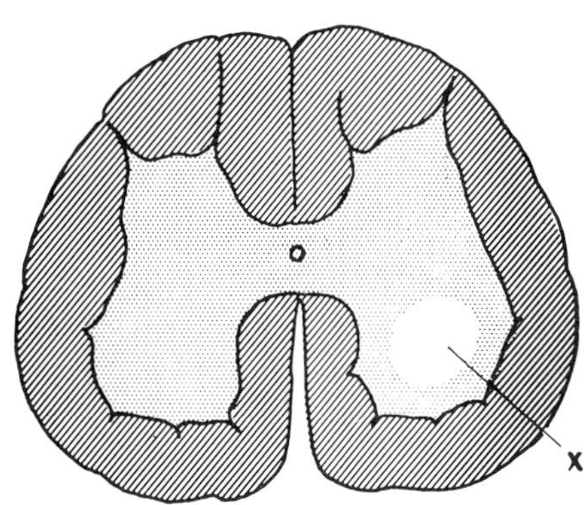

Fig. 19-29. Damage, **X**, to the anterior column of the cord caused by poliovirus.

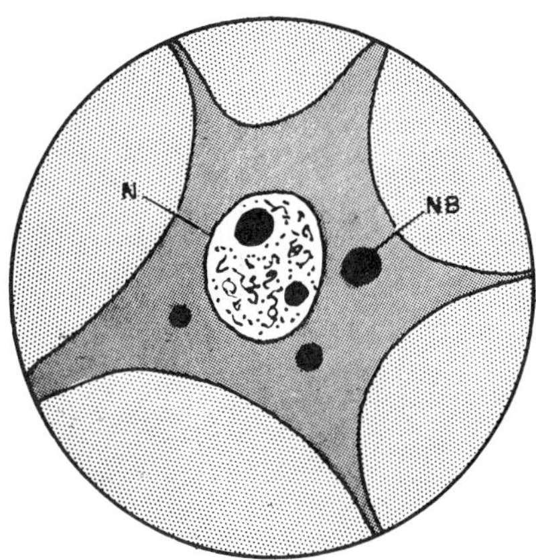

Fig. 19-30. Neuron from the brain of a rabid animal showing Negri bodies, **NB**. **N** is the nucleus.

where from 70 to 90 percent effective in preventing paralytic poliomyelitis. But the oral *attenuated* vaccine (Sabin) has now been shown to produce even better results.

Rabies. Rabies, or *hydrophobia,* is perhaps the most vicious disease of the nervous system. The virus, present in the saliva of rabid animals, is introduced into the tissues as the result of a bite or stratch. Although dogs cause most cases of rabies among human beings, cats, foxes, wolves, skunks, squirrels, bears, and bats are also occasionally responsible.

From the portal of entry the virus travels along the nerves to the spinal cord and then on to the brain. Here it multiplies and invades the vital areas; in "unprotected" persons death is *always* the result. At autopsy, engorged vessels, tiny diffuse areas of hemorrhage, and nerve cell destruction are seen. Characteristically, the neurons in certain areas show cytoplasmic structures called *Negri bodies* (Fig. 19-30), the presence of which represents a definitive diagnosis.

Clinical highlights include an early period of mental depression, fever, and restlessness followed by fanatic excitement and painful spasms in the larynx and throat. Indeed, since an attempt to drink precipitates these spasms, the victim shuns fluid (hence, the term *hydrophobia*).

Any bite or scratch, particularly about the head or on unprotected surfaces (clothing affords some protection), demands immediate attention, for, as indicated, there is no *treatment* for rabies. The wound should be laid open and repeatedly washed with soap and water. This simple but vital procedure enhances bleeding and kills the exposed virus. In the event the animal is known to be rabid or cannot be found, *immediate* vaccination is indicated. Otherwise, the animal is caged and observed by a veterinarian for at least 10 days. If during this time the animal shows signs of the infection, immunization is started by giving both hyperimmune serum and rabies vaccine. *All severe bites,* regardless of the condition of the animal at the time of exposure, call for immediate immunization. Finally, *licks of abraded skin* are to be considered in the same light as actual bites.

Herpes zoster. Herpes zoster, or shingles, is an infection of the central nervous system with cutaneous manifestations. The details of this particular disease were presented earlier (p. 184).

Psychiatric disorders. For the sake of completeness and because one half of the hospital beds in this country are occupied by victims of mental disease, it seems proper that we should at least attempt to classify and define the major psychiatric disorders.

Psychiatry is the branch of medicine that deals with disorders of the *psyche,* or our conscious and unconscious mental life. Basically, such disorders fall into two major categories—those caused by or associated with *damage* of brain tissue and those of psychogenic origin *without* demonstrable physical cause. Mental disorders of the first category can be ameliorated or sometimes even completely corrected by treatment of the underlying organic cause; mental disorders of the second category, however, require the special talents of psychiatry in addition to those of physical medicine.

Mental disorders of psychogenic origin are classified, according to one scheme, into four subcategories: (1) psychoneurotic disorders, (2) psychotic disorders, (3) psychosomatic disorders, and (4) personality disorders.

Psychoneurotic disorders. Psychoneurotic disorders, or *neuroses,* are relatively mild abnormalities in which the symptoms play some compensative or protective role in the patient's mental life. However, and this is important, the neurotic's behavior remains more or less intact. Also, his emotions, thoughts, and impulses seem strange and foreign even to himself.

Characteristic of all forms of neurosis is anxiety. Indeed, the various defense mechanisms employed by the neurotic patient in coping with his anxiety are the basis of the various recognized types of the illness. Hysterical blindness, for example, may occur at the moment a person witnesses an overwhelming act of violence, as when a mother sees a car run over her child.

Psychotic disorders. Psychotic disorders, or *psychoses,* are more profound and far-reaching and the aberrations are more prolonged than in neuroses. There is disintegration of the personality, and the conscious ego is unable to distinguish effectively between the real and the unreal. The two major psychotic categories are schizophrenic reaction and manic-depressive reaction.

The schizophrenic reaction, or *schizophrenia* (formally, dementia praecox), represents cleavage of the mental functions. Characteristically, there are progressive withdrawal from the environment and deterioration of emotional response. In simple terms we may consider the disorder to arise from a personality structure that is unable to meet the demands of adjustment. It is rather startling to learn that over half the population of the public mental hospitals suffer from some form of schizophrenia. Since there is a growing body of evidence that the disorder stems from some sort of biochemical defect, a chemical cure may prove to be an attainable goal.

In the manic-depressive reaction the patient experiences alternating periods of mania and depression. Some patients, however, experience only one phase of the illness; that is, they are either elated or depressed. The manic phase is characterized by verbosity, singing, shouting, frenzied dancing, and the like. The depressive phase may range all the way from downheartedness to frank stupor in which the patient fails to respond to external stimuli. Studies indicate that both hereditary and environmental factors are etiologic possibilities.

Psychosomatic disorders. The realization that mental processes can inflict bodily harm is one of the outstanding developments of modern medicine. In a word, psychosomatic disorders are personality situations in which the defense against anxiety is expressed through the viscera which, as we well know, are innervated by the autonomic nervous system. Since the functions of the central and autonomic nervous systems are integrated, it is not difficult to understand how emotional conflict in the former can physiologically trigger the latter. The upshot is excessive autonomic stimulation and malfunctioning internal organs.

Perhaps the most common psychosomatic disorder is the proverbial "nervous breakdown." In this condition the body becomes overstimulated and extremely tense because of excessive sympathetic bombardment. Another potentially serious variety is peptic ulcer. Whereas the normal gastric mucosa releases just enough juice to deal with digestion, the "psychosomatic mucosa" (as a result of too much parasympathetic stimulation) pours out so much juice that a hole is eaten in the stomach wall. Other commonly encountered psychosomatic complaints include palpitation of the heart, hypertension, constipation, and diarrhea. In each instance the symptoms can be explained by autonomic activity.

Personality disorders. Personality disorders include developmental defects in the personality structure. Since there are no acute mental or emotional symptoms, a person with such a condition may pass through life without realizing his basic problem. Ineptness, poor judgment, social incompatibility, overconsciousness, and sexual deviation are all examples of this category.

Alcoholism. In the United States there are at least two million pathologic drinkers. Moreover, recent studies show that about

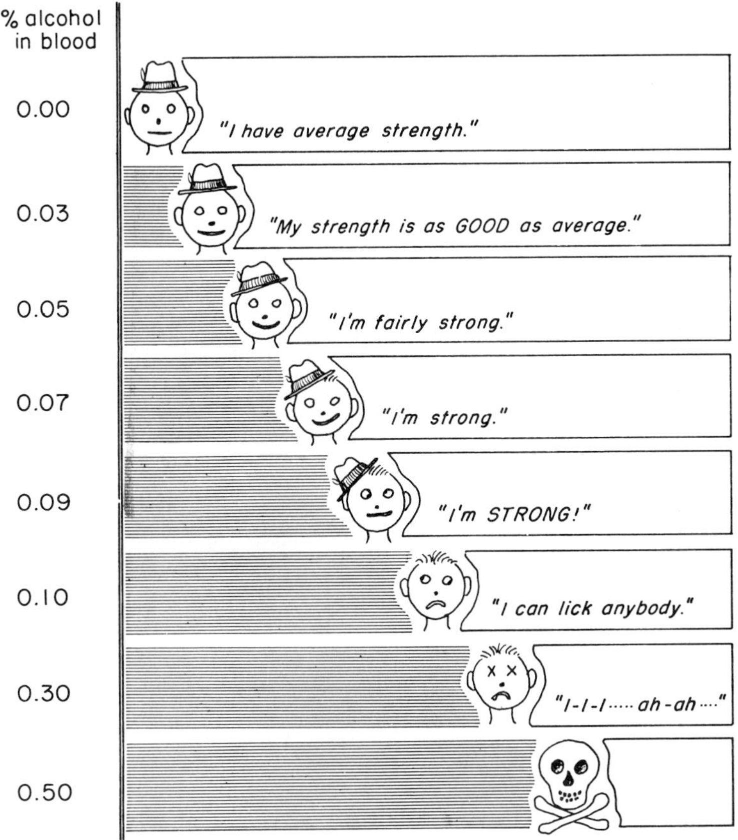

Fig. 19-31. Cerebral effects of alcohol. (From Brooks, S. M.: Basic facts of pharmacology, ed. 2, Philadelphia, 1963, W. B. Saunders Co.)

10 percent of the first-admission patients to mental hospitals belong to the alcoholic category.

In the pursuit of that "wonderful feeling" (Fig. 19-31) many normal persons not infrequently drink until intoxicated. However, relatively few become alcoholics; those who do are persons with personality disorders. Without alcohol, these individuals find it difficult to mingle with people socially and they feel inferior. Generally, they are anxious, immature, and insecure. Alcoholism, therefore, is a form of mental disease that demands the best in the way of both medical and psychiatric treatment.

Questions

1. What is the function of the neurolgia?
2. How does one distinguish between an axon and a dendrite?
3. Describe the structure of the perikaryon.
4. Of what value is chromatolysis in the study of the nervous system?
5. Describe the regeneration of a nerve fiber.
6. How are neurons classified on the basis of structure? On the basis of function?
7. Distinguish between a receptor and an effector.
8. What is a tract?
9. What are the essential features of the membrane theory?
10. Explain the manner in which a nerve impulse originates and runs along a nerve fiber.
11. How would you demonstrate the all-or-none law?
12. How would you demonstrate wave summation?
13. What is meant by the refractory period?
14. Compare the impulse velocity of a myelinated and a nonmyelinated nerve fiber.
15. Describe the parts and function of a simple reflex.
16. Distinguish between divergence and convergence.
17. What is meant by an ipsilateral reflex arc?
18. Explain the difference between the central inhibitory state and the central excitatory state.
19. How are reflexes classified?
20. Cite several good examples of a conditioned reflex.
21. Describe the gross anatomy of the spinal cord.
22. Discuss the structure and function of the gray matter of the spinal cord.
23. Describe the meninges.
24. Name some of the more important spinal tracts and state their function.
25. How can one tell from its name whether a tract is motor or sensory?
26. Describe the structure of a typical spinal nerve.
27. What is a plexus?
28. Distinguish among the terms *sulcus, gyrus,* and *fissure.*
29. Distinguish between an associational tract and a commissural tract.
30. What is the function of the corpus callosum?
31. Discuss the structure and function of the corpus striatum.
32. What is the function of the somesthetic area of the cerebrum?
33. State the function of the pyramidal tracts.
34. Compare spastic paralysis and flaccid paralysis relative to etiology.
35. Locate and state the function of the thalamus.
36. Locate and state the function of the hypothalamus.
37. Give the location, structure, and function of the mesencephalon.
38. What is the metencephalon?
39. Describe the gross anatomy of the cerebellum and briefly discuss its functions.
40. Give the location, structure, and function of the medulla oblongata.
41. What would be the result of injury to the fifth cranial nerve?
42. Most nerves are "mixed." Explain.
43. Describe the structure and function of the cerebral ventricles.
44. Compare the anatomy of the sympathetic and parasympathetic nervous systems.
45. Compare the purpose of the two autonomic systems.
46. Explain how fear can "dry" the mouth.
47. Explain why miosis and excessive salivation occur during sleep.
48. When a solution of atropine sulfate is instilled in the eye, mydriasis results. Explain the mechanism of action.
49. Explain the mechanism of action of miotic drugs.
50. What is meant by the terms *adrenergic* and *cholinergic?*
51. Compare the physiologic effects of acetylcholine and norepinephrine.
52. The use of cholinergic drugs by asthmatic patients is potentially dangerous. Why?
53. Discuss what happens when the nerve impulse arrives at the myoneural junction of a parasympathetic fiber.

54. Discuss unconsciousness relative to cause and treatment.
55. Discuss epilepsy relative to cause, clinical picture, and therapy.
56. Compare cerebral palsy and multiple sclerosis.
57. A cerebrovascular accident of the right hemisphere results in hemiplegia of the left side. Explain.
58. Describe the pathogens commonly encountered in meningitis.
59. Describe the morphology and staining characteristics of *Neisseria meningitidis*.
60. Discuss the cause, clinical picture, treatment, and prevention of poliomyelitis.
61. State the cause, diagnosis, and treatment of rabies.
62. Distinguish between psychoses and neuroses.
63. What is "dementia praecox?"
64. Cite three commonly encountered psychosomatic disorders and account for the signs and symptoms.
65. Discuss alcoholism relative to the underlying cause(s) and treatment.

Chapter 20

The eye

The eyes are the organs of vision. They are spherical in shape (about 1 inch in diameter), with a clear circular window (the cornea) in front to permit the entrance of light. The optic nerve, which issues from the posterior pole of the eyeball, carries impulses from the retina (the light-sensitive tissue of the eye) to the brain. Except for the small area that is exposed anteriorly the eye is enclosed in a bony socket of the skull (the orbital cavity, or orbit) and, as further protection, embedded in the loose fat that "lines" the orbital cavity.

Inserted about the circumference of the eyeball are six small muscles that originate at the back part of the orbit. By their contractions they permit the eye to turn and roll about in its fatty bed. Other structures associated with the eye include the eyelids, the lacrimal glands, and the lacrimal ducts.

COATS OF THE EYE

The eyeball is composed of three coats—outer, middle, and inner (Fig. 20-1). The outer or *sclerotic* coat (sclera), the tough white supporting tunic composed of dense fibrous tissue, covers the entire eyeball except in front, where it becomes the cornea. Part of the sclera is seen as the white of the eye. The middle or *choroid* coat (the choroid) is a dark brown vascular layer that nourishes the retina and lens. Anteriorly, in the vicinity behind the cornea, this coat becomes the *iris* and the *ciliary body.*

Retina. In a sense the retina, the innermost coat, is the heart of the eye, for it is here that light is converted into nerve impulses that make their way to the brain via the optic nerve. This highly specialized structure, formed by the "expansion" of the optic nerve, consists of ten microscopic layers, of which the pigment layer is the outermost and the layer of nerve fibers the innermost. The layer of *rod* and *cone* cells adjacent to the pigment layer is now known to be the light-sensitive layer of the retina. The biochemistry of this particular layer has been explored in great detail and has yielded much to our knowledge of vision (p. 364).

Macula lutea. The macula lutea (yellow spot) is an oval depression on the retina temporal to the entrance of the optic nerve and the retinal blood vessels (Fig. 20-2). In the center of this area is a tiny depression (about 0.5 mm. across) called the *fovea centralis.* It is upon this

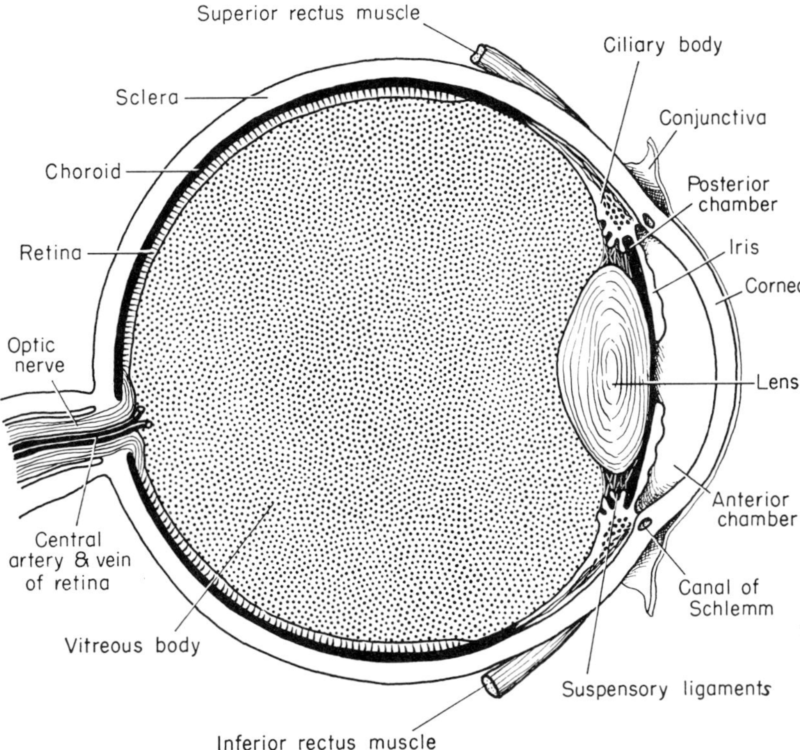

Fig. 20-1. Section through the eye showing the major anatomic features.

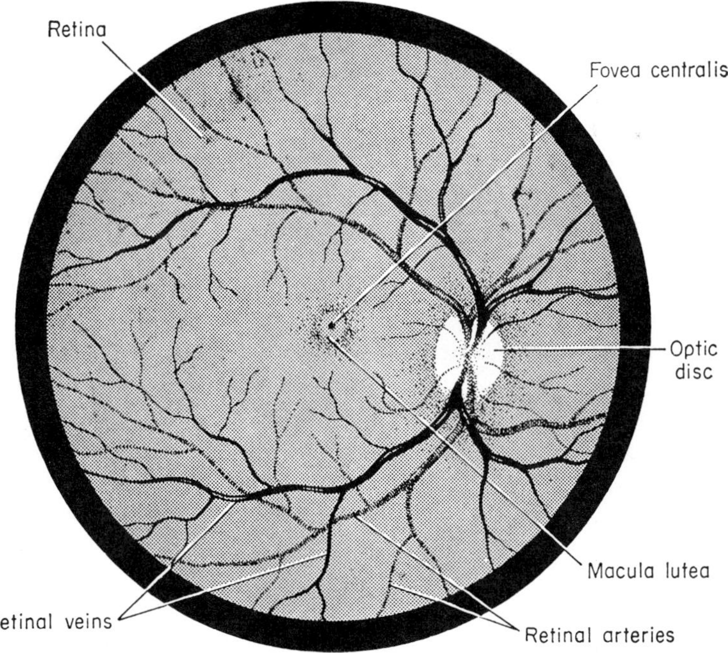

Fig. 20-2. Fundus (eyegrounds) of the right eye as seen with the ophthalmoscope.

tiny spot that the eye bends its every effort to focus the objects of the outside world, because here the retina is the most sensitive to daylight and color. The fovea centralis is made up exclusively of cone cells, but farther and farther from the fovea centralis the cones progressively decrease and the rods progressively increase.

These facts can be vividly demonstrated by two simple experiments. If we focus our eyes on a single object, say the tip of a pencil, other objects not in the line of vision become vague and colorless. This is because only the object that we are concentrating on is striking dead center at the fovea centralis. All other objects in the visual field are forming images peripheral to the "retinal bull's-eye." The second experiment is best performed out-of-doors at night. Looking up at the heavens, one will discover that more stars come into view when the eyes are moved to the side than when they are fixed straight ahead. This shows that the rods, which are more sensitive to dim light (night light) than the cones, are concentrated in the retinal periphery, away from the fovea centralis.

Optic disc. The optic disc, a white spot in the fundus medial to the macula lutea, corresponds to the entrance of the optic nerve (Fig. 20-2). Since there is no retina in this area, it is actually a "blind spot" (Fig. 20-3).

Cornea. The cornea, the transparent structure of the anterior part of the eye, may be considered a derivative of the sclerotic coat. Although it is as clear as glass, microscopic examination discloses a heterogeneous structure. As a matter of fact, four layers are recognized: the outer corneal epithelium (continuous with the conjunctiva), the substantia propria, the elastic propria, and the endothelium of the anterior chamber, in that order.

Fig. 20-3. Demonstrating the blind spot. With the left eye closed, hold the figure about 12 inches in front of the right eye and, focusing on the white disc, slowly move the book toward the eye until the cross disappears. When this occurs, the image of the cross falls upon the optic disc, or blind spot.

Iris. The iris, the colored doughnut-shaped structure behind the cornea, derives from the choroid coat. It is composed of smooth muscle arranged in such a manner that the *pupil*—the hole in the doughnut—narrows or widens, depending upon whether the circular fibers or the radial fibers are contracted. Two delicate nerves, the constrictor and the dilator, innervate the circular and radial muscles, respectively. In strong light the constrictor nerve (a *parasympathetic* nerve) predominates, producing constriction of the pupil (*miosis*); in dim light the dilator nerve (a *sympathetic* nerve) predominates, producing dilatation of the pupil (*mydriasis*). Thus, the iris controls the amount of light that enters the eye, much like the diaphragm of a camera. Also, when looking at near objects, the pupils narrow to sharpen the image (p. 394).

Ciliary body. The ciliary body, also a structure derived from the choroid coat, is situated about the interior periphery of the iris (Fig. 20-1). It is composed of the ciliary muscle and the ciliary process, the latter giving rise to the suspensory ligament that inserts into the capsule enclosing the lens. The engineering is such that contraction of the ciliary muscle pulls the ciliary process slightly *forward*, thereby *relieving* tension on the suspensory ligament and the "squeeze" on the lens. The lens, being elastic, now assumes a more convex shape. Conversely, when the ciliary muscle relaxes, the ciliary process *falls back, increasing* the tension on the capsule and compressing the lens. As we shall see, this "thinning" and "thickening" of the lens permits the eye to focus upon far and near objects, respectively.

Lens. The lens, or crystalline lens, is a glass-clear biconvex elastic disc suspended behind the iris (Fig. 20-1). As already explained, it is enclosed in a transparent capsule and held in position by the suspensory ligament. The lens serves as the major element in focusing (p. 393).

Cavities. The eyeball is divided into the *anterior* and the *posterior* cavities. The latter is the larger of the two and is filled with a clear jellylike substance called the *vitreous humor* (Fig. 20-1). The anterior cavity, which lies before the lens, is subdivided into the anterior and posterior *chambers.* The former is the space between the cornea and the iris, and the latter is the space behind the iris. As shown in the illustration, they are interconnected via the pupil and are filled with a watery fluid called the *aqueous humor.*

Canal of Schlemm. The canal of Schlemm is a tiny channel that circumscribes the cornea (Fig. 20-1). The aqueous humor, produced by filtration from the capillaries in the ciliary body and iris, enters the canal via the *trabecular meshwork* (Fig. 20-10). The importance of this drainage system in glaucoma will be discussed later in this chapter.

MUSCLES

The eyes are equipped with a marvelous muscular system. The *intrinsic* muscles, that is, the smooth muscles in the ciliary body and iris, have been discussed previously. The *extrinsic* muscles are of the skeletal type and are under voluntary control. These six muscles, which originate in the bone of the orbit and insert into the sclera, include the superior rectus, inferior rectus, lateral rectus, medial rectus, superior oblique, and inferior oblique (Fig. 20-4). The desired movement of the eye is accomplished by the reciprocating action of the opposing muscles. For example, if we wish to look up, the superior rectus muscles are contracted and the inferior rectus muscles are relaxed; the opposite occurs when we look down.

Whereas the intrinsic muscles are inner-

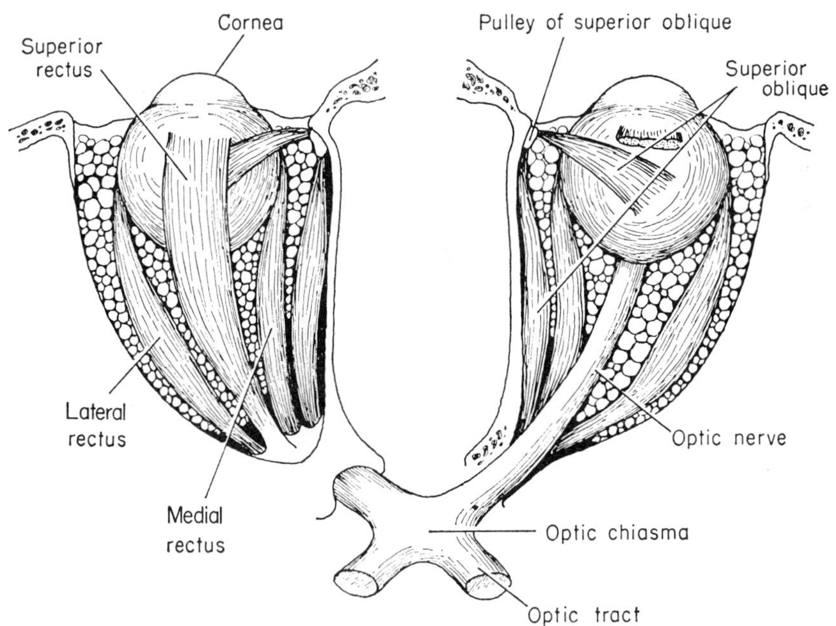

Fig. 20-4. Diagram showing four of the six extrinsic muscles. The inferior rectus and inferior oblique muscles are situated below the eyeball. (Redrawn from Tuttle, W. W., and Schottelius, B. A.: Textbook of physiology, ed. 16, St. Louis, 1969, The C. V. Mosby Co.)

vated by *autonomic* fibers (of the third and fourth cranial nerves), the extrinsic muscles receive *somatic* fibers (via the third, fourth, and sixth cranial nerves).

ACCESSORY STRUCTURES

Aside from the eyeball proper and its associated extrinsic muscles, there are certain accessory structures that have to do with the workings of the eyes. These include the eyelids, the lacrimal apparatus, and the eyebrows.

Eyelids. The eyes are protected in front by the eyelids, or *palpebrae,* two movable folds of skin containing skeletal muscle and a border of thick connective tissue (the tarsal plate), from which project the eyelashes. There are a number of small sweat and sebaceous (meibomian) glands in the lids that empty by minute openings along the free margin. Though we generally consider the eyelashes a cosmetic element, they do serve as a valuable device against the entrance of foreign bodies.

The inside surfaces of the eyelids are lined with a transparent mucous membrane, the *conjunctiva,* which also continues over the surface of the eyeball. Any inflammation of this membrane, a fairly common occurrence, is referred to as *conjunctivitis.*

The upper and lower eyelids join at the corners to form an angle called the *canthus* (the inner or medial canthus and the outer or lateral canthus). The opening between the lids, the *palpebral fissure,* extends between the canthi. It is of interest that the width of the fissure ordinarily determines the apparent size of the eye. In other words, "those great big beautiful eyes" are due not to the size of the eyeballs but to the fact that the eyelids are naturally held wide apart. Conversely, the person with "small eyes" owes this feature to a narrow palpebral fissure.

Lacrimal apparatus. The lacrimal apparatus is composed of the lacrimal glands, lacrimal ducts, lacrimal canaliculi, lacrimal sacs, and nasolacrimal ducts (Fig. 20-5). The glands reside in a depression of the frontal bone at the upper, outer margin of the orbit. Several short ducts, the lacrimal

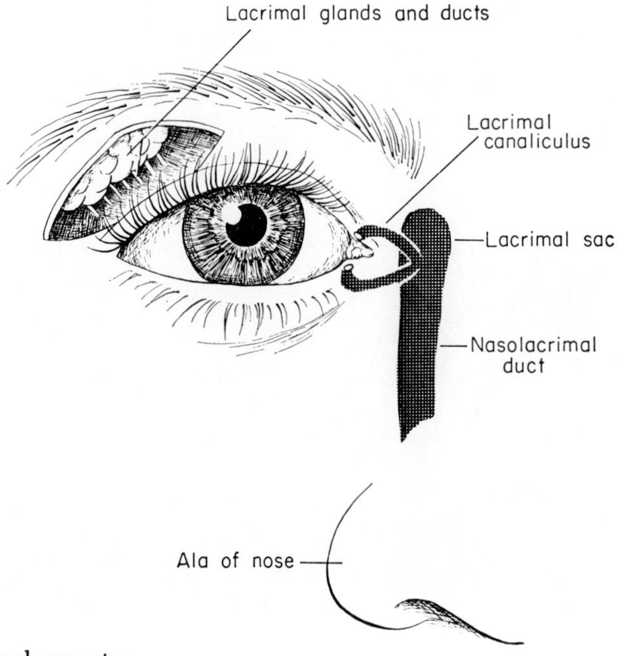

Fig. 20-5. Lacrimal apparatus.

ducts, lead the tears from these glands onto the surface of the conjunctiva. In addition to moistening the exterior part of the eye and lubricating the eyelids, the tear secretions wash down any debris upon the surface into the conjunctival trough, or sac, between the lower lid and the eyeball. As soon as the secretions start to accumulate, they are drained away into the inferior nasal meatus of the nose via the lacrimal canaliculus, the lacrimal sac, and the nasolacrimal duct, in that order.

We are unhappily reminded of this unique drainage system during a "head cold." As a result of nasal inflammation, the nasolacrimal ducts become plugged and squeezed, thereby obstructing the flow of tears into the nose and producing watering of the eyes.

Crying, of course, is something else again. We can only speculate concerning its purpose. Perhaps crying occurs because sorrowful experiences are often allied with danger and the body is mustering all its defenses; that is, the tears are called forth to wash out and refresh the eye for "come what may."

FOCUSING

Vision, or the act of seeing, results from the reception of nerve impulses at the visual areas of the cerebral cortex. These impulses are sent out by the rods and cones of the retina, in response to light, and carried to the brain via the optic nerve. In order for this precious experience to be meaningful, however, light rays must be *focused* upon the retina. Essentially, this entails three separate physical acts—refraction, constriction of the pupil, and convergence. Let us consider each one of these in some detail.

Refraction. Refraction, or the bending of light rays, occurs when light passes from one medium into another (p. 39). In the case of the eye, light rays are refracted three times: at the anterior surface of the cornea, at the anterior surface of the lens, and at the interface of the posterior surface of the lens and vitreous humor. In

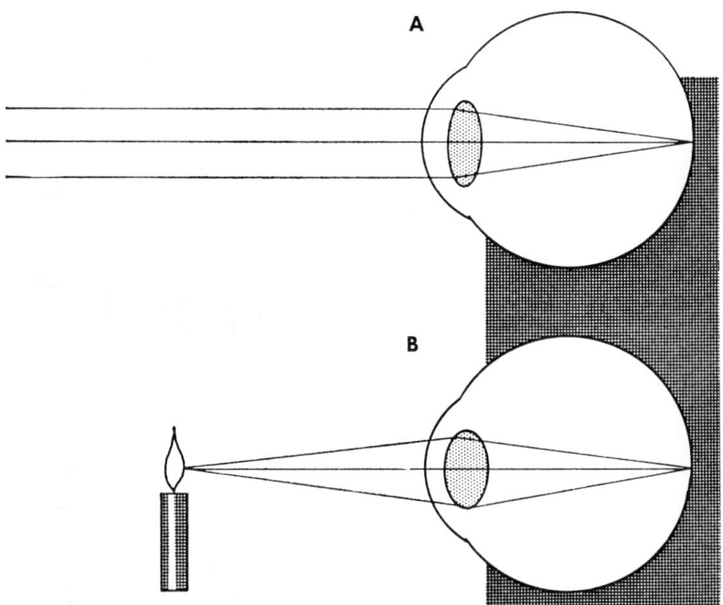

Fig. 20-6. Adjustment of the lens of the eye to far, **A,** and near, **B,** objects. Note the change in convexity.

the normal eye the aforementioned refracting mechanisms are of such "strength" that an object 20 feet or more away forms a clear image upon the retina. In other words, for distant focusing the relaxed eye is "all set to see" (Fig. 20-6).

In order to form clear images of objects at a distance of less than 20 feet, however, the refractive power of the eye must be increased to bend the parallel and divergent rays that impinge upon the cornea. (Light rays from distant objects, it will be recalled, p. 39, are parallel.) Since the degree of divergence increases rapidly as the object comes closer to the eye, the degree of refraction must increase to bring the rays into focus. Indeed, if an object is too close to the eye it cannot be focused at all.

The eye (Fig. 20-6), but not the camera (Fig. 20-7), can increase its refractive power for near vision by *accommodation*, that is, by increasing the convexity of the lens. As explained earlier, this is accomplished by contraction of the ciliary muscle. In this connection it is interesting to note that with age the lens becomes less elastic and therefore less able to focus *near* objects, an occurrence referred to as *presbyopia*.

Constriction of pupil. The iris serves the eye in two ways. First, it protects the retina against bright light by constricting the pupil. Second, it aids in the focusing of near objects, also by constricting the pupil. The former response can be demonstrated by shining a light into the eyes and the second by watching the pupils of a subject who is focusing on the tip of a pencil as it is brought toward the eyes. Conversely, in dim light and in distant focusing the pupils enlarge.

The reason that the size of the pupil varies with the intensity of light is quite obvious. It is equally obvious in near vision, too, if we remember that the more peripheral divergent rays cannot be focused; that is, by "constricting these rays out," the sharpness of the focus is enhanced.

Convergence. Although we see with both eyes (*binocular* vision), we do not see double images (*diplopia*). This is because when we train our eyes on an object,

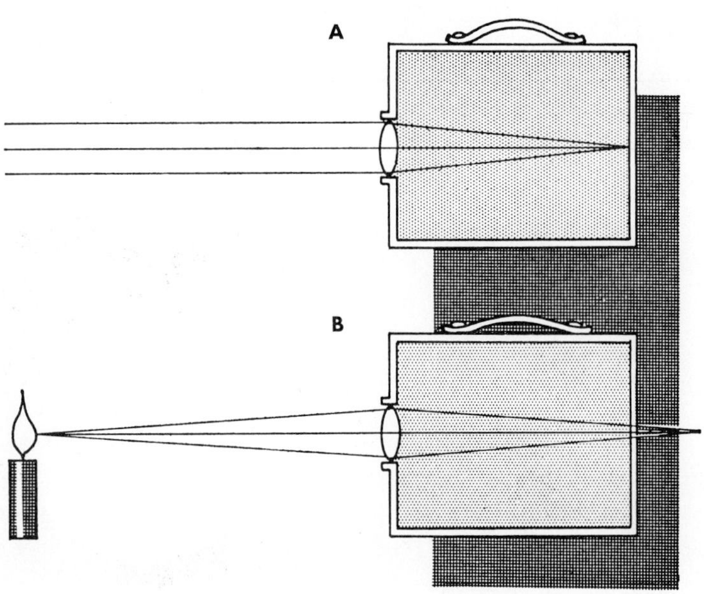

Fig. 20-7. Illustration showing a lens of fixed convexity (such as that of a camera) focusing on far, **A**, and near, **B**, objects. (Compare with Fig. 20-6.)

the two images fall on corresponding parts of the retina. This is true whether we are looking at a distant object or at a near object. Obviously, the nearer the object, the more the eyes must converge. Convergence is effected by contraction of the *medial* rectus muscles and by relaxation of the lateral rectus muscles. Proper focusing and vision, therefore, depend upon keen functional balance between these antagonistic extrinsic muscles.

A simple experiment will vividly demonstrate what has been said: While focusing on a single object, if one of the eyeballs is gently pressed in, two objects appear. This is because the image in the disturbed eyeball falls on a different or noncorresponding part of the retina.

VISUAL PATH

The fibers from the rods and cones gather together at the optic disc and leave the eyeball as the *optic* or *second* cranial nerve. The two nerves then curve medially and meet just above the pituitary gland at the *optic chiasm* (Fig. 20-4). Here there is a 50 percent decussation of fibers; that is, those from the medial half of the retina cross over to the optic nerve on the opposite side, while the fibers from the lateral portion pass directly into the optic tract on the same side. The fibers now continue on to the *visual areas* of the two occipital lobes via the *lateral geniculate body* (of the thalamus) and the *superior colliculi* (of the midbrain). Thus, each occipital lobe "sees with both eyes," or, turned around, each eye "sees with both lobes." This unique feature explains the rather peculiar visual disturbances resulting from injury or damage to the brain.

CHEMISTRY OF VISION

The emission of nerve impulses by the retinal rods and cones results from photochemical reactions within these microscopic structures. It has now been established that dim light vision is caused by the extreme photosensitivity of a substance in the rods called *rhodopsin,* or *visual purple,* a material derived from a protein called *scotopsin* and a carotenoid called *retinene,* the latter being an aldehyde derived from vitamin A. In bright light, rhodopsin is bleached into these two components and therefore is "nonoperational"; in dim light they are resynthesized into the active molecule. Perhaps the most significant thing is that vitamin A serves as a raw material for vision, for without this vitamin the rods cannot synthesize retinene, and without retinene there can be no rhodopsin. Indeed, the earliest sign of vitamin A deficiency is *night blindness,* or *nyctalopia.*

In regard to color, the Young-Hemholtz theory has recently been shown to be correct—to wit, there are *three* types of cones, each containing a photosensitive pigment responsive to a primary color (red, green, or blue). Thus, we experience red, green, and blue when the red, green, and blue cones, respectively, are stimulated by the corresponding frequency (p. 39). Other color experiences result from an interplay of the cones. Yellow, for example, is due to stimulation of equal numbers of green and red cones and a very few blue cones. The sensation of white apparently results when the three types of cones are stimulated equally.

VISUAL ACUITY AND OPTICAL DEFECTS

If at 20 feet a person can barely read letters that are barely readable at that distance to all persons with normal vision, his visual acuity, or "eyesight," is said to be 20/20. If, on the other hand, a person is barely able to read letters at 20 feet that are barely readable at 40 feet to all persons with normal vision, his visual acuity is said to be 20/40. Worse yet, if a person is barely able to read letters at 20 feet that are barely readable at 100 feet to all persons with normal vision, his visual acuity is 20/100, and so on. The more common optical defects that relate to visual acuity are discussed below.

Astigmatism. Astigmatism, probably the most common defect of the eye, is a condition characterized by "blemished" vision; that is, instead of light rays hitting the retina in sharp focus, they spread out over a more or less diffuse area (Fig. 20-8). As a matter of fact, the word *astigmatism* (of Greek origin) means without point.

Astigmatism is due to an unevenness in the surface of either the cornea or the lens, sometimes both. In geometric terms this means that the radius of curvature in one plane is longer or shorter than the radius at right angles to it. Consequently, the rays passing through the plane of greater curvature are refracted more than the rays passing through the other plane. The result is two focal points instead of one.

Because the cornea and lens are never optically perfect, most of us experience some degree of astigmatism. If this were not true, stars would appear as small bright dots instead of star-shaped bodies (that is, bright centers with radiating short lines). The reason that stars twinkle, by the way, involves the constant rapid movement of the eyeballs, making the radiating lines shift upon the retina. The natural imperfection of the refractive apparatus of the eye also explains why a light in the darkness appears to come to the eye in radiating beams.

To correct astigmatism, the oculist prescribes glasses that correct the unevenness of the corneal and lens surfaces; that is, the convexity of each lens in the glasses is increased or decreased to compensate for the defect in the corresponding diameter, or meridian, of the eye.

Myopia. Myopia, or *nearsightedness,* is an eye condition in which the focus falls in *front* of the retina (Fig. 20-9). To put the image on the retina where it belongs, the myopic person must look at an object at closer range than the emmetropic person. To remedy the defect, the ophthalmologist prescribes glasses with concave lenses that diverge the light rays hitting the cornea just enough to force the focus back upon

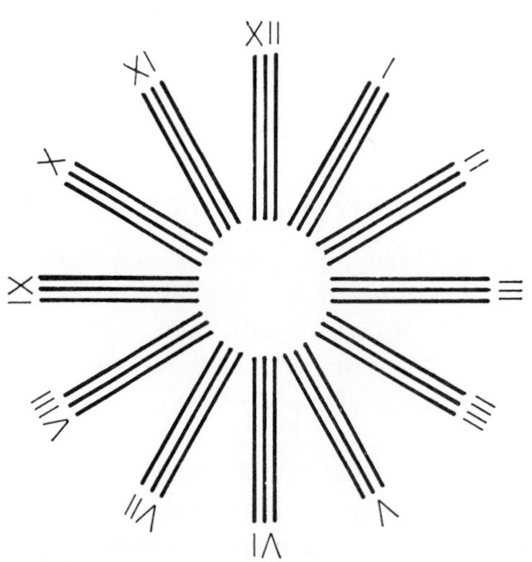

Fig. 20-8. To the normal eye, all the black lines of the chart appear to be of the same intensity. To the astigmatic eye, some will appear darker than others.

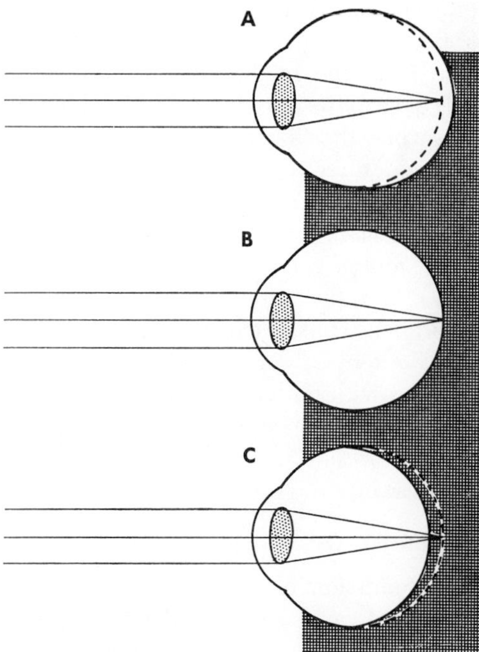

Fig. 20-9. Diagram to illustrate nearsightedness, **A,** normal sight, **B,** and farsightedness, **C.**

the retina. The cause of myopia may be either that the refractive power of the eye is too great or that the eyeball is too long (Fig. 20-9).

Hyperopia. In contrast to the myopic eye, the hyperopic eye sees objects most clearly at far range; that is, hyperopia, or *hypermetropia,* is *farsightedness.* Thus, instead of the focus falling before the retina, as in myopia, it falls *behind* it (Fig. 20-9). The usual cause of hyperopia is a flattened lens or cornea (with a consequent loss of refractive power) or an eyeball that is too short. To correct the condition, convex lenses are prescribed to concentrate the light rays and cause the focus to retreat to the retina.*

Color blindness. Color blindness is the inability to distinguish differences in color; it is generally partial and is seldom, if ever, complete. Usually hereditary and rarely seen in women, the condition is said to affect about 8 percent of all men. In *dichromatism,* the most common variety, the person does not see red or green but only yellow and blue or combinations thereof. Apparently, the retinas of such persons lack the pigments that are sensitive to these fundamental colors. Since color blindness may lead to serious accidents in driving and in all occupations in which colored signals are used, it is of the greatest importance that the condition be detected at an early age.

Glaucoma. Glaucoma, the leading cause of blindness in this country, results from faulty drainage of aqueous humor (p. 391). Because the inflow and outflow of the fluid are normally balanced, the result is a rise in the *intraocular* pressure, sometimes four times the average range (14 to 25 mm. Hg). Indeed, the affected eye may feel as hard as a marble.

In the acute condition there is intense pain, fogged vision, and lights ringed with halos, whereas in the chronic condition, in which the pressure rises over long periods of time, the symptoms are transitory and mild. In either circumstance, however, the prolonged elevation of pressure ultimately destroys the optic nerve.

The drainage difficulty resides at the

*The refractive power, or strength, of a lens is expressed in diopters (D). A lens that can focus parallel light rays to a point 100 cm. behind it is arbitrarily given a strength of 1 D. Lenses with shorter focal distances—that is, those with greater refractive power—are above 1 D. For example, a lens with a focal distance of 50 cm. has a refractive power of 2 D (100/50 = 2); a lens with a focal distance of 20 cm. is 5 D, and so on.

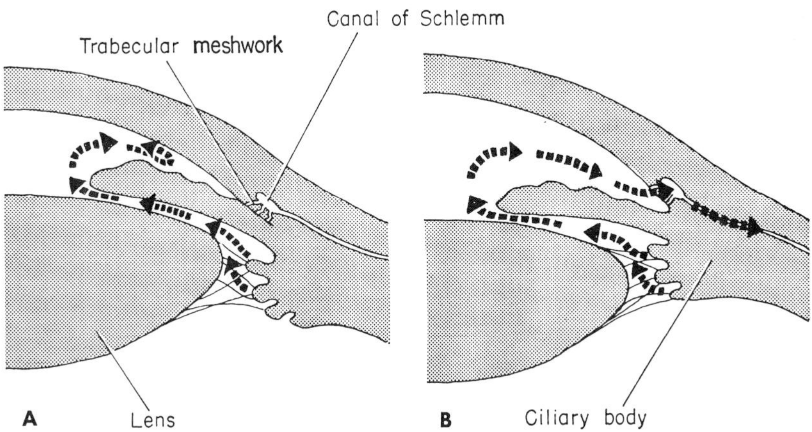

Fig. 20-10. Glaucoma. **A,** In angle-closure glaucoma the base of the iris prevents the flow (arrows) of the aqueous humor into the trabecular meshwork because of narrow angle. **B,** Normal flow into the canal of Schlemm via the trabecular meshwork. In open-angle glaucoma the angle is normal (as in **B**) but the trabecular meshwork is occluded.

periphery of the anterior chamber (p. 391) in the angle between the cornea and the iris. Here, as shown in Fig. 20-10, a spongy network of fibers, the so-called *trabecular meshwork,* affords a series of microscopic channels that extend from the anterior chamber to the *canal of Schlemm.* Through this meshwork the aqueous humor drains into the canal of Schlemm and finally returns to the blood via the veins in the sclera.

In *angle-closure* glaucoma the space between the cornea and iris is less than average, so that when the pupil dilates somewhat, the thickened iris closes off the narrowed angle (Fig. 20-10). Consequently, the outflow of fluid stops and the pressure begins to rise. In *open-angle* glaucoma, on the other hand, the primary trouble is in the trabecular meshwork itself; that is, although the angle is normal (open), the tiny channels for some reason have become narrowed or clogged. But the end result is the same—poor drainage and increased intraocular pressure.

The standard approach to acute glaucoma is the use of *parasympathomimetic* drugs (for example, *pilocarpine*) to reduce the size of the pupil. This procedure "thins out" the iris at the periphery, thereby enlarging the angle and facilitating drainage into the trabecular meshwork. A more recent medicinal, Diamox, improves the acute condition by inhibiting the production of aqueous humor.

Drugs, of course, do not correct the underlying factors, and because of the very nature of the disease, a cure must come by way of surgical intervention. Great hope in this area has arisen chiefly from an operation called *peripheral iridectomy,* a procedure whereby a tiny piece is snipped from the edge of the iris. This permits the aqueous humor to pass *directly* from the posterior chamber to the anterior chamber instead of going through the pupil. Since the roundabout way (through the pupil) causes the pressure in the posterior chamber to be normally slightly *higher* than in the anterior chamber, the iris is always pushed a little forward normally, *narrowing* the angle. The effect of the operation, then, is to equalize the pressure in the two chambers, "straighten" the iris, widen the angle, and facilitate drainage, in that order. In early pure angle-closure glaucoma, peripheral iridectomy can sometimes effect a complete cure; in the open-angle form a modified operation is helpful. However, in the latter variety of glaucoma, ophthalmologists usually rely upon drugs alone, particularly if the patient responds and there is no further visual loss.

Cataract. A cataract is an opacity of the lens or its capsule. The so-called *developmental* cataracts seen in young persons result from infection of the mother in the first trimester of pregnancy, or they may be hereditary. *Degenerative* cataracts, on the other hand, occur in elderly persons (*senile* cataracts) and in persons exposed to excessive radiation and heat. The senile variety makes up the bulk of all cases. When there is considerable impairment of vision, operative removal of the lens is essential.

Tumors. The main tumors of the eye are the *retinoblastoma* in children and the *malignant melanoma* in persons past middle age. The retinoblastoma is a gray, soft tumor of the retina that may invade the vitreous humor and often the entire eyeball. In the final stages it works its way along the optic nerve and extends to the cranial cavity. In addition to mechanical damage, there is necrosis and hemorrhage.

The melanoma is a black tumor that starts in the choroid, iris, or ciliary body and later projects into the eyeball and tissues surrounding the eye. As in the case of other malignant growths, metastases may occur, particularly in the liver.

Less common tumors include the myoma, the neurofibroma, and the angioma.

Infections of the eye. The tissues and

various structures of the eye are fertile ground for a variety of pathogens. The more common infections include *hordeolum,* or *sty* (involvement of one or more sebaceous glands of the eyelids); *blepharitis* (involvement of the margin of the eyelids); *conjunctivitis* (involvement of the conjunctiva); *keratitis* (involvement of the cornea); and *iritis* (involvement of the iris). Gonorrheal conjunctivitis in the newborn infant (commonly referred to as *ophthalmia neonatorum*) is easily preventable by the instillation of two drops of 1 percent silver nitrate in each eye at the time of delivery.

Questions

1. Describe the general features of the eyeball.
2. Describe the structure of the retina.
3. Describe the workings of the iris.
4. Explain how the ciliary body controls the convexity of the crystalline lens.
5. Compare the anterior and posterior chambers of the eye.
6. Discuss the extrinsic muscles and the manner in which they move the eyeball.
7. Discuss the function of the eyelids and meibomian glands.
8. Describe the structure and function of the lacrimal apparatus.
9. Why do the eyes water during a severe head cold?
10. Discuss in detail the manner in which the eye refracts and focuses light rays.
11. Explain why we see only a single image even though we have two eyes.
12. Even though one eye is closed, we see by both cerebral hemispheres. Explain.
13. Explain why nyctalopia is an early sign of vitamin A deficiency.
14. Discuss color vision.
15. Why does a blue shirt appear black when viewed in red light?
16. Compare the rods and cones.
17. We "see" with the brain. Explain.
18. Why do most of us have some degree of astigmatism?
19. What is the cause of hypermetropia? How is it corrected?
20. What is dichromatism?
21. In the examination of the eye the ophthalmologist uses mydriatic drugs. Explain the action of such agents.
22. Why do the pupils enlarge during excitement?
23. Discuss the cause and treatment of glaucoma.
24. Why must glasses be worn following a cataract operation?
25. Discuss the prophylaxis of ophthalmia neonatorum.
26. Explain why our night vision is temporarily impaired if we are dazzled by the headlights of an oncoming car.
27. If a person has 20/15 vision, what does this mean?

Chapter 21

The ear

The ear is the receptor of sound and the "seat of balance." In order to understand these activities, we must first look into the structural details.

OUTER EAR

The three subdivisions of the ear include the outer, middle, and inner ear—and we shall start with the first. The outer or external ear comprises the *auricle,* or *pinna,* and the *auditory canal* (Fig. 21-1). The former structure, familiar to one and all as the "ear," is composed of an irregular plate of elastic cartilage covered with skin. It varies considerably in size and shape, usually being larger in the male than in the female. Though a considerable number of muscle fibers are attached to the auricle, modern man has all but lost the ability to "wiggle" his ears.

The auditory canal is a bent tube, a little more than 1 inch long, which leads from the auricle to the eardrum. There is cartilage in its outer third and bone constitutes the remainder. Characteristically, the skin over the cartilaginous portion contains hairs and special glands that secrete *cerumen,* a waxlike material commonly referred to as earwax. The auditory canal is also supplied with a large number of sensory fibers from certain cranial nerves.

MIDDLE EAR

The middle ear (Fig. 21-1) is a small chamber within the temporal bone separated from the external ear by the eardrum, or *tympanum* (less correctly, the tympanic membrane), a thin, translucent disc composed of fibrous tissue. The back of the chamber communicates with the mastoid air cells through a tiny opening and the front of the chamber communicates with the *eustachian* tube, a passageway leading to the *nasopharynx.* The inner wall is composed of bone, except for the *oval* and *round* windows which communicate with the inner ear. The *footplate* of the *stapes* fits over the oval window and a fibrous disc fits over the round window (Fig. 21-4). The entire chamber is lined with a mucous membrane continuous with that which lines the mastoid air cells and nasopharynx. Tiny muscles are attached to the ear bones (below), and all the soft structures mentioned receive sensory fibers.

Ossicles. There are three ear bones, or ossicles, in each ear—aptly named the *malleus* (hammer), the *incus* (anvil), and the

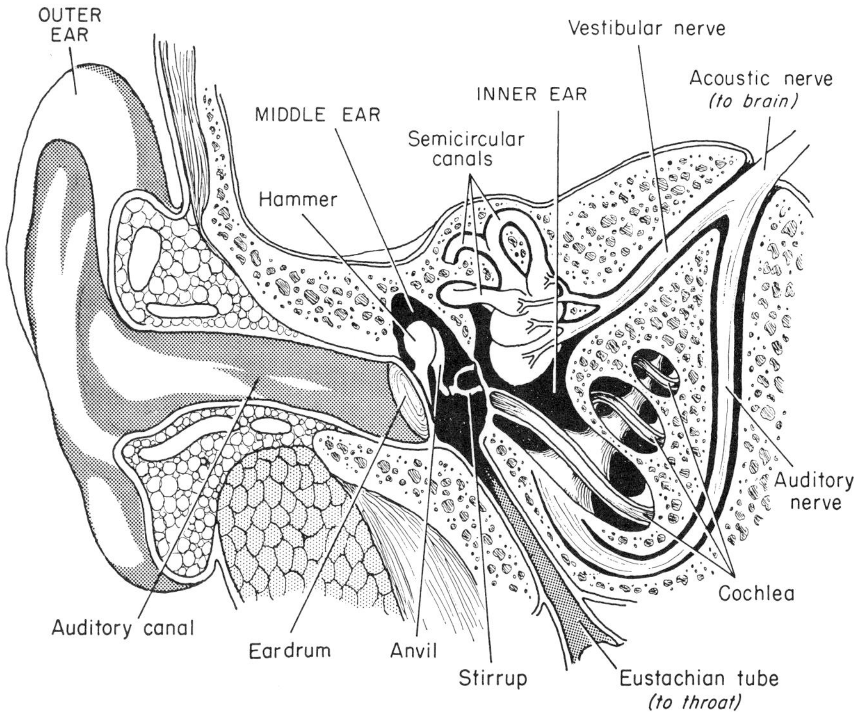

Fig. 21-1. The ear. (The auditory nerve is also called the cochlear nerve.)

stapes (stirrup). These tiny irregular bones extend across the chamber from the tympanum to the oval window in the order mentioned; that is, the malleus articulates with the incus, and the latter articulates with the stapes. In this manner, tympanic vibrations (produced by sound waves) are transmitted across the middle ear to the oval window and thence to the inner ear.

INNER EAR

The inner ear consists of the *osseous labyrinth* and *membranous labyrinth.* The latter is a soft structure composed of two small sacs—the *utricle* and the *saccule*—the *three semicircular canals,* and the *membranous cochlea* (Fig. 21-2).

A watery fluid, the *endolymph,* fills the membranous labyrinth and a similar fluid, the *perilymph,* fills the space between the membranous labyrinth and the osseous labyrinth. These fluids serve the dual purpose of cushioning the soft structures and conducting sound waves from the middle ear to the *organ of Corti,* the actual receptor of sound.

Cochlea. The *osseous* cochlea is divided by the *vestibular* membrane (Reissner's membrane) and the *basilar* membrane into three spiral tubes called *scalae:* the scala vestibuli, the scala media, and the scala tympani (Fig. 21-3). The scala vestibuli communicates with the middle ear via the oval window which, as stated before, is secured by the footplate of the stapes. The scala tympani is secured by the round window and the scala media—which is actually the *membraneous cochlea*—is sealed off from the middle ear by bone (Fig. 21-4).

Organ of Corti. Upon the delicate basilar membrane rest receptor cells supplied with nerve fibers from the *auditory* or *cochlear nerve* (Fig. 21-3). These cells, which are long and slender and stand on end, in most instances are capped by a row of hairlike processes. This collection of cells is known

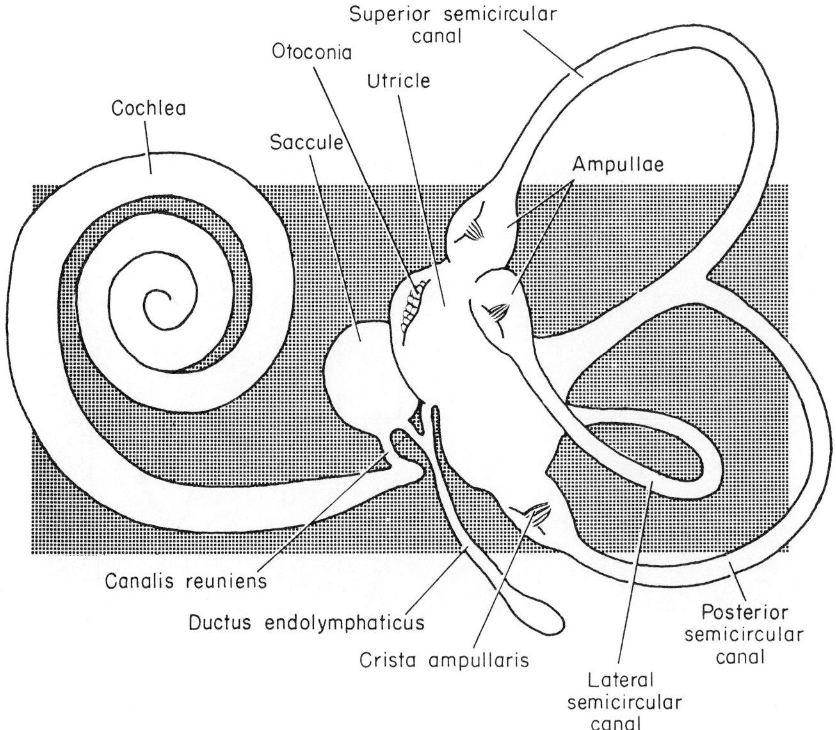

Fig. 21-2. The membranous labyrinth. (The ductus endolymphaticus is shown pulled down.) (Adapted from Best, C. H., and Taylor, N. B.: The human body, ed. 3, New York, 1956, Holt, Rinehart & Winston, Inc. By permission.)

as the organ of Corti. Overlying this structure and touching the hairs is a veillike tissue called the *tectorial membrane,* whose motion in the endolymph somewhat resembles a long string of seaweed waving in the water.

Semicircular canals. The semicircular canals include the three sickle-shaped, fluid-filled membranous tubes of the labyrinth that communicate with the utricle (Fig. 21-2). They are at right angles to each other and form a swelling (the *ampulla*) at one end just before entering the utricle.

Within the ampullae are special rotary receptors called *cristae,* that is, groups of hair cells with their hairlike processes embedded in a gelatinous covering (the *cupula*). The cristae are supplied with sensory nerve fibers that convey impulses to the brain via the vestibular portion of the acoustic nerve. The function of the semicircular canals will be discussed later in the chapter.

Utricle. The utricle is the fluid-filled membranous sac, situated within the *vestibule* of the osseous labyrinth, that communicates with the three semicircular canals. Inside are special "gravity receptors" constructed of hair cells with calcareous bodies (the *otoliths*) attached to the hairlike processes. Because of their weight, the otoliths pull upon the hairs with a force that depends upon the position of the head. Sensations from these cells are transmitted to the brain via the *vestibular* nerve.

Saccule. The saccule, a much smaller sac than the utricle, also resides within the vestibule and communicates with both the utricle and the membranous cochlea. Although its function is not definitely

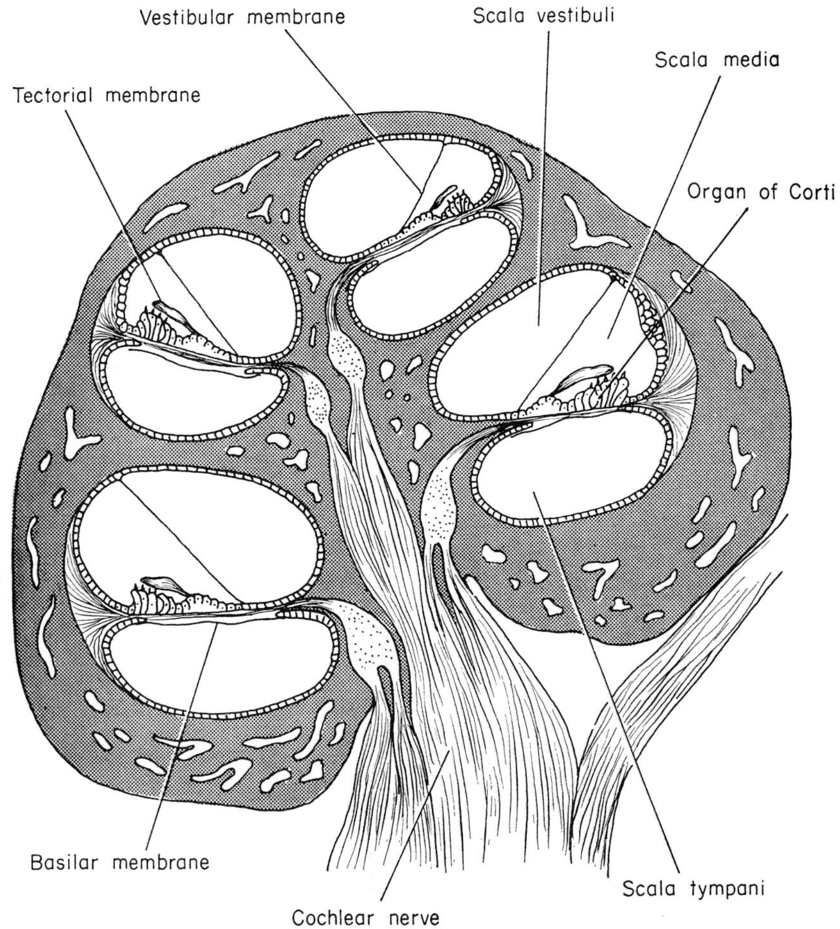

Fig. 21-3. Cross section of the cochlea showing the scalae and the organ of Corti. (Modified from Guyton, A. C.: Function of the human body, Philadelphia, 1959, W. B. Saunders Co.)

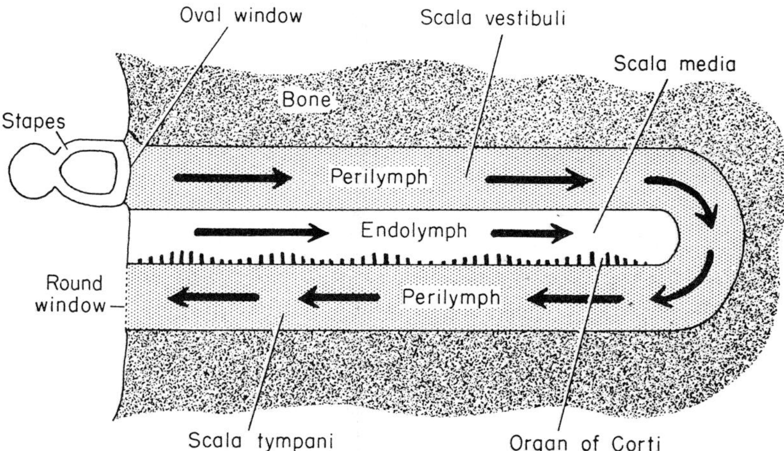

Fig. 21-4. Diagram of the basic relationship between the osseous and membranous cochlea. (After Williams; modified from Anthony, C. P.: Textbook of anatomy and physiology, ed. 7, St. Louis, 1967, The C. V. Mosby Co.)

known, most authorities believe that in some way it is associated with maintenance of balance.

HEARING

To the musician, the sense of hearing is his most precious experience; for others, it is at least next to vision in importance. The mechanics of the ear and the cerebral mechanisms responsible for the experience of sound are indeed one of nature's greatest engineering feats. As a matter of fact, the more one knows about the mechanics of sound, the more phenomenal the sense of hearing becomes. For instance, a sound wave with a pressure of only one ten-billionth of one atmosphere* can provoke an audible sensation!

To understand the salient features of hearing, we must begin with the sound waves (p. 29) funneled into the auditory canal by the pinna. (Here, of course, we do not do as well as the dog because of our inability to "prick up our ears" and aim them in the direction of the sound.) When sound waves reach the end of the canal, the tympanum is set in vibration and, in turn, so are the hammer, anvil, and stirrup. Thus, across the middle ear sound is conducted as vibrating bone. At the footplate of the stapes (at the oval window) the vibrations are conveyed to the perilymph in the scala vestibuli and thence throughout the fluid in the scala media and scala tympani. As a consequence of these fluid vibrations, the basilar membrane is caused to vibrate, thereby moving the hair cells of the organ of Corti against the tectorial membrane. This "tapping" and "tickling" of the hairs initiates electrical impulses in the hair cells that are then conducted to the auditory center located in the temporal lobe of the cortex. And as we know, it is here that we experience the sense of hearing. Just how the brain does this, of course, is a moot question.

*One atmosphere is the pressure of the air at sea level.

Pitch. Several theories have been proposed to explain pitch, but the idea of *sympathetic resonance* is now generally considered the accepted explanation. According to this theory, first proposed by Helmholtz, the 24,000-odd delicate cross fibers of the basilar membrane, instead of vibrating *en masse*, vibrate in groups; that is, the longer fibers near the top of the cochlea vibrate, or resonate, in sympathy (p. 30) with the lower-pitched sounds, while the shorter fibers at the bottom resonate "in tune" with the higher-pitched sounds. (As a matter of fact, if the 1½-inch basilar membrane were to be removed and laid out flat, we would have a microscopic string instrument.) Thus, the theory holds that a sound of a given pitch will set off certain basilar fibers which, in turn, will tap certain hair cells which, in turn, will trigger certain nerve fibers which, in turn, will excite a certain region in the auditory center.

The human ear is not sensitive to sound waves with a frequency of less than 16 or more than 20,000 cycles per second. It is most sensitive to sound vibrations between 500 and 5000. Cats and dogs pick up sound waves far above this range. The human voice ranges between 100 and 800 cycles per second, and musical instruments between 30 and 4000 cycles per second.

Eustachian tube. Were it not for the eustachian tube running from the nasopharynx to the middle ear (p. 400), our hearing would be impaired. By allowing the air pressure on both sides of the eardrum to be equalized, the structure is not pushed in, as would be the case if air were not allowed to enter the middle ear chamber. A stretched, pushed-in eardrum, as we can well appreciate, does not vibrate the way it should.

We become acutely aware of the function of the tube when we go from one air pressure to another, as in a sudden ascent or descent in an elevator or airplane. This is because the pressure in the middle ear does not adjust instantly to external pressure. The condition is easily remedied by swallowing several times in quick succession, for it is only when we swallow that the eustachian tubes open.

SENSE OF BALANCE

Because the semicircular canals lie in three different planes at right angles to one another, the muscles are immediately activated to maintain proper balance, or equilibrium, should the entire body or the head be quickly rotated about any axis. If the body is spun about a vertical axis, as in a swivel chair, the semicircular canals in the horizontal plane will be particularly stimulated; that is, receptors, or cristae, in the ampullae of these two structures will be bent because of the inertia of the endolymph. At the instant the motion begins the receptors turn with the body while the endolymph stands still. As a consequence, the bent hair cells release nerve impulses over the vestibular fibers going to the balance centers in the brain whereby we experience the sensation of motion; too, reflexes are initiated that effect the appropriate movement of the head and limbs.

The sensation of rotation, however, is experienced only in the first few seconds; prolonged rotation, if smooth, does not provoke the sensation. The reason is that the endolymph loses its resting inertia and moves with the receptors; thus, the latter will not be bent or stimulated. When rotation stops, however, the endolymph continues to move, once again bending and stimulating the receptors. Interestingly, this time the sensation of rotation is in the opposite direction because the hair cells are bent in the opposite direction.

Working hand in hand with the semicircular canals in maintenance of equilibrium and position are the receptors in the utricle. However, while the semicircular receptors are triggered by rotation, the utricle receptors are triggered by the position of the head, or gravity. That is, when the head is placed in various positions, the otoliths resting upon the hair cells, because of their weight, pull in different directions with varying degrees of tension. This triggers nerve impulses which, upon arrival in the brain, effect the appropriate muscular movements to "right the body." The coordinating mechanism of this so-called *righting reflex* resides within the *cerebellum.* The efficiency of this reflex is dramatically illustrated by holding a kitten a few feet above a soft surface and allowing it to fall —back downward. In a flash it turns in midair and lands upon all four feet in perfect balance.

DISEASES OF THE EAR

The ear is subject to a number and variety of injuries, obstructions, infections, and abnormalities. The more common of these will be discussed.

Conduction deafness. Deafness is lack or loss, complete or partial, of the sense of hearing. Conduction deafness is due to some defect in the sound-conducting system, that is, the auditory canal, eardrum, ear bones, and eustachian tube. In children most cases of conduction deafness result from the presence of excessive lymphoid tissue in and about the eustachian tube opening in the nasopharynx. This interfers with proper ventilation of the middle ear, thereby upsetting the normally equalized pressures on either side of the eardrum. As a result, tympanic vibrations are inhibited and hearing is impaired. The treatment usually recommended is surgical removal of the lymphoid obstruction.

In adults the usual cause of conduction deafness is *otosclerosis,* especially in women. This is a chronic disease characterized by the formation of spongy bone in the osseous labyrinth and ossification of the annular ligament by which the stapes footplate is attached to the circumference of the oval window. The result, once again, is poor vibration and impaired hearing. A dramatic and usually successful surgical procedure is the stapes mobilization or stapes substitution operation.

Perceptive deafness. Perceptive deafness results from disorders of the auditory nerve, cerebral pathways, or auditory center. The etiologic factors may be infection, tumors, psychogenic disturbances, injuries, and certain drugs (for example, quinine and streptomycin), to name a few. Treatment is directed at the underlying cause, and every attempt is made to eradicate the cause. If the condition is irreversible, careful rehabilitation (hearing aid, lip reading, and the like) is essential.

Tinnitis. Tinnitis is an annoying symptom characterized by hissing, ringing, buzzing, thumping, whistling, or roaring in the ears. The underlying cause can be "almost anything." It could be an infection, drug intoxication, obstruction of the external auditory canal, obstruction of the eustachian tube, or a dental disorder. When this symptom "presents," therefore, the physician must consider every possibility in searching for the answer.

Infection. From the standpoint of a general threat to health, infection (particularly the acute form) is probably the most serious ear condition. Infection of the outer ear (*otitis externa*) involves the auricle and/or auditory canal. Since the area is relatively easy to reach, administration of appropriate anti-infective drugs usually effects a swift cure.

Otitis media, or middle ear infection, however, is always potentially dangerous. Although almost any pathogen can incite an infection in the area, the most commonly encountered pathogens include certain hemolytic streptococci, pneumococci, staphylococci, *Corynebacterium diphtheriae, Pseudomonas aeruginosa, Mycobacterium tuberculosis,* and *Escherichia coli.* Often the infection is secondary and follows in the wake of scarlet fever, measles, mumps, pneumonia, and influenza. The principal danger is *mastoiditis* (infection of the mastoid antrum and cells), which not infrequently complicates acute purulent otitis media. Mastoiditis may lead to infection of the brain and sudden death.

Questions

1. Describe the anatomy of the external ear.
2. Describe the anatomy of the middle ear.
3. Distinguish between the membranous and osseous labyrinths.
4. What is the organ of Corti?
5. Describe the structure and function of the semicircular canals.
6. Describe the structure and function of the utricle and the saccule.
7. Starting with when sound waves strike the tympanum, describe the mechanism of hearing.
8. What is meant by pitch?
9. What is the function of the eustachian tube?
10. Distinguish between conduction deafness and perceptive deafness.
11. What is tinnitis?
12. Describe the righting reflex.
13. What is meant by sympathetic resonance?
14. Discuss the more common infections of the ear.
15. What is cerumen?

Chapter 22

The endocrine system

The endocrines are small *ductless* glands distributed throughout the body (Fig. 22-1) that manufacture miraculous chemical regulators called *hormones*. In contrast to the exocrines, or duct glands, the endocrines release their secretions into the blood. In the present chapter we shall discuss the anatomy of these glands, the nature and action of their hormones, and the disorders occasioned by under (*hypo-*) and over (*hyper-*) secretion.

PITUITARY GLAND

The pituitary gland, or *hypophysis,** a tiny gland that lies in the *sella turcica* of the sphenoid bone, is divided into two completely separate parts—the anterior lobe, or *adenohypophysis,* and the posterior lobe, or *neurohypophysis* (see Fig. 19-17, p. 368). The latter portion is connected to the hypothalamus by a stalk that permits neurohormonal control of pituitary function.

Hormones of anterior lobe. The insignificant-looking anterior lobe secretes at least six known hormones that profoundly affect in one way or another just about all the activities in the body. Since five of these potent regulators act indirectly through endocrine structures situated elsewhere, the pituitary has been quite accurately dubbed the "master gland."

Growth hormone. The growth hormone, or *somatotropin,* by increasing the synthesis of cellular elements, stimulates the development and enlargement of all the tissues. Although it is released in highest concentrations during preadolescence, the anterior lobe never completely curtails its manufacture.

One of the causes of *dwarfism* is an insufficient output of the growth hormone. The degree of underdevelopment, of course, will depend upon the extent of the insufficiency. *Gigantism,* on the other hand, usually results from a tumor of the acidophilic cells of the anterior lobe during preadolescence, resulting in an increased output of the growth hormone and a tremendous enlargement of all parts of the body (Fig. 22-2). If the tumor occurs after adolescence, however, when most of the bones have "fused," the skeleton grows in thickness instead of length—and disproportionately. The result in this instance is not gigantism but *acromegaly.* Characteristically, the lower jaw, nose, lips, hands, and feet become tremendously enlarged.

*More formally, hypophysis cerebri.

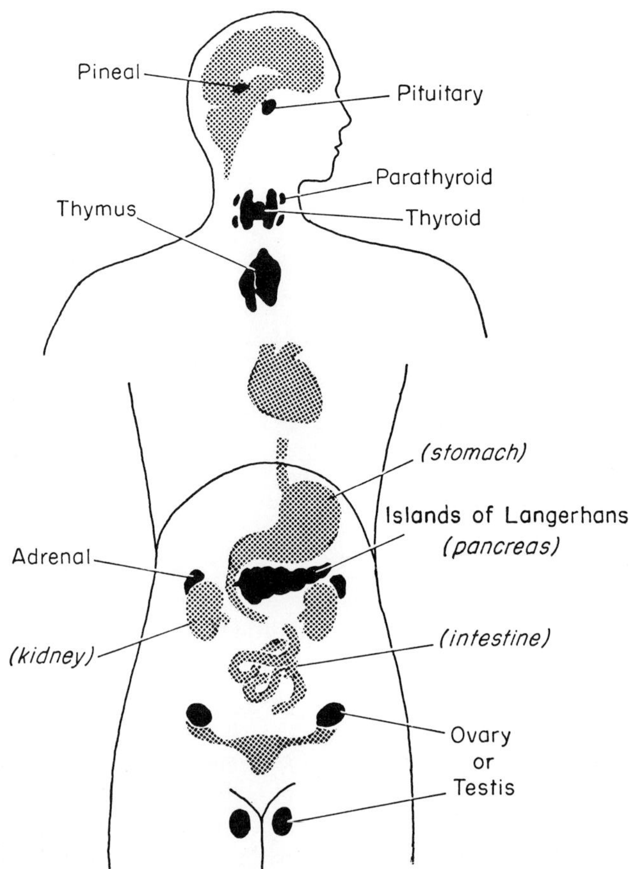

Fig. 22-1. Endocrine glands.

Thyrotropic hormone. The thyrotropic hormone, or *thyrotropin,* stimulates growth and multiplication of the cells in the thyroid gland and their secretion of the all-important hormone *thyroxine.* We shall have much to say about both hormones later in the chapter in the discussion of the thyroid gland.

Adrenocorticotropic hormone. The adrenocorticotropic hormone, or ACTH, acts upon the adrenal cortex (in much the same fashion as the thyrotropic hormone acts upon the thyroid) to stimulate release of the *adrenocortical hormones.* The details will be considered in our discussion of the adrenal glands later in this chapter.

Gonadotropic hormones. As indicated by the term, the gonadotropic hormones are concerned with sexuality. Those of prime concern are the *follicle-stimulating hormone* (FSH), the *luteinizing hormone* (LH), and the *luteotropic hormone (*LTH). In the female, FSH stimulates development of the follicles in the ovaries, bringing about maturation of the ova and the release of *estrogens,* the female hormones. In the male, FSH stimulates development of the testes, thereby promoting the manufacture of sperm. The luteinizing hormone causes rupture and release of the ovum from the follicle in the female (Chapter 23), and in the male (where it is called the *interstitial cell–stimulating hormone,* or ICSH) the hormone stimulates the testes to secrete *testosterone,* the male hormone (p. 426). Although the function of the luteo-

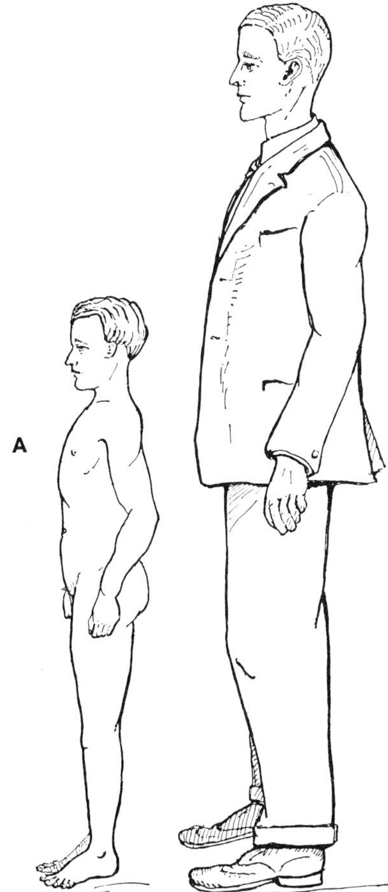

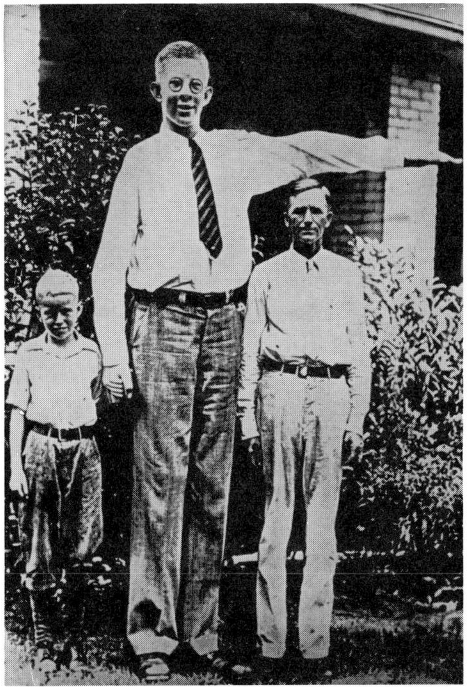

Fig. 22-2. **A,** Midget type of drawfism due to pituitary deficiency. Dwarf is 21 years of age. His body proportions are those of a 12-year-old boy, with a relatively large head. His sexual and mental development are normal. The man on the right is about average height. **B,** An example of gigantism. The boy in the center, 13 years of age, is 7 feet 5 inches tall and weighs 290 pounds. He is shown with his father and brother, who are of normal size. (From Best, C. H., and Taylor, N. B.: The human body, ed. 4, New York, 1963, Holt, Rinehart & Winston, Inc.)

tropic hormone in the male is unknown, in the female it stimulates release of *progesterone* by the corpus luteum and aids in production of milk by the glands in the breasts (Chapter 23). For the latter reason, the hormone is often called *prolactin.*

Melanocyte-stimulating factor. This hormone—generally referred to as MSH—acts upon the melanocytes in the skin in such a way as to increase pigmentation. The overproduction of the hormone, as in Addison's disease, causes darkening of the skin.

Hormones of posterior lobe. In response to stimulation of certain areas in the anterior hypothalamus, the posterior lobe releases two hormones—vasopressin and oxytocin. The actual *synthesis* of these hormones, however, takes place in the *hypothalamus.* Once formed, they migrate (as beadlike droplets) down the connecting fibers leading to the neurohypophysis.

Vasopressin. Vasopressin, or the *antidiuretic hormone* (ADH), has two actions: it contracts smooth muscle, particularly in the blood vessels (thereby elevating blood pressure) and, most important, it stimulates the *reabsorption* of water from the distal tubules in the kidney (Fig. 22-3). This renal mechanism is the principal means that the body has of conserving water (hence, the expression *antidiuretic*) and regulating the concentration of the extracellular compartment. One theory holds that ADH is released when the so-called *osmoreceptors* of the anterior hypothalamus are stimulated by an increased osmotic pressure of the plasma and interstitial fluid. As indicated earlier, the receptor cells transmit impulses to the posterior pituitary, bringing about the release of ADH, and the latter, by cutting down the production of urine, conserves water and reduces the concentration of the extracellular solutes. This mechanism will operate until the osmotic pressure is reduced to normal and the osmoreceptors are no longer stimulated.

When the posterior pituitary function is inhibited, the body will start to lose prodigious amounts of water via the urine. This strange derangement, referred to as *diabetes insipidus,* is also marked by voracious appetite, weakness, and emaciation.

Oxytocin. Oxytocin acts upon the uterine musculature, causing more forceful contractions. Even so, most indications are that the hormone does not play a significant role in labor (physiologically, that is). Thera-

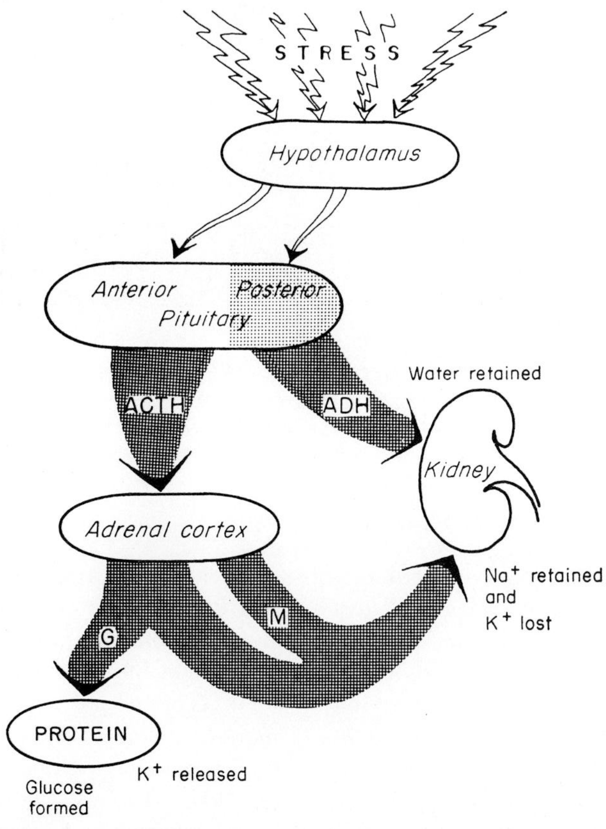

Fig. 22-3. Effect of stress upon body water and ions. **G** and **M** are glucocorticoids and mineralocorticoids, respectively. Aldosterone (a mineralocorticoid) is also released independently of ACTH. (From Brooks, S. M.: Basic facts of body water and ions, ed. 2, New York, 1968, Springer Publishing Co., Inc.)

peutically, however, the physician uses Pitocin (a commercial form of oxytocin) to induce labor and control postpartum hemorrhage (Chapter 23).

Another rather interesting action of oxytocin is its effect upon the alveoli and milk ducts of the breasts, causing them to contract and release milk. Experiments show that the stimulus for this release arises in response to sucking.

THYROID GLAND

The thyroid is a comparatively large endocrine gland situated beneath the muscles of the neck at the anterior juncture of the larynx and the trachea (p. 266). It consists of two lateral masses, or lobes, connected at the midline by a bar of tissue called the isthmus. Histologically, the gland is seen as a mass of follicles, each of which is lined with a single layer of epithelium and filled with an amorphous material called *colloid* (Fig. 22-4). Chemically, the latter is composed of *thyroglobulin,* a conjugated protein from which the hormones *thyroxine* (tetraiodothyronine) and *liothyronine* (tri-iodothyronine) are released in response to the thyrotropic hormone of the anterior pituitary. The follicle cells synthesize thyroxine, generally considered the chief hormone, according to the "summarized" reaction shown at the bottom of the page. A more recently discovered thyroid hormone is *calcitonin,* an agent we shall discuss in the section on the parathyroid glands (p. 192).

The relationship between the thyroid and the adenohypophysis is a good example of *negative feedback,* to use an engineering expression. To wit, as the concentration of circulating thyroxine begins to drop, the adenohypophysis is thereby *stimulated* and the output of thyrotropin is increased; as a consequence, the thyroxine output increases, which in turn *inhibits* the output of thyrotropin. The upshot and purpose of this feedback mechanism, of course, is to maintain steadiness in the concentration of circulating thyroid hormones.

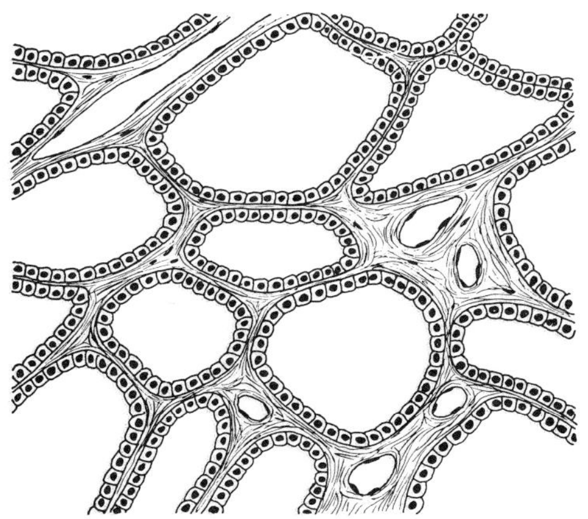

Fig. 22-4. Thyroid gland as seen under the microscope. The large spherical sacs, or vesicles, are filled with colloid.

As needed, thyroxine is gradually released to the blood, where it forms a loose complex with the circulating plasma proteins. From the latter it enters the interstitial fluids and finally the cells. Here it increases the rate of metabolism and thereby enhances the activities of all tis-

$$2\left[\mathrm{HO{-}C_6H_4{-}CH_2{-}CHNH_2{-}COOH}\right] + 4\mathrm{I} \longrightarrow$$

Tyrosine

$$\mathrm{HO{-}C_6H_2I_2{-}O{-}C_6H_2I_2{-}CH_2{-}CHNH_2{-}COOH} + \text{Alanine}$$

Thyroxine

sues, organs, and systems. Some idea of the potency of the hormone can be gained when one realizes that lack of it can drop the metabolic rate to as low as −50! An excess, on the other hand, can elevate the rate to about three times normal. The mechanism of the effects of thyroxine remains something of a mystery, at least where the particulars are concerned.

Hyperthyroidism. Hyperthyroidism refers to the condition resulting from overproduction of thyroid hormones. The cardinal signs and symptoms include an enlarged thyroid *(goiter)*, loss of weight, nervousness, and tachycardia. Also, because the tissues are literally being burned out, there are degenerative changes, particularly of heart muscle. Commonly, hyperthyroidism is accompanied by *exophthalmos* (protrusion of the eyes), a condition resulting from hypertrophy and edema of the orbital tissue. The basal metabolic rate (BMR) is always elevated, and the *protein-bound iodine* (PBI) is above normal. The latter is now considered one of the most accurate diagnostic tests of thyroid function.

The usual methods employed in the treatment of hyperthyroidism include surgical removal of part of the gland and administration of drugs (for example, propylthiouracil) to inhibit synthesis of the hormones. More recently, radioactive iodine (I^{131}) has been used with striking success. Since iodine is almost completely absorbed by the gland, a high dose of radiation is delivered precisely at the spot where it is needed.

Hypothyroidism. Since hypothyroidism results from lack of thyroid hormones, the pathologic picture is physiologically opposite that of hyperthyroidism. The usual features include a low BMR and PBI, mental sluggishness, myxedema, cold dry skin, coarse hair, deep voice, and generalized retardation. Occasionally, there is a goiter, which represents the attempt of the gland to "compensate" for its deficiency. The mechanism is believed to be as follows: A low PBI calls forth an increased output of thyrotropic hormone, and, as we know, the latter causes the thyroid gland to enlarge. Even though the gland continues to grow larger and larger, however, this growth is to no avail for it (the gland) has lost its ability to produce thyroxine in sufficient amounts to meet the needs of the body.

When hypothyroidism occurs congenitally, the body and mind fail to develop properly and the result is a pathetic creature called a cretin *(cretinism)*. Hypothyroidism, when acquired later in life (the adult form), is referred to as *myxedema*. It should be appreciated, however, that there are degrees of hypothyroidism and therefore instances in which the signs of a deficiency are subtle (for instance, poor skin and hair, poor academic performance, and the like). This means that the physician must rely upon such diagnostic tests as the BMR and the PBI, particularly the latter.

Treatment of hypothyroidism is highly specific, effective, and dramatic. It involves the use of thyroid extract, which is prepared by drying and powdering the glands removed from cattle, sheep, and hogs. The yellowish powder, usually referred to in medicine as "thyroid," contains a large amount of the hormone and is readily absorbed by the intestinal mucosa. Preparations of the pure hormones such as Synthroid and Cytomel are also available.

Endemic goiter. In areas of the world in which there is a deficiency of iodine in the soil and food, the population at large will be afflicted with endemic goiter unless the element is added to the diet. Because of the wide use of "iodized salt" (that is, regular salt containing a trace of some iodide), this disorder is now rare in the United States. The mechanism of the enlargement concerns elaboration of excessive amounts of the thyrotropic hormone which, as explained previously, is secreted in response to a deficiency of thyroxine, in this instance occasioned by lack of iodine. As before, this enlargement represents a mode of compensation. As a matter of fact, the compensation is usually good enough to maintain a normal BMR.

PARATHYROID GLANDS

The parathyroids, four tiny glands embedded in the posterior aspect of the thyroid, secrete a hormone called *parathormone* that stimulates the release of calcium from bone into the blood and inhibits reabsorption of phosphate by the kidney. The purpose of the body in doing this, of course, is to maintain a steady concentration of calcium ions in the extracellular fluid (p. 346). A severe drop in [Ca^{++}] can cause tetany and sudden death. Fortunately, almost any factor that serves to decrease calcium stimulates production of parathormone.

Hypoparathyroidism. Although an occasional person develops hypoparathyroidism, the most common cause of this disorder is the inadvertent removal of the parathyroids during thyroidectomy. When this happens, tetany develops in a day or two. Treatment includes administration of parathormone and/or a suitable salt of calcium.

Hyperparathyroidism. Quite rarely, a parathyroid gland may develop a tumor and start pouring out excessive amounts of the hormone. The result is decalcification, soft bones, and kidney stones (p. 334). Sometimes the bones become so weak and brittle that they break under the slightest amount of pressure or tension. Treatment is surgical removal of the tumor.

Calcitonin. As its name indicates, *calcitonin* has to do with the metabolism of calcium. It is secreted by the thyroid gland and, to a much less extent, the parathyroid glands. In startling contrast to the parathyroid hormone, calcitonin stimulates the calcification of bone and thereby the removal of calcium from the blood. No one knows for sure just exactly how this is done, but it could be that the hormone stimulates osteoblastic activity. It is known, though, that the hormone is released by the thyroid in response to an increase in blood calcium. Thus, the parathyroid hormone and calcitonin work together in keeping the Ca^{++} titer "in balance."

ADRENAL GLANDS

The two adrenal glands are elongated, flattened bodies situated at the top of each kidney. The outer portion of the gland, the *cortex,* secretes an array of hormones collectively referred to as the *adrenocortical* hormones; the inside of the gland, the *medulla,* secretes *epinephrine* and *norepinephrine.* Since these vital hormones produce such a variety of physiologic effects, we shall discuss each category in some detail.

Adrenocortical hormones. The adrenocortical hormones* are very much alike chemically (Fig. 22-5) but quite different physiologically. For this reason, they are divided into three categories: mineralocorticoids, glucocorticoids, and androgens. (Since the latter are produced in insignificant amounts in the healthy gland, they are normally of little physiologic concern.)

Mineralocorticoids. The principal mineralocorticoids are *desoxycorticosterone* and *aldosterone,* especially the latter. These hormones are so named because they control the extracellular concentrations of sodium and potassium by their action upon the distal renal tubes: they stimulate the reabsorption of sodium and *inhibit* the reabsorption of potassium. Also, in the process, large amounts of water are returned to the blood along with the sodium ions. One of the major effects of all this, aside from conservation of sodium (which the body needs in appreciable amounts) and excretion of potassium (which is needed only in minute amounts), is the maintenance of blood volume.

---

*Also called adrenocorticoids, adrenocorticosteroids, or simply corticosteroids.

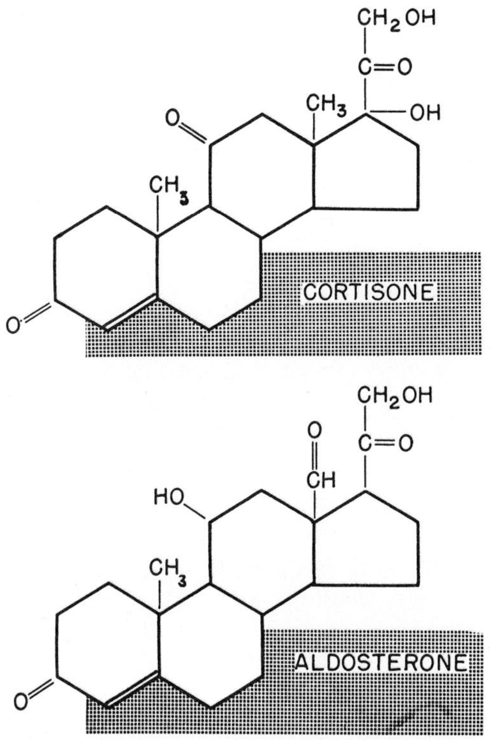

Fig. 22-5. Structural formulas for two corticosteroids. Cortisone is a glucocorticoid, and aldosterone a mineralocorticoid.

The body sees fit to increase the output of the mineralocorticoids in three instances —(1) when the extracellular concentration of sodium starts to fall; (2) during periods of physical stress when an increased blood pressure is generally desirable; and (3) when there is a drop in blood pressure. Just how this is mediated is not known for certain, but it could be that a low $[Na^{+}]$ triggers the adrenal cortices directly or indirectly (via ACTH), perhaps in both ways. In the case of stress, perhaps ACTH is the important avenue (Fig. 22-3). In regard to the drop in blood pressure, the general feeling is that the mechanism centers about the kidney enzyme *renin.* Specifically, renin converts a plasma globulin into *angiotensin I* which, in turn, is converted (by an unknown enzyme) into *angiotensin II*—an agent that stimulates the adrenal cortices to produce aldosterone. (As pointed out on p. 336, angiotensin II also causes vasoconstriction.)

Glucocorticoids. The adrenal cortices secrete a number of glucocorticoids that have a pronounced effect upon the metabolism of protein, fat, and carbohydrate. To a lesser extent, they act upon inorganic metabolism much in the same manner as the mineralocorticoids. From the data currently available, hydrocortisone (cortisol) appears to be the chief hormone of this category.

In some fashion, which is not yet completely understood, the glucocorticoids cause breakdown of protein into amino acids and assist transport of these acids across the cellular membrane into the extracellular compartment. In a word, then, these hormones "mobilize protein." The purpose of such drastic chemical measures is not difficult to understand in light of the fact that the output of the glucocorticoids is greatly increased during periods of physical stress (infection, exposure, trauma, and the like); that is, by having amino acids immediately available, distressed areas can use them to repair protoplasmic damage, to synthesize new cytoplasmic elements, and to provide energy. Also (and this is a key point), the increased concentration of amino acids in the blood provides the liver with the raw materials to make glucose *(gluconeogenesis).* Because nerve cells cannot survive without glucose, gluconeogenesis is especially important during stress. Indeed, the ability of the glucocorticoids to elevate the concentration of blood glucose was their first discovered action (hence, the expression *glucocorticoids*).

Fats are handled in much the same manner, being split into fatty acids for energy and other emergency needs. But unless these acids are used up right away, acidosis may result.

Stress response. The increased output of the adrenocortical hormones in response to stress, first emphasized by Selye, represents the body's "call to arms." As we have learned, these hormones provide the tissues, organs, and systems with emergency materials—amino acids, fatty acids, glucose, sodium, and water. In a very general way, we can say that the mineralocorticoids attend to fluid and electrolyte balance and the glucocorticoids to energy and tissue resistance.

Just how stressful situations stimulate the production of the adrenocortical hormones is not known with certainty, but strong evidence points to the sympathetic nervous system as the "alarm." As we know, this system is most active in times of emergency, and many authorities believe that sympathetic impulses and/or epinephrine trigger the release of ACTH which, in turn, stimulates the adrenal cortices (Fig. 22-3). However, recent experiments show that these hormones can also be released independently of ACTH.

Hypoadrenocorticism. If the adrenal cortices atrophy or are damaged by disease, hyposecretion of adrenocortical hormones (hypoadrenocorticism) results. Commonly known as *Addison's disease,* hypoadrenocorticism leads to death in a very short time unless it is treated. The immediate threat to life is the *loss* of sodium and *retention* of *potassium.* Excess potassium is toxic, and the loss of sodium (and the water that it carries away with it) reduces the extracellular compartment in general and the blood volume in particular. Interestingly, simply taking extra amounts of salt will prolong life somewhat by replacing the lost sodium.

The full treatment of hypoadrenocorticism includes, in addition to salt, administration of desoxycorticosterone and one of the many synthetic glucocorticoids now available (for example, Meticorten). The former corrects the electrolyte and fluid disturbance, and the latter corrects the low state of metabolism and bolsters resistance.

Hyperadrenocorticism. Excessive secretion of the adrenocorticoids by the adrenal cortices usually occurs as a result of a tumor of the adrenal cortex; in rare cases it is due to a tumor of the pituitary gland. In the former instance, the overactivity results from an increase in cortical tissue; in the latter, the cortices are overstimulated by excess ACTH.

The major repercussions include edema (due to retention of salt and water), hypertension (due to the increased blood volume), loss of weight and weakness (due to gluconeogenesis), and masculinization (due to excess androgens). When these effects occur simultaneously, the syndrome is referred to as *Cushing's disease.* Treatment usually involves surgical removal of the tumorous growth.

Corticosteroids. The term *corticosteroids,* or simply *steroids,* is commonly applied to the various synthetic drugs that are chemically and pharmacologically related to the adrenocortical hormones, particularly the glucocorticoids. Cortisone (17-hydroxy-11-dehydrocorticosterone) was the first glucocorticoid to be used clinically. Although it proved to be a "wonder drug," its considerable side effects stimulated the search for drugs that did not have such drawbacks. Today a number of derivatives that pretty much circumvent the disadvantages of the parent drug are available.

Considering the wide and profound metabolic effects that the corticosteroids produce, it is not difficult to appreciate their ability to ameliorate a great many diverse disorders. In addition to their effectiveness in the treatment of hypoadrenocorticism, the corticosteroids frequently produce dramatic results in the treatment of rheumatoid arthritis, rheumatic fever, gout, allergies, inflammatory eye conditions, and many heretofore fatal skin diseases.

In addition to the corticosteroids, the physician sometimes employs the adrenocorticotropic hormone (ACTH). As we might expect, its clinical effects closely parallel those of the corticosteroids.

Epinephrine. In emergency situations

the adrenal medulla secretes epinephrine (commonly called adrenaline) and a closely related hormone called norepinephrine (or noradrenaline). Since these hormones are also released at sympathetic nerve endings (p. 376), we can readily see that the adrenal medulla functions to intensify sympathetic bombardment. Apparently, then, the body employs these two means together for defense and protection.

An injection of epinephrine does many things—all uniquely designed to prepare the body for "fight or flight." It elevates the blood pressure, widens the pupils, dilates the bronchioles, decreases peristalsis, stimulates glycogenolysis, and constricts all vessels *except* those in the coronary system and muscles. The effects of norepinephrine are similar but not identical. Upon blood pressure, for example, this hormone exerts a much more pronounced action. Whereas epinephrine elevates pressure chiefly by increasing cardiac output, norepinephrine does so via vigorous vasoconstriction. As a matter of fact, norepinephrine is now considered a drug of choice in the treatment of shock. On the other hand, epinephrine is the drug of choice in the treatment of acute asthma.

Pheochromocytoma. Pheochromocytoma is a chromaffin cell tumor of the adrenal medulla that results in release of excessive amounts of epinephrine and norepinephrine. Hypertension, together with its associated manifestations, is the main symptom. Characteristically, the rise in blood pressure is intermittent, an "attack" ranging anywhere from a few minutes to several hours. The condition is remedied by surgical removal of the tumor.

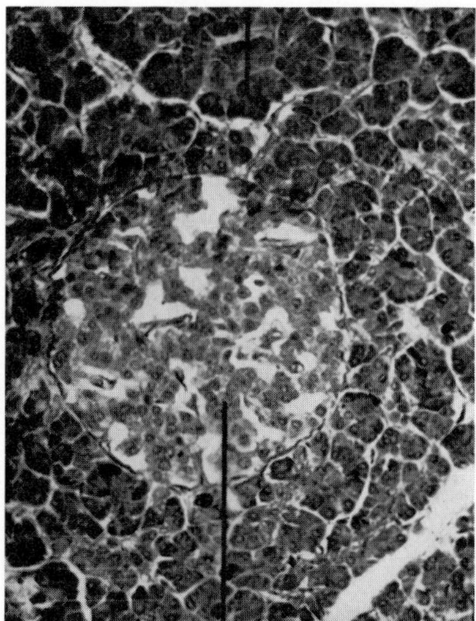

Fig. 22-6. Photomicrograph of human pancreas. (From Bevelander, G.: Essentials of histology, ed. 5, St. Louis, 1965, The C. V. Mosby Co.)

PANCREAS AND INSULIN

Because of the millions of diabetic persons whose lives depend upon insulin, there can be little question that it is the most important hormone used in medical practice. Before this miraculous substance was isolated by Banting and Best in 1923, there was little that diabetic patients could do but starve and wait for the inevitable. Today, the outlook for patients with diabetes is almost as good as for persons with normal metabolism.

Insulin is a relatively simple protein produced in the pancreas (p. 298) by the *beta cells of the islands of Langerhans* (Fig. 22-6). Like other hormones, it enters the blood directly. The release of insulin by these cells probably results from the direct action of excess glucose (*hyperglycemia*). As a matter of fact, the *glucose tolerance test* (Fig. 22-7) is an important tool for determining the functional ability of the pancreas. The test is performed by giving an oral dose of glucose and then taking blood samples at specified intervals. Whereas the blood glucose level in a nondiabetic person will rise to somewhere around 145 mg. per 100 ml. and return to the normal value (around 90 mg. per 100 ml.) in about 2 hours, that of the diabetic patient may run well over 300 mg. per 100 ml. and not return to normal for several hours.

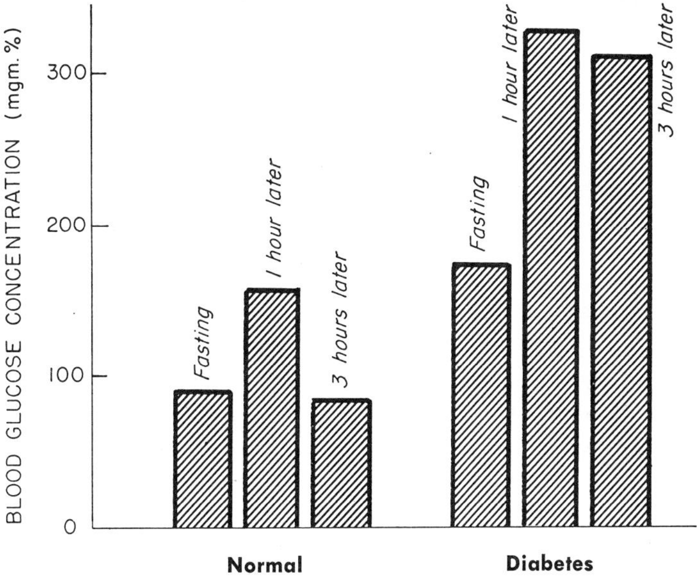

Fig. 22-7. Comparison of the blood glucose levels following ingestion of 50 gm. of glucose by a normal subject and by a diabetic subject.

The glucose tolerance test shows in a most dramatic way that insulin causes glucose to disappear from the blood. The big question, of course, is *how* it does this. Though it is handy and actually not very wrong to say that insulin "burns" glucose, the physiologist wants to know the molecular details. Herein lies one of the great biochemical hunts of our time. This may prove to be a highly surprising quest, too, for the "simplest" explanation appears to be answering more questions than the elaborate theories, most of which are concerned in one way or another with the enzymes of biologic oxidation.

The latest research points to the cell membrane as the chief site of activity. In brief, it is held that the hormone accelerates the transfer of glucose through the cell membrane and into the cell (p. 36). Amazingly, this one single action could indeed account for the major effects of insulin. In the first place, it explains the rapid uptake of glucose by the tissues and its disappearance from the blood. In the second place, it explains the wasting away of tissue in the diabetic patient; that is, since glucose cannot enter the cells (because of a lack of insulin), fat and protein must be sacrificed for the fire. As for *glycogenesis,* or conversion of glucose into glycogen by the liver (p. 308), this cannot take place if glucose is unable to enter the hepatic cells.

In summary, then, the cell membrane explanation seems to fit the facts quite well. However, we cannot, at this time at least, accept it as the last and only word on insulin. Ancillary mechanisms must also be considered, particularly in light of the fact that the hormone exhibits a variety of biochemical activities in the test tube. Glucokinase, for example, a key enzyme in the metabolism of glucose, is "facilitated" by insulin.

Diabetes. Though diabetes mellitus is most conveniently viewed as a disease caused by lazy or incapacitated islands of Langerhans, recent findings—including the fact that some diabetics have *high* circulating levels of insulin—disclose a much more elaborate pathology. Other endocrine glands may be involved; insulin may circulate in a bound, inactive form; immunologic factors may be involved; and so on.

Also there is a great mass of clinical data linking the disease to obesity and heredity. Indeed, in 25 percent of the patients there is a family history of diabetes. Other conditions associated with the development of the disease include certain infections, pancreatic tumors, and even trauma. And in animals the feeding of certain chemicals, namely, alloxan, incites diabetes by a demonstrable destruction of beta cells.

The signs and symptoms of diabetes mellitus are referable in the main to the failure of the body to utilize glucose. These include hyperglycemia, glycosuria, polydipsia, polyphagia, polyuria, weakness, and loss of weight. From the facts previously presented, the student should have little difficulty in figuring out the relationship of excess glucose to these derangements.

Diabetic coma is the immediate threat to life, but once again we go back to glucose. Without sugar, the cells are forced to burn fats, and when fats are burned in excess, *keto acids* (namely, acetoacetic and β-hydroxybutyric acids) are formed. These intermediate products of fat metabolism, which are normally metabolized in the Krebs cycle, accumulate in the blood and produce *acidosis* (p. 345). Unless treated with insulin, the patient will lapse into coma and die.

Diagnosis. Persistent *glycosuria* (sugar in the urine) is presumptive evidence of diabetes. The diagnosis, however, rests largely upon the blood sugar level and glucose tolerance test.

Testing of the urine for glucose is a simple but highly useful procedure. It serves as a screening test for the disease and is a speedy way for the patient to "gauge his insulin." Although there are several modifications, the basic laboratory test depends upon reduction of Cu^{++} to Cu^{+} by glucose. The latter ion then couples with oxygen to form cuprous oxide (Cu_2O), a *red* precipitate, disclosing not only the presence of glucose but also, depending upon the color change (Cu^{++} is blue), its concentration. For use by the patient, test papers (for example, Tes-Tape) are available that undergo a color change incident to the action of glucose oxidase.

Treatment. The treatment of diabetes centers upon the character of the diet and the administration of exogenous insulin, both of which must be tailored to the severity of the disturbance and the needs of the patient.

From the various forms of insulin available, the physician selects the appropriate preparation. These vary with respect to both duration of action and presence of foreign protein. Crystalline zinc insulin (CZI), for example, has a quick onset and short duration of action (4 to 6 hours); on the other hand, protamine zinc insulin (PZI) and NPH insulin have a delayed onset and much longer duration of action. We can easily see that CZI is the preparation of choice in an emergency situation and that the latter agents are better for a mild case of diabetes in which sustained action represents the most desirable feature. A more recent long-acting form of insulin called *Lente Iletin* has the outstanding advantage of being free of foreign protein and therefore less likely to cause allergic reactions.

The need to administer insulin by injection long ago sparked the search for an oral preparation. To some degree, this search has borne fruit, for there are now available several drugs (for example, *Orinase*) that make it possible to control certain types of diabetes without using insulin. Although these drugs have their shortcomings and are not infrequently ineffectual, there is the prospect that development of the ideal drug may someday be realized. These agents, which bear no chemical relationship to the hormone, act by *stimulating* the beta cells. In this connection it is interesting to note that in cases in which the drugs are *not* effective the beta cells have probably lost their ability to make insulin, which apparently is not so in the cases in which they are effective.

Hyperinsulinism. Hyperinsulinism may result from either an overdose of injected hormone or oversecretion as caused by a pancreatic tumor involving the beta cells. In either instance the upshot is *hypoglycemia.* Since nerve cells must receive a constant supply of glucose for proper metabolism, the repercussions of a low blood sugar are ominous. The initial effects are characterized by excitement and, if the deprivation is severe, convulsions. Later these subside and the patient lapses into coma. Paradoxically—and of prime clinical significance—is the fact that the coma of hyperinsulinism mimics diabetic coma. Not infrequently the physician must tax his diagnostic skills to tell whether the diabetic patient in coma has taken too much or too little insulin. Diabetics, of course, are always on guard against hyperinsulinism and carry a piece of candy or other sweet to take at the very first sign of intoxication.

The advent of insulin shock in the treatment of certain forms of mental illness was a milestone in psychotherapy. There are some authorities who still believe that this mode of therapy yields better results than electric shock and even more recently developed procedures. Insulin shock is produced by injecting just enough of the hormone to produce a few moments of unconsciousness. Just exactly how it benefits the higher mental processes is a good but moot question. Perhaps it erases the fresh neural paths forged by impulses that have gone astray.

Glucagon. Whereas the beta cells in the island tissue elaborate insulin, it is indeed interesting to learn that the *alpha* cells secrete a hormone called glucagon, a polypeptide of known amino acid structure. By increasing the activity of phosphorylase, the enzyme that initiates the first step in *glycogenolysis,* glucagon, causes the liver to release glucose to the blood. Apparently, the hormone is released by the pancreas during those times when the tissues are in immediate need of extra glucose.

Recently, glucagon was introduced into medical practice as an antidote in hyperinsulinism. Since only a very small dose of the hormone is required, and since it can be given simply by an injection under the skin (subcutaneously), it is vastly superior to intravenous glucose for use outside the hospital.

OVARY

In girls at the age of about 12 years the anterior pituitary starts to release the follicle-stimulating hormone (FSH) and the luteinizing hormone (LH). As shall be explained in some detail in the next chapter, these agents stimulate the development of the ovaries and cause them to release *estrogens* and *progesterone.* As soon as the effects of these hormones become manifest, we say that puberty has commenced.

Estrogens. The estrogens are steroid substances secreted by the cells of the *graafian* follicle in response to stimulation by the follicle-stimulating hormone. *Estrone* and *estradiol,* particularly the second substance, are the principal members of the group. Their chemical structure differs little from that of progesterone and the male hormone.

Besides stimulating growth of the sex organs, the estrogens are responsible for the development and maintenance of the so-called *secondary sex characteristics,* that is, distribution of body fat and hair, breasts, texture of skin, and character of voice. The role that they play in the menstrual cycle is discussed in Chapter 23.

Undersecretion of estrogens (*hypogonadism*) results in retardation of the sex organs and secondary characteristics. This may be due to either a primary deficiency or lack of the follicle-stimulating hormone. Excessive secretion of hormones (*hypergonadism*), on the other hand, is characterized by sexual precocity. This may result from a tumor of either the ovary or the anterior pituitary. Hypogonadism is treated with estrogens (natural or synthetic) and hypergonadism by surgical intervention.

Progesterone. Progesterone is a steroid released by the *corpus luteum* (Chapter 23) in response to the LH and LTH hormones of the anterior pituitary. Its known effects include inhibition of uterine muscle, "preparation and maintenance" of the lining of the uterus, development of the breasts, and suppression of ovulation in the latter half of the menstrual cycle. These features are taken up in more detail in Chapter 23.

As with estrogens, there is a lack of progesterone in hypogonadism and an excess in hypergonadism. Therefore, the manifestations of these two derangements stem from the combined effects of both hormones. Hypogonadal disorders, for example, amenorrhea, are treated with synthetic progesterone or its derivatives, often in combination with estrogens.

TESTIS

The interstitial tissue of the testis secretes a variety of male hormones collectively referred to as *androgens.* Testosterone, the chief androgen, is closely related chemically to progesterone. Androgens are required for development of the male sex organs and secondary sex characteristics and, in conjunction with FSH, for maintenance of spermatogenesis. In addition, they inhibit the pituitary gland, stimulate the synthesis of protein, and cause the retention of potassium and phosphate. When injected into the female, androgens suppress menstruation and lactation and "tranquilize" uterine activity.

The output of male hormone in the fetus is stimulated by chorionic gonadotropin secreted by the placenta. At birth, however, the testes become dormant and remain so until puberty, at which time the *interstitial cell–stimulating hormone* (ICSH) of the adenohypophysis stimulates them to produce androgens. (ICSH is identical to the LH of the female.) In the event of hyposecretion the male characteristics fail to develop. Castration, for example, causes atrophy of the penis and accessory structures.

DIGESTIVE HORMONES

A number of hormones are called into play in the digestive process (Fig. 22-8). The most important of these are briefly described.

Gastrin. Certain protein factors in food stimulate the stomach mucosa to secrete gastrin which, in turn, provokes the release of gastric juice. This hormone is chemically and physiologically related to the ubiquitous *histamine* (p. 115). (At one time they were thought to be the same.) Among other pronounced effects, both agents provoke a copious flow of gastric juice. Indeed, an injection of histamine is sometimes given in order to secure a sample of the juice for gastric analysis.

Secretin. When acid chyme enters the duodenum, it causes certain cells in the mucosa to release a hormone called secretin. Once in the blood, secretin stimulates the pancreas to form *pancreatic juice* and the liver to form *bile.* This is one of the ingenious ways in which these two organs are apprised of the presence of food in the intestine and of the urgent need for digestive juices.

Pancreozymin. Pancreozymin is a duodenal enzyme also released into the blood in response to acid chyme. As indicated by its name, it induces the secretion of pancreatic juice. However, in contrast to secretin, which provokes chiefly water and sodium bicarbonate, pancreozymin stimulates chiefly the elaboration of digestive *enzymes.*

Cholecystokinin. Bile is forced into the duodenum by contraction of the gallbladder. This action is initiated by a hormone called cholecystokinin that is released by the duodenal mucosa in response to food (especially foods rich in fat such as cream

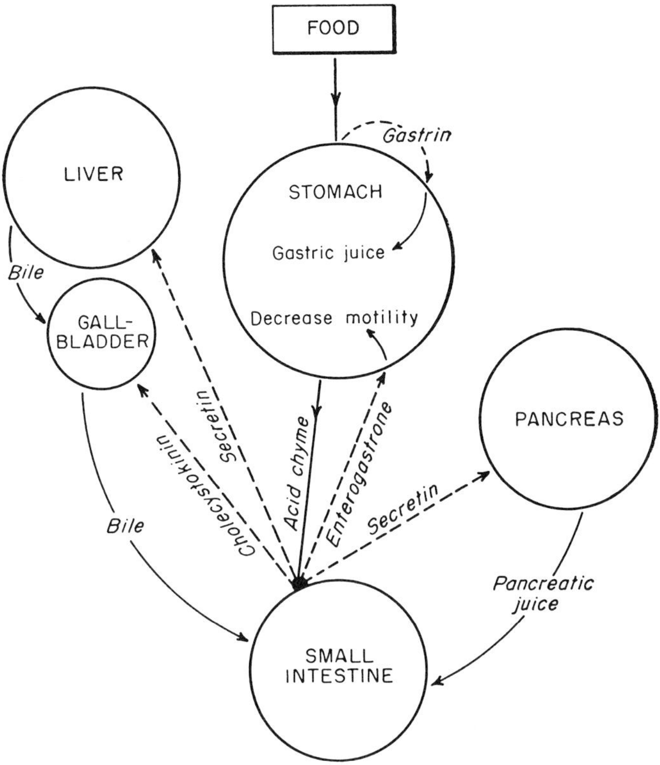

Fig. 22-8. Digestive hormones. (See text.) (From Brooks, S. M.: Basic facts of general chemistry, Philadelphia, 1956, W. B. Saunders Co.)

and egg yolk). This response is one of direct action of the hormone upon the musculature within the wall of the gallbladder.

Enterocrinin. Intestinal juice is called forth by a number of factors, one of which is hormonal. Several hormones, collectively referred to as enterocrinin, are released by the mucosa and are carried to the intestinal glands via the bloodstream. It is believed that these agents are especially important in determining the character of the juice; for example, protein provokes peptidases and carbohydrate provokes carbohydrases.

Enterogastrone. When fat-bearing food enters the duodenum, the mucosa releases enterogastrone. This hormone travels to the stomach via the bloodstream, where it decreases gastric secretion and motility.

PINEAL GLAND

The pineal gland, a tiny (about a tenth of a gram) white structure, shaped somewhat like a pine cone and buried nearly in the center of the brain, is, like the thymus, slowly yielding its secrets to the techniques of present-day biochemistry and neurophysiology. In the rat, at least, it now appears that the pineal is a neuroendocrine *transducer*—that is, a gland which converts nervous input into hormonal output. Specifically, the pineal manufactures a potent hormone called *melatonin* that slows the estrus or sex cycle. Moreover, sympathetic bombardment of the gland (as a consequence of impulses relayed from the retina upon stimulation by light) inhibits the output of the hormone and thereby accelerates estrus. Thus, the current view is that the pineal is a true "biologic clock" that regulates sexuality in mammals—and perhaps the timing of menstrual cycles in human beings. Future developments are obviously awaited with much enthusiasm.

Questions

1. Locate and describe the structure of the hypophysis.
2. Why is the pituitary called the "master gland"?
3. Compare acromegaly and gigantism.
4. Discuss the action of the gonadotropic hormones.
5. Compare the action of vasopressin and oxytocin.
6. What is Pitocin?
7. What is the cause and treatment of diabetes insipidus?
8. What are osmoreceptors?
9. What is thyroglobulin?
10. Distinguish between myxedema and cretinism.
11. Discuss the function of thyroxine.
12. Discuss the treatment of hyperthyroidism.
13. Distinguish between simple goiter and toxic goiter.
14. What is endemic goiter?
15. Discuss the use of thyroid extract.
16. How does the parathyroid hormone control the [Ca^{++}] of blood?
17. What is the immediate cause of tetany? What is the treatment?
18. Compare the glucocorticoids and mineralocorticoids.
19. What is the relationship of stress to adrenal function?
20. Why are drugs such as cortisone often contraindicated in diabetes mellitus?
21. What is the relationship of ACTH to the adrenal cortices?
22. What is the effect of stress upon fluid balance?
23. A characteristic finding in Addison's disease is hyperkalemia. Explain.
24. Discuss the etiology, signs, symptoms, and treatment of Cushing's disease.
25. Compare the effects of epinephrine and norepinephrine.
26. What is a pheochromocytoma?
27. What is the mechanism of action of insulin?
28. Why does insulin have to be injected?
29. Describe the glucose tolerance test.
30. What is the mechanism of action of Orinase and the other "oral insulins"?
31. Explain the etiology of diabetic acidosis.
32. Explain the color change of Benedict's solution occasioned by the presence of sugar.
33. Compare the action of protamine zinc insulin and crystalline zinc insulin.
34. State the action of estradiol, progesterone, and testosterone.
35. Excess histamine might cause a gastric ulcer. Explain.

Chapter 23

Reproduction

In this chapter we shall explore in some detail the structure and function of the male and female sexual apparatus and the development and birth of the human being.

MALE SYSTEM

The reproductive apparatus in the male includes the testes, seminal ducts, seminal vesicles, glands (prostate and bulbourethral), urethra, and penis (Fig. 23-1). These structures will be discussed in the order named, and in studying them the student should make full use of the illustrations.

Testes. The testes, the primary male sex organs (*gonads*), are ovoid bodies enclosed in the *scrotum,* a cutaneous pouch suspended from the pubic and perineal regions. In the fetus, however, they lie within the lower abdominal cavity until about 2 months before birth, at which time they descend into the scrotum. In the event the testes do not descend, sterility results, for human spermatozoa cannot properly develop or thrive unless their environment is below body temperature, as it is in the scrotum.

The interior of the testis is divided by fibrous partitions into a number of wedge-shaped lobes, each containing one to three convoluted *seminiferous tubules* (Fig. 23-2). These tortuous structures unite to form a series of straight ducts that immediately unite in plexiform fashion to form the *rete testis.* From this plexus emerge other ducts that ultimately unite into a long, single, convoluted duct called the *epididymis.* This structure, situated on the posterior aspect of the testis, gives rise to the *vas deferens.* This tube, also called the ductus deferens and the seminal duct, ascends the posterior border of the testis, enters the abdominal cavity, and travels several inches before joining the seminal vesicle.

Seminal vesicles. The seminal vesicles are two coiled tubes with sacculated walls situated just behind the lower portion of the bladder. As stated in the preceding paragraph, each joins a vas deferens and in so doing gives rise to the *ejaculatory duct,* a short tube that passes through the prostate gland to join the prostatic urethra.

Glands. The glands include the prostate and the bulbourethral (Cowper's) gland. The prostate is about the size of a walnut and surrounds the neck of the bladder and the urethra. Its median and two lateral lobes are composed partly of glandular

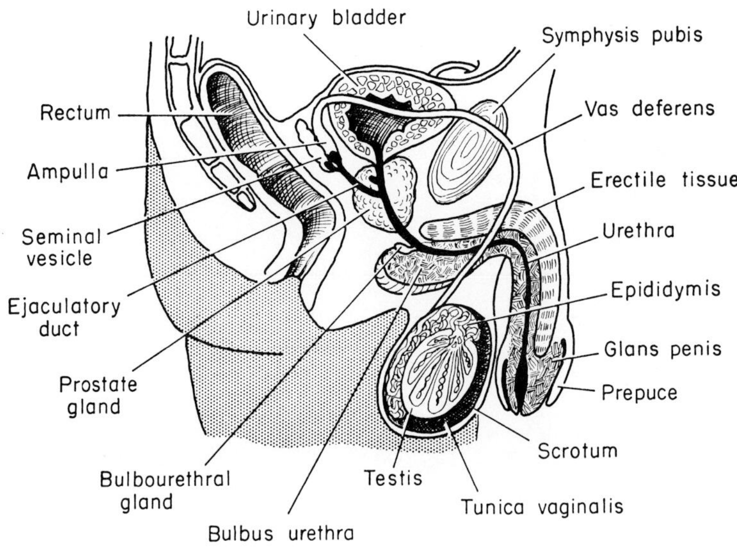

Fig. 23-1. Male reproductive system in longitudinal section.

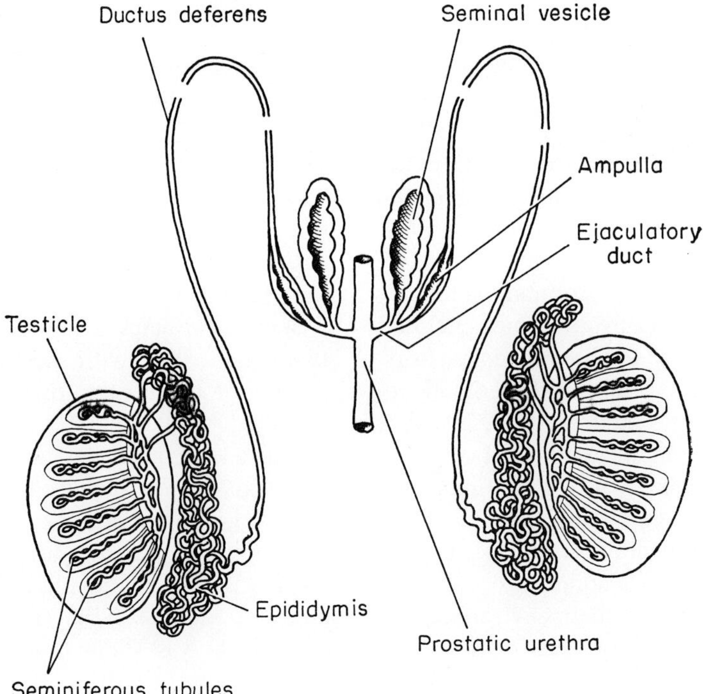

Fig. 23-2. Diagram of the male reproductive "duct system."

matter and partly of muscular fibers, the latter encircling the urethra. The two bulbourethral glands lie near the bulb of the *corpus spongiosum* and send out ducts into the posterior section of the *cavernous urethra.* Both glands secrete a thin fluid that enters into the formation of semen.

Urethra. The male urethra is a membranous tube that conveys urine and semen to the surface; it extends from the neck of the bladder to the urinary meatus and measures about 8 inches in length. The urethra is divided into three parts on the basis of the structures through which it passes (Fig. 23-1): the *prostatic,* the *membranous,* and the *cavernous* (or spongy) portions. About the membranous portion is a band of circular striated muscle fibers, the *external sphincter,* which remains contracted except during micturition (p. 333).

Penis. The penis, the male organ of copulation, has three divisions—the *root,* the *body,* and the extremity, or *glans penis.* The root is attached to the descending portions of the pubic bone by the crura, or extremities, of the corpora cavernosa. The body, the major portion of the structure, consists of the two parallel *corpora cavernosa* and the *corpus spongiosum* beneath (Fig. 23-3). Through the latter passes the urethra. The glans penis is covered with mucous membrane and is ensheathed by the foreskin, or prepuce.

Semen. The collective purpose of the structures just described is to produce and deliver semen to the female.

Semen, the whitish fluid ejaculated in copulation, is composed of male sex cells, or *spermatozoa,* suspended in the nutrient secretions contributed by the prostate, seminal vesicles, and Cowper's glands. The spermatozoa arise from the cells of Sertoli lining the seminiferous tubes (see spermatogenesis, p. 164) and are conveyed to the epididymis through the complex system of channels mentioned earlier. Here they assemble, mature, and await discharge.

Copulation. Copulation, or *coitus,* is the sexual union between male and female, accomplished when the erect penis inserted in the vagina ejaculates semen. Erection results from parasympathetic nerve stimuli that cause the spaces in the spongy or erectile penile tissue (corpora cavernosa

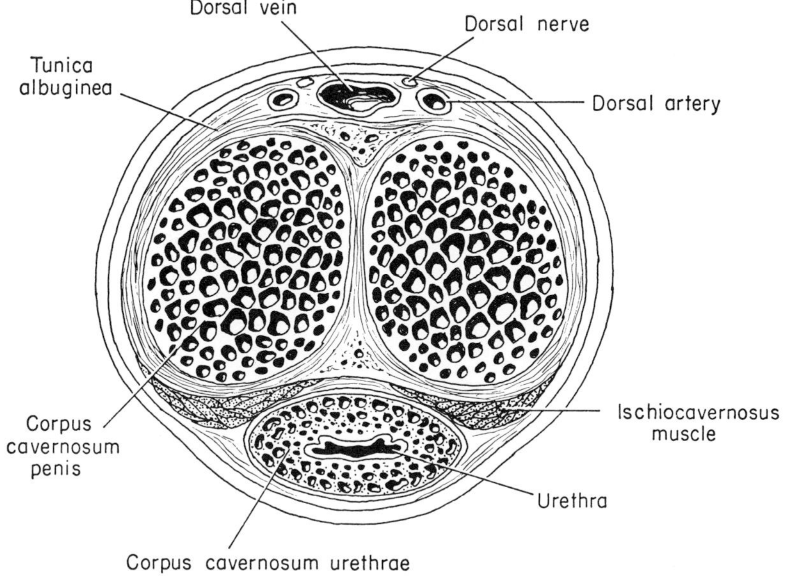

Fig. 23-3. Penis in cross section. (W.R.U. museum specimen C338.) (Modified from Francis, C. C : Introduction to human anatomy, ed. 5, St. Louis, 1968, The C. V. Mosby Co.)

and corpus spongiosum) to dilate with blood and the venous outlets simultaneously to contract. In this fashion the erectile tissue is expanded by increased blood pressure. Ejaculation is the convulsive contraction of the epididymis, vasa deferentia, and seminal vesicles, propelling semen through the urethra. The amount of semen varies from 3 to 7 ml.

Male hormone. In order for the gonads, accessory structures, and secondary sex characteristics to develop, the male hormone testosterone must be present. The particulars about this key substance were presented in Chapter 22.

FEMALE SYSTEM

The female reproductive system consists of the ovaries, the uterine tubes, the uterus, the vagina, and the vulva (Fig. 23-4).

Ovaries. The ovaries, or female gonads, each about the size and shape of an almond, are located in a shallow depression on the lateral wall of the pelvis (one on each side) and are connected with the posterior surface of the *broad ligament* (Fig. 23-5). The infundibulopelvic ligament, a fold of peritoneum that passes from the pelvic wall to the ovary, carries blood vessels and nerves.

Histologically, the ovary is made up of about fifty thousand ova-containing follicles embedded in connective tissue referred to as the *stroma.* Whereas the fetal ovary and ovaries of children consist almost entirely of immature follicles, in the sexually mature female some of these develop into the *mature graafian follicle* (Fig. 23-6). This does not occur until the time of puberty because the follicle-stimulating hormone (FSH) of the hypophysis is not available until then. Of special interest also is the fact that only the mature follicle can produce hormones (p. 408) and discharge its ovum.

Uterine tubes. The uterine (or *fallopian*) tubes are two long slender tubes that run from the upper lateral angle of the uterus to the region of the ovary of the same side (Fig. 23-5). They are attached to the broad ligament by the mesosalpinx, and they enlarge into a funnel-shaped mouth called the *infundibulum.* The rim of the latter structure is formed into fringelike extensions called *fimbriae.* To propel along the ova passed into the infundibula, the mucosa of the tubes is equipped with cilia and the walls with smooth muscle.

Uterus. The uterus is the hollow, muscular, pear-shaped organ that houses the

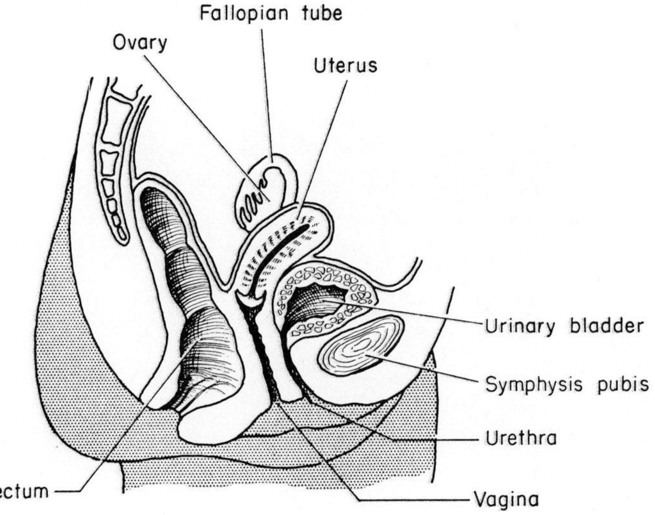

Fig. 23-4. General outline of the female reproductive system.

embryo and fetus. It is about 3 inches long and has a broad, flattened body above and a narrow, cylindrical part called the *cervix* below. The rounded portion that passes above the openings of the fallopian tubes is referred to as the *fundus*. The organ is anchored to the pelvic walls, rectum, and bladder by the broad ligaments, the round ligaments, the uterosacral ligaments, and the vesicouterine ligaments. As shown in Fig. 23-5, the uterine cavity opens into the vagina below through the mouth or cervical os.

The walls of the uterus are formed of smooth muscle (the *myometrium*), and its lining is made of a very special mucous membrane called the *endometrium*. As we shall see presently, the latter tissue plays a key role in the reproductive process.

Vagina. The vagina, the curved, musculo-

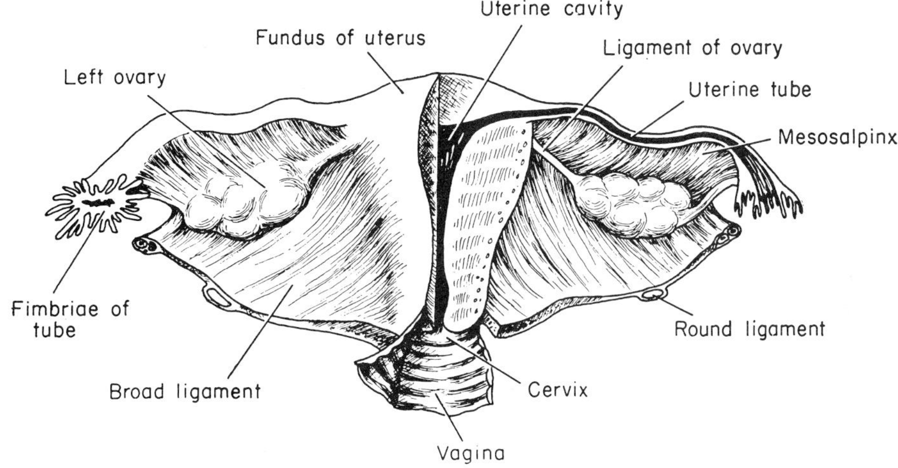

Fig. 23-5. Posterior view of uterus and allied structures. (Modified from Francis, C. C : Introduction to human anatomy, ed. 5, St. Louis, 1968, The C. V. Mosby Co.)

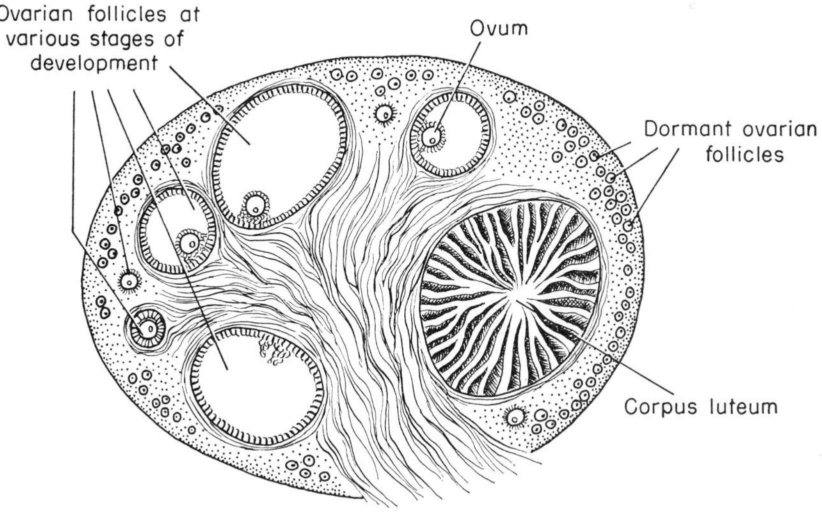

Fig. 23-6. Section through the cat ovary. (After Schrön; modified from Tuttle, W. W., and Schottelius, B. A.: Textbook of physiology, ed. 15, St. Louis, 1965, The C. V. Mosby Co.)

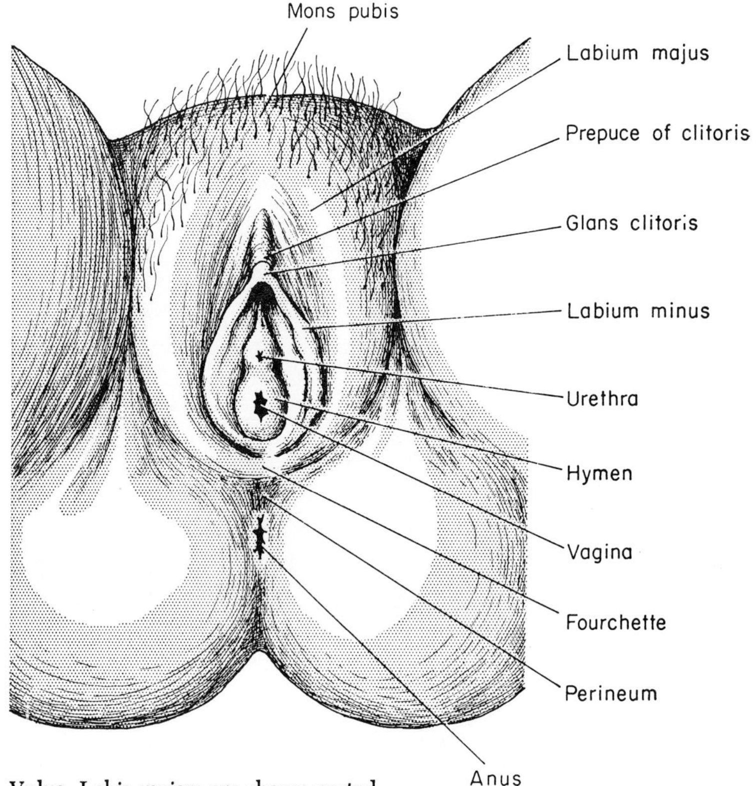

Fig. 23-7. Vulva. Labia majora are shown parted.

membranous canal leading from the vulva to the cervix, receives the erect penis in copulation. It is lined with stratified squamous epithelium, and its walls are composed of an inner circular and an outer longitudinal layer of smooth muscle. In the virgin the vaginal orifice is partly closed by a fold of mucous membrane called the *hymen.* As a consequence of intercourse and parturition, this structure is only fragmentary in the nonvirgin. Often the condition of the hymen upon vaginal examination has medicolegal significance in cases of rape.

Vulva. The vulva, the external female genitals, consists of the mons pubis, the labia majora, the labia minora, the vestibule, and the clitoris (Fig. 23-7). The *mons pubis,* or mons veneris ("mount of Venus"), is a cushionlike, rounded prominence overlying the symphysis pubis. After the age of puberty, this area becomes covered with hair.

The *labia majora* (sing., *labium majus*) are the two large folds of skin and fatty tissue that extend backward and downward from the mons pubis to within about 1 inch of the anal opening. The skin of the labia majora contains hair follicles and sebaceous glands. Medial to and lying under the cover of these structures are the *labia minora* (sing., *labium minus*), two smaller folds of mucous membrane extending backward from the clitoris. The labia minora do not contain hair follicles but have many glands and blood vessels. The cleft between them leads into the *vestibule,* the slight recess containing the vaginal and urethral orifices.

The *clitoris,* the small elongated body situated at the anterior angle of the vulva, corresponds to the penis in the male. It

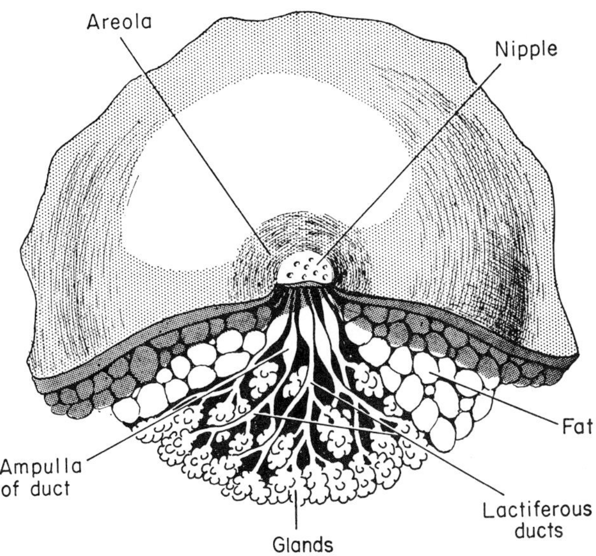

Fig. 23-8. Structure of the breast.

is composed of erectile tissue and becomes hard and erect upon sexual stimulation.

Mammary glands. The mammary glands, or breasts, are the milk-secreting organs in the female (Fig. 23-8). They are composed of glandular tissue organized into some twenty lobes, and the latter are organized into lobules. The lobes are partitioned by connective tissue, and the whole mass is embedded in a variable but large amount of fatty tissue.

At its center the breast is surmounted by the nipple—a small, dark, conical structure composed of erectile tissue. The lactiferous ducts (one from each lobe) meet here and open to the exterior upon its surface. About the nipple is a circular area of pigmented skin known as the *areola.*

Before the age of puberty the mammary glands are composed mostly of connective tissue, but with the onset of puberty the ducts and glandular tissue undergo rapid development. This hyperplastic activity stems from the activity of the female hormones (p. 419). Estrogens stimulate development of the duct system, and progesterone stimulates the alveoli (the basic milk-secreting units of the gland). This is especially true during pregnancy, when these hormones reach high levels.

Lactation. The secretion of milk by the breasts (lactation) is provoked chiefly by *prolactin,* the lactogenic hormone of the anterior pituitary. It is believed that the sudden drop in progesterone concentration at the end of pregnancy brings about the release of prolactin, since the former hormone is known to inhibit production of the latter. Finally, the act of sucking plays a role via *oxytocin* (p. 409). This hormone does not increase the production of milk, but it does enhance its release by contracting the smooth muscle in the alveoli and milk ducts. Sucking is probably not the only stimulus, however. Indeed, music in the stable is said to facilitate the milking of cows.

Milk. For the first 6 months of life human milk provides all the materials necessary for proper growth. Although human milk is noticeably low in iron, the newborn infant has absorbed enough of this mineral in utero to meet the needs of the first year or so. Like cow's milk, human milk is low in vitamin D, and for this reason the infant's diet should be supplemented. Human milk and cow's milk are very much alike except for the concentration of protein and sugar (Table 23-1).

An often overlooked fact is that, aside from nutrition, milk also provides the offspring with immunologic protection; that is, the glandular tissue in the breasts extracts antibodies as well as nutrients from the mother's blood. This is a form of passive immunity (p. 154) that will carry the infant through the first few months in his new microbe-infested world. After this time the infant must weather infection "alone."

Table 23-1. Human milk vs. cow's milk (percent composition)

	Human	Cow
Water	88.5	87.2
Fat	3.3	3.5
Lactose	6.5	4.9
Protein	1.4	3.5
Electrolytes	0.3	0.9

Menstrual cycle. The periodic discharge of blood from the vagina (*menstruation*) is only one phase of a tremendously interesting "hormonal clock" whose mainspring is situated in the anterior pituitary.

Somewhere between the ages of 10 and 14 years, the anterior pituitary begins to secrete, among other hormones, three gonadotropins: the follicle-stimulating hormone (FSH), the luteinizing hormone (LH), and the luteotropic hormone (LTH). The follicle-stimulating hormone causes a few of the immature follicles to grow and

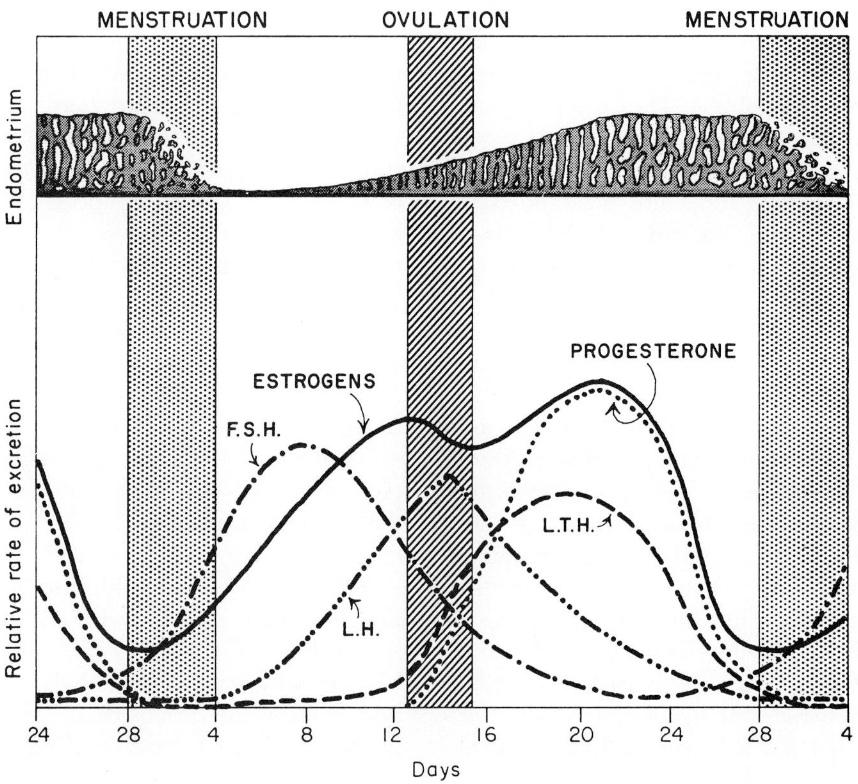

Fig. 23-9. Menstrual cycle in graphic form. **FSH,** Follicle-stimulating hormone; **LH,** luteinizing hormone; **LTH,** luteotropic hormone.

release estrogens, one of the two major types of female sex hormones (Fig. 23-9). A few days following the release of FSH, the pituitary starts putting out LH, which increases the rate of follicular growth and secretion even more. Finally, one of the follicles becomes so large that it ruptures, expelling its ovum into the abdominal cavity. When this happens, the follicular cells (still under the influence of LH) increase in size, become fatty and yellow, and thereby become a structure called the *corpus luteum* (Fig. 23-6).

A few days following the release of LH, the pituitary gland sends forth its third gonadotropin—LTH. This hormone further enhances the growth of the corpus luteum and, in addition, causes it to secrete large quantities of both estrogens and progesterone. The former hormones cause the endometrium to grow in thickness (Fig. 23-9), and the latter enhances endometrial blood flow and nutrient secretion. The purpose of the body in doing this, of course, is to provide a suitable environment in which the fertilized ovum can grow.

If, indeed, fertilization does occur, the developing ovum itself becomes an endocrine gland and releases a gonadotropic hormone that sustains the corpus luteum throughout pregnancy. This is most fortunate, for the pituitary produces LTH for only about 2 weeks. Thus, when fertilization *does not* occur, the corpus luteum undergoes involution, and the output of estrogens and progesterone is brought to a halt. As a consequence, the endometrium degenerates and sloughs off into the uterine cavity, the necrotic debris—measuring about 50 ml.—containing blood, serous exudate, and dead endometrial cells.

Following menstruation, the endometrium is once again a thin "anemic" lining. Soon, however, it begins to thicken in the manner just described, and the cycle starts anew.

With these facts in mind, the student should carefully study the graphic representation of the cycle as presented in Fig. 23-9. In addition to distilling the information already discussed, the illustration gives the arithmetic data for the statistical female —that is, a cycle of 28 days, menstruation lasting 4 days, and ovulation occurring on the fourteenth day. By convention (and note this especially), the cycle begins and ends on the *first* day that the menses appears.

Period of fertility. Since the ovum can be fertilized by a sperm cell only during the 24-hour period following ovulation, and since the sperm cell can live in the vaginal canal usually for no more than 24 hours, it stands to reason that fertilization cannot ordinarily occur unless there is intercourse either shortly before, during, or shortly after ovulation. Because ovulation in most instances occurs on or about the fourteenth day of a 28-day cycle, the meeting of the ovum and sperm is statistically most likely to occur somewhere around the thirteenth, fourteenth, or fifteenth day. Although many women have cycles as short as 20 days and as long as 40 days, it appears that ovulation still follows a rather definite schedule—14 days *before* menstruation. For example, if a woman has regular cycles, let us say of 33 days' duration, ovulation will occur on about the nineteeth day ($33 - 14 = 19$).

In the event that man and wife desire to prevent conception, these facts and figures are useful and usually dependable in the presence of *regular* cycles. Obviously, when the cycles are erratic (for example, 28 days one time, 20 the next, 35 the next, and so on), ovulation cannot be predicted with any degree of accuracy. In the so-called *rhythm method* of birth control the average of several successive cycles is computed and, as explained before, the number 14 is subtracted from this average to derive the day of ovulation. Now if abstinence is observed for the 5 days preceding and the 5 days following the calculated day of ovulation, fertilization will almost never occur. Once again, this method is not applicable to *erratic* menstrual cycles.

It should be stressed that at this time there is no absolute method of birth control short of total abstinence and sterilization. It is quite possible, however, that chemists may yet synthesize the "perfect" drug to prevent ovulation. Such an agent, of course, to be of real value, would have to be inexpensive and nontoxic in addition to being 100 percent effective. The so-called "contraceptive pill" we hear so much about is an estrogen-progestin* combination that inhibits ovulation via its inhibitory effect on the output of the follicle-stimulating hormone. The pill is certainly effective but not cheap and, more important, it is not without adverse effects, some of which may prove serious.

Menopause. In the average woman at about the age of 45 years the follicles no longer secrete their hormones in full amounts, and the monthly cycles cease. This is termed the menopause. Aside from the not always pleasant fact that this period of one's life signals advancing years, the menopause is not infrequently accompanied by distressing signs and symptoms —nervousness, headache, "hot flashes," and the like. Since the syndrome is usually benefited by estrogenic therapy, there is good reason to believe that the sudden drop in hormone output is the underlying cause of the menopausal symptoms. Psychosomatic factors undoubtedly play a role, perhaps the major role in some instances.

Copulation. The female's role in intercourse is to cause the male to reach an orgasm by providing the appropriate mental and physical environment. In particular, the act is enhanced by the swelling of the erectile tissue about the vaginal opening and the secretion of large quantities of mucus by the two small Bartholin glands situated just inside the vagina on either side. The tight but distensible and lubricated opening thus provided intensifies the stimulation resulting from the to-and-fro movement of the penis in the vaginal canal.

The bulk of the stimuli leading to the female climax stems from the movement of the penis against the clitoris. The climax itself is characterized by an exotic sensation and rhythmic peristalsis-like contractions of the uterus and fallopian tubes. The latter effect serves to hasten along the ejaculated semen into the upper reaches of the fallopian tubes. Although the act reaches its highest emotional development when the male and female experience the climax at the same time, this is by no means a prerequisite for successful fertilization. Indeed, at the proper time in the menstrual cycle fertilization may be accomplished via artificial insemination.

REPRODUCTIVE PROCESS

The normal charge of semen deposited in the vagina generally contains from 150 to 300 million spermatozoa per cubic centimeter of fluid. Traveling at a speed of about 1 foot per hour, most will arrive in the upper reaches of the fallopian tubes in a little over a half hour. In order for fertilization to occur, the sperm must encounter the fresh ovum either here or in the abdominal cavity before the ovum enters the tube. An encounter elsewhere is generally of no avail, for by the time the ovum reaches the uterus, it has acquired an armor of mucus.

It is quite surprising to learn that a sperm count below fifty million generally results in infertility, although many pregnancies have occurred with sperm counts of this magnitude. In view of the fact that it takes but one single sperm to "do the job," this is something of a phenomenon. There is good evidence, however, for believing that a galaxy of spermatozoa are needed to secrete sufficient amounts of the enzyme hyaluronidase to remove the *corona*

*As used nowadays, *progestin* is the term applied to the various brands of synthetic progesterone (and is so used here).

radiata, a relatively thick barrier of cells surrounding the ovum. (The enzyme does this by digesting away the protein that links these cells together.) Once the barrier is removed, a single sperm enters the ovum and a new life begins. To ensure against an abnormal chromosome number, one sperm cell—and only one—is admitted; that is, the membrane of the ovum "shuts the door" to the millions of others outside. Just how the ovum accomplishes this feat remains a moot question.

Embryology. The marvels that follow fertilization are awesome and tantalizingly complex. To think that a single cell can develop into a trillion-celled being capable of reading this sentence is indeed the mystery of life. All that most of us can do is to observe what happens and record the events—and this is, in itself, no mean task. As a matter of fact, for fear of not seeing the forest because of the trees (and, moreover, because of time and space limitations), we shall here touch only upon the highlights of human embryology.

Morula. As the sperm enters the ovum, its tail drops off (Fig. 23-10) and its head swells into the male pronucleus, the original nucleus of the egg being called the female pronucleus. The two nuclei, each containing the *haploid* number of twenty-three chromosomes (p. 164), then fuse into the forty-six chromosome *zygote,* the cell destined to be the new individual. In about 24 hours the zygote undergoes the first cleavage (division) and continues to do so every 12 to 15 hours thereafter. By the time the fertilized structure reaches the uterus (in about a week's time), the segmented mass, now called the morula, contains in the vicinity of twenty-five cells. However, it is still barely visible to the unaided eye.

Blastula. As growth continues, the new cells arrange themselves in such a way that a cavity forms within the mass, with a cluster of cells (the *inner cell mass*) projecting into the cavity. This hollow-ball structure is called the blastula and the cavity within is called the *blastocoele.*

The cells forming the outer layer of the blastula are referred to en masse as the *trophoblast* (or *trophectoderm*). The trophoblast secretes proteolytic enzymes that digest away a tiny bit of the endometrium, and then its cells phagocytize the digested products. In this fashion the blastula implants itself into the uterine wall and in the process derives its sustenance. By the end of 2 weeks we find the blastula completely embedded within the endometrium and the trophoblastic cells rapidly growing and dividing. Soon they and the adjacent cells start to form the fetal membranes. The *chorion,* the outer membrane, sends out thousands of microscopic projections called *villi* that invade the surrounding mucosa and lay the groundwork for the *placenta,* the cakelike mass within the uterus that will establish communication between the mother and the child via the umbilical cord (p. 438).

While this is going on outside, drastic changes are taking place in the inner cell mass. Two cavities have appeared in the mass, and a new layer of cells (the *mesoderm*) has grown over the original lining of the blastocoele, passing between the two new cavities. The cavity closest to the trophoblast, called the *amniotic* cavity, is destined to house the embryo, which has not yet appeared; the outer cavity, called the *yolk sac,* serves no purpose in man and will ultimately degenerate and disappear.

Embryonic disc. The three-layered plate of cells running between the amniotic cavity and the yolk sac, aptly referred to as the embryonic disc, now becomes the crucial area of development. This is where the miracles of nature in general and biochemistry in particular form the embryo.

The *ectoderm,* the outermost of the three primary germ layers of the disc, will evolve into the skin, the nervous system, the external sense organs, and the mucous mem-

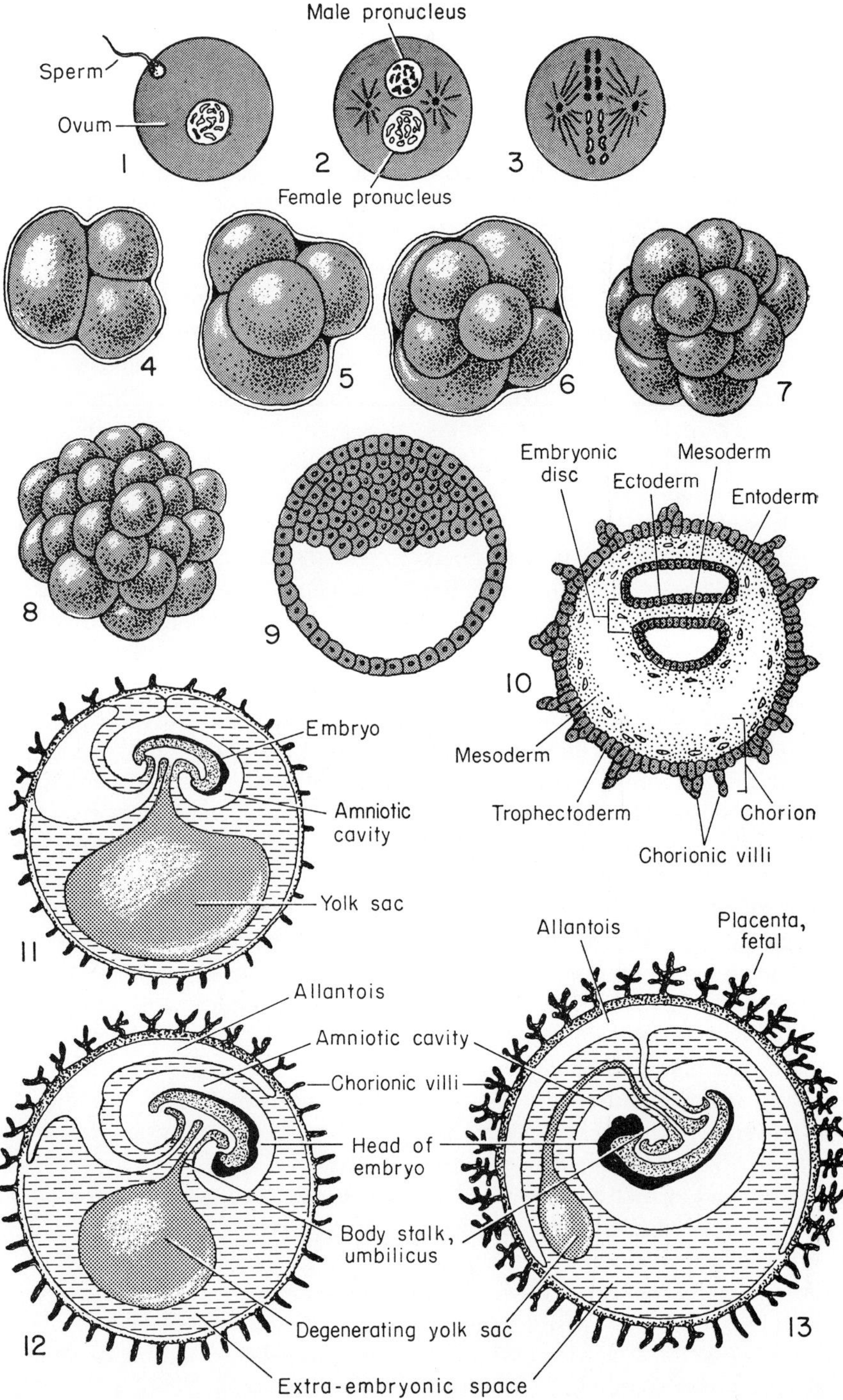

Fig. 23-10. Embryologic highlights of mammalian gestation from the time of fertilization, **1**, to the development of the fetal placenta, **13**. Stages **8** and **9** are called the morula and the blastula, respectively. (**11** to **13** adapted from Woodruff, L. L.: Animal biology New York, 1961, The Macmillan Co.)

brane of the mouth and anus; the *mesoderm,* the middle layer, will evolve into the connective tissues, muscles, blood vessels, *sex organs,* and epithelium of the pleura, pericardium, peritoneum, and kidney; and the *endoderm* (or *entoderm*), the innermost layer, will evolve into the epithelium of the pharynx, respiratory tract, gastrointestinal tract, bladder, and urethra. Some idea of how these transformations take place in the early stages can be obtained by a close study of the diagrammatic sections shown in Fig. 23-10.

Sex. In each human somatic cell, two of the forty-six chromosomes are concerned with sex. When two so-called X chromosomes appear together following gametic union, the result is a female individual; when an X and Y chromosome are together, the result is a male. It stands to reason, then, that all ova will carry an X chromosome, whereas half the sperm cells carry an X chromosome and the other half a Y chromosome. Thus, when an X sperm cell fertilizes an ovum, the offspring is a girl; conversely, when a Y sperm cell fertilizes an ovum, the offspring is a boy. Since it is the father who carries the odd chromosome, he should by no means blame the mother in the event the sex of the offspring is not to his liking.

Twinning. In the event that two or more ova instead of the customary one are released and are fertilized simultaneously, *fraternal* twins result. Identical twins, on the other hand, result from a single fertilized ovum that has split one or more times into cell masses that develop into separate but identical offspring. In the instance of *quintuplets* there are four such divisions prior to implantation.

Placenta. Though the embryo naturally "steals the show" throughout gestation, we should not forget that it is the placenta that makes intrauterine life feasible. As shown in Fig. 23-11, this structure is essentially a mass of blood sinuses formed by the placental septa. Into these sinuses extend chorionic projections from the fetal portion of the placenta, each covered with an astronomical number of microscopic villi containing blood capillaries.

Maternal blood flows in and out of these sinuses by means of a well-channeled sys-

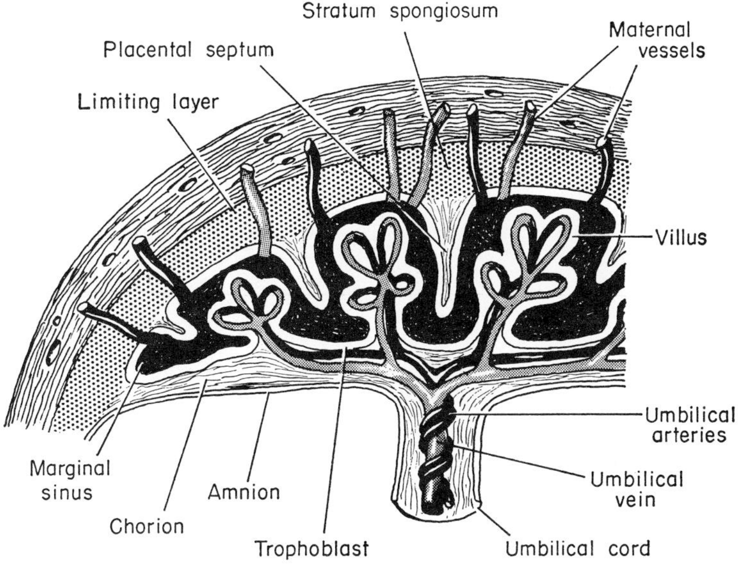

Fig. 23-11. Gross structure of the placenta. (After Gray; modified from Guyton, A. C.: Function of the human body, Philadelphia, 1959, W. B. Saunders Co.)

tem of vessels derived from the uterine wall. Fetal blood is led into the villi via the two umbilical arteries and is then led back via the umbilical vein. As the blood courses through the villi, nutrients are absorbed and waste products are excreted. This is largely effected through simple *diffusion;* that is, since the concentration of oxygen and nutrients is greater on the maternal side of the placental barrier, these materials "flow" from the mother to the offspring. By the same token, fetal wastes (carbon dioxide, urea, and the like) diffuse from the villi into the blood sinuses, whence they are removed by the mother's excretory organs.

Placental hormones. Aside from serving as a food source and purifier, the placenta also secretes hormones, without which pregnancy cannot continue. Earlier it was pointed out that when fertilization occurs the *corpus luteum,* which normally degenerates at the end of each menstrual cycle, is maintained by *gonadotropin* secreted by the developing ovum (at first by the trophoblast and later by the chorionic membrane). However, after about the fourth month of pregnancy, the chorionic gonadotropin concentration drops to low levels, and the corpus luteum ceases to be stimulated sufficiently to produce the necessary high levels of estrogens and progesterone. At this time the placenta takes over the job and pushes the concentration of these hormones to well over fifty times their peak value during nonpregnancy.

The female hormones are especially vital during pregnancy. In brief, the estrogens thicken the uterine musculature, greatly enhance the uterine blood supply, enlarge the breasts, and facilitate embryonic development. Progesterone relaxes the uterine musculature until the time of birth, aids the development of the endometrium, prevents ovulation, and produces an alveolar arrangement of cells in the breast to make ready for milk production and secretion.

Membranes. There are two membranes surrounding the fetus—the *amnion* and the *chorion* (Fig. 23-12). The amnion, the in-

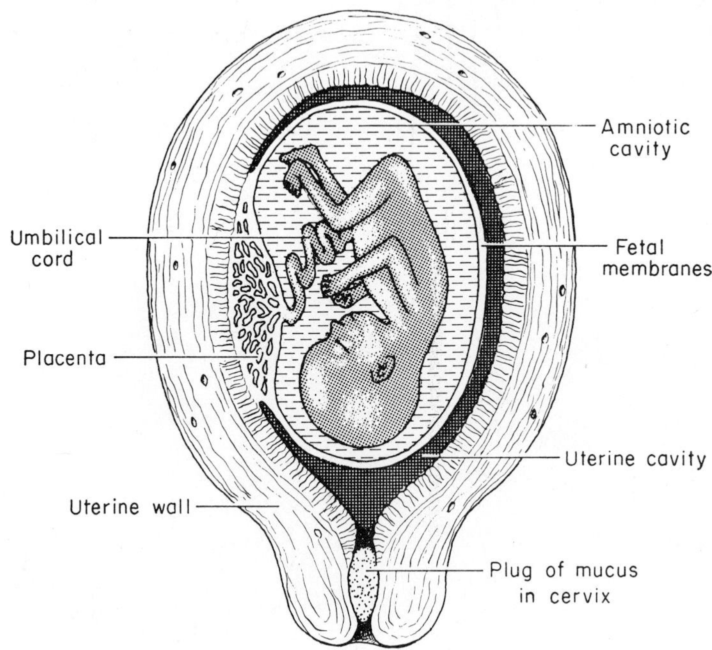

Fig. 23-12. Fetus in utero. (Modified from Guyton, A. C.: Function of the human body, Philadelphia, 1959, W. B. Saunders Co.)

nermost membrane, is a thin transparent tissue that encloses the so-called amniotic cavity, and in order to equalize and cushion the pressures bearing upon the fetus, nature has filled this cavity with a watery liquid referred to as the amniotic fluid.

The chorion, the thick outermost membrane, is actually composed of two layers—an outer ectoderm and an inner mesoderm. The portion of the chorionic surface that gives rise to the villi and forms the embryonic and fetal placenta is called the *chorion frondosum.* The remaining surface, called the *chorion laeve,* is membranous and smooth.

Fetal circulation. Because the fetus has no need for its liver or lungs, the blood flow through these organs is cut to a minimum via three shunts—the *ductus venosus,* the *foramen ovale,* and the *ductus arteriosus* (Fig. 23-13). The ductus venosus runs straight through the liver and carries blood from the umbilical vein and portal vein directly into the inferior vena cava, thereby shutting off most of the blood supply of the liver. The blood, on reaching the heart, now bypasses the nonaerated lungs by flowing through the foramen ovale, the opening between the atria, and the ductus arteriosus. The former shunts part of the blood returning to the right atrium into the left atrium and thereby cuts down on the amount passing into the right ventricle and pulmonary artery. Considerable blood, however, does pass into the artery, and it is for this reason that a second shunt—the ductus arteriosus—directs most of the right ventricular blood directly into the aorta.

Other major features of the fetal circulatory system are the three vessels composing the umbilical cord—*the umbilical vein* and *the two umbilical arteries.* The vein carries fresh blood from the placenta to the fetus, and the arteries return "poor" blood from the fetus to the placenta. A substance called *Wharton's jelly,* a soft pulpy type of connective tissue, constitutes the protective matrix about these vessels as they pass through the cord.

Fetal growth. The fetus grows by leaps

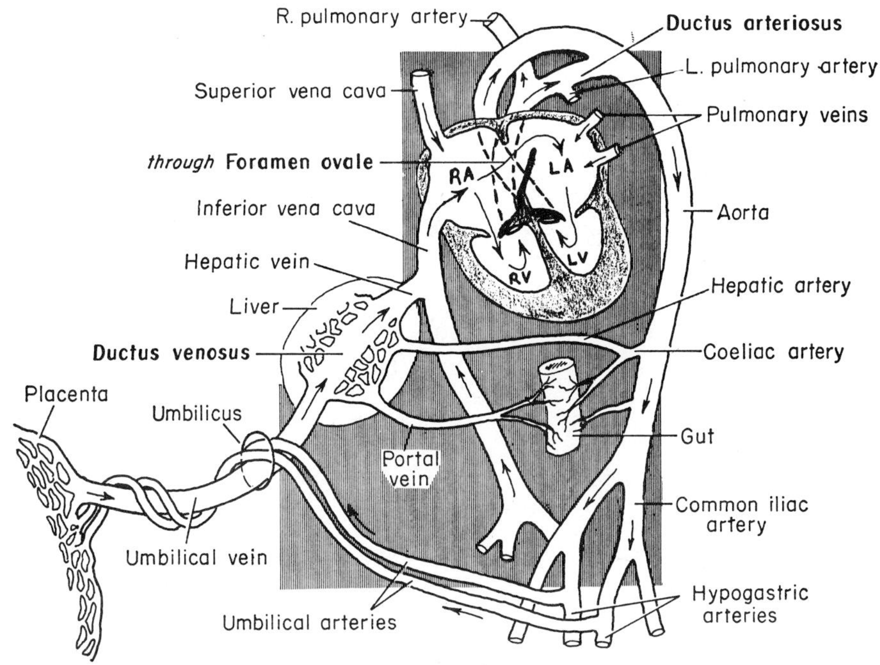

Fig. 23-13. Circulation of blood in the fetus. **RA,** Right atrium; **RV,** right ventricle; **LA,** left atrium; **LV,** left ventricle.

and bounds and in a unique fashion ("multiplying by division"). Metabolizing prodigious amounts of nutrients supplied by the mother's blood, it evolves from an average weight of 1 ounce at 3 months to an average weight of 7 pounds at the time of birth. The bulk of this terrific increase in weight occurs during the last 3 months of pregnancy (Table 23-2).

Maternal physiology. Pregnancy is by no means confined to the explosive anabolic happenings within the amniotic cavity. The mother, too, undergoes tremendous change. Her metabolism is accelerated, her tissues retain excess fluid (about 3 quarts), and last, but by no means least, she gains an average of about 20 pounds (fetus, 7 pounds; uterus, 2 pounds; placenta and membranes, 2½ pounds; breasts, 2 pounds; fat and extra fluid, 6½ pounds). However, if all goes well throughout pregnancy and during delivery, these anatomic and physiologic alterations reverse themselves in an amazingly short period of time. Indeed, there is good reason to believe that a normal pregnancy strengthens the body.

Parturition. The duration of pregnancy averages 280 days from the beginning of the last menstrual period; about 90 percent of all births occur within a week before or after this figure. Although there is still no unanimous agreement on the mechanism or mechanisms behind such precise timing, there is good reason to believe that the placental hormones play the principal role. The support of this view stems from the changes in their concentrations that occur a month or so prior to birth. Progesterone, which inhibits uterine motility, begins to decrease, whereas estrogens, which enhance motility, begin to increase. As a consequence, the myometrium becomes progressively more active as the fetus approaches the end of its intrauterine life. Also, the fetus grows larger and larger, and this in itself aids in stimulating uterine contraction.

Table 23-2. Growth of the embryo

Age (weeks)	Length (inches)	Weight
8	1	1/10 ounce
12	4	1 ounce
20	10	12 ounces
28	14	2 pounds
36	18	5 pounds
40	20	7 pounds

Thus, uterine activity steadily increases during the last 2 months of pregnancy, finally terminating in intense rhythmic contractions a few hours before birth. The period from the onset of these terminal contractions until delivery is referred to as labor, or parturition.

The duration of labor usually runs between 8 and 18 hours. In the *first* stage the *cervix is dilated* and, generally, the amniotic membrane is torn, causing expulsion (the "show") of the amniotic fluid. During the *second* stage the powerful contractions push the baby through the birth canal and out into the "brave new world." The *third* stage is actually an anticlimax—the expulsion of the *afterbirth* (fetal membranes and placenta). As soon as the child is born, that is, at the end of the second stage, the umbilical cord is tied and cut.

The pulling away of the placenta from the uterine wall leaves a wide area of bare, oozing vessels and accounts for the considerable bleeding that accompanies parturition. Though the loss of a pint or so of blood (the usual amount) is well tolerated and is actually provided for by the mother's enhanced supply, larger losses are obviously dangerous. This is why the physician often administers *oxytocic* drugs. Such agents cause the uterus to "clamp shut," thereby closing dilated blood vessels and facilitating clotting.

Pregnancy tests. Gonadotropin, the hormone produced by the trophoblast shortly after implantation, appears in the urine and may be detected by its action on the mammalian ovary and on the gonads of various amphibia. The original test, the *Aschheim-Zondek* (A-Z) test, depends upon development of hemorrhagic follicles in the ovaries of immature female white mice. However, six injections of urine must be made over a period of 2 days. In the *Friedman test* the mature female rabbit is used.

The simplest and most accurate biologic pregnancy test utilizes the South African toad *(Xenopus laevis)*. Concentrated urine (1 ml.) is injected into the dorsal lymph sac, and if a sufficient concentration of chorionic gonadotropin is present, ovulation occurs and myriads of eggs are extruded in 8 to 16 hours. The toad test is 96 to 100 percent accurate. Since the South African toad is expensive and occasionally difficult to procure, many laboratories now use the American male frog *Rana pipiens* as the test animal. In this version of the test 5 ml. of urine is injected into the dorsal or lateral lymph sac. The presence of spermatozoa in the urine of the frog after 2 to 4 hours is interpreted to indicate a positive test. This test has proved to be about 95 to 96 percent accurate and entirely satisfactory in most laboratories.

Recently a number of in vitro tests have been developed (available commercially as Gravindex, Pregnosticon, and UCG Test, to name a few). While each differs in procedure, all are based on the use of antihuman chorionic gonadotropin serum derived from rabbits that have been caused to produce antibodies against human chorionic gonadotropins.

DISEASES OF THE REPRODUCTIVE SYSTEM

The reproductive apparatus in both sexes is subject to a number of functional, organic, and infectious disorders. In this section we shall discuss the basic points of the more common of these.

Diseases of the male. The bulk of the diseases afflicting the male reproductive system are focused upon the testes, prostate gland, and urethra. As indicated, these derangements may be infectious or noninfectious.

Cryptorchidism. Cryptorchidism is a condition in which the testes fail to descend into the scrotum and remain within the abdominal cavity. True cryptorchidism is usually bilateral and may be due to a hormonal deficiency. Generally, however, there is partial descent, with only one testis being affected. The cause here is usually some type of mechanical obstruction. Cryptorchidism is serious because the testes are more subject to injury, tumors, and developmental failure. If bilateral, the condition may lead to sterility.

Cryptorchidism is best treated surgically before the age of 5 years. If the physician has decided that the condition is hormonal, he administers an injection of chorionic gonadotropin, the hormone that normally effects the descent of the testes. In the event that the difficulty is mechanical, the obstruction is remedied surgically. Although the testes may descend by themselves up to the age of about 13 years, spermatogenesis is generally inhibited past the age of 7 years.

Prostatism. After the age of 60 years, approximately one fourth of all men experience prostatism, or enlargement of the prostate. As a result, the urethra, which passes through the gland, becomes narrowed and urinary obstruction, a most serious situation, occurs. Generally, the underlying cause is benign hypertrophy, cancer, or fibrosis. The last named is frequently a sequel to infection. Although mild cases are successfully treated with antibiotics and estrogens, moderate to severe obstruction requires surgical intervention.

Sterility. Inability of the male to effect fertilization may be caused by inhibited spermatogenesis (due to absence of the testes, cryptorchidism, hypogonadism, or overradiation), obstruction of the seminal tract, or some form of impotence. The

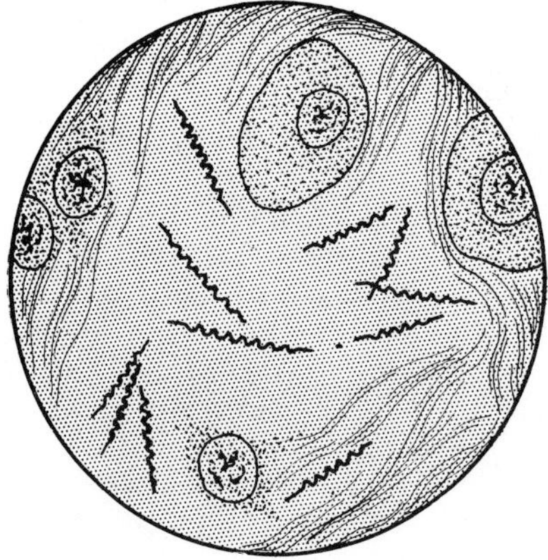

Fig. 23-14. *Treponema pallidum* in tissue.

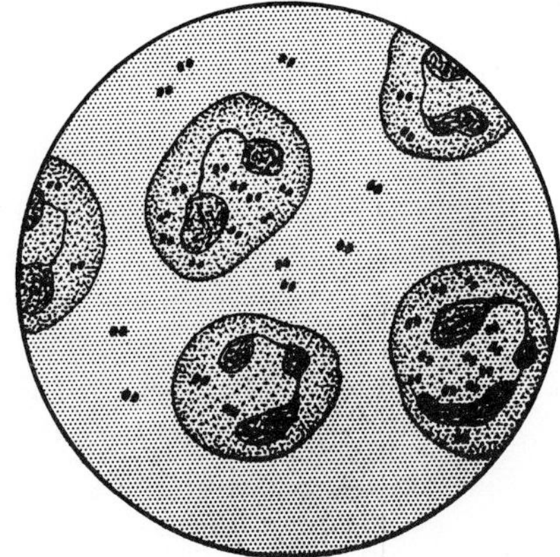

Fig. 23-15. *Neisseria gonorrhoeae* in pus. Note that many organisms have been ingested by the white cells.

treatment of the condition centers about correction of the underlying cause. In obstruction, for example, surgery is indicated.

Syphilis. Syphilis, the chief venereal disease and one of the most vicious infections of man, is caused by the microorganism *Treponema pallidum* (Fig. 23-14). Except for the congenital variety, syphilis is almost always contracted through sexual intercourse; the male passes it to the female, or vice versa.

The first or primary stage of the infection is characterized by the appearance of the *chancre,* a hard, painless papule that develops at the portal of entry (p. 130). This lesion eventually becomes a reddish ulcer covered with a yellowish discharge that finally clears up, leaving the patient asymptomatic. The spirochetes, however, are still present and multiplying in the tissues. In 8 weeks or so the second stage (secondary syphilis) begins. The principal pathologic features here include fever, reddish brown skin eruptions, mucous patches in the mouth, alopecia, and pain in the head and joints. These signs disappear, and once again the victim may appear free of disease—in some cases for years. The final blow—the third, or tertiary, stage—eventually arrives and slowly consumes the body. Since the terminal lesions are omnipresent, the cause of death can be just about anything. Usually, however, the heart fails or a vessel ruptures, producing fatal hemorrhage.

The pathologic picture just described *does not* hold true if treatment has been instituted. Indeed, if massive doses of penicillin are given in the primary or early secondary stage, the prognosis is excellent. Treatment is generally less successful in the last stage, however, because the damage has already been done. In other words, the spirochetes must be killed at the earliest possible moment if the tissues are to escape permanent injury.

The main laboratory tests for syphilis include dark-field microscopic examination, serologic tests, spinal fluid tests, and x-ray examination. The dark-field procedure is the best tool for diagnosis of early lesions. For the asymptomatic phases of the infection, serologic tests are the most useful. Among others, these include the Kolmer complement-fixation test, VDRL flocculation test, treponema immobilization (TPI) test, indirect fluorescent antibody (IFA) test, and direct fluorescent antibody (DFA) test. Spinal fluid tests are essential for the diagnosis and treatment of neurosyphilis, and x-ray examination is helpful in the diagnosis of bone and cardiovascular involvement.

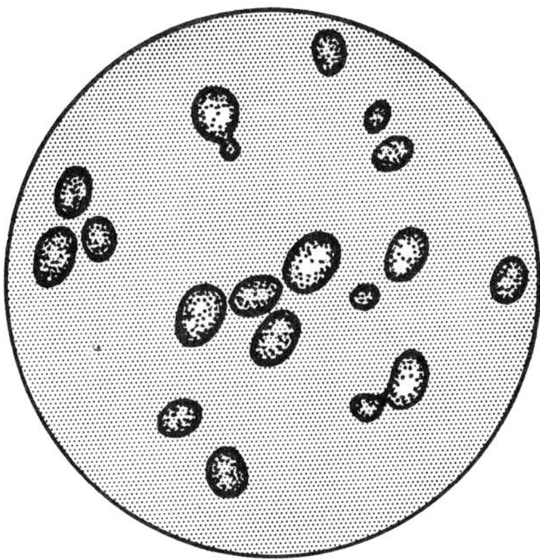

Fig. 23-16. *Candida albicans.*

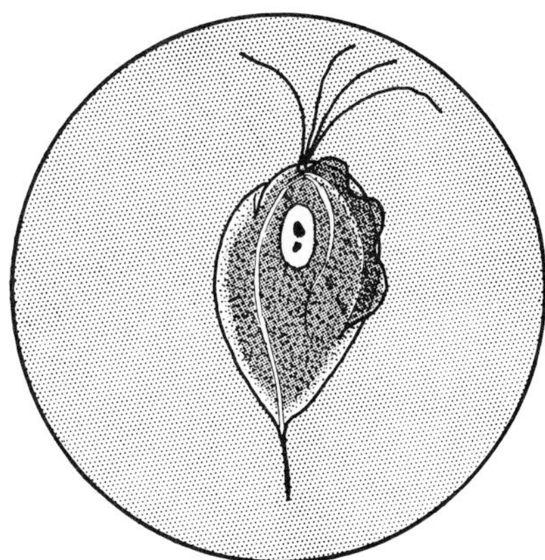

Fig. 23-17. *Trichomonas vaginalis.*

Gonorrhea. Gonorrhea, a venereal infection second only to syphilis in importance, is caused by the gram-negative diplococcus *Neisseria gonorrhoeae* (Fig. 23-15). Aside from the congenital form, almost all cases of gonorrhea are contracted via sexual intercourse. The infection starts as a severe local inflammation of the genital mucosa and, if untreated, spreads to the accessory structures in both sexes. Also, advanced invasion of tissues frequently leads to arthritis and endocarditis. The treatment of choice is administration of large doses of penicillin. As a preventive measure against gonorrheal conjunctivitis (*ophthalmia neonatorum*), a 1 percent solution of silver nitrate is instilled in the eyes of the newborn infant.

Diseases of the female. The principal diseases of the female reproductive system include the infectious and noninfectious disorders affecting the vagina, uterus, ovaries, and breasts.

Infection. Besides syphilis and gonorrhea, there are several other infections to which the female is subject, particularly vaginitis and mastitis. Vaginitis, or inflammation of the vaginal canal, may be caused by a variety of pathogens—bacteria, yeasts, and protozoa. The more common invaders are staphylococci, streptococci, *Candida albicans* (Fig. 23-16), and *Trichomonas vaginalis* (Fig. 23-17). This condition, marked by pain and purulent discharge, is generally treated locally with antibiotics or specific anti-infective agents. In the treatment of trichomonas vaginitis the drug *mitronidazole* (Flagyl) has 100 percent cure rate.

Mastitis, or inflammation of the breasts, is frequently a severe infection characterized by redness and tenderness over the involved area. The causative organism is usually *Staphylococcus aureus,* which gains entrance during the course of lactation or infection elsewhere in the body. In most instances the infection readily yields to specific antibiotic therapy.

Diseases of uterus. The major organic lesions of the uterus are the leiomyoma (fibroid), a benign tumor, and adenocarcinoma, a malignant growth that starts in the endometrium. Both tumors, especially the latter, demand prompt investigation and surgical or radiologic treatment.

The more common functional disorders of the uterus include amenorrhea, dysmenorrhea, and abnormal uterine bleeding. Amenorrhea refers to the abnormal cessation of menstruation; dysmenorrhea means painful menstruation. Since these derangements are actually signs of some underlying disturbance, the physician must direct treatment to the latter. For example, if the etiology is associated with hormonal deficiency, as it often is, hormones are prescribed.

Complications of pregnancy. Pregnancy not uncommonly assumes pathologic proportions—nausea and vomiting, abortion, eclampsia, and the like. While some degree of nausea and vomiting "is to be expected" and usually proves anything but serious, pernicious vomiting (*hyperemesis gravidarum*) is a real problem and often demands hospitalization. In some cases of severe vomiting, liver damage and hemorrhagic retinitis may occur. Treatment entails administration of intravenous fluid to remedy dehydration and supply calories and the use of such antiemetic drugs as pyridoxine (p. 326) and prochlorperazine (Compazine).

Abortion, or the interruption of pregnancy prior to the period of fetal viability, may be spontaneous or induced. An induced (or therapeutic) abortion is done for either reasons of health or the likelihood of a defective baby. Spontaneous abortion may be due to embryonal abnormalities, acute infectious diseases, uterine abnormalities, severe injury, or dysfunction of the thyroid, ovary, or pituitary gland.

Eclampsia is a disorder of unknown etiology, usually occurring during the first pregnancy or with twins, and is characterized by hypertension, edema, convulsions, and albuminuria. Usually it may be prevented by adequate prenatal care, with careful attention to diet and salt restriction. When the full-blown disease process occurs, it may cause death of the fetus, of the mother, or of both. Treatment includes measures to lower blood pressure, to increase blood flow and oxygenation of vital tissues, and to secure an adequate urinary output. Eclampsia is cured only by delivery.

TERATOLOGY

Teratology is the division of embryology and pathology that deals with abnormal development and congenital malformations. The various possible etiologic factors fall into three categories: *environmental, genetic,* and *multifactorial* (environmental plus genetic). And then there are those abnormalities that cannot be traced to any environmental or genetic factor, but instead appear to be simply the result of the statistical probability that a certain small fraction of embryos will fail to develop properly.

Teratogens. Currently much concern and research is being directed in the area of teratogens, that is, specific environmental agents causing congenital malformations. Teratogens known to be effective against the human embryo include irradiation, thalidomide, carbon monoxide, rubella virus (p. 184), and *Toxoplasma gondii.*

Metabolic diseases. Perhaps the most outstanding development in functional pathology has been the finding that certain diseases are the result of a metabolic defect incident to a lack of a specific enzyme system.

Phenylketonuria. Phenylketonuria is a hereditary disease marked by mental retardation and the presence of *phenylpyruvic* acid in the urine, the latter being readily detected by ferric chloride (which produces a green color in urine containing the substance). The disease has an incidence of about one case in each twenty-five thousand births. Quite interestingly, it is rare among Jews and has never been seen among pure Negroes. Painstaking research has shown that the underlying defect stems from a deficiency of *phenylalanine hydroxylase,* an enzyme needed to convert the amino acid phenylalanine into tyrosine. Provided that a newborn baby with the disease is maintained on a low phenylalanine diet, brain damage can be averted.

Galactosemia. This is a hereditary disorder of carbohydrate metabolism characterized by vomiting, diarrhea, jaundice, poor weight gain, cataracts, cirrhosis, and mental retardation. Here the defect arises from a deficiency of the enzyme *galactose l-phosphate uridyl transferase.* The disease is easily diagnosed (urine is positive to Benedict's test but negative to glucose oxidase test) and is easily treated through exclusion of lactose and galactose from the diet for at least 3 years while the central nervous system is developing.

Chromosomal diseases. Unearthed in recent years were cytologic facts of great interest to clinical medicine—the association of certain disease states with abnormal numbers of chromosomes. Heretofore puzzling and unexplained developmental anomalies are now giving way to chromosome analysis, and already three clinical states have been identified: Klinefelter's syndrome (forty-seven chromosomes), Turner's syndrome (forty-five chromosomes), and mongolism (forty-seven chromosomes). These will be discussed in the next chapter.

Questions

1. Describe the testis.
2. Describe the structure of the seminal vesicles, prostate gland, and urethra.
3. Describe the structure of the penis.
4. What is semen?
5. Explain the mechanism of erection.
6. Discuss the action of the male hormone.
7. Describe the histology of the ovary.
8. Describe the structure of the uterus and uterine tubes.
9. Describe the vulva.
10. Discuss the anatomy and physiology of the mammary glands.
11. Discuss the role of the gonadotropic hormones in the menstrual cycle.
12. Compare the action of estradiol and progesterone.
13. What is the rhythm method of contraception?
14. What is meant by the menopause?
15. Describe the process of fertilization.
16. Outline the major events in the development of the embryo.
17. What is the embryonic disc?
18. How do you explain the difference between identical and fraternal twins?
19. Describe the anatomy and physiology of the placenta.
20. What is the function of the ductus venosus, the foramen ovale, and the ductus arteriosus in fetal circulation?
21. Describe the birth process.
22. Discuss the various pregnancy tests.
23. Why does cryptorchidism lead to sterility?
24. Discuss syphilis relative to cause, diagnosis, treatment, and prevention.
25. Discuss gonorrhea relative to cause, diagnosis, treatment, and prevention.
26. Consulting other sources, write up the highlights of the thalidomide tragedy; include etiology, pathology, statistics, and the like.
27. During 1964 epidemics of German measles occurred. What have statistics shown relative to the teratologic aspects?
28. Why must infants with galactosemia be placed on a lactose-free diet?
29. Discuss the diagnosis and treatment of phenylketonuria.
30. Define the following terms: idiogram, autosomal, gonad, follicle, erectile tissue, androgen, trophoblast, gonadotropin, diffusion, hypogonadism, alopecia, yeast, enzyme, and galactose.

Chapter 24

Basic genetics

When *red-eyed* fruit flies of "pure stock" (that is, flies that produce only red-eyed offspring) are mated with *brown-eyed* fruit flies of pure stock, *all* the offspring are *red-eyed.* Now, if these red-eyed *hybrids* are mated to one another, about three quarters of the offspring are red-eyed and the rest brown-eyed. And if these brown-eyed flies are mated *among themselves,* only *brown-eyed* offspring are produced.

This in a nutshell is the essence of *mendelian genetics,* a concept that stands next to Darwin's theory of evolution in biologic significance. Prior to the time of Gregor Mendel—and indeed for almost a half century after his historic paper of 1866—it was thought that heredity was a blending process, much like the mixing together of different kinds of paint. What Mendel did (using garden peas) was to show that heredity is of a *particulate* nature. In the case of our fruit flies this means that "red particles" and "brown particles" associate *but are not changed* by said association in the hybrids.

THE GENE

These hereditary particles Mendel called *factors;* today we call them genes. Each *chromosome* is composed of hundreds and hundreds of genes, and each gene carries a genetic or hereditary message. Further, such messages come in pairs, as do the chromosomes that contain them. Again, referring to the fruit fly, when a sex cell carrying a red gene unites with a sex cell carrying a brown gene, the resulting zygote gives rise to an organism carrying a red gene and a brown gene in every one of its *body* cells. Only in the eyes, however, is the influence of these genes manifest. Moreover, only the red gene has a noticeable effect; hence, the red gene is said to be *dominant* and the brown gene *recessive.* Brown eyes—a recessive trait—occurs only in the *absence* of the dominant gene or, saying the same thing another way, *both* recessive genes must be present to produce a recessive trait.

Sometimes a gene is only *partially* dominant. For example, in some flowers a cross between a red and a white produces *pink hybrids.* Thus, in this particular instance you can tell a hybrid just by looking at it, whereas in fruit flies, hybrid red eyes are just as red as those of the pure stock. The inheritance of eye color in fruit flies is an example of *complete* dominance.

Alleles. Two genes that alter a characteristic in *contrasting ways* are said to be alleles of each other; that is, the red gene is an allele of the brown gene and vice versa. Alleles occupy the same position, or *locus,* on corresponding (*homologous*) chromosomes. Further, whereas body cells carry alleles in pairs, sex cells carry only one of the partner alleles. For example, in the fruit fly the body cells carry two eye color genes: two red, two brown, or one brown and one red. The sex cell carries *either* a red gene *or* a brown gene.

Genotype vs. phenotype. The particular set of genes present in the cells of an organism is called its genotype, and the actual physical appearance of an organism is called its phenotype. In other words, the phenotype is an expression of the genotype. But not to be forgotten is the fact that individuals with the same phenotype *do not* necessarily have the same genotype. For example, a red-eyed fruit fly may have either two red genes per cell *or* one red gene and its brown allele. On the other hand, *all* brown-eyed fruit flies do indeed have the same genotype relative to this trait.

Homozygous vs. heterozygous. More or less hand in hand with the expressions genotype and phenotype go homozygous and heterozygous. By homozygous we refer to an organism possessing a pair of alleles for a given trait that are of the *same* kind; on the contrary, by heterozygous we refer to an organism possessing a pair of alleles of unlike genes. Thus, red-eyed fruit flies may be *either* homozygous *or* heterozygous, whereas brown-eyed fruit flies are always homozygous.

Multiple alleles. It is now known that a given locus on a chromosome may be occupied by more than two kinds of alleles. For example, the four major blood groups —A, B, AB, and O—relate to *three* kinds of *alleles* (that is, A, B, and O). In any given individual, however, only *one pair* of alleles are involved. Phenotype A blood stems from the genotype AA or AO (O is recessive); phenotype B blood stems from genotype BB or BO (O is recessive here too); phenotype O blood stems from genotype OO; and phenotype AB blood stems from genotype AB. We note in the latter blood group phenotype, incidentally, that A and B alleles display *no* "dominant relationship" to each other. This situation is also known to obtain among alleles associated with other characteristics.

LINKAGE AND CROSSING OVER

Mendel noted that certain traits tend to be inherited together and today we know the reason why. In brief, these so-called "linked traits" arise from a linear series of genes *linked* together on the *same* chromosome; that is, as the chromosome is passed on and on in the reproductive process, so too are its constituent linked genes. Sometimes, however, such genes become "unlinked," and this is due to what is called "crossing over." This occurs during gametogenesis when paired chromosomes twist around each other and cause breaking—the broken pieces then fusing back together the *wrong way;* thus, crossing over amounts to a *mutual exchange* of genes between homologous chromosomes. For example, if a chromosome containing genes A, B, C, and D—in that sequence—crosses over with its partner chromosome—with genes a, b, c, and d—the result might be the *new* chromosomes ABcd and abCD.

DEFECTIVE GENES

Some genes carry the wrong chemical information and result in structural or metabolic defects. Those that kill the organism in utero are know as *lethal* genes. Some lethal genes are dominant and some are recessive. So-called "dominant recessive lethals" are recessive lethal genes that produce noticeable deleterious effects even in the heterozygous condition. A true recessive lethal produces no effects whatsoever in the heterozygous condition. Diseases and

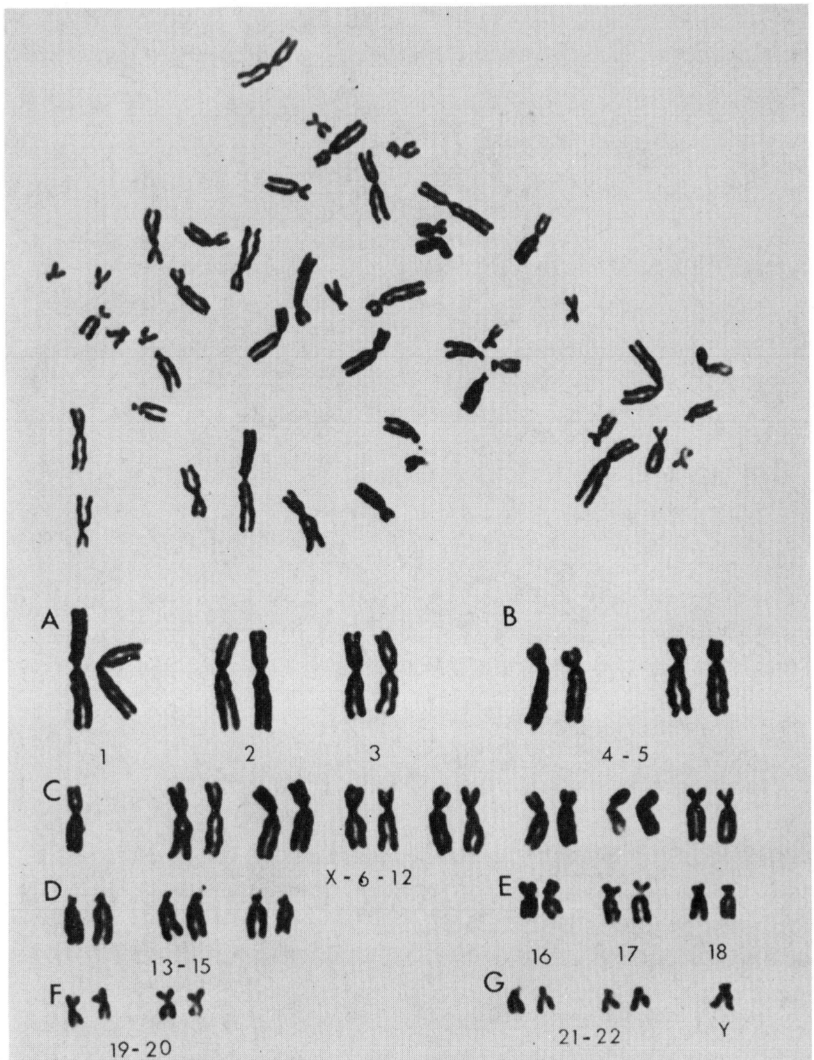

Fig. 24-1. Karyotype of normal human chromosomes. (From Rowley, J. D.: J.A.M.A. **207**:914, 1969.)

disorders stemming from defective genes include, among many others, *brachydactyly, Huntington's chorea, Tay-Sachs disease, hemophilia* (p. 256), *erythroblastosis fetalis* (p. 252), *phenylketonuria* (p. 442), *galactosemia* (p. 442), and *red-green color blindness.*

SEX (AUTOSOMES AND HETEROSOMES)

As pointed out earlier, sex is an inheritable trait involving the so-called sex or X and Y chromosomes (p. 439). These two chromosomes are formally known as heterosomes; all the other chromosomes are known as autosomes. Each human *somatic* or body cell contains twenty-two pairs of autosomes and one pair of heterosomes, that is, forty-six chromosomes altogether (the *diploid* number). A formal arrangement of these chromosomes, called a *karyotype,* is shown in Fig. 24-1. Each sex cell, of course, contains twenty-three chromo-

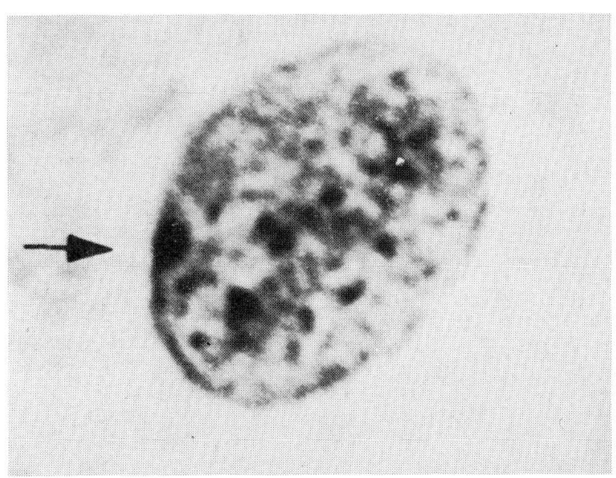

Fig. 24-2. The dark body in the nucleus (indicated by the arrow) is the now famous Barr body. Since it represents two X chromosomes, its presence is proof of femaleness. (From Rowley, J. D.: J.A.M.A. **207**:914, 1969.)

somes (the *haploid* number). The X chromosome carries "female genes" and the Y chromosome carries "male genes," the upshot being that 2 X's produce a female, whereas an X and Y produce a male. Apparently, then, the Y chromosome is a more potent genetic force than the X chromosome inasmuch as it takes only the *single* chromosome to induce maleness. In instances where there is doubt as to an individual's sex a simple test is now available to establish genetic sex based on the presence or absence of so-called Barr bodies (Fig. 24-2).

In the process of gametogenesis the diploid number of chromosomes is *reduced* by *meiosis* to the haploid number. Thus, each human ovum carries twenty-two autosomes and one X heterosome; each human sperm carries twenty-two autosomes and either one X *or* one Y heterosome. On the average, therefore, half the sperm cells carry the X heterosome and half carry the Y heterosome, which means in practice that the chances for a baby being either a boy or a girl amount to a fifty-fifty proposition.

CHROMOSOMAL DISORDERS

Sometimes during gametogenesis things do not come off the way they should and the sex cells end up with too few or too many chromosomes. Mongolism (Down's syndrome) results when a normal sperm cell fertilizes an ovum carrying *twenty-four* chromosomes (p. 443). Thus, the body cells of the ensuing individual carry a *triple* dose of one of the kinds of *autosomes,* a condition called *trisomy* (as contrasted to the *normal* condition of the *double* dose, or *diploidy*). Chromosomal disorders involving *heterosomes* include the *metafemale* (XXX), *Turner's syndrome* (XO; that is, only one X chromosome), and *Klinefelter's syndrome* (XXY). In conditions such as Turner's syndrome where there is a *single* dose of one of the kinds of chromosomes in the body cells, the term *monosomy* is used.

SEX-LINKED TRAITS

The Y heterosome in man apparently carries no genes other than those relating to maleness; the X heterosome, however, carries an array of genes *other* than those relating to femaleness. Understandably, then, certain traits are "sex linked," a phenomenon that is exquisitely underscored in red-green color blindness (the inability to distinguish between red and green). The gene involved here (let us call it "little c") is *recessive,* meaning that it does not cause color blindness in association with the *normal* gene ("big C"). This means that although a Cc female does not exhibit color blindness, she nonetheless is a *carrier.* The female is color blind only when two "little c's" occur together. In the male, however, it takes but one "little c" to cause color blindness because the Y heterosome carries no overriding gene.

By way of example, let us suppose a normal man (CY)—that is, he has the "big C" on the X chromosome—marries a carrier (Cc). Half the sperm would carry "big C" and half (the "Y sperm") would carry no genes relating to the trait. In contrast, half the ova would carry "big C" and half would carry the "little c." As shown in Fig. 24-3, there are four possible offspring com-

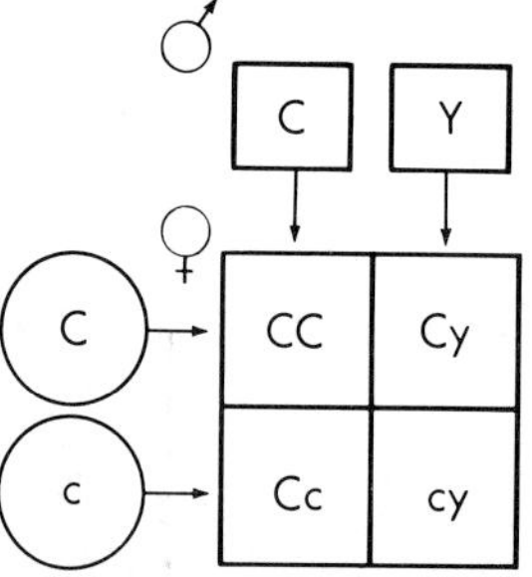

Fig. 24-3. Possibilities of color blindness in the children of a normal father, **CY**, and a carrier mother, **Cc**. (See text.)

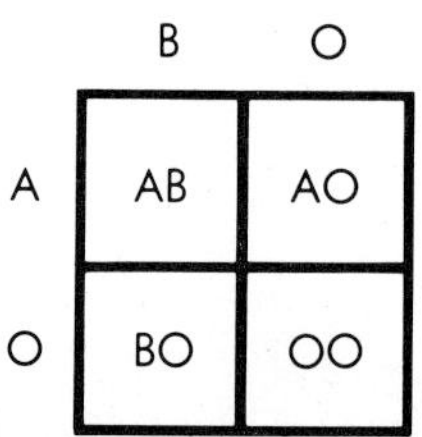

Fig. 24-4. Possible blood types in the children of parents heterozygous for blood types A (**AO**) and B (**BO**). (See text.)

binations: *normal female* (CC), *carrier female* (Cc), *normal male* (CY), and *colorblind male* (cY). Thus, among the boys resulting from such a marriage there would be a fifty-fifty chance of color blindness; among the girls there would be no color blindness, but there would be a fifty-fifty chance of the carrier state.

Exactly the same situation obtains in the sex-linked disease of *hemophilia,* where the abnormal gene (call it "little h") is *recessive* to the normal gene ("big H"). Thus, HY and HH stand for the normal male and female, respectively; hY and hh stand for the male and female hemophiliac, respectively; and Hh stands for the female carrier.

THE PUNNETT SQUARE

To predict the genetic character of the offspring of parents of known genotypes, we may use algebra or, thanks to the geneticist R. C. Punnett, the so-called Punnett square. Actually, we have already used the "square" in the solution of color blindness (Fig. 24-3); that is, all one need do is draw a block of squares and "interact" the sex cells (indicated at the top and at the side) so as to produce a zygote in each square. For example, if a man heterozygous for type A blood marries a woman heterozygous for type B blood, then the possible blood types of the offspring would be as shown in Fig. 24-4.

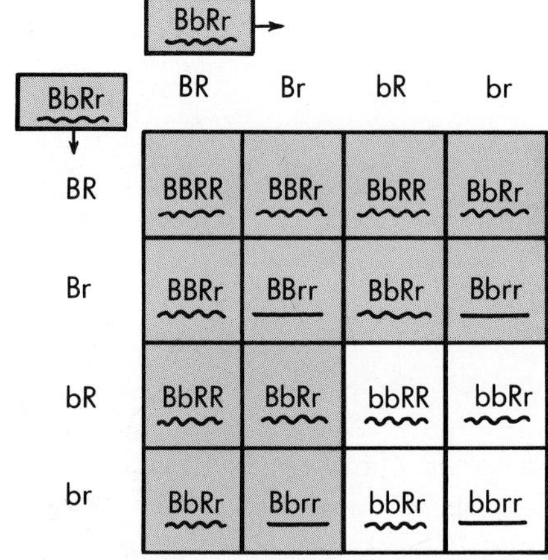

Fig. 24-5. Possible offspring in the matings between guinea pigs heterozygous for a black rough coat, **BbRr.** (**BR**, **Br**, **bR**, and **br** are male and female gametes; wavy lines represent rough coats; straight lines represent smooth coats.)

A more involved situation is shown in Fig. 24-5. Here we see the possibilities of the interaction of sex cells carrying *two* kinds of traits—*color* (black or white) and *texture* (rough or smooth) of the coats of guinea pigs. Specifically, the square predicts the offspring in the matings of a pair of guinea pigs hybrid for black and rough coats; that is, they have the genotype BbRr and produce the sex cells BR, Br, bR, and br (black, B, is dominant over white, b, and rough, R, is dominant over smooth, r). In sum, the square tells us that the offspring will be *in the ratio* of nine black-rough to three black-smooth to three white-rough to one white-smooth.

MUTATIONS

Upon rare occasion genes may undergo a sudden change in character, a change that will be *inherited* if it occurs in the sex cells. This we call mutation, and the new genetic individual that exhibits the trait we call the *mutant*. For the most part, mutations are *recessive* and *undesirable,* and the reason why they are undesirable is that in most instances a given species already represents perfection through the *natural selection of prior mutations*. That is to say, evolution employs the mutation mechanism to make the best possible fit between a species and its environment—but once the right fit has been found, any subsequent alteration can only be for the worse, or neutral at best. The big exception, of course, is an environmental change that proves disadvantageous to the previously perfected species and thereby affords room for improvement.

A great jump in genetic thinking came in 1927 when Herman J. Muller showed that exposure to x rays induced mutations in fruit flies. Since that time all sorts of physical and chemical agents have been found to be *mutagenic*. (The agents themselves are called *mutagens*.) Understandably, man's great genetic problem at the moment is just exactly how much damage is being caused by the increasing use of ionizing rays and radioactive materials, not to mention radioactive fallout. Of course, we are all now greatly aware of the ominous possibilities and this in itself affords some degree of hope for our genetic future. Moreover, there is good reason to believe that man may one day control his genetic destiny through biologic engineering.

HEREDITY AND ENVIRONMENT

One of the most important things for the beginning student to *unlearn* is that a gene *always* does just exactly what it is supposed to do. This is not true because in actual practice the genotype represents *potential* not *realization*. A given gene does indeed carry the blueprint for a certain trait, but in order for this trait to be realized, environmental factors are most certainly involved. And by environment we mean every single influence that a gene encounters from within and without. Above all, there is the influence of *other* genes—those that have the power to turn a gene "on" or "off." In rabbits, for example, gene B (the gene for black) operates only in the presence of so-called gene C. In regard to the "outside environment," there are examples galore, some of which are of medical concern. It is said that 10 percent of the general population carry the gene for epilepsy, yet only one in twenty of these individuals ever develops the condition. Again, the individual who carries the gene for diabetes often fails to develop the disease if he is the type who avoids sweets and fats. Thus, when such genes are known to exist, the door to prevention of the development is clearly indicated.

THE CODE

From former chapters we know that the thing we call a gene is composed of *deoxyribonucleic* acid (DNA). More specifically, a gene is a segment of the filamentous DNA molecule about 450 *nucleotides** in length. This *master* chemical message is transcribed into a 450-nucleotide segment of *messenger* RNA which, in turn, directs the synthesis of *amino acids into protein*. As we well know, protein is the very essence of protoplasm in

*A DNA nucleotide consists of one so-called "*base*" (adenine, guanine, cytosine, or thymine), one *sugar* (deoxyribose) group, and one phosphate group. A RNA nucleotide differs only in respect to the base *uracil* (which replaces thymine) and the sugar *ribose* (which replaces deoxyribose). *Adenine* always links up with *thymine*—or *uracil*—and *guanine* always links up with *cytosine*. In this fashion the DNA message is both perpetuated and transcribed. (See Fig. 5-7, p. 124.)

general and *enzymes* in particular. Indeed, there is much experimental proof that a *single gene* directs the synthesis of a *single enzyme* (the so-called "one gene one enzyme" theory). Certain disorders in man, for instance, have been traced to the lack of a single enzyme and a single defective gene.

It has now been shown that a *nucleotide triplet* (referred to as a *codon*) spells out a specific amino acid. Thus, the 450-nucleotide gene—via messenger RNA—strings together a protein molecule containing 150 amino acid units. The central point in all this is that DNA uses its *nucleotide alphabet* and *codon words* to write thousands of different *protein sentences,* all of which combine to compose a living theme.

Questions

1. What is meant by a hybrid?
2. In a trait produced by a dominant gene, is it possible to tell the difference between hybrids and pure stock?
3. What is meant by partial dominance?
4. Mendel showed that for each trait there are two contrasting factors, one dominant and the other recessive. Discuss this statement in the framework of present-day genetics.
5. What is the essential difference between somatoplasm and germ plasm?
6. An individual that displays a trait's recessive expression is generally of pure stock. Explain.
7. Distinguish between chromatin, chromosomes, and genes.
8. What is the derivation of the term *allele?*
9. What are homologous chromosomes?
10. Alleles occupy corresponding loci. Explain.
11. Organisms with the same genotype have the same phenotype ("other things being equal"), but the reverse may or *may not* be true. Explain.
12. Pure stocks are homozygous; hybrids are heterozygous. Explain.
13. The idea of multiple alleles goes way beyond classic mendelism. Explain.
14. Crossing over makes for variety, whereas linkage (of genes) does not. Explain.
15. The "one gene one enzyme" theory of genetics is exquisitely demonstrated by such a metabolic disorder as galactosemia. Explain.
16. What do you think might be done in the year 2001 about the problem of defective and lethal genes?
17. In gametogenesis the diploid number becomes reduced to the haploid number. Explain.
18. What is reduction division?
19. A recessive gene on the X chromosome in the male becomes dominant. Explain.
20. How do you account for the genotypes of individuals with Klinefeller's syndrome and Turner's syndrome?
21. Distinguish among the terms *trisomy, diploidy,* and *monosomy.*
22. For some species at least, the statement that mutations are usually harmful (or at best neutral) *did not apply* 100 million years ago. Explain.
23. What, if any, were the genetic effects of the radioactivity released in the bombings of Hiroshima and Nagasaki?
24. What precautions are taken among those who work with ionizing rays and radioactive materials?
25. On a basis of molecular biology, how do mutagens produce mutations?
26. DNA is composed of only four *kinds* of nucleotides. How then do you account for the very large number of genes?
27. Somatic mutations are not inheritable. Explain.
28. How do you account for the fact that a mutated gene may not make its presence known for some time to come?
29. What are the Rh possibilities in the offspring of heterozygous Rh-positive parents? What are the possibilities when the man is "heterozygous Rh positive" and the wife Rh negative?
30. What are the possibilities of hemophilia in a match between a normal man and his carrier wife? What are the possibilities in a match between a hemophiliac male and a normal female?
31. If a baby has type O blood and the mother type A blood, then Mr. X with type AB blood could not be the father. Explain.

General references

Allen, A. C.: The kidney, ed. 3, New York, 1962, Grune & Stratton, Inc.

Anthony, C. P.: Textbook of anatomy and physiology, ed. 7, St. Louis, 1967, The C. V. Mosby Co.

Arey, L. B.: Developmental anatomy—a textbook and laboratory manual of embryology, ed. 7, Philadelphia, 1965, W. B. Saunders Co.

Beaver, W. C., and Noland, G. B.: General biology, ed. 7, St. Louis, 1966, The C. V. Mosby Co.

Besson, P. B., and McDermott, W., editors: Cecil-Loeb textbook of medicine, ed. 11, Philadelphia, 1963, W. B. Saunders Co.

Best, C. H., and Taylor, N. B.: The human body, ed. 5, New York, 1963, Holt, Rinehart & Winston, Inc.

Bevelander, G.: Essentials of histology, ed. 5, St. Louis, 1965, The C. V. Mosby Co.

Bland, J. H.: Disturbances of body fluids, ed. 3, Philadelphia, 1962, W. B. Saunders Co.

Bloom, W., and Fawcett, D. W.: A textbook of histology, ed. 8, Philadelphia, 1962, W. B. Saunders Co.

Boyd, W. C.: Fundamentals of immunology, ed. 3, New York, 1956, Interscience Publishers, Inc.

Brachet, J.: The cell, vol. 2, New York, 1961, Academic Press, Inc.

Brooks, S. M.: Basic facts of general chemistry, Philadelphia, 1956, W. B. Saunders Co.

Brooks, S. M.: Basic facts of medical microbiology, ed. 2, Philadelphia, 1962, W. B. Saunders Co.

Brooks, S. M.: Basic facts of pharmacology, ed. 2, Philadelphia, 1963, W. B. Saunders Co.

Brooks, S. M.: Basic facts of body water and ions, ed. 2, New York, 1968, Springer Publishing Co., Inc.

Brooks, S. M.: Biology simplified, New York, 1968, Barnes & Noble, Inc.

Burdon, K. L., and Williams, R.: Microbiology, ed. 6, New York, 1968, The Macmillan Co.

Burrows, W.: Textbook of microbiology, ed. 19, Philadelphia, 1968, W. B. Saunders Co.

Cable, E. J., Getchell, R. W., Kadesch, W. H., Poppy, W. J., and Crull, H. E.: The physical sciences, ed. 4, Englewood Cliffs, N. J., 1959, Prentice-Hall, Inc.

Cannon, W. B.: The wisdom of the body, ed. 2, New York, 1963, W. W. Norton & Co., Inc.

Carpenter, P. L.: Microbiology, ed. 2, Philadelphia, 1967, W. B. Saunders Co.

Dameshek, W.: Morphologic hematology, New York, 1947, Grune & Stratton, Inc.

Darlington, G. D., and Davenport, C. F.: Applied pathology, ed. 2, Philadelphia, 1954, J. B. Lippincott Co.

De Coursey, R. M.: The human organism, ed. 2, New York, 1961, McGraw-Hill Book Co.

Dorland's illustrated medical dictionary, ed. 24, Philadelphia, 1965, W. B. Saunders Co.

Francis, C. C : Introduction to human anatomy, ed. 5, St. Louis, 1968, The C. V. Mosby Co.

Gardiner-Hill, H.: Modern trends in endocrinology, ed. 2, New York, 1961, Grune & Stratton, Inc.

Gardner, E.: Fundamentals of neurology, ed. 3, Philadelphia, 1958, W. B. Saunders Co.

Garven, H. S. D.: A student's histology, Baltimore, 1957, The Williams & Wilkins Co.

Gebhardt, L. P., and Anderson, D. A.: Microbiology, ed. 3, St. Louis, 1965, The C. V. Mosby Co.

Geldard, F. A.: Human senses, New York, 1953, John Wiley & Sons, Inc.

Goodman, L. S., and Gilman, A.: The pharmacological basis of therapeutics, ed. 3, New York, 1965, The Macmillan Co.

Goss, C. M., editor: Gray's anatomy of the human body, ed. 27, Philadelphia, 1959, Lea & Febiger.

Guyton, A. C.: Textbook of medical physiology, ed. 3, Philadelphia, 1966, W. B. Saunders Co.

Guyton, A. C.: Function of the human body, ed. 3, Philadelphia, 1967, W. B. Saunders Co.

Ham, A. W., and Leeson, T. S.: Histology, ed. 5, Philadelphia, 1965, J. B. Lippincott Co.

Hardin, G.: Biology: its principles and implications, ed. 2, San Francisco, 1966, W. H. Freeman & Co. Publishers.

Harris, R. S.: Vitamins and hormones, vol. 15, New York, 1957, Academic Press, Inc.

Kimber, D. C., Gray, C. E., Stackpole, M. A., and Leavell, C. E.: Anatomy and physiology, ed. 14, New York, 1961, The Macmillan Co.

King, B. G., and Showers, M. J.: Human anatomy and physiology, ed. 5, Philadelphia, 1963, W. B. Saunders Co.

Kleiner, I. S., and Orten, J. M.: Biochemistry, ed. 7, St. Louis, 1966, The C. V. Mosby Co.

Levine, S. A.: Clinical heart disease, ed. 5, Philadelphia, 1958, W. B. Saunders Co.

Linksz, A.: Physiology of the eye. Vision, vol. 2, New York, 1952, Grune & Stratton, Inc.

Mason, A. S.: Introduction to clinical endocrinology, Springfield, Ill., 1957, Charles C Thomas, Publisher.

Merck index, ed. 8, Rahway, N. J., 1968, Merck & Co., Inc.

Pelczar, M. J., and Reid, R.: Microbiology, ed. 2, New York, 1965, McGraw-Hill, Book Co.

Porter, E. L.: Fundamentals of human reproduction, New York, 1948, McGraw-Hill Book Co.

Ranson, S. W., and Clark, S. L.: Anatomy of the nervous system, ed. 19, Philadelphia, 1959, W. B. Saunders Co.

Reith, E. J., et al: Textbook of anatomy and physiology, New York, 1964, McGraw-Hill Book Co.

Robbins, S.: Textbook of pathology, ed. 2, Philadelphia, 1962, W. B. Saunders Co.

Rogers, T. A.: Elementary human physiology, New York, 1961, John Wiley & Sons, Inc.

Ruch, T. C., and Patton, H. D.: Physiology and biophysics, ed. 19, Philadelphia, 1965, W. B. Saunders Co.

Selle, W. A.: Body temperature, Springfield, Ill., 1952, Charles C Thomas, Publisher.

Semat, H.: Fundamentals of physics, ed. 3, New York, 1957, Holt, Rinehart & Winston, Inc.

Slabough, W. H., and Butler, A. B.: College physical science, Englewood Cliffs, N. J., 1958, Prentice-Hall, Inc.

Smith, A. L.: Principles of microbiology, ed. 6, St. Louis, 1969, The C. V. Mosby Co.

Spalteholz, W.: Atlas of human anatomy, ed. 16, New York, 1967, F. A. Davis Co. (Revised by R. Spanner.)

Steen, E. B., and Montagu, A.: Anatomy and physiology, vols. 1 and 2, New York, 1959, Barnes & Noble, Inc.

Szent-Gyorgyi, A.: Chemical physiology of contraction in body and heart muscle, New York, 1953, Academic Press, Inc.

Tuttle, W. W., and Schottelius, B. A.: Textbook of physiology, ed. 16, St. Louis, 1969, The C. V. Mosby Co.

Weisz, P. B.: Elements of biology, ed. 2, New York, 1965, McGraw-Hill Book Co.

Wiggers, C. J.: The physiology of shock, New York, 1950, Commonwealth Fund.

Wohl, M. G., and Goodhart, R. S.: Modern nutrition in health and disease, ed. 2, Philadelphia, 1959, Lea & Febiger.

Glossary

abdomen that portion of the body between the thorax and pelvis.
abduction withdrawal of a part from the midline.
abscess localized collection of pus in a cavity formed by degeneration of tissue.
absolute temperature centigrade temperature added to 273 degrees algebraically.
absorption the taking up of fluid or other substances by the mucous membranes.
acapnia diminished carbon dioxide in the blood.
acceleration the rate of change of velocity.
acetabulum the large cup-shaped cavity on the lateral surface of the hip.
acetone bodies ketone compounds (for example, acetone) that appear in the blood in diabetes.
acetylene series hydrocarbons that contain a triple bond.
Achilles tendon the tendon that attaches the gastrocnemius muscle to the heel bone.
acid a compound that furnishes hydrogen ions or donates protons.
acid fast a term applied to bacteria that retain a stain even though treated with acid alcohol.
acidosis acidemia, or lowered blood bicarbonate.
acquired immunity any type of immunity that is not inherited.
acromegaly an enlargement of bones of the face and extremities caused by an excess of the growth hormone.
acromion outmost projection (of the spine) of the scapula.
actinomycosis an infection caused by *Actinomyces bovis*.
active immunity production of antibodies by a person's own body.
acute sudden, sharp, and severe.
addition a reaction between an unsaturated compound and some element whereby the element "adds" on at the double bond.
adduction the act of drawing toward the midline.
adenohypophysis anterior pituitary.
adenoids hypertrophy of the pharyngeal tonsil.
adenoma a benign epithelial tumor with a gland-like structure.
adenosine triphosphate a high-energy compound of the cell.
adhesion the attraction of unlike molecules.
adipose fatty; fat.
adrenal gland an endocrine gland located on the top of the kidney.
adrenaline another name for epinephrine, the hormone of the adrenal medulla.
adrenergic pertaining to sympathetic nervous system.
adventitia tunica externa.
Aedes aegypti a species of mosquito that transmits the yellow fever virus.
aerobe a microbe that requires oxygen.
afferent neuron a neuron that carries impulses to the central nervous system.
agar a dried mucilaginous substance derived from seaweed.
agglutination the clumping of cells.
agglutinins antibodies that cause agglutination.
agonist the prime mover (muscle); a muscle opposed to another (antagonist).
agranulocytosis an acute disease marked by leukopenia and ulcerative lesions of the mucous membranes.
albuminuria the presence of albumin in the urine.

alcohol an organic compound containing one or more hydroxyl (OH) groups.
aldehyde an organic compound containing a —CHO group.
algae thallophytes that contain chlorophyll.
alicyclic cyclic organic compounds that resemble the paraffins.
alkali a strong soluble base, for example, NaOH; physiologically, any body chemical that neutralizes acid.
alkalosis an alkalemia, or increased blood bicarbonate.
allantois an extraembryonic membrane.
alleles different forms of the "same" gene.
allergen an antigen that provokes an allergy.
allergy a hypersensitive state acquired through exposure to a particular allergen.
allotropism a condition in which an element exists in two or more forms.
alveolus tiny cavity or space, for example, the alveoli of the lung.
ameba a protozoan belonging to the class Rhizopoda.
amebiasis a protozoiasis caused by *Entamoeba histolytica.*
amenorrhea cessation of menstruation.
amino acids a carboxylic acid containing one or more amino ($-NH_2$) groups.
amnion an extraembryonic membrane that immediately encloses the embryo.
ampere the unit of intensity of an electric current.
amphiarthrosis an articulation permitting little motion.
amphitricate bacilli equipped with flagella at both ends.
amphoteric exhibiting both acidic and basic properties.
ampulla a flasklike dilatation of a tubular structure.
amylase any starch-digesting enzyme.
amylopsin pancreatic amylase.
anabolism the synthesis of nutrients into protoplasm; constructive metabolism.
anaerobe an organism that does not require oxygen.
anaphylaxis an exaggerated allergic reaction (especially in animals) to a foreign substance.
androgen a male hormone.
anemia a condition in which the blood is deficient in either quantity or quality.
anesthesia loss of feeling or sensation.
aneurysm a blood-filled sac formed by the dilatation of the walls of an artery or vein.
angina a suffocating pain.
angina pectoris paroxysmal thoracic pain usually resulting from myocardial anoxia.
angstrom unit of wavelength equal to 10^{-8} cm.
anhydrous without water.
anion a negative ion.
anode a positive electrode.
Anopheles a genus of mosquito that transmits malaria.
anorexia lack of appetite.
anoxemia lack of oxygen in the blood.
anoxia lack of oxygen.
antagonist a muscle that acts in opposition to another (agonist).
anterior situated in front of.
antibiotic an agent produced by one microorganism that inhibits or kills another microorganism.
antibody a specific immune substance present in the blood.
anticoagulant a drug that interferes with the clotting mechanism.
antigen an agent that provokes (in the body) the production of antibodies.
antiseptic an agent that inhibits microorganisms.
antiserum a serum that contains antibodies.
antitoxin an antibody that neutralizes a toxin.
antrum a cavity or chamber within a bone.
anuria absence of excretion of urine from the body.
anus the outlet of the rectum.
aorta the largest artery of the body.
apex a pointed extremity.
apnea transient cessation of breathing.
aponeurosis sheet of white fibrous tissue serving mainly as an investment for muscle.
apoplexy a condition caused by acute vascular lesions of the brain, such as hemorrhage, thrombosis, or embolism.
appendectomy the removal of the appendix.
aqueous containing water.
arachnoid delicate, weblike membrane of the meninges.
Archimedes' principle a submerged or floating body is buoyed up by a force equal to its weight.
areola a dark circular area.
armature the movable part of a dynamo or motor, consisting of coils of wire around an iron core.
Arnold sterilizer a device that sterilizes by free-flowing steam.
arteriole a microscopic artery.
arteriosclerosis loss of elasticity, thickening, and hardening of the arteries.
artery a vessel that carries blood away from the heart.
arthrosis a joint or articulation.
articulation a joint.
aseptic sterile.
asexual having no sex.
asphyxia suffocation.
asthma recurrent attacks of paroxysmal dyspnea caused by constriction of bronchioles.
astigmatism defective curvature of the refractive surfaces of the eye.
atelectasis incomplete expansion of lung at birth.
atherosclerosis a condition of the arteries marked

by deposits of yellowish fatty plaques in the intima.

atlas the first cervical vertebra.

atom smallest "practical unit" of an element.

atomic number the number of protons in the nucleus.

atomic theory theory that all matter is composed of basic units called atoms.

atomic weight the weight of an atom compared to carbon-12.

atrium (pl., **atria**) the upper chambers of the heart.

atrophy diminution in size.

attenuated weakened.

auricle the atrium of the heart.

auscultation listening for sounds in the body.

autoclave a device that sterilizes by steam under pressure.

autonomic nervous system the functional division of the nervous system that supplies the glands, heart, and smooth muscles.

autosome any chromosome not related to sex.

avitaminosis vitamin deficiency.

Avogadro's law under the same conditions, equal volumes of gases contain the same number of molecules.

Avogadro's number 6.02331×10^{23} (the number of molecules contained in 1 mole of any substance).

axilla the armpit.

axis a line about which any revolving body turns.

axon the efferent fiber of a nerve cell.

bacillary dysentery severe enteritis caused by bacteria of the genus *Shigella.*

bacillus a rod-shaped bacterium.

bacteriolysin an antibody that causes the dissolution of bacteria.

bacteriophage a virus that destroys bacteria.

Bang's disease a disease of cattle caused by *Brucella abortus.*

barometer an instrument used to measure atmospheric pressure.

baroreceptor a receptor sensitive to changes in pressure.

Barr body the characteristic dark spot present in the nucleus of female somatic cells.

basal metabolism the lowest level of energy expenditure.

base a chemical that furnishes OH^- ions; a proton acceptor (Brönsted).

basophil a granulocyte whose granules and nucleus take a basic stain.

BCG vaccine a vaccine against tuberculosis prepared from attenuated tubercle bacilli.

beta rays high-speed electrons.

bile the greenish yellow secretion of the liver.

bilirubin a red pigment of bile.

biliverdin a green pigment of bile.

biotin a member of the vitamin B complex.

biuret test a test for protein.

blastomycosis chronic systemic mycosis caused by *Blastomyces dermatitidis.*

blastula an early stage in the development of the embryo produced by cleavage.

bleeding time the duration of the bleeding that follows puncture of the earlobe (about 3 to 5 minutes).

boil a furuncle; a circumscribed area of inflammation of the skin and subcutaneous tissue containing a central core.

bond the linkage between atoms.

botulism a severe type of food poisoning caused by *Clostridium botulinum.*

Bowman's capsule the invaginated proximal portion of the nephron tubule.

Boyle's law provided that the temperature remains constant, the volume of a gas is inversely proportional to the pressure.

bradycardia abnormal slowness of the heartbeat.

broad-spectrum antibiotic an antibiotic effective against a wide variety of pathogenic microbes.

bronchioles the smallest air tubes (lung).

bronchitis inflammation of the bronchi.

bronchus an air tube (lung).

Brönsted theory theory that acids are proton donors and bases are proton acceptors.

brownian movement the dancing motion of particles suspended in a fluid.

brucellosis an infection caused by *Brucella abortus, Br. suis,* or *Br. melitensis.*

budding an asexual mode of reproduction in yeasts.

buffer an agent that resists a change in pH.

bundle of His the neuromuscular bundle located in the wall of the interventricular septum of the heart.

bursa a fluid-filled sac or pouch, usually lined with a synovial membrane.

calorie a small calorie is the amount of heat required to raise the temperature of 1 gm. of water 1° C.; a large Calorie, or kilocalorie, equals 1000 small calories.

calyx a recess of the pelvis of the kidney.

cancellous spongy (for example, bone).

canthus the angle formed by the meeting of the upper and lower eyelids.

capillaries the minute vessels that connect the arterioles and venules.

capsule a gelatinous covering that surrounds a bacterium.

carbohydrate a class of organic compounds containing the starches and sugars.

carbonate a salt of carbonic acid.

carbonyl group the organic radical —C=O.
carboxyl group the —COOH group that occurs in nearly all organic acids.
carbuncle inflammation of the subcutaneous tissue terminating in slough and suppuration and accompanied by marked systemic symptoms.
carcinoma a malignant new growth made up of epithelial tissue.
caries decay of a bone.
carpus wrist.
catalyst an agent that alters the speed of a reaction but remains unchanged in the process.
cataract an opacity of the eye lens or its capsule.
catarrh inflammation of a mucous membrane with a free watery discharge.
cathode the negative electrode.
cation a positive ion.
cauda equina the name given to the bundle of spinal nerves issuing from the lower portion of the spinal cord.
caudal toward the tail.
cecum the pouch at the proximal end of the large intestine.
cell a microscopic circumscribed mass of protoplasm containing a nucleus.
cellulose an indigestible carbohydrate forming the basic framework of most plant structures.
centimeter a unit of length in the metric system; 0.3937 inch.
central nervous system the brain and spinal cord.
cerebellum the division of the brain immediately below the occipital lobes of the cerebrum.
cerebrum the two great hemispheres forming the upper and larger portions of the brain.
cerumen the waxlike material found in the external meatus of the ear; earwax.
cervix neck or any necklike part.
chancre the primary lesion of syphilis.
Charles' law provided that the pressure remains constant, the volume of a gas is directly proportional to the absolute temperature.
chemotherapy the treatment of disease using chemicals.
Cheyne-Stokes respiration abnormal breathing in grave diseases in which the respirations increase progressively in depth and vigor to a maximum, then diminish again, and finally cease.
chickenpox a dermotropic virus infection.
chloride a salt of hydrochloric acid.
cholecystitis inflammation of the gallbladder.
cholera an acute infectious disease caused by *Vibrio comma.*
cholesterol a fatty steroid alcohol present in all animal fats and oils.
cholinergic pertaining to the parasympathetic nervous system.
cholinesterase the enzyme that hydrolyzes acetylcholine into acetic acid and choline.
chordae tendineae the cords that attach the heart valves to the papillary muscle.
chromatin the easily stained network of fibrils within the nucleus.
chromosome dark-staining, rod-shaped bodies that appear in the nucleus at the time of mitosis.
chronic long continued.
chyle lymph containing absorbed fat.
chyme partially digested food as it leaves the stomach.
cilia microscopic hairlike processes.
cisterna chyli an enlargement at the base of the thoracic duct.
class the main division of a phylum.
Clostridium a genus of anaerobic, sporebearing, gram-positive bacilli.
coal tar a product obtained by the destructive distillation of coal.
coccus a spherical bacterium.
cochlea the spiral-shaped structure that forms part of the inner ear.
codon the segment (or nucleotide triplet) of the DNA molecule that specifies a certain amino acid.
coenzyme the less specific part of an enzyme.
collagen the chief supportive protein of the skin and connective tissue.
colloid a state in which minute particles of one substance are dispersed throughout some other substance.
colony an isolated group of bacteria on a solid culture medium.
compartment a theoretical division of the water of the body.
complemental air the volume of air that can be inspired over and above the normal volume.
compound a substance composed of two or more elements in a definite proportion.
concentrated solution one which contains a relatively large amount of solute.
concha(e) the bony plates of the nasal cavity.
condyle a rounded projection of a bone.
congenital existing at or before birth.
conjunctivitis inflammation of the conjunctiva.
convex rounded or elevated surface.
corium the true skin, or dermis.
cornea the transparent portion of the eyeball.
coronal refers to a plane parallel to the long axis of the body.
cortex the outer part of an organ.
costal pertaining to the ribs.
covalence the sharing of electrons.
cretinism a condition caused by a congenital lack of thyroid secretion.
crystalloid a compound that forms a true solution.
culture a growth of microorganisms.
cyanosis bluing of the skin, usually due to lack of oxygen.

cyst any sac, normal or otherwise, filled with a liquid or semisolid.
cystitis inflammation of the bladder.
cytology the study of cells.
cytoplasm the protoplasm of a cell exclusive of the nucleus.

dark-field microscope an optical microscope modified to permit lateral lighting of the specimen.
deamination removal of the amino group ($-NH_2$) from an amino acid.
deciduous shedding at a certain stage of growth (for example, deciduous teeth).
decussation crossing over.
defecation elimination of wastes from the intestine.
deglutition swallowing.
dehydration removal of water.
deltoid the deltoid muscle.
dendrite an afferent nerve process (also, dendron).
density mass per unit volume.
dentin the main part of the tooth under the enamel.
dermatitis inflammation of the skin.
dermatome area of skin supplied with afferent nerve fibers by a single posterior spinal root.
dermatomycosis fungal infection of the skin.
dermis true skin (also, corium).
dermotropic having an affinity for the skin.
destructive distillation heating of a substance out of contact with air.
dextrose glucose.
diabetes mellitus a metabolic disease caused by a deficiency or deactivation of insulin.
dialysis the separation of a crystalloid and a colloid by means of a semipermeable membrane.
diapedesis the passage of blood cells through the wall of the intact capillary.
diaphragm the muscular sheath between the thorax and the abdomen.
diaphysis the shaft of a long bone.
diarthrosis freely movable joint.
diastole relaxation of the heart between contractions.
Dick test a skin test to determine susceptibility to scarlet fever.
Dick toxin a toxin produced by the pathogen *Streptococcus pyogenes.*
diencephalon the portion of the brain between the cerebrum and the midbrain.
diffusion the spreading out of particles.
digestion the conversion of food into assimilable molecules.
diphtheria a severe infection caused by *Corynebacterium diphtheriae.*
diplococcus cocci that occur in pairs.
diploid number the number of chromosomes in a "body cell" (in man, 46).
diplopia double vision.
direct current a current that flows in only one direction and has polarity.
disaccharide a sugar with the formula $C_{12}H_{22}O_{11}$.
disinfectant an agent that kills pathogens.
disinfection the destruction of pathogenic organisms.
distillation the heating of a liquid and condensation of its vapors.
diuretic a drug that increases the production of urine.
diverticulum outpouching of the intestine.
dorsal in back of; posterior.
droplet infection transmission of an infection via minute particles of sputum.
duodenum the first portion (12 fingerbreadths in length) of the small intestine.
dura mater the outermost layer of the meninges.
dwarf an abnormally undersized person.
dynamic equilibrium a reversible reaction.
dyne a unit of force.
dysentery an acute enteritis, especially of the colon.
dyspnea labored breathing.
dystrophy faulty nutrition.

ectoderm the outermost germ layer.
ectoparasite a parasite that lives on the surface of the body.
eczema an inflammatory skin disease with vesiculation.
edema the accumulation of fluid in the tissues.
efferent neuron one that carries an impulse away from the central nervous system.
electrocardiography the graphic recording of the heart's action potentials.
electrolysis decomposition of a compound by means of an electric current.
electrolyte a compound that, in solution, conducts an electric current.
electron a negative particle of electricity.
electron theory the theory that the atom is composed of three basic particles—electrons, protons, and neutrons.
electron volt a measure of energy.
electrophoresis the migration of colloidal particles to an electrode.
electrostatics the study of static electricity.
electrovalence the loss or gain of electrons.
element a substance composed of like atoms.
elephantiasis edematous swelling of the legs or genitals caused by the presence of filarial worms in the lymph vessels.
embolism the sudden blocking of an artery or vein by a clot brought by the bloodstream.
embryo an organism in the early stages of development (especially before the third month).

emphysema the presence of air in the intra-alveolar tissue of the lungs.
emulsion a colloidal system of one liquid dispersed in another liquid.
encephalitis inflammation of the brain.
endemic prevalent in a particular area.
endemic typhus fever a rickettsial disease transmitted from rat to man by the bite of the rat flea.
endocrine gland a ductless gland.
endoderm the innermost germ layer of the embryo (entoderm).
endolymph the fluid contained in the membranous labyrinth of the inner ear.
endometrium the inner lining of the uterus.
endospore a spore within the bacterial cell.
endosteum the lining of the medullary cavity of long bones.
energy ability to do work.
enteric pertaining to the intestine.
enterokinase an enzyme of the small intestine that converts trypsinogen into trypsin.
enzyme an organic catalyst.
eosinophil a granulocyte whose granules are readily stained by eosin.
epidemic attacking many people in a given region at the same time.
epidermis the outer layer of skin.
epididymis a group of coiled tubules continuous with the seminiferous tubules of the testis.
epinephrine adrenaline.
epiphysis the end of a long bone.
epithelium a basic tissue that forms the epidermis and lines the ducts and hollow organs.
equivalent weight the atomic weight of an element divided by its valence.
erepsin a mixture of proteolytic enzymes produced by the intestinal glands.
erythema a pathologic redness of the skin.
erythrocyte a red blood cell.
esterification the reaction between an alcohol and an acid forming an ester and water.
estrogen a female sex hormone.
ethylene series a series of hydrocarbons whose members contain a double bond.
etiology study of the cause of disease.
eupnea normal respiration.
exocrine glands glands that have ducts.
exotoxin a toxin released by a living bacterium.
extension stretching out.
extracellular compartment fluids located outside the cells.

facultative anaerobe a microbe that lives best in the presence of oxygen but can live in its absence.
family main division of an order.
fascia the tissue that binds organs or parts of organs together.
fauces the space bounded by the soft palate, tongue, and tonsils.
feces the material excreted from the rectum.
fetus the unborn mammalian organism at a later stage of development, especially after the second month.
fibrin protein threads that form the framework of the clot.
fibrinogen a protein of the blood plasma.
fission the splitting of atomic nuclei.
fissure a cleft or groove (for example, fissure of the brain).
flaccid lax and soft.
flagellum a whiplike process of a microbe.
flexion bending.
follicle a very small sac containing a secretion.
fomite a contaminated object.
fontanel a membranous spot in the infant's skull.
foramen an opening.
fossa a depression; a cavity.
fractional distillation separation of liquids by distillation.
frambesia an infection caused by *Treponema pertenue.*
frequency the number of cycles or vibrations per second.
FSH follicle-stimulating hormone.
fundus base.
fungicide an agent that destroys fungi.
fungus a mold (Fungi, a subphyllum of the thallophytes).
furuncle a boil.

gallbladder a muscular sac, contiguous with the liver, that stores and concentrates bile.
galvanometer a sensitive instrument for measuring weak electric currents.
gamete a sex cell.
gametogenesis the development of gametes.
gamma globulin the fraction of the blood that contains the antibodies.
gamma rays one of three types of rays emitted by radioactive substances; similar to but more penetrating than x rays.
ganglion a collection or mass of nerve cells.
gas gangrene a morbid infection caused by several species of the genus *Clostridium.*
gastritis inflammation of the stomach.
gastrocnemius the calf muscle.
gel a semisolid colloid.
gene a hereditary unit of the chromosome.
genitals the reproductive organs.
genotype a cell's genetic constitution.
German measles a dermotropic virus infection characterized by a rash.

germicide an agent that kills germs (microbes).
gigantism abnormal growth caused by excessive secretions of the anterior lobe of the hypophysis.
gingivitis inflammation of the gums.
glaucoma an eye disease characterized by elevated intraocular pressure.
glomerulus a coiled mass of capillaries within Bowman's capsule of the kidney.
glossitis inflammation of the tongue.
gluconeogenesis formation of glucose from protein or fat.
glucose dextrose ($C_6H_{12}O_6$).
glycogen a carbohydrate, $(C_6H_{10}O_5)_n$, formed in the liver and muscle from glucose.
glycogenesis formation of glycogen from glucose.
glycogenolysis the breakdown of glycogen into glucose.
glycosuria the presence of sugar in the urine (also, glucosuria).
goiter an enlargement of the thyroid gland.
gonadotropin a hormone of the anterior pituitary that stimulates the sex glands.
gonads sex glands.
gonorrhea a venereal disease caused by *Neisseria gonorrheae.*
graafian follicle an ovarian follicle.
gram a unit of weight in the metric system.
gram negative taking the counterstain when stained according to Gram's method.
gyrus a convolution of the cerebral cortex.

half-life time required for a given mass of radioactive element to lose half of its radioactivity.
halogens the elements fluorine, chlorine, bromine, and iodine.
haustrum the recess made by the sacculations of the colon.
hemiplegia paralysis of one side of the body.
hemoglobin the oxygen-carrying substance of red blood cells.
hemoglobinuria presence of hemoglobin in the urine.
hemolysis destruction of red cells.
hemophilia a sex-linked hereditary blood disease characterized by a prolonged bleeding time.
hemopoiesis formation of blood.
hemorrhage loss of blood from the vessels.
heparin an anticoagulant present in many tissues, especially the liver.
hernia protrusion of a loop of the intestine or of another organ through an abnormal opening.
herpes simplex cold sore.
herpes zoster shingles.
heterosome a sex chromosome.
heterozygous when the genes of a pair of alleles are not the same.
histamine a chemical agent that is thought to account for certain allergies.
histology the study of tissues; tissue anatomy.
histoplasmosis systemic mycosis caused by *Histoplasma capsulatum.*
homeostasis a tendency toward uniformity in the internal environment of the organism.
homozygous the genes of a pair of alleles are the same.
hormone a chemical produced by an endocrine gland that influences the activity of other organs.
hyaluronidase an enzyme that dissolves the intercellular cement of tissue.
hybrid an organism that is heterozygous for one or more traits.
hydrolysis a chemical reaction involving water.
hydrophobia rabies.
hydrostatic pertaining to a liquid in a state of equilibrium.
hymen a membrane partially covering the orifice of the vagina.
hyperemia an excess of blood in any part of the body.
hyperglycemia an excess of sugar in the blood.
hyperkalemia excess potassium in the blood.
hypermetropia farsightedness.
hypernatremia excess sodium in the blood.
hyperopia farsightedness.
hyperplasia an increase in the number of cells.
hyperpnea abnormally rapid breathing.
hypertension high blood pressure.
hyperthyroidism overactivity of the thyroid gland.
hypertonic solution a solution that has a greater osmotic pressure than another solution with which it is compared.
hypertrophy overgrowth.
hypervolemia abnormally high blood volume.
hypochondrium the region under the cartilages of the ribs.
hypogastric under the stomach.
hypokalemia deficiency of potassium in the blood.
hyponatremia deficiency of sodium in the blood.
hypoparathyroidism decreased activity of the parathyroid glands.
hypophysis the pituitary gland.
hypothalamus part of the diencephalon.
hypoxia oxygen deficiency.

idiogram a diagrammatic representation of a chromosome complement or karyotype.
ileum the distal portion of the small intestine.
immunity resistance to disease.
inclusion bodies intracellular lesions of viral origin.
incubation period the period between the entrance of the pathogen and the first manifestation of infection.
infarct an area of necrosis due to lack of blood.
infectious hepatitis a severe infection of the liver caused by a virus.
infectious mononucleosis a viral infection charac-

terized by an increase in abnormal leukocytes.
inferior lower.
influenza acute catarrhal inflammation of the respiratory tract caused by a virus.
infundibulum the stalk of the pituitary gland.
inguinal of the groin.
insertion the attachment of a muscle to a bone at the more freely movable end.
insulin the chief hormone secreted by the islands of Langerhans.
intercellular between the cells.
interstitial fluid intercellular fluid.
intima the innermost of the three coats of a blood vessel.
intracellular within the cell.
ion a charged particle.
iris the colored circular muscle of the eye behind the cornea.
ischemia local and temporary deficiency of blood.
islands of Langerhans cells of the pancreas that secrete insulin.
isotonic said of solutions that have the same osmotic pressure.
isotopes elements that have the same atomic number but different atomic weights.

jaundice a disease characterized by yellowing of the skin.
jejunum the second portion of the small intestine.
jugular pertaining to the neck.

karyokinesis mitosis.
karyotype the chromosomal characteristics of an individual presented as an arrangement of metaphase chromosomes of a single cell and arranged in pairs in descending order of size.
keratin the chief protein of the epidermis.
ketones organic compounds containing the carbonyl (CO) group.
kidney the excretory organ that forms urine.
kilogram the metric unit of weight (equal to 2.2 pounds).
kinetic referring to motion; kinetic energy.
Klebs-Löffler bacillus the common name for *Corynebacterium diphtheriae.*
Kline test a precipitation test for syphilis.
Koch's postulates criteria that establish the causal relationship between an infection and its etiologic agent.
Koplik's spots small bluish white spots with a reddish areolar present on the lining of the mouth during the prodromal stage of measles.
kymograph an instrument (usually a smoked drum) used to record physiologic activity.
kyphosis hunchback.

lactase an enzyme that acts upon lactose.
lacteals lymph vessels of the small intestine.
lactose a disaccharide sugar ($C_{12}H_{22}O_{11}$) present in milk.
larynx the "voice box."
latent syphilis the asymptomatic stage of syphilis.
lateral of or toward the side.
leprosy an infectious disease caused by *Mycobacterium leprae.*
lesion a pathologic change in tissue.
leukemia a fatal disease marked by leukocytosis and enlargement and proliferation of the spleen, lymph glands, and bone marrow.
leukocytosis an increase in the number of leukocytes.
leukopenia a reduction in the number of leukocytes.
lichen a symbiotic combination of fungi and algae.
lipase a fat-splitting enzyme.
lipids fatty substances.
liter the unit of volume in the metric system.
lobar pneumonia inflammation of one or more lobes of the lung.
loin the part of the back between the thorax and pelvis.
lumbar pertaining to the loin.
lumen the space within a tube.
lymph the watery fluid that circulates through the lymphatic system.
lysis dissolution of cells.
lysosome an organelle containing digestive enzymes.

macrophage a large phagocytic cell of the reticuloendothelial system.
maltase an enzyme that converts maltose into glucose.
mammary pertaining to the breasts.
manubrium top part of the sternum.
matrix intercellular material.
meatus passageway.
medial toward the midline.
mediastinum the space in the middle of the thorax.
medulla the central part of a gland or organ.
medulla oblongata the portion of the brain just above the spinal cord.
meiosis cellular division in which the chromosome number is halved; also called reduction division.
meninges the membranes covering the brain and spinal cord.
menopause the cessation of menstruation at the close of the reproductive period.
mesencephalon the midbrain.
mesenchyme embryonic connective tissue.
mesentery the large expanse of tissue that anchors the intestine to the posterior abdominal wall.
mesoderm the middle germ layer of the embryo.
metabolism the sum total chemical processes of life.

metacarpus the part of the hand between the wrist and the fingers.
metatarsus the part of the foot between the tarsus and the toes.
meter the metric unit of length (equal to 39.371 inches).
micron 0.001 mm. (1/25000 inch).
milliequivalent one thousandth of an equivalent; abbreviated mEq.
mitochondria minute bodies in the cytoplasm of the cell charged with respiratory enzymes.
mitosis cell division by means of which the two daughter cells receive the same number of chromosomes as the parent cell.
mitral the left atrioventricular heart valve.
mole the molecular weight expressed in grams.
monosaccharide a simple sugar ($C_6H_{12}O_6$).
mucus a slimy, clear fluid secreted by mucous membranes.
mutation an inheritable altered gene.
myelin the fatlike substance forming the sheath around certain nerve fibers.
myocardium heart muscle.
myxedema a condition of hypothyroidism in the adult.

necrosis death of a circumscribed portion of tissue.
Negri bodies inclusion bodies that appear in the brain tissue of rabid animals.
neoplasm a tumor.
nephritis inflammation of the kidney.
nephron the physiologic unit of the kidney.
nephrosis any disease of the kidney, particularly one marked by degenerative changes in the tubules.
neurohypophysis the posterior pituitary.
neuron a unit of nerve tissue.
neutralization the reaction between an acid and a base forming a salt and water.
neutrophil a granulocyte that stains with neutral dyes.
normal saline a 0.9 percent solution of NaCl.
nutrient a substance essential for life.

olfactory pertaining to the sense of smell.
omentum a fold of peritoneum attached to the stomach.
ophthalmia neonatorum gonorrheal conjunctivitis of the newborn infant.
opsonins antibodies that facilitate phagocytosis.
optically active said of a compound that in solution rotates the plane of polarized light.
organ of Corti the receptor of hearing located in the cochlea.
organism a living thing.
os bone; mouth or orifice.
osmosis the passage of water through a semipermeable membrane separating two solutions, the chief flow being from the less dense to the more dense solution.
ossification the formation of bone.
otitis media inflammation of the middle ear.
ovary the female sex gland.
oviduct the uterine or fallopian tube.
ovulation the release of the ovum from the ovary.
ovum the female sex cell.
oxidation the loss of electrons.
oxide a compound of oxygen and another element.
oxytocin a hormone of the posterior pituitary gland that stimulates contraction of the uterus.

pancreas a digestive gland located in the loop of the duodenum.
pandemic a worldwide epidemic.
paralysis loss of motor function.
parasite an organism that lives upon another living organism.
parasympathetic nervous system the autonomic fibers that originate in the lower part of the brain and the sacral portion of the cord.
parathyroids four tiny glands located on the posterior surface of the thyroid.
parietal pertaining to the wall.
parotitis inflammation of the parotid glands; mumps.
parturition childbirth.
passive immunization the injection of immune sera.
pasteurization destruction of pathogens by the use of moderate heat; milk is pasteurized by heating at 143° F. for 30 minutes.
pathogen a disease-producing microbe.
pellagra avitaminosis caused by lack of nicotinic acid.
pelvis the cavity in the lowest part of the trunk; basin or basinlike structure.
periodic table an arrangement of the elements according to their atomic numbers.
periosteum membranous covering around bone.
peripheral away from the center.
peristalsis the wormlike movement by which the alimentary canal propels its contents.
peritoneum the serous membrane that surrounds the organs and lines the abdominal cavity.
peritonitis inflammation of the peritoneum.
pertussis whooping cough, caused by *Bordetella pertussis*.
Petri dish a shallow covered glass dish used for solid culture media.
Peyer's patches oval elevated areas of lymphoid tissue in the mucosa of the small intestine.
pH a measure of acidity (or alkalinity) equal to the logarithm of the reciprocal of the amount of hydrogen ion (in grams) in a liter of solution.
phagocytosis the engulfing and destruction of microbes and other foreign particles by granulo-

cytes, macrophages, and certain other cells of the reticuloendothelial system.

pharynx that part of the ailmentary canal that connects the mouth and esophagus.

phenol coefficient a number that expresses the germicidal action of an agent compared to phenol.

phenotype an organism's physical appearance.

phosphate salt of phosphoric acid.

phylum the primary division of the plant or animal kingdom.

pia mater the innermost membrane of the meninges.

pituitary gland the endocrine gland that lies beneath the brain in the sella turcica of the sphenoid bone.

placenta the membranous structure that provides for exchange of nutrients and wastes between the blood of the mother and the fetus.

plasma the fluid portion of the blood.

plasmolysis rupturing of the cell wall resulting in escape of protoplasm.

plasmoptysis swelling of the protoplasm of the cell due to an excessive intake of water.

platyhelminthes a phylum of the animal kingdom comprised of parasitic flatworms.

pleomorphism indefinite morphology.

pleura the serous membrane that lines the thorax and covers the lungs.

plexus a network of nerves, veins, or lymphatics.

pneumonia inflammation of the lungs.

poliomyelitis a neurotropic virus infection characterized by fever, sore throat, headache, vomiting, and stiffness of the muscles—often with paralysis.

polymerization the building up of large molecules from smaller molecules.

polysaccharide carbohydrates having the general formula $(C_6H_{10}O_5)_n$.

posterior situated behind or toward the rear.

progesterone one of the hormones produced by the corpus luteum.

prone lying with the face downward; of the hand, having the palm turned downward.

prostate the male gland that surrounds the base of the urethra.

proteins polymers of amino acids.

proton a positively charged particle of the atomic nucleus.

protoplasm the matter of living cells.

protozoa one-celled animals.

proximal nearest; opposite of distal.

psittacosis a viral infection of birds and man (also called parrot fever).

psychic pertaining to the mind.

ptyalin salivary amylase.

puberty the age at which the reproductive organs become functional.

purulent pus forming.

pyelitis inflammation of the pelvis of the kidney.

pyemia generalized septicemia with pus-forming lesions.

pyloris the opening of the stomach into the duodenum.

pyramidal tracts the cerebral motor fibers extending into the spinal cord.

Q fever a pneumotropic rickettsial infection.

quadriceps four-headed (muscle).

quarantine to isolate because of suspected contagion.

rabies a fatal neurotropic virus infection; hydrophobia.

radical a group of two or more elements that act as a unit.

radioactivity the spontaneous emission of alpha, beta, and gamma rays.

reactor a device that houses a controlled chain reaction.

reflection the turning back of a light ray from a surface that it does not penetrate.

refraction the bending of a light ray as it passes from one medium into another.

refractory period the period of reduced irritability.

rennin a milk-coagulating enzyme of the gastric juice.

resonance the intensification of a sound by means of a cavity.

reticuloendothelial system the tissue of the spleen, lymph nodes, bone marrow, and liver engaged in phagocytosis.

retina the nerve coat of the eye.

riboflavin one of the vitamins of the B complex.

ribosome cytoplasmic granules composed of protein and ribonucleic acid.

rickettsiae microscopic rod-shaped obligate parasites.

roentgen the international unit of intensity of x rays or gamma rays.

rubella German measles.

rubeola measles.

rugae folds or wrinkles on the inside of the stomach.

sagittal pertaining to a plane that divides the body into right and left portions.

saprophyte an organism that lives on dead organic matter.

saturated compound a compound without double bonds between carbons.

scarlet fever an infection caused by *Streptococcus pyogenes* and marked by generalized erythema.

Schick test a test to determine susceptibility to diphtheria.

Schultz-Charlton test a diagnostic test for scarlet fever.
scrotum the pouch that contains the testes.
scrub typhus a severe rickettsial infection; tsutsugamushi disease.
scurvy a condition due to lack of vitamin C.
sebum the secretion of the sebaceous glands.
secretin an intestinal hormone that stimulates the pancreas and liver.
seminal vesicle a secretory gland of the male reproductive system.
septic sort throat severe pharyngitis caused by *Streptococcus pyogenes*.
septicemia the presence and active multiplication of bacteria in the blood.
serum plasma minus fibrinogen.
sign an objective manifestation of disease.
smallpox a severe dermotropic virus infection.
soap a metallic salt of a fatty acid.
soft chancre a venereal disease caused by *Haemophilus ducreyi*.
solute that which is dissolved in the solvent.
solvent the liquid in which another substance is dissolved.
specific gravity the ratio of a given weight of a substance to the weight of an equal volume of water.
spermatozoa male sex cells; sperm.
sphincter a muscle that closes an orifice.
spirometer an instrument for determining the volume of expired air.
staphylococci cocci that occur in bunches.
starch a polysaccharide that forms a purple color with iodine.
sterilization the killing or removal of all microorganisms and their spores.
sternum the breastbone.
streptococci cocci that occur in chains.
stye inflammation of a sebaceous gland of the eyelid.
subarachnoid space the space between the arachnoid membrane and the pia mater.
subcutaneous under the skin.
sucrase an enzyme that converts sucrose to glucose and fructose.
sudoriferous secreting sweat.
sugar a sweet, white, crystalline, water-soluble carbohydrate.
supination turning the palm upward.
symbiosis living together.
sympathetic nervous system that portion of the autonomic system whose fibers originate in the thoracic and lumbar portions of the spinal cord.
symphysis pubis the place where the pubic bones join together.
synapse the junction between the terminal endings of one neuron and the dendrites of another.
synarthrosis an immovable joint.
syndrome a typical set of conditions that characterize a disease.
synovia the fluid found in joint cavities, bursae, and tendon sheaths.
systole the contracting of the heart chambers.
temperature the intensity of heat.
testes the male reproductive glands.
testosterone the chief male sex hormone.
tetanus an acute infectious disease caused by a toxin elaborated by *Clostridium tetani*.
tetany a syndrome marked by muscle twitching, cramps, and convulsions; caused by hypocalcemia.
thrombus a blood clot formed within the heart or blood vessels.
thrush an infection of the mucous membranes of the mouth caused by *Candida albicans*.
thymus an endocrine gland in the upper chest; present in the infant but absent in the adult.
thyroid the endocrine gland located in the neck just below the thyroid cartilage.
thyroxine a hormone of the thyroid gland.
tidal air the volume of air inspired or expired during quiet breathing.
toxin a poisonous agent of plant or animal origin.
toxoid a neutralized toxin.
tuberculin test a skin test used in the diagnosis of tuberculosis.
tuberculosis an infection caused by *Mycobacterium tuberculosis*.
tularemia an infection caused by *Pasteurella tularensis*.
tympanum the eardrum.
typhoid fever a severe enteric infection caused by *Salmonella typhosa*.

umbilicus the navel.
undulant fever brucellosis.
unsaturated compounds those that have double or triple bonds.
urea the chief nitrogenous urinary waste.
ureter the duct that conveys urine from the kidney to the bladder.
urethra the passageway through which urine leaves the bladder.
urethritis inflammation of the urethra.
urticaria hives.
uterus the pear-shaped muscular organ of the female in which the fetus develops.
uvula the posterior tip of the soft palate.

vaccine a preparation made from a killed or attenuated pathogen.
vagina the passageway from the uterus to the vulva.
valence the combining power of an element.
varicella chickenpox.

vas deferens the duct that carries sperm from the testis to the ejaculatory duct.

vasopressin a hormone of the posterior pituitary that stimulates the absorption of water from the renal tubules.

vector a line that represents both magnitude and direction.

vector (animal) an insect or arachnid that transmits infection.

vein a vessel that conveys blood to the heart.

ventral the front (of the body).

venule a very small vein.

vertebrae the bones of the spinal column.

vesicle a circular elevation of the skin containing a clear watery fluid.

villi microscopic fingerlike projections of the intestinal mucosa.

Vincent's angina trench mouth.

virus an ultramicroscopic obligate parasite.

viscus an internal organ.

vitamin an essential nutrient present in foods in very small amounts.

volt the unit of electrical pressure.

vulva the female external genitals.

Wassermann test a complement-fixation test used in the diagnosis of syphilis.

water balance the proper distribution of water between the intracellular and extracellular compartments of the body.

wavelength the distance from the top of one wave to the top of the next.

Weil-Felix test an agglutination reaction used to diagnose rickettsial infections.

white matter nerve tissue composed of myelinated nerve fibers.

whooping cough pertussis.

Widal test an agglutination test used in the diagnosis of typhoid fever.

x rays electromagnetic radiations of great penetrating power.

xanthoproteic test a test for protein (a yellow color is produced when concentrated nitric acid is added).

yeasts fungi characterized by large oval cells.

yellow fever a viral infection of the liver transmitted by the *Aedes aegypti* mosquito.

Ziehl-Neelsen stain a method for doing the acid-fast stain.

zona pellucida the transparent layer surrounding the ovum.

zymase an enzyme mixture in yeast that converts glucose into alcohol and carbon dioxide.

zymogen an inactive precursor of an enzyme.

zygote the fertilized ovum.

Index

Numbers in italics designate pages with illustrations and tables.

C

G

J

K